American Nursing
A History

Fourth Edition

American Nursing
A History

Philip A. Kalisch, PhD

Professor
Division of Acute, Critical, and Long-Term Care Programs
School of Nursing
University of Michigan
Ann Arbor, Michigan

Beatrice J. Kalisch, EdD, RN, FAAN

Director
Division of Nursing Business and Health Systems Programs
School of Nursing
University of Michigan
Ann Arbor, Michigan

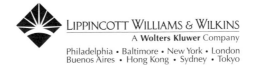

LIPPINCOTT WILLIAMS & WILKINS
A **Wolters Kluwer** Company
Philadelphia • Baltimore • New York • London
Buenos Aires • Hong Kong • Sydney • Tokyo

Senior Acquisitions Editor: Patricia Casey
Editorial Assistant: Dana Irwin
Production Editor: Danielle Litka
Senior Production Manager: Helen Ewan
Art Director: Carolyn O'Brien
Manufacturing Manager: William Alberti
Indexer: Victoria Boyle
Compositor: TechBooks
Printer: Quebecor-World

4th Edition

9 8 7 6 5 4 3 2 1

Library of Congress Cataloging-in-Publication Data
Kalisch, Philip Arthur.
    American nursing : a history/Philip A. Kalisch, Beatrice J. Kalisch.—4th ed.
        p. ; cm.
    Rev. ed. of: The advance of American nursing. 3rd ed. c1995.
    Includes bibliographical references and index.
    ISBN 0-7817-3969-1 (alk. paper)
    1. Nursing—United States—History. I. Kalisch, Beatrice J., 1943– II. Kalisch, Philip
 Arthur. Advance of American nursing. III. Title.
    [DNLM: 1. History of Nursing—United States. WY 11 AA1 K14ab 2004]
    RT4.K34 2004
    362.1′73′0973—dc21
                                                        2003054517

Care has been taken to confirm the accuracy of the information presented and to describe generally accepted practices. However, the authors, editors, and publisher are not responsible for errors or omissions or for any consequences from application of the information in this book and make no warranty, express or implied, with respect to the content of the publication.

The authors, editors, and publisher have exerted every effort to ensure that drug selection and dosage set forth in this text are in accordance with the current recommendations and practice at the time of publication. However, in view of ongoing research, changes in government regulations, and the constant flow of information relating to drug therapy and drug reactions, the reader is urged to check the package insert for each drug for any change in indications and dosage and for added warnings and precautions This is particularly important when the recommended agent is a new or infrequently employed drug.

Some drugs and medical devices presented in this publication have Food and Drug Administration (FDA) clearance for limited use in restricted research settings. It is the responsibility of the health care provider to ascertain the FDA status of each drug or device planned for use in his or her clinical practice.

LWW.com

To Philip Peter Kalisch and Melanie Jean Kalisch

The U.S. health care system is in a time of great change. Increasingly broader health concerns are influencing how nurses are educated and practice. Since the publication of the 3rd edition back in 1995, few subjects have generated more interest, more debate, or more activity than our nation's health and health care delivery system. The nation has seen its health bills consume 14 percent of the gross national product, or one seventh of the economy, on an annualized basis, at the amount of $1 trillion, 400 billion. However, there are interesting paradoxes:

- Most Americans have access to unparalleled, state-of-the-art health care and are satisfied with the treatment and nursing care they receive.
- People from all over the world come to the United States in search of the most advanced medical procedures and technologies.
- Our nursing and medical education systems produce some of the world's finest nurses, physicians, and scientists.
- The United States is the world's recognized leader in biomedical and nursing research. For example, we have made remarkable progress toward unlocking the mysteries of the human genome.

At the same time, however, 40 million Americans are without health insurance, and another 30 million Americans do not have adequate health insurance. Our morbidity and mortality rates do not compare favorably to countries that expend half the amount on health care that the United States does. We have seen the reemergence of preventable diseases such as polio and measles, the continuation of devastating but preventable disabilities caused by various carcinogenic substances, lead poisoning, the return of tuberculosis, and an explosion of sexually transmitted diseases. In addition, we perceive new threats of the results of bioterrorism and the use of biological weapons of war.

Consumers are understandably confused or ambivalent: thankful for but expecting and demanding that high-technology subspecialty care be available when they need it, yet also concerned about their ability to afford and obtain general care that attends to their health as well as their diseases. In addition, the quality of delivery of health care in all settings is increasingly compromised by an inadequate number of registered nurses along with an aging nursing force that is significantly dissatisfied with the working conditions and compensations available.

Solving today's health care and nursing problems is tied closely to a comprehension of the past performance of the health care industry and the nursing profession. The purpose of this book is to place nursing's past in a broader social, cultural, and economic context.

As practitioners of the caring arts and sciences, nurses have immense capacity to assist people in confronting and addressing the inevitable health problems that come with everyday life and aging. While this book is largely a history of nursing in the United States, it explores the impact of the profession on American society, and it is our hope that the work helps elucidate the manner in which nursing and society have interacted generally and provides perspective on key health care issues of the early 21st century.

The 4th edition of a textbook is a learning experience for any author. We have been fortunate to have very helpful and concerned users of the first three editions on both the faculty and student sides of the podium, as well as active practicing nurses. We hope the improvements in the 4th edition reflect their helpful comments.

A critical thread throughout the work is America's investment in nursing services, education, and research, and the important partnership between the government and the profession that has strongly supported its advancement. The hospital industry, which has been at the core of nursing in the United States for more than 130 years, has been a key factor in the development of nursing as well. One trend we highlight in Chapter 22 is the movement toward increasing consumer involvement in health care decision making, which we expect to accelerate in the next few years.

What challenges will we face in the years to come, and what forces will affect our lives, our health, and our health care system—as well as nursing—in the year 2010? If we can take a clue from the past, the challenges are likely to be significant and, at least to some degree, unpredictable. Therefore, we look to the future grounded in a rich past and are confident that whatever lies ahead, nursing will be there to play its essential part in finding solutions, answering questions, and guiding decision makers in the effort to improve the quantity and quality of health care, both in the United States and worldwide.

Finally, as we move 4 years into the new millennium, it is clear that we as a nation are broadening our perspective on health. Until recently, biomedical understanding of disease and the definition of health as "the absence of disease" provided the fundamental framework in which modern medicine, and to a large degree nursing, evolved. The curative model of medical care supported by nursing predominated. The curative model narrowly focused on the goal of cure, that is, the eradication of the cause of an illness or disease. Although cure is unquestionably an appropriate goal, other goals, many of which are drawn from the rich repository of nursing theory, are important as well: restoring functional capacity; relieving pain and suffering; promoting health; preventing illness, injury, and untimely death; and caring in humane fashion for those who cannot be cured.

In conclusion, this book helps students appreciate the history and complexity of nursing and the U.S. health care system; develops a framework, past and present, for assessing current and emerging issues in health care; facilitates learning about the rapidly changing structure of health care delivery and financing; and, most importantly, facilitates understanding of and background on how changes in the health care system affect students' education, their patients and clients, and their careers. We look forward to the results achieved by both the practicing nurses of today and the students who are preparing to practice tomorrow.

Philip A. Kalisch and Beatrice J. Kalisch

CONTENTS

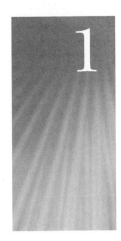

FROM HIPPOCRATES TO FLORENCE NIGHTINGALE: THE BIRTH OF MODERN NURSING

Nursing is as old as humanity, although the origins of the profession as we know it today go back less than 1½ centuries. The word *nurse* is a reduced form of the Middle English *nurice*, which was derived, through the Old French *norrice*, from the Latin *nutricius* (nourishing). In Roman mythology, the goddess Fortuna, in addition to her usual function as goddess of fate, was also worshipped as Jupiter's nurse (Fortuna Praeneste) and was prayed to for hygiene in the public baths (Fortuna Balnearis). The earliest evidence in the prehistoric record shows that people sought to acquire a knowledge of pain-relieving remedies and to discover additional means of preventing disease. Nursing roles also developed in the desire to alleviate human suffering.

DAWN OF CIVILIZATION

Primitive peoples looked on natural phenomena as the work of the gods. The sun crossed the heavens in the chariot of Apollo. Wind blew as the breath of a god. Storms and earthquakes registered the anger of gods or demons. Sicknesses with intense suffering revealed the presence of some evil spirit in possession of the sufferer. In an effort to scare away this malevolent spirit, friends of the sufferer, wearing hideous masks and making terrifying noises, danced about him. Wearing an amulet, setting up horrible images about the camp, or making offerings and sacrifices would ward off troublesome spirits. Usually, primitive peoples revered medicine men, who possessed the "magic" necessary to drive away the evil spirits, appease the offended demons, or intercede with the gods on behalf of those afflicted with illness.

Ancient civilizations considered the fine arts and the knowledge of healing as compatible pursuits. Not surprisingly, then, in the earliest societies the priests served as physicians. This was true in Babylon, Egypt, Israel, and Greece. In classical mythology, Apollo, often associated with the arts of music and poetry, is the god who first teaches humans the art of medicine. Apollo, brightest of the ancient Greek gods, presided over music, archery, prophecy, healing, and the care of animals and young growing creatures; from the 5th century B.C., he was identified with the sun.

Apollo's sexual union with a mortal woman produced the god Aesculapius. Abandoned by his mortal mother, the child was raised by the wise centaur, Cheiron, who taught him the intricacies of healing. Aesculapius developed the healing art to perfection, a blessing to suffering mortals. Jupiter destroyed the wondrous healer, however, for attempting to revive the dead. Later worshipped by the Romans as the god of medicine, Aesculapius had temples erected in his honor beside mineral springs, on wooded mountains where invigorating air restored the sick, and in other healthful locations. Traditionally, Hygeia and Panacea, daughters of Aesculapius, were among the earliest temple attendants. These temples became sanitariums where the priests of Aesculapius acquired skill in treating disease. Known as Asclepieia, the sanitariums appeared throughout the classical world, with a famous one located at Cos.

A typical later reference to the myth of Aesculapius was succinctly rendered by the Elizabethan poet Thomas Watson:

> *In time long past, when in Diana's chase,*
> *A bramble bush prickt Venus in the foot,*
> *Olde Aesculapius healpt her heavie case,*
> *Before the hurte had taken any roote.*[1]

In the Victorian era, an English painter, Thomas Poynter, vividly depicted this scene in a large painting. In that work, Aesculapius sits on the honeysuckle-covered porch of his house, which faces a garden in which a fountain plays softly and soothingly. The gate in the garden wall leads to his temple, seen partly through a grove of large ilex trees. Venus, attended by the Three Graces, leans on one of them for support as she shows Aesculapius her wounded

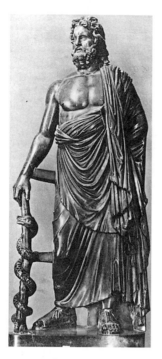

Aesculapius.

foot. Behind Aesculapius stands Hygeia, holding a small box of medicines. One of the Graces holds out her hand, hastening an attendant who fetches water from the fountain. Doves and sparrows, sacred to Venus, flit about; a serpent, the physician's special attendant, twines round Aesculapius' staff.

In Egypt, the primary responsibility for treating disease belonged for a long time to the priesthood. As indispensable mediators between the gods and humans, priests—and especially those of the goddess Sekhmet—held an exalted social rank. For the people of ancient Egypt, personal health intertwined with security, and security meant keeping the gods, the spirits, and the dead appeased. This accounts for the multitude of precautionary measures taken by Egyptians at every juncture of their daily lives. They would refuse to embark on any journey without choosing a date to coincide with the permitted days. As an additional protection, the Egyptians took care to adorn themselves with apotropaic symbols: amulets to ward off accidents or sickness.

Four thousand years ago, Egyptian physicians and nurses possessed an abundant pharmacopoeia with which to cure the ill. The Ebers Papyrus lists more than 700 remedies for ailments from snakebites to puerperal fever. The Kahun Papyrus (circa 1850 B.C.) prescribed suppositories apparently used for contraception. The tomb of an Eleventh Dynasty queen yielded a medicine chest containing vases, spoons, dried drug compounds, and medicinal roots. Because the composition of prescriptions reflected a curious mixture of medicine and magic, the concoctions thought most repulsive were believed to provide the most efficacious remedies. Lizard's blood; swine's ears and teeth; putrid meat and fat; tortoise brains; old books boiled in oil; milk of a lying-in woman; water of a chaste woman; lice; and excreta of men, donkeys, dogs, lions, and cats are examples of some of the ingredients. The nauseous substances found so frequently in the Egyptian pharmacopoeia were intended to sicken and drive out the intruding spirit responsible for the disease. Egyptian concoctions, therefore, used strong offensive ingredients directed

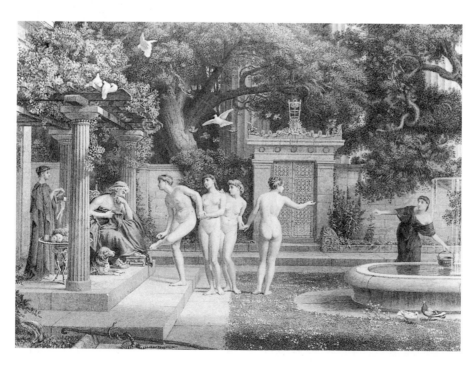

A Visit to Aesculapius.

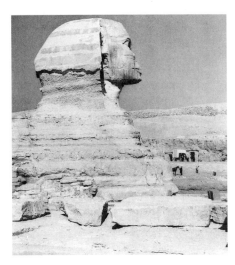

In ancient Egypt, the priesthood assumed responsibility for treating disease.

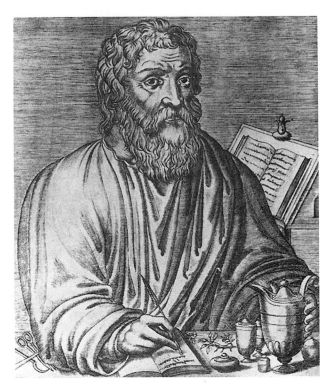

Hippocrates.

not against the sick person but against the hostile power whose prolonged presence could be fatal.

GREEK AND ROMAN ERA (460 B.C.–A.D. 476)

In ancient Greece, Hippocrates of Cos (460–370 B.C.), "the father of medicine," emphasized the rational treatment of sickness as a natural rather than god-inflicted phenomenon. Hippocrates systematically arranged the oral and written teachings on remedies and diseases, which had once been the secrets of priests, into a textbook of medicine used widely for centuries thereafter. He recognized the fundamental truth that making accurate observations of and drawing general conclusions from actual phenomena form the basis of sound medical reasoning.

The notion most persistent and most damaging to the practice and theory of medicine was the doctrine of the four humors, first elaborated by Empedocles of Acragas (493–433 B.C.). A philosopher as well as a physician, Empedocles readily incorporated his cosmologic ideas into his medical theory. He believed that the same four elements, or "roots of things," of which the universe was supposedly made, had to be found in humans and in all animate beings. Empedocles, following ancient, mythical teachings, considered a human being to be a microcosm, a small world within the macrocosm, or great world. The four humors of the body—blood, bile, phlegm, and black bile—corresponded to the four elements of the world—fire, air, water, and earth. Depending on the predominating humor, a person was either sanguine, choleric, phlegmatic, or melancholic.

This doctrine gave rise to a fallacious though seemingly rational system of medicine that for centuries superseded the practical art of medicine of the Hippocratic school. Treatment was aimed at restoring the appropriate balance of humors, through the control of their corresponding elements, by the manipulation of two sets of opposite qualities: hot and cold, wet and dry. Fire was hot and dry, air was hot and wet, water was cold and wet, and earth was cold and dry. If a man had a fever he needed more cold; if he had a chill he needed more heat. Because these theories bore practically no relation to actual physiology, medical practice based on them was rarely, if ever, effective.

Another outstanding figure in the development of Greek science was Aristotle (384–322 B.C.), who demonstrated the hearts of animals as the origin of the blood vessels. Because religious bans forbade the touching of the dead human body, however, this new knowledge lay dormant. Theophrastus of Lesbos (372–288 B.C.), a pupil of Aristotle, followed the example of his master in the study of natural history by arranging and systematizing plants, rather than delving into the human body. Ignorance, rooted in the doctrines of Empedocles, continued for several centuries until the anatomic discoveries made by Galen of Pergamum (A.D. 129–199).

Aristotle had distinguished the arteries from the veins, but he had considered the arteries to be air vessels. Galen refuted this theory by demonstrating that the arteries, when opened, always gushed blood. He profited from this knowledge by tying the arteries for the purpose of stopping hemorrhage. He also displayed insight through his accurate assessment of the human skeleton and the organs of motion, and he

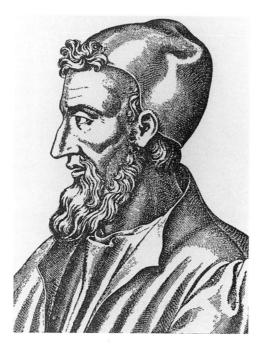

Galen.

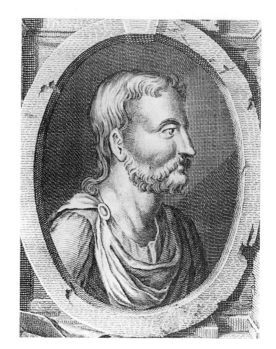

Celsus.

identified the muscular filaments, blood vessels, and nerves. Through experiments on animals, he detected the spinal marrow, the nerves of the brain, and the nerves of sensation and motion. Galen enumerated and classified the nerves into pairs and groups and even discovered several of the ganglia. He recognized the natural division of the human body into cavities and was familiar with the locality and appearances of the chief organs. Indeed, his knowledge of particular body structures was generally so correct that it formed the basis for most subsequent anatomic classification. He made careful dissections of animals, including an elephant, and is known to have imprudently attributed peculiarities of pigs or monkeys to the human organism. As personal physician to the emperor Marcus Aurelius, he established a school in Rome and wrote a huge work, largely polemic, whose surviving pages are still impressive. He was the last of the great physicians of antiquity.

Little advance in nursing or medicine occurred during the rise and fall of the Roman Empire. Nursing practice remained in the hands of well-meaning relatives and friends, for the most part, although with the spread of Christianity came an increased association of nursing with religion. Roman physicians such as Celsus (53 B.C.–A.D. 7) relied heavily on Greek medicine.

After A.D. 300, the advance of medical knowledge ground to a halt with the gradual collapse of the empire. Three centuries later, medical knowledge had practically disappeared in the Western world. Although copies of the works of Hippocrates and Galen were extant, few could read and understand them. Thus, the embryo of medical and nursing theory died in western Europe, a victim of the disintegration of classical civilization.

BYZANTINE AND ISLAMIC INFLUENCES (476–1096)

In the Eastern Roman, or Byzantine, Empire, the knowledge of medicine and nursing did not sink as low as it did in the West. Constantinople survived successive attacks by the Turks and preserved its libraries, and its Greek-speaking inhabitants had a high regard for learning, which they zealously pursued when conditions permitted. Elsewhere, the Arabs, an able people whose ancestors had lived at the edge of all the great Mediterranean civilizations, fostered a respect for erudition. Once firmly in control of a vast empire, the Muslims supported learning. The great caliphs had camel caravans laden with Greek and Latin books brought to Baghdad, where they engaged Nestorians, Jews, and Persians to translate these works into Arabic. This knowledge was disseminated through the new schools that arose in Baghdad, Cairo, and, ultimately, in Cordova, in Spain.

In western Europe, scientific medicine survived the Dark Ages chiefly through the efforts of Jewish physicians who translated Greek and Arabic medical treatises into Latin and who circulated Greco-Arabic medical knowledge throughout Christendom. About 1060, Constantinus Africanus (1030–1087) brought a cargo of Islamic medical treatises to Salerno and, with the aid of his translations of Greek and Arabic medical works, spurred the revival of medicine in Italy. Ideally situated to take advantage of such external influences, the famous school of Salerno remained the leading medical institution in western Europe until the 12th century. There women studied nursing and obstetrics; *Mulieres Salernitanae* were probably midwives trained at the school. One of the most famous Salernitan products is an early 12th-century obstetric treatise by a midwife named Trotula, entitled *Trotulae curandarum aegritudinum muliebrum (Trotula on the Cure of Diseases of Women)*.

FIGHTING MALE NURSES OF THE CRUSADES

During the 11th century, the attention of western Europe turned to the Holy Land. In about 1050, European merchants secured permission from the Muslim ruler of Egypt to build a hospital in Jerusalem for receiving and sheltering Christian pilgrims who had fallen ill during visits to the Holy Land. This hospital was dedicated to St. John, and the nursing duties were performed by Benedictine monks under the leadership of a man named Gerard. After the capture of Jerusalem by the Crusaders in 1099, a number of wealthy nobles, having witnessed the excellent nursing care given to wounded Christians, endowed the hospital with land in Europe and in the Holy Land.

When some of the crusaders observed the outstanding patient care provided by the Hospital of St. John, they decided to join its nursing force. As the battle for the Holy Land raged back and forth in later years, the hospital workers organized into a separate military-nursing order: The Knights Hospitalers of St. John of Jerusalem. Gerard became grand master of the order, drew up a code of rules, and introduced as a uniform for the brethren the well-known black robe with a white Maltese cross that later became a familiar sight on the battlefields of the Holy Land. Organized into a hierarchy of knights, priests, and serving brothers, the Knights took oaths of poverty, humility, and chastity and followed a democratic constitution under which the major decisions were determined by vote.

The Hospitalers soon became famous and highly esteemed, providing thousands of pilgrims and crusaders in the Holy City with hospitality and care. Each year they increased their possessions, wealth, and network of hospitals and commanderies, and they attracted large numbers of recruits. In time, besides performing works of nursing and charity, the Hospitalers, many of whom were monks and priests, undertook to defend the Holy Land by becoming soldiers as well. Gradually, the order developed into a full-fledged fighting force, although its paramount activity continued to be that of caring for the pilgrims, the sick, and the poor.

The next religious military order founded was that of the Knights Templars in 1118, followed in 1190 by the third and most famous, the Knights of the Teutonic Order. After they had been summoned to help fight the pagan Prussians in 1225, the Teutonic Knights concentrated increasingly on military pursuits. The Knights Hospitalers, conversely, never lost sight of their nursing duties. A less important and ill-fated order was founded especially for knights who had contracted the dreaded disease of leprosy endemic in the Near East: the Knights Hospitalers of St. Lazarus, whose grand master was always a leper.

For nearly 2 centuries, from 1096 to 1291, successive waves of Europeans swept down on the Levant, first to retake the Holy Land from the Muslims and later to protect it from reconquest. They came in the tens of thousands: pilgrims, mercenaries, children, small companies of men at arms following their feudal lords, and even whole armies. As an instrument of papal foreign policy, the Crusades were designed to secure the Holy Land and to protect the pilgrim routes. They also proved useful in channeling the aggressive energy of warring and often lawless nobles into a war outside the confines of Europe.

Throughout the Crusades, the Templars and the Hospitalers played the dominant role in military and religious activities. The finest fighting force in the Holy Land, in battle after battle they deployed in positions of honor: Templars on the right, Hospitalers on the left. Large numbers of women formed a separate chapter of the Hospitalers, and they soon helped found scores of additional hospitals under the auspices of the Hospitaler Dames of the Order of St. John of Jerusalem.

In the Holy Land, the 13th century witnessed the ever growing wealth and pretensions of the Templars

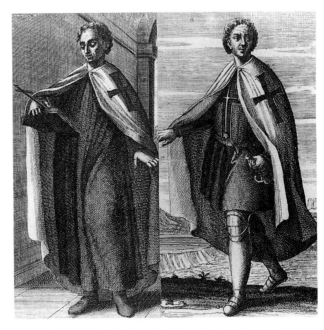

Members of the Knights Hospitalers of St. Lazarus.

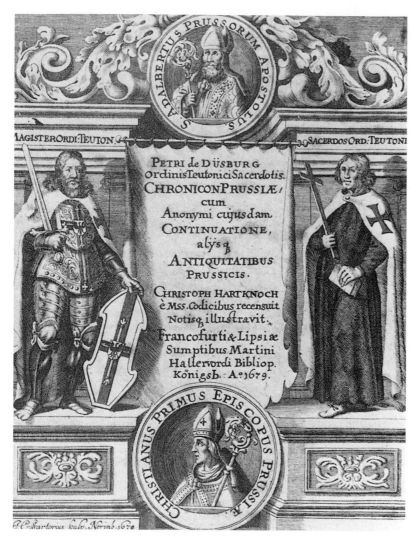

Dual functions of the military religious orders of the Crusades.

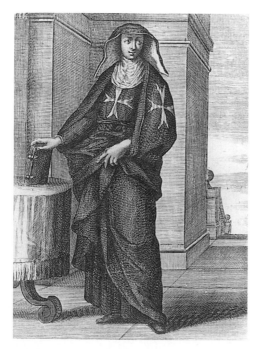

Hospitaler Dame of the Order of St. John of Jerusalem.

and Hospitalers, their ferocious rivalry, and a series of military disasters for the Knights. Gradually, control of the conquered territories slipped from their hands. While important hospitals, almshouses, preceptories, and commanderies were built and soon flourishing in France, Germany, Spain, and England, and while the Knights in high offices of the great orders appeared at the courts of leading princes and churchmen, the unity of Christendom overseas, already riddled by internal dissension, began to crumble under Islamic counteroffensives. The Hospitalers remained in the Mediterranean as Christendom's front-line defense against the Muslim threat; the Knights of the Teutonic Order withdrew to found a state of their own in northern Europe; and knights of other religious military orders continued to fight the Muslims outside the Holy Land.

After the Hospitalers had been expelled from the Holy Land by the Turks, they annexed the island of Rhodes in 1309. When Rhodes fell to the Turks in 1530, the Hospitalers obtained Malta from the Holy Roman Emperor. One of the best descriptions of the nursing activities of the Knights in the Malta Hospital is recorded in the diary of British naval chaplain

Henry Teonge, who visited Malta aboard the H.M.S. *Assistance* in 1674: "The Hospital is a vast structure, wherein the sick and wounded lye. This so broade that twelve men may with ease walke abreast up the midst of it; and the bedds are on each syde, standing on four yron pillars with white curtens and vallands, and covering, extremely neate, and kept cleane and sweete . . . " Almost everyone who visited the Hospital commented on its cleanliness and that the Knights themselves attended the patients. Throughout these centuries, although known primarily for their incessant warfare against the Muslims, the Knights Hospitalers continued to perform their original and foremost function: nursing.

MEDIEVAL MEDICINE AND NURSING (1096–1438)

Early in the 14th century, the medical school of Salerno was surpassed by that of Bologna, due to the latter's revival of human dissection. In 1315, Mondino de Luzzi (1270–1326), a professor at Bologna, wrote an illustrated account of dissections he had performed on the bodies of two women. This work became the bible of anatomy students for the next 250 years. De Luzzi was the first to add illustrations to anatomic descriptions. His dissection, however, was scarcely less crude than that practiced by the ancients. "Beneath the veins of the forearm," he remarked, "we see many muscles and many large and strong cords to which it is not necessary to attend in the anatomy of such a corpse."

The corpse was used only as a teaching aid and not as a source of anatomic knowledge. Anatomic dissections became a regular part of the curriculum in most medical schools, however, and a standard procedure was developed. The cadaver was laid on a table, around which the students clustered. The actual dissection was performed by a demonstrator (often a surgeon) while the professor on his high lecture platform read from Galen.

Students abruptly disregarded any anatomic evidence that conflicted with Galen's statements, despite the mental gymnastics necessary in making the facts of anatomy conform with that revered authority. Certain corpses were thus considered "defective" when they failed to uphold Galen's speculations. De Luzzi insisted that the best corpse for the purposes of dissection was one that had been dried in the sun for 3 years.

The religious orders revived the embryo of nursing during the Middle Ages. St. Benedict's Rule decreed that every monastery have a hospital, and although care for the ailing was at first directed mainly toward members of the order, workers on church-owned estates were eventually included. The masses, however, still had to depend on their womenfolk for treatment and care during illness.

The increase in the tempo of hospital founding during the 12th and 13th centuries can be attributed to monastic and papal reform movements then taking place and to an accompanying upsurge of intense religious feeling. The oldest actual hospital in Europe was probably the Hôtel Dieu in Lyons, founded about 542 by Childbert I, king of France. The famous Hôtel Dieu in Paris was founded about 652 by St. Landry, bishop of Paris. The oldest hospital in Italy is believed to be Santa Maria della Scala in Sienna, established in 890. During the Middle Ages, charitable institutions, hospitals, and medical schools multiplied, and popes, princes, and priests exemplified their devotion to the religious sentiment of the age by personally nursing the sick and the wounded.

Hôtels Dieu for the sick and aged were developed as a result of the institution of religious nursing orders. These orders commonly followed the Rule of St. Augustine; as the most lenient of the monastic rules, it particularly suited men and women who had a hard nursing task to perform in addition to their prescribed religious ritual. In France, *chanoinesses hospitalières* were assigned to serve the Hôtel Dieu in Abbeville (1158) and in Beauvais (1158), for the Hôtel Dieu Saint Gervais (1177), and for the Hôtel Dieu Saint Oppostune in Paris (1188). The Ordre Hôspitalier du Saint-Espirit was founded in Montpellier about 1195 to tend for the sick, the poor, foundlings, pilgrims, and strangers; by 1198 it had established six or seven daughter houses. Funds were solicited by traveling brethren who displayed relics to the faithful in churches.

More than 700 hospitals were founded in England between the Norman conquests and the middle

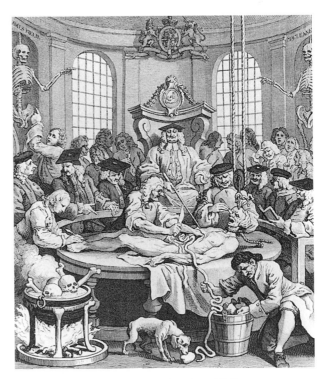

Anatomic dissection circa 1750.

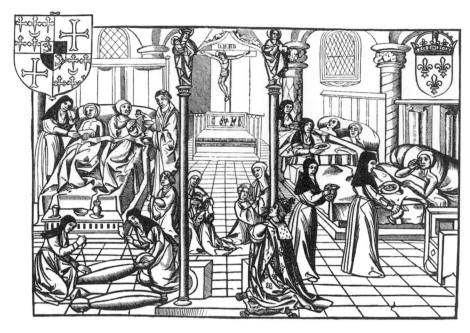

Ward scene circa 1500.

of the 16th century. This number is surprisingly large given that the population of the country never exceeded 4 million. Of course, many of them were not really hospitals as we know them today. Their name indicated their primary function; it was derived from the Latin word *hospitalis*, meaning being concerned with *hospites*, or guests, and guests were any persons who needed shelter. Some of the hospitals were, therefore, erected for the use of pilgrims and other travelers; others were really almshouses, intended chiefly for the poor and the aged. Nevertheless, a considerable number of them provided accommodation where the sick could receive care and even some primitive form of treatment for their ailments. Because seldom cured, lepers usually became permanent inmates, and becoming a patient in a leper hospital was almost like entering a monastery.

Other orders were created to provide hospital service to those suffering from certain diseases: the Lazarites looked after lepers, and the Antonites cared for those afflicted with skin diseases. In France alone, by the end of the reign of St. Louis (1226–1270), an estimated 800 Lazarite houses tended to lepers. By the middle of the 14th century, the diocese of Paris alone had 59 such houses. They comprised small, separate dwellings for the lepers and a modest house for the nurses who looked after them.

Like the infirmaries of monasteries, the monastic Hôtels Dieu were built on a churchlike plan of nave and transept with an altar at the head of the building. The great hospital hall at Angers, nearly 200 ft long and more than 70 ft wide, was remarkable for its tall columns and high-pitched vaults, for its 16 windows, and for its light and elegant proportions. The male patients occupied the right aisle, the female patients occupied the left, and the middle aisle was kept empty. A cloister opened off the great hall and led to a small frescoed chapel. Nearby were large barns for the hospital and quarters for the staff. Approximately 40 nursing sisters provided nursing care, with 25 men to help them and two canons to serve the chapel.

By the mid-13th century a new type of hospital began to develop in Italy. Its first example was Santa Maria Nuova in Florence, founded in 1286 by Folco Portinari. In 1334 a new men's department was built, in which the four wards radiated in a cruciform manner from a central altar—the east-west wards were much shorter than the north-south wards. Later, an east-west ward for women was added. Lay brothers looked after the men, and lay sisters attended the women.

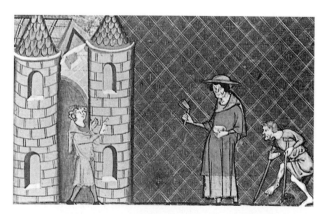

Lepers were so stigmatized that special hospitals were founded for them.

HOSPITAL WORK IN THE 15TH CENTURY

In the 15th century, Florence had 35 hospitals, each generously supported by public and private donations. Some hospitals were notable examples of architecture, and some of their halls were adorned with inspiring works of art. Martin Luther later described several of these hospitals:

> In Italy the hospitals are handsomely built, and admirably provided with excellent food and drink, careful attendants, and learned physicians. The beds and bedding are clean, and the walls are covered with paintings. When a patient is brought in, his clothes are removed in the presence of a notary who makes a faithful inventory of them, and they are kept safely. A white smock is put on him, and he is laid on a comfortable bed, with clean linen. Presently two doctors come to him and servants bring him food and drink in clean vessels. . . . Many ladies take turns to visit the hospitals and tend the sick, keeping their faces veiled, so that no one knows who they are; each remains a few days and then returns home, another taking her place. . . . Equally excellent are the foundling asylums of Florence, where the children are well fed and taught, suitably clothed in a uniform, and altogether admirably cared for.[2]

The Hospital of the Innocents at Florence has two outstanding claims to fame: as the first home of Europe to care for deserted infants and for the Della Robbia infant reliefs across the front of the hospital portico.

When Brunelleschi designed the building for the institution, which started its career of benevolence in 1444, he left circular frames in the arches of the long arcade, so that some fitting decoration might later adorn the spandrels. Among the many shops that produced artworks in the Florence of that day was one set up by the Della Robbia family. Luca Della Robbia, founder, was the originator of an exceptional kind of glaze that, combined with clay, was known to the trade as "Robbia Ware." Enameled terracotta (baked earth) became the specialty of the Della Robbias. Altar pieces, panels, medallions—works great and small but all of purest design and color—were turned out by the Florentine artist and his assistants. Luca's right-hand man was Andrea, his nephew. Andrea, although not so gifted in conceiving large ornate pieces, excelled in small designs with exquisite detail and worked almost exclusively in terracotta. Andrea must have been very much gratified when, in 1466, he was asked to fill the empty space awaiting decoration on the facade of the Hospital of the Innocents. He knew that this home of waifs, dedicated to the tiny martyrs of Herod's sword, had passed through dire vicissitudes. Some of its little charges had starved to death when the treasury ran empty. This mournful incident inspired Andrea to create infant figures so embued with pathos that no one looking at them could resist their helpless appeal. Soon after the medallions were finished, rich merchants endowed the hospital, and the merciful work went on, continuing even to this day.

Early European hospitals were more like hospices or homes for the aged. The sick belonged to a group of helpless individuals including paupers, pilgrims, travelers, orphans, and the aged, for whom Christian charity provided food and shelter. Usually the sick were received for the purpose of ministering to their physical and spiritual needs until they were well enough to return to work. Nursing was handled by various religious orders.

In a typical hospital of the 1400s, the daily work of the nurses began at 5:00 a.m., when, after rising and washing, they went downstairs to church service. Then the sister nurses went about their work in

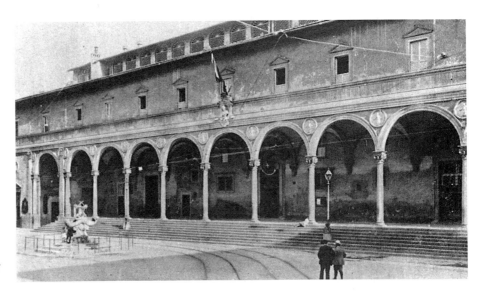

Hospital of the Innocents at Florence.

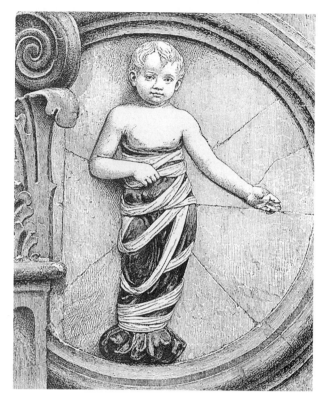

Medallion of Infant by Della Robbia.

covered by a counterpane of heavy gray cloth draped over both sides.

Sister nurses could not witness childbirths, help with gynecologic examinations, or even diaper male babies. Close contact with male patients, such as administering enemas, was also prohibited, as was the care of patients suffering from venereal diseases. Servants performed these tasks. Most medicines were derived from herbs, but were often combined with such offensive substances as urine, animal excreta, and powdered earthworms.

PLAGUE AND PESTILENCE

During the Middle Ages, a series of horrible epidemics, including St. Anthony's fire (erysipelas), leprosy, typhus, and bubonic plague, ravaged the civilized world. The Black Death was one of the names given to the bubonic plague, which devastated Europe, Asia, and Africa in the 14th century. Characterized by acute inflammation of the lungs, burning sensations, unquenchable thirst, and inflammation of various parts of the body, the Black Death derived its name from the black spots symptomatic of the circulatory arrest and putrefactive decomposition evident in one of its stages on the skin and in the inflamed parts.

The first plague epidemic flared up in A.D. 540 during the reign of the Byzantine emperor Justinian. This outbreak lasted 60 years and inflicted a catastrophe equivalent to any nuclear holocaust. The English historian Edward Gibbon states in *The History of the Decline and Fall of the Roman Empire* that the estimated death toll of 100 million is a figure "not wholly inadmissible." The plague leaped, wrote a contemporary chronicler, "to the ends of the hospitable world" beginning at the seaports and spreading inland.

areas such as the laundry, the wards, and the hall for admittance. When the patients awoke, each sister would make the rounds with a basin in one hand and a towel in the other. Each bed, a straw-filled mattress suspended on cords stretched from four corner posts, held at least two and in many cases three patients. The patient lay with his or her head encircled by a piece of rolled linen. The bed was

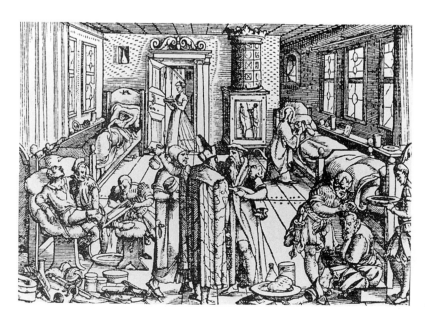

Sixteenth-century Frankfurt hospital ward.

The most fatal and widespread plague epidemic, believed to have originated in China about 1340 to 1345, spread to nearly all parts of the known world. Advancing westward, it invaded Persia, Arabia, North Africa, and Palestine; carried over caravan routes, it proceeded along the coasts of the Mediterranean and Black seas, arrived in Constantinople about 1347, and by means of sailing vessels eventually reached the seaports of Italy. From so many foci of contagion it soon established itself in Europe by sweeping in one great wave over Italy, Austria, Germany, France, and finally England in 1348.

In China, perhaps 13 million people perished from the plague, while in the rest of Asia it claimed nearly 24 million lives. A moderate estimate places the number who perished in Europe at 25 million, contributing to a total of more than 60 million deaths. In many parts of Europe, only one fourth of the population survived, and in some places too few remained to bury the dead. Hardly anyone afflicted by the plague survived the third day of the attack. The black spots and tumors sealed a doom that even the best of physicians and nurses were powerless to avert. So great loomed the fear of contagion that parents deserted their plague-stricken children, family ties dissolved, and the sick died alone. Ships overtaken by the epidemic, their decks strewn with dead, putrefying bodies, drifted unmanned through the North, Black, and Mediterranean seas.

Professors at the University of Paris attributed the outbreak of the plague to the astrologic conjunction of Saturn, Jupiter, and Mars in the house of Aquarius on March 20, 1345, at 1:00 p.m. The conjunction of

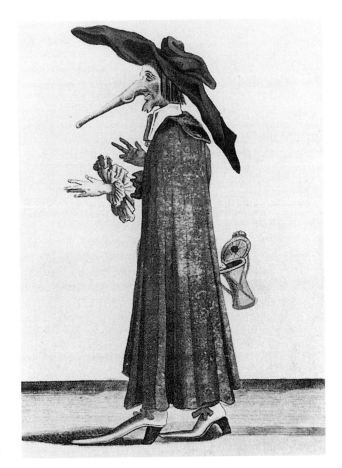

Costume of a plague physician.

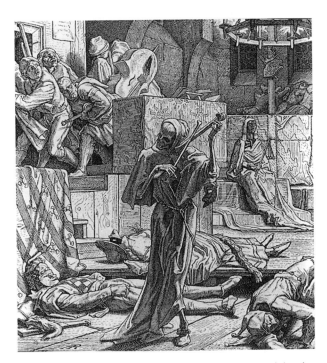

Horrific epidemics killed millions and unraveled the social order.

Saturn and Jupiter dictated death and disaster; that of Mars and Jupiter brought forth pestilence. The cataclysmic epidemic was thus believed to have been duly ordained by the heavens, and mankind was helpless against it.

More often, people blamed the atmosphere for the spread of disease, especially between seasons, when it was warm and moist and when sudden, radical changes in temperature were most common. Once contagion broke out, nothing could stop it. Epidemics that started at the end of winter usually lasted until the heat of summer, at which point they gave way to other diseases, such as malaria. Plague and puerperal fever dispatched victims quickly, especially in the towns, with their narrow streets and closely packed houses. There, epidemics took the greatest toll.

CHANGING CONCEPTS OF DISEASE AND MEDICINE

Traditionally, illness was regarded as a foreign element that lodged in the bodies of the sick and had to be expelled—a concept partly based on the belief in magic. In this view, exorcism of an affliction constituted effective treatment in cases of unjustified bodily invasion of the pious. Diseases came to be ascribed not to external agents invading the body but rather to internal imbalances of the four humors. Thus, diseases did not exist as separate entities: There were only diseased states of the body. Few medicines were derived from mineral sources because the ancient Greek philosophers and the medieval scholars were not greatly interested in chemical substances or properties, even though some chemical problems had been studied by alchemists during late antiquity and in the Middle Ages. A few of these alchemists became interested in the application of alchemy to medicine. This interest culminated in the work of Paracelsus (1493–1540), a Swiss physician who attempted to develop a new medical science by combining medicine with alchemy. Throughout the ages, alchemy had involved the practice of chemical crafts and mysticism.

Paracelsus rejected the belief that physical health was determined by the four constitutional humors. He devised the theory that the human body was essentially a chemical system composed of the two principal elements of mercury and sulfur, plus a third, salt. Salt had been recognized earlier as a fundamental substance, but it was not generally regarded as a basic chemical until the time of Paracelsus. In his opinion, disease was caused by an imbalance of the principal elements, just as the physician-followers of Empedocles believed that diseases arose from a lack of harmony among the humors. According to Paracelsus' theory, however, the balance could be restored not by organic remedies but by mineral medicines. The followers of Paracelsus were distinguished from the Galenic

school by their use of chemical compounds in medical practice. No doubt they killed many patients, but in so doing they learned through experimentation. Largely by accident, they soon discovered a number of useful drugs that added to their chemical knowledge.

THE RENAISSANCE (1438–1660)

The revival of learning during the Renaissance spurred the advance of medicine. Ambroise Paré (1510–1590), a barber surgeon of Paris, began his successful career as surgeon to Marshal de Monte in 1536. Freed from the confines of ancient dogma that had for centuries enveloped medicine in superstitious blindness, Paré was determined to observe things for himself and to accept only the evidence derived from personal experience. In his opinion, medical practice based on accurate observation would surpass the fallacious doctrines of the ancients. Paré revived Galen's method, long in disuse, of tying the blood vessels to stop hemorrhaging. He was probably the first to use ligatures instead of cauterization after amputations. Hitherto, gunshot wounds, which had been considered poisonous, had been treated by the application of boiling oil, hot pitch, or a red-hot iron. After observing that wounds not treated in such a severe fashion were more likely to heal, Paré rejected these drastic methods.

In 1543, a Flemish physician, Andreas Vesalius (1514–1564), published an elaborate treatise on surgery and anatomy. Because this work, based on his experience in numerous dissections, dared to refute Galen, it was violently attacked and Vesalius' findings hotly disputed. Not until 6 decades later, in the time of the English physician William Harvey (1578–1657), who discovered the process by which the heart keeps the blood circulating throughout the body, was the scientific spirit of Vesalius reaffirmed. The methodology of Harvey's research exemplified the new, analytical principle of induction, a process in which data were carefully collected and considered.

Three and a half centuries have elapsed since William Harvey proved that

Philip Theophrastus PARACELSUS *He died at Saltzburge An.º Dom: 1540. aged 47 yeares.*

Paracelsus.

> the blood does pass through the lungs and the heart by the pulse of the ventricles, and is driven in and sent into the whole body, and does creep into the veins and porosities of the flesh, and through them returns from the little veins into the greater, from the circumference to the center, from whence it comes at last into the Vena Cava, and into the ear of the heart in so great abundance, with so great flux and reflux, from hence through the veins hither back again, so that it cannot be furnished by those things which we do take in, and in a far greater abundance than is competent for nourishment. It must be of necessity concluded that the blood is driven into a round by a circular motion and creatures, and that it moves perpetually; and

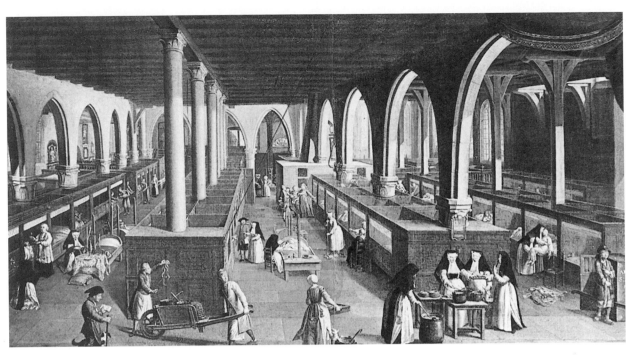

Sick ward of St. John's Hospital, Belgium 1778.

hence does arise the action and function of the heart, which by pulsation, it performs; and lastly, that the motion and pulsation of the heart is the only cause.[3]

Thus did Harvey expound his great discovery. Before Harvey, physicians knew that arteries and veins contained blood but believed that the blood ebbed and flowed "like the human breath." For centuries, people accepted this fundamental error without question. Harvey upset prevailing dogma by demonstrating the heart to be both a muscle and a pump.

The idea that the liver was the center of the circulatory system and that the human heart and blood

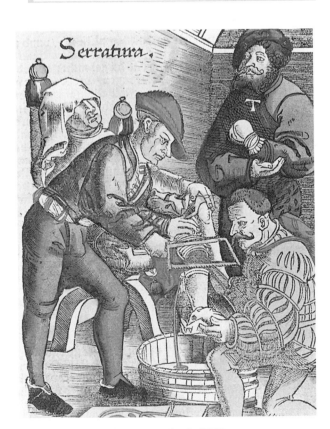

Leg amputation in 1540.

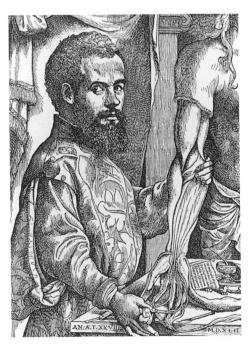

Andreas Vesalius, father or scientific anatomy.

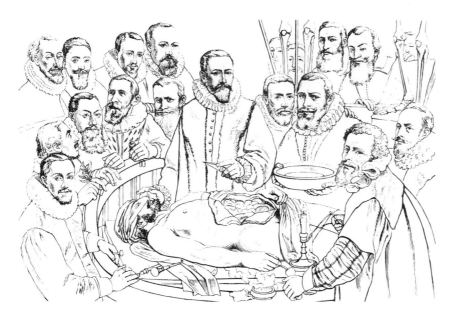

Evisceration in an early anatomy class.

possessed a metaphysical virtue reigned for more than 14 centuries before the time of Harvey. During all these centuries, Galen remained the undisputed authority of medicine, with only a faint dissenting voice here and there. Such men as Servetus and Vesalius did, with great temerity, dare to question the current ideas. But it devolved on Harvey to free medicine from ancient dogma and superstition and to place it on a rational, scientific basis.

Harvey also undertook remarkable advanced research in embryology. In his *De generatio animalium* (1651), he affirmed that every living creature originates in an egg (*ex ovo omnia*), thus opposing the Aristotelian theory of preformation: that the development of the animal is directed by formal, final causes. For Harvey, mechanical causes alone accounted for development. Thus the fetus grows by epigenesis: the progressive development of initially undifferentiated parts.

René Descartes (1596–1650), the most influential thinker of his generation, carried these ideas still further. The human and animal organism becomes a machine acting through movement in geometric space. The soul is a thinking substance, united with but not the same as a machine, which is an extended substance. The living body is thus subjected entirely to the laws of inanimate matter.

For centuries before Harvey, certain axioms, improperly called "principles," had been placed at the head of all medical treatises and taken as medical canon. By the beginning of the 17th century, however, scientific discoveries had finally begun to refute the fallacies of the ancients. By using the inductive process, Francis Bacon (1561–1626) soon devised what would come to be known as the scientific method.

17TH- AND 18TH-CENTURY HOSPITALS

Throughout Europe, the average life span remained wretchedly short. People married at very early ages, and widows aged 15 and younger abounded in every town. The high mortality rate accounted for the prestige of the "graybeards," who were accorded places of honor for having passed the age of 40 in a society characterized by early death. The high birth rate could not compensate for the brevity of life—about 20 years.

The slums of the growing cities contributed to a rate of infant mortality that was sometimes as high as 50%. In London, 58% of all children died before their 5th birthday, and abandonment of infants was common. Between 1771 and 1777, nearly 32,000 infants were admitted to the Paris Foundling Hospital

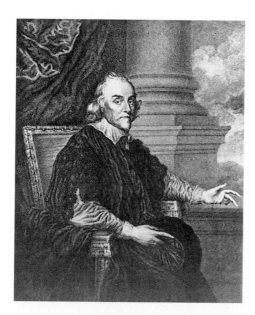

William Harvey.

at the rate of 89 per day; 80% died before the age of 1 year. The spread of dry nursing—replacement of the breast by the bottle—contributed greatly to infant mortality in the 18th century. Sir Hans Sloane estimated the death rate of bottle-fed infants to be three times that of breast-fed infants. Unsterilized dry feeding became especially popular among the French upper class, until the publication of Rousseau's *Emile* in 1762 made breast-feeding fashionable. Some progress was evident, however. In Geneva, the average life span increased from 21.21 years in the 16th century to 25.67 years in the 17th century and to 33.62 years in the 18th century.

Physicians in the 18th century were generally positivistic, insisting on fact and description. They began to use the Oriental method of inoculation against the dreaded disease smallpox after Lady Mary Wortley Montagul had reported its use in Constantinople. At the end of the century, the English physician Edward Jenner began to prescribe vaccination against smallpox by means of infectious matter from the milder cowpox.

Giovanni Battista Morgagni, by comparing the anatomic findings revealed by postmortems with a clinical history of the patient, laid the theoretical basis for the anatomic localization of disease in his *De sedibus et causis morborum* of 1761. Bichat developed Morgagni's ideas and originated the idea of tissue.

A clearer conception of organic lesions changed the notion of disease, and the realization spread that not all diseases indicated general disorders and that a localized lesion could best be treated locally by the surgeon. Surgery and obstetrics had been scorned for centuries, but in the 18th century these two disciplines began to make up for lost time. In England, France, Holland, and Italy, surgeons of great skill began to appear. But not until the 19th century, with the discovery and application of narcosis and asepsis, was surgery to make its greatest advances and take full advantage of the anatomic conception of disease.

For many complex reasons, physicians grew increasingly concerned about hospitals and hospital conditions, thus causing the gradual development of hospital medicine. Hospitals could not satisfy the need for institutional care. Though greater in number, their quality declined and mortality remained high between 1737 and 1748. The Hôtel Dieu in Paris received 251,178 patients, of whom 24% died. The demands made on this "Mansion of God" led to its putting three, four, five, or even six persons in each bed. Max Nordau wrote the following description of a late-18th-century hospital:

> In one bed of moderate width lay 4, 5, or 6 sick persons beside each other, the feet of one to the head of another. . . . In the same bed lay individuals inflicted with infectious diseases beside others only slightly unwell; on the same couch, body against body, a woman groaned in the pains of labor, a nursing infant writhed in convulsions, a typhus patient burned in the delirium of fever, a consumptive coughed his hollow cough, and a victim of some diseases of the skin tore with furious nails.[4]

The year 1788 saw the publication of a valuable study on hospitals, *Mémoires sur les hôspitaux de Paris*,

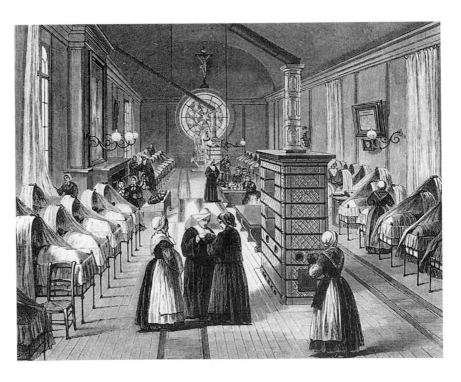

Foundling Hospital, Paris early 1800s.

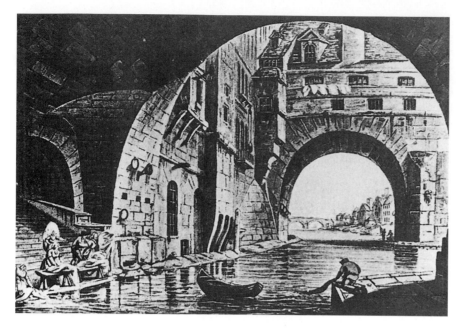

Hotel Dieu; river entrance, about 1710.

by French surgeon J. R. Tenon. Informative and well organized, the book contained ample statistical tables and a colorful narrative, including unsavory passages on hospital latrines. The description of the operating room, in which those who were to be operated on the next day lay beside those who had been operated on that morning, was especially terrifying.

Although thousands were admitted into hospitals, in times of pestilence thousands more were turned away and died in the streets. Milton's description of a contemporary hospital serves as an appropriate commentary:

> *Immediately a place*
> *Before his eyes appeared, sad, noisome, dark;*
> *A lazar-house it seemed, wherein were laid*
> *Numbers of all diseased—all maladies*
> *Of ghastly spasm, or racking torture, qualms*
> *Of heart-sick agony, all feverous kinds,*
> *Convulsions, epilepsies, fierce catarrhs,*
> *Intestine stone and ulcer, colic pangs,*
> *Demoniac phrensy, moping melancholy,*
> *And moon-struck madness, pining atrophy,*
> *Marasmus, and wide-wasting pestilence,*
> *Dropsies and asthmas, and joint-racking rheums.*
> *Dire was the tossing, deep the groans; Despair*
> *Tended the sick, busiest from couch to couch;*
> *And over them triumphant Death his dart*
> *Shook, but delayed to strike, though oft invoked*
> *With vows, as their chief good and final hope.[5]*

In England, John Howard's *Account of the Principal Lazarettos in Europe* appeared in 1789 and contained plans of and remarks about lazarettos in Marseilles, Genoa, Leghorn, and Spezia, as well as a lengthy commentary on hospital conditions in London and in some of the provinces. Howard's remarks mixed praise with criticism. He noted that in London Hospital "there are no cisterns for water; the vaults are often offensive. . . . Medical and chirurgical are together. . . . In a dirty room in the cellar there is a cold and a hot bath which seemed to be seldom used." Of St. Bartholomew's Hospital, Howard commented, "The wards . . . were clean . . . the windows were open." Of St. Thomas' Hospital, "The wards are fresh and clean . . . there were not water closets." Of St. George's, "The kitchens . . . are underground and were neither neat nor clean. A good old coal bath, but not used." Of Bethlehem (Bedlam), "There is no separation of the calm and quiet from the noisy and turbulent, except those who are changing theirselves. To each side of the house there is only one vault: very offensive." Of St. Luke's, "This noble hospital was neat and clean."[6]

CARE OF THE SICK IN COLONIAL AMERICA

Meanwhile, across the Atlantic in the British colonies of America, hospital care was no better. During the 17th and 18th centuries, the colonies had almshouses and pesthouses, but proper hospitals did not yet exist. Hospitals for contagious diseases, called pesthouses, were erected in most of the major cities, not so much out of humane motives but rather to protect the public from the spread of infectious diseases, which often broke out among immigrants during the long voyage from Europe.

The medical profession could offer little help against rampant disease and sickness. Patients often underwent such crude forms of treatment as bleeding and purgatives, which actually aggravated illnesses. Medicine in America lagged behind that in Europe, with colonial physicians in general poorly educated.

They usually acquired their skills not in colleges and hospitals but as apprentices to those already engaged in practice. After taking a short course of readings in medical books, a young man might then ride out with an older physician to gather herbs and run other errands for him. In this way, he would be initiated into the mysteries of healing. At the end of his term of apprenticeship, with this inadequate training, he was turned loose on the public. Fees were small, and frequently he had to engage in some other occupation on the side, most commonly the barber's trade.

A few colonial physicians received a regular medical education in Great Britain, mainly at the University of Edinburgh, and by the end of the 18th century, 117 Americans had graduated from this university. Two medical schools had been established in America by the end of the colonial period: the Medical College of Philadelphia in 1765 (later affiliated with the University of Pennsylvania) and the medical department of King's College in New York City in 1767. Consequently, by 1770 a handful of first-class physicians and surgeons were practicing in America. Except for a few religious orders, however, nursing remained in the hands of the uneducated.

Average life expectancy at birth was estimated to be only 35 years. Plagues presented a constant nightmare. Smallpox, which afflicted about one person in five—including the heavily pockmarked George Washington—was especially dreaded. A crude form of inoculation was introduced in 1721 despite the objections of many physicians and a few clergymen who opposed "tampering with the will of God." Powdered toad was a favorite prescription for smallpox, and sanitation was primitive.

During the 18th century, yellow fever caused perhaps 41,000 deaths in New Orleans, 10,000 in Philadelphia, and 3400 in New York. "Bring out your dead!" was the daily cry of the drivers of the death wagons. Dr. Benjamin Rush, the foremost physician of the time, believed that the Philadelphia epidemic of 1793 arose from the fumes of a coffee shipment that had spoiled on the docks, and although he noted that mosquitoes were numerous that summer, he failed to realize their significance. In 1797 he observed that one patient had developed the fever after smoking a cigar and that wind direction seemed to have had some influence on the number of persons infected.

MORTALITY OF THE CITY,

November 1, 1801, to December 31, 1802, inclusive.

BY JOHN PINTARD.*

[The following Report is believed to be the first regular, official enumeration of the deaths and interments in this city:]

1801.	Adults.	Children.	Not Mentioned.	Total.	1802.	Adults.	Children.	Not Mentioned.	Total.
Nov....	54	67	17	138	June....	30	42	23	95
Dec....	48	55	44	147	July....	44	72	17	133
1802.					August..	54	169	25	248
Jan....	57	84	23	164	Sept....	55	88	12	155
Feb....	64	116	12	192	Oct.....	65	65	14	144
March..	67	117	45	229	Nov....	49	61	28	138
April...	52	71	21	144	Dec.....	88	72	5	165
May....	51	62	10	123	Total.	773	1141	296	2215

The causes of death were reported as from—

Abscess	3	Childbed	27
Abscess on Brain	1	Child Distemper	1
Apoplexy	6	Chin Cough	9
Ascites	1	Colic	1
Asthma	5	Colic, Painter's	1
Bite of Mad Dog	1	Cold	15
Breaking Out	1	Cold after Measles	1
Burns	10	Complication of Diseases	1
Cancer	5	Convulsions	15
Carbuncle	1	Complaint in Stomach	1
Casualties	26	Cramp in Stomach	3

* N. Y. Medical Repository, vi., 444.

Consumption	395	Measles	131
Debility	20	Mortification	2
Decay	27	Nervous Affection	1
Decline	37	Old Age	51
Derangement	2	Palsy	18
Diarrhœa	5	Phthisis Pulmonalis	54
Dropsy	53	Peripneumony	8
Dropsy in Breast	1	Pleurisy	24
Dropsy in Head	13	Quinsy	1
Drowned	27	Rash	1
Drunkenness & Intemperance	11	Rheumatism	1
Dysentery	24	Rickets	1
Epilepsy	2	Rupture	1
Fever	19	St. Anthony's Fire	2
Fever, Bilious	7	Scrophula	3
Fever, Hectic	1	Scurvy	1
Fever, Intermitting	6	Small Pox	108
Fever, Malignant	3	Sore Throat	7
Fever, Nervous	15	Sore Leg	1
Fever, Putrid	5	Spasms	1
Fever, Scarlet	17	Sprue	19
Fever, Slow	2	Stoppage	1
Fever, Yellow	1	Stoppage on Lungs	1
Fits	139	Still Born	7
Flux	8	Sudden Death	39
Found Dead	1	Swelling	1
Fracture	1	Suicide	9
Fistula	1	Syphilis	7
Gravel	3	Teething	30
Hives	45	Thrush	1
Hydarthrus	1	Typhus	2
Jaundice	13	Vomica	2
Inflammation	8	Vomiting Blood	2
Inflammation in Bowels	14	Vomiting and Purging	10
Inflammation in Lungs	7	Ulcers	5
Influenza	1	Whooping Cough	15
Inward Gathering	1	Whooping Cough and Measles	7
Killed and Murdered	4	Worms	31
Lax	77	Worm Fever	5
Lethargy	1	Diseases not mentioned	498
Lingering Illness	2		
Lockjaw	4	Total	2,215
Mania	1		

Mortality report for New York from November 1, 1801, to December 31, 1802.

FIRST HOSPITALS IN AMERICA

Hospitals developed slowly in the 13 colonies. In 1751, the first hospital deserving the name was founded in Philadelphia at the suggestion of Benjamin Franklin. To justify its construction, he maintained that the public had a duty to provide the same quality of care for the poor, friendless, sick, and mentally ill inhabitants native to Philadelphia as was afforded to newly arrived immigrants. A petition written by Franklin and presented to the Pennsylvania Assembly in 1751 prompted a bill authorizing the establishment of the Pennsylvania Hospital, passed the same year. Popular subscription raised nearly $14,000 to erect the building, and the colony appropriated an additional $10,000. The second colonial hospital was New York Hospital (Table 1-1),[7] founded in 1770 under a charter granted by George III at the request of several New York physicians seeking to prevent the spread of infectious diseases by sailors and immigrants. Due to the outbreak of the Revolutionary War, however, the hospital did not open until 1791.

These early general hospitals reflected French and English organization. Patients too poor to afford a private physician could pay small sums for their hospital care. Part-time staffs of physicians served without remuneration to increase their experience and reputations through hospital affiliations. Each of the early colonial hospitals had an agreement with a nearby medical school to permit teaching in the hospital wards. The important teaching positions in the school were usually held by members of the hospital staff. The original hospitals were privately managed and funded by public subscription, generous gifts and bequests from wealthy families, and financial support provided by contributions from the colonial governments.

The first hospital in the colonies for treatment of the mentally ill was established in Philadelphia as a department of the Pennsylvania Hospital in 1752. A second such institution was founded at Williamsburg, Virginia, in 1773, and a third, the Friends' Hospital

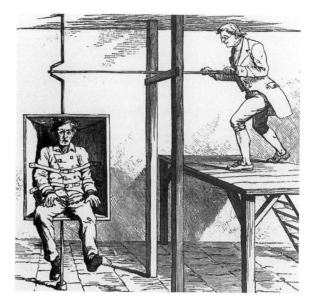

Rotating swing used in hospitals for the mentally ill, circa 1820.

near Philadelphia, in 1817. Forms of treatment for mental patients ranged from the cruel to the absurd, such as the frequent use of the rotating swing. By 1840, the United States had only eight hospitals for the mentally ill, the overflow being confined to poorhouses and prisons.

The admission list of the Pennsylvania Hospital for the Insane for the year 1842 reveals the nebulous state of mid-19th-century psychiatric diagnosis (Table 1-2).[8]

Dorothea Dix, a frail, soft-spoken, middle-aged schoolteacher from New England, almost single-handedly wrought a revolution in the field of mental health care. Infinitely compassionate, she journeyed thousands of wearisome miles to investigate existing conditions in mental institutions and to appeal to state legislatures for improved treatment of the insane. Despite the powerful public prejudice against women in medicine, she succeeded in obtaining improved facilities and better-trained attendants.

Dix's petition to Congress on June 27, 1848, which requested a land grant to be used for the relief and support of care for the mentally disturbed, reveals the results of her travels and research on the subject:

> At A__, in the cell first opened, was a madman. The fierce command of his keeper brought him to the door, a hideous object: matted locks, an unshorn beard, a wild, wan countenance, disfigured by vilest uncleanness; in a state of nudity, save the irritating incrustations derived from that dungeon, reeking with loathsome filth. There, without light, without pure air, without warmth, without cleansing, absolutely destitute of everything securing comfort or decency, was a human being—forlorn, abject, and disgusting,

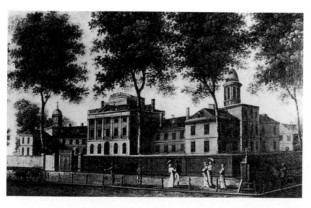

Pennsylvania Hospital, Philadelphia.

TABLE 1-1 Patients Admitted to and Discharged From New York Hospital, January 1795 to December 1803

DISEASE	TOTAL ADMITTED	CURED	RELIEVED	SENT TO ALMSHOUSE	DISORDERLY	ELOPED*	DIED	REMAINING DECEMBER 1803
1. Syphilis	1,201	882	79	8	65	75	50	42
2. Ulcer	640	396	81	10	9	86	29	29
3. Fevers	475	322	29	3	3	12	100	6
4. Rheumatism	365	264	40	10	8	10	10	23
5. Pneumonia	265	185	15	—	1	11	42	11
6. Mania	216	108	45	15	5	16	16	11
7. Tuberculosis	179	25	12	1	—	1	137	3
8. Fracture	126	93	10	1	6	2	13	1
9. Dysentery	120	70	4	1	3	1	36	5
10. Wounds	108	82	8	1	4	5	6	2
11. Frost	105	80	10	1	3	2	8	1
12. Dyspepsia	103	66	13	1	—	2	14	7
13. Ascites	86	42	10	1	2	4	25	2
14. Contusion	77	62	5	1	2	2	4	1
15. Diarrhea	66	42	6	—	—	2	12	4
16. Catarrh	60	45	4	—	1	4	4	2
17. Puerperal fever	47	36	4	1	1	—	—	5
18. Burn	47	31	3	—	—	1	11	1
19. Palsy	45	20	10	1	1	1	7	5
20. Ophthalmia	41	25	6	1	2	7	—	—
21. Abscess	40	20	6	2	—	—	9	3
22. Gonorrhea	37	22	1	1	1	7	2	3
23. Smallpox	28	19	—	—	—	1	8	—
24. Tumors	27	19	3	—	1	2	1	1
25. Anasarca (dropsy)	24	13	—	—	—	1	8	2
26. Scrofula	24	16	4	—	1	1	—	2
27. Scurvy	23	15	4	—	1	3	—	—
28. Dislocations	21	17	1	2	—	1	—	—
29. Herpes	21	11	6	1	1	1	1	—
30. Cancer	20	11	4	2	—	—	2	1
31. Epilepsy	18	8	3	1	1	1	4	—
32. Calculus	16	11	1	—	—	—	4	—
33. Hoemoptoe	16	9	—	1	—	—	5	1
34. Cataract	15	8	5	1	—	1	—	—
35. Jaundice	15	9	1	—	1	—	4	—
36. Cholera	14	9	—	1	—	—	4	—
37. Amenorrhea	13	6	1	—	—	4	2	—
38. Measles	13	10	—	—	—	—	3	—
39. Painter's colic	12	7	1	—	—	1	3	—
40. Hepatitis	11	6	1	—	—	1	3	—
41. Hernia	11	4	2	1	—	1	3	—
42. White swelling	9	6	3	—	—	—	—	—
43. Erysipelas	8	6	1	—	—	1	—	—
44. Ischuria	8	5	2	—	—	—	1	—
45. Menorrhagia	8	5	3	—	—	—	—	—
46. Sarcocele	8	6	1	—	—	—	—	1
47. Asthma	6	3	—	—	—	—	3	—
48. Apoplexy	6	2	—	—	—	—	4	—
49. Concussion	6	4	—	—	1	—	—	1
50. Hysteria	6	4	1	—	—	1	—	—
51. Hemorrhage	6	5	1	—	—	—	—	—
52. Ringworm	6	5	1	—	—	—	—	—
53. Constipation	5	3	—	—	—	—	2	—
54. Cynanche	4	4	—	—	—	—	—	—
55. Hydrothorax	4	2	—	—	—	1	1	—
56. Lumbar abscess	4	1	1	—	—	—	2	—
57. Pyrosis	4	2	—	—	—	2	—	—
58. Vertigo	4	3	1	—	—	—	—	—
59. Aneurism	3	1	1	—	—	—	—	1

(continued)

TABLE 1-1   Patients Admitted to and Discharged From New York Hospital, January 1795 to December 1803 (Continued)

DISEASE	TOTAL ADMITTED	CURED	RELIEVED	SENT TO ALMSHOUSE	DISORDERLY	ELOPED*	DIED	REMAINING DECEMBER 1803
60. Fluor albus	3	3	—	—	—	—	—	—
61. Rickets	2	1	—	—	—	—	1	—
62. Splenitis	3	2	—	—	—	—	1	—
63. Vermes (worms)	3	2	—	—	—	—	1	—
64. Enteritis	2	2	—	—	—	—	—	—
65. Film	2	1	1	—	—	—	—	—
66. Hypochondriasis	2	2	—	—	—	—	—	—
67. Saint Vitus' dance	1	—	1	—	—	—	—	—
68. Convulsion	1	1	—	—	—	—	—	—
69. Gout	1	1	—	—	—	—	—	—
70. Hydrocele	1	1	—	—	—	—	—	—
71. Hydrocephalus	1	—	—	—	—	—	1	—
72. Incurvated spine	1	1	—	—	—	—	—	—
73. Shingles	1	1	—	—	—	—	—	—
74. Tetanus	1	—	—	—	—	—	1	—
Total	4,935	3,211	426	70	124	275	608	177
Percentage	100	65	9	1	3	6	12	4

*Left the hospital without being discharged.

it is true, but not the less a human being—nay more, an immortal being, though the mind was fallen in ruins, and the soul was clothed in darkness. . . .

At R__, and M__, and L__, and B__, were repetitions of the like dismal cells, heavy chains and balls, and hopeless sufferings. After my visit to L__, I found one of the former inmates at the hospital in the charge of Dr. Brigham. He bore upon his ankles the deep scars of fetters and chains, and upon his feet evidence of exposure to frost and cold.

At E__, the insane were confined in cells crammed with coarse, dirty straw, in the basement, dark and damp. "They are," said the keeper, "taken out and washed (buckets of water thrown over them) and have clean straw, once every week."

In H__, were many furiously crazy. Several of the women were said to be the mothers of infants, who were in an adjoining room pining with neglect, and unacknowledged by their frantic mothers. . . .

Do you turn with inexpressible disgust from these details? It is worse to witness the reality. Is your refinement shocked by these statements? There is but one remedy: the multiplication of well-organized hospitals; and to this end, creating increased means for their support.[9]

Although Congress eventually enacted legislation based on Dix's plea for aid to the mentally ill, President Franklin Pierce vetoed the bill as an unwarranted intrusion by the federal government into purely state matters.

The Pennsylvania Hospital of Philadelphia, the New York Hospital, and the Massachusetts General Hospital in Boston, situated in the three largest cities of the country, furnish the best examples of hospital construction in the United States in the early 19th century. Designs followed the block plan and buildings resembled large barns. Although hospitals appeared in most of the important coastal cities and in inland locations, such as Cincinnati (1821), Pittsburgh (1847), Buffalo (1845), and

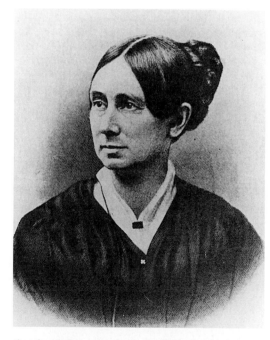

Dorothea Lynde Dix, reformer in the field of mental health care.

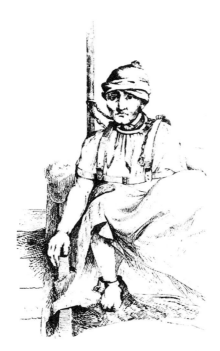

Manner in which William Norris was confined.

Rochester (1847), most facilities were housed in large buildings converted into temporary quarters. Later, as a result of the increase in population and wealth of the communities they served, many of these institutions built more suitable facilities.

During the 1850s, the Massachusetts General Hospital began construction of three pavilion wards, each a separate building accommodating about 30 patients. With high ceilings and good ventilation, they were generally well planned. In the belief that in 20 years the wards would become so contaminated that it would be unsafe to continue to house patients in them, buildings were constructed of wood so they could be easily torn down and replaced.

The pavilion-type hospital developed from the idea that it was necessary to segregate patients and to replace buildings frequently. It represented a great improvement over the old block plan by providing fresh air, sunlight, and ample space for each patient. It was also expected to prevent gangrene and infectious diseases, which were believed to be airborne and the result of poor ventilation, but this reasoning was soon disproved. Occupying large areas and costly to construct, heat, and maintain, the pavilion-type hospital persisted because it represented an excellent means of providing the patients with light, air, and space.

SLOW MEDICAL ADVANCES

By 1850, although nearly 100 years had passed since the first general hospital had been established in the United States, the public still regarded hospitals as institutions for the accommodation of strangers and the sick poor—in other words, as places for the care rather than the cure of patients. No self-respecting woman ever thought of having her baby in a public hospital. Conditions in some of these institutions, notably in the surgical wards, defied description. A mid-19th-century student might think his teacher to be excessively fussy if he prohibited spitting in the wards. Infection and cross-infection were frequent. Several diseases became so common in hospitals that they were known as "hospital diseases": erysipelas, pyemia, septicemia, and gangrene. Before the discovery of antisepsis, a surgeon often prided himself on the condition of his blood-encrusted apron, the degree of filth indicating to some extent his experience. Nurses in these pioneer hospitals were normally drawn from the tough, charwoman class, which regarded nursing as distasteful drudgery rather than as a humanitarian calling.

Surgery, although improved by an increased knowledge of anatomy, dealt chiefly with physiologic emergencies such as fractures, amputations, and superficial growths. Patients in surgical operations were ordinarily tied down and sometimes braced with a stiff shot of whiskey. The surgeon then sawed or cut with breakneck speed, undeterred by the shrieks of his patient. Even if the operation seemed a success, the patient had little hope of surviving the inevitable postsurgical "hospitalism," the term applied to a variety of septic infections virtually endemic in hospital wards. Hospitalism was fatal in about one of every three surgical patients. Committing surgical patients to hospitals came to be regarded as almost tantamount to signing their death certificates in advance.

In the period before the Civil War, medical standards declined, unable to keep pace with the demands of a fast-growing population for more trained physicians. Medical schools usually conferred

TABLE 1-2 Pennsylvania Hospital for the Insane, 1842			
ADMISSIONS	**MEN**	**WOMEN**	**TOTAL**
Ill health of various kinds	22	24	46
Intemperance	20	0	20
Loss of property	17	6	23
Dread of poverty	2	0	2
Disappointed affections	2	4	6
Intense study	5	0	5
Domestic difficulties	1	5	6
Fright at fires	2	3	5
Grief—loss of friends	4	16	20
Intense application to business	2	0	2
Religious excitement	8	7	15
Want of employment	9	0	9
Use of opium	0	2	2
Use of tobacco	2	0	2
Mental anxiety	4	1	5
Unascertained	73	50	123
Total	173	118	291

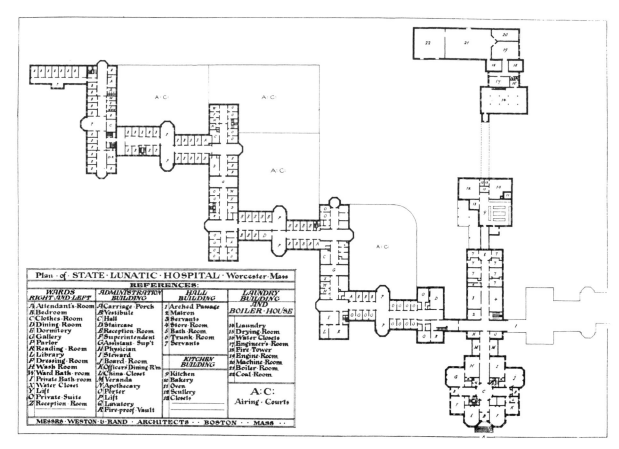

Pavilion-type hospital at Worcester, MA.

full degrees on completion of annual courses of 4-months' duration over a 2-year period. First- and second-year students attended the same lectures each year. Regular attendance was not required, and examinations were generally cursory. A common saying was that "a boy who is unfit for anything else must become a doctor." It was hoped that medical students would spend the months between the two lecture courses in practical observation of patients with their preceptors and in some study and review of what they had listened to during the first term. The University of Virginia Medical School, considered to be one of

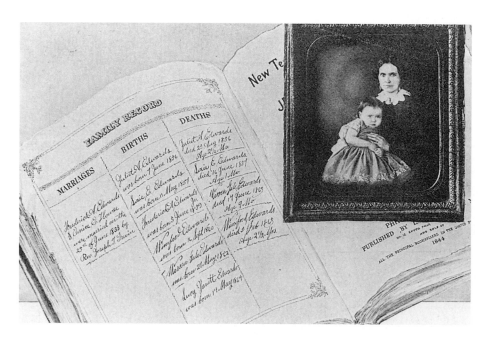

Early death was common in the mid-19th century.

the best in the country, was actually giving *two* courses of lectures in the same calendar year, with little time in between.

With such inadequate training, physicians often aggravated rather than alleviated disease. Emetics, purgatives, and bleeding remained the three mainstays among the therapeutic treatments of the typical mid-century practitioner. Bloodletting, the prevailing cure for most ailments, contributed to the death of Zachary Taylor in 1850. After consuming iced milk and chilled cucumbers on a hot Fourth of July, the president came down with gastroenteritis, which his physicians diagnosed as cholera morbus. They drugged, bled, and blistered the president for 5 days until he finally succumbed to the standard practices of mid-19th-century medicine.

Normally, a physician attempted to treat a limited variety of diseases, and his chief bedside problem concerned the proper portion of medicine. In addition to the favored use of calomel, medicines most frequently given were quinine, jalap, and occasionally opium (laudanum).

Until the late 19th century, brandy and whiskey were favorite remedies for many of the severe febrile illnesses. The treatment of such prevalent diseases as typhus, puerperal fever, and septic conditions required large quantities of alcohol: a patient might be dosed with a whole quart of whiskey within 24 hours. Whiskey was considered so valuable in the treatment of pneumonia that one distinguished New York physician famous for his diagnostic ability in pulmonary diseases declared that if given a choice between using all the drugs of the pharmacopeia *without* whiskey or using whiskey *without* all the drugs of the pharmacopeia for the treatment of pneumonia, he would choose the latter alternative, confident that whiskey alone would save far more of his patients. Medical textbooks of the 1860s recommended brandy and whiskey for the treatment of many diseases, and medical lectures extolled the virtues of their use.

QUACK DOCTORS AND SELF-MEDICATION

One hindrance to good health was the use of patent medicines and fake remedies. Americans placed much faith in folk medicines. For example, some believed that whooping cough should be treated by hanging a bag of live groundbugs around the patient's neck, or the patient might be advised to eat the shed skin of a snake or hens' eggs obtained from a person whose name had not been changed by marriage. According to popular belief, a vegetable-free diet protected against cholera, a horse chestnut in one's pocket healed piles (hemorrhoids), and mercury chloride served as a universal balm.

In 1854, S. S. Fitch boasted that 100,000 copies of his *Health Almanac* had been sold in 6 years: Fitch, who claimed to be a medical doctor, sold a wide variety of patent medicines through the mail. Offering to diagnose any ailments described in letters written to him, he would, on receipt of the money requested, forward his secret-formula medicines. Directions for the use of all 20 were the same:

> Begin with one-quarter of the smallest dose printed on each box or bottle.
> If using two or more medicines, mix the doses together, if to be taken at or near the same time of day.
> Increase one or two drops of each daily, until you arrive at the full doses, if no inconvenience is previously felt.

President Zachary Taylor fell victim to mid-19th-century medical practice.

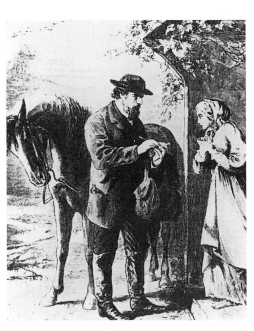

The country physician typically concocted his own medications.

Shake each bottle before using.
For each distinct disease you have, use the medicine directed for it. The medicines do not injure each other, and used as directed will not injure any one. For their effects see the letters in this Guide.
Consult me as soon as possible, either by letter or personally, and I will give you all needful advice.[10]

Fitch advertised one of his more popular concoctions as follows:

Nervine

In almost every case of chronic disease the nerves become weak, and something is required to sooth and strengthen them, and to prevent sinking and debility, and wasting of the nervous system. In all of these cases the Nervine is an invaluable medicine, and should be faithfully used. Begin with three drops, and increase one drop a day until you get up to fifteen drops, which is as much as is generally useful. You may then suspend its use for four days, that it may not lose its effect. It is highly useful, and assists the effects of other medicines. I feel as if I could not cure consumption without it. It is most useful in consumption, heart disease, liver complaint, dyspepsia, costiveness, diarrhea, bronchitis, neuralgia, rush of blood to the head, confusion in the head, restlessness, rheumatism, and all humors, kidney disease, female complaints, piles, scrofula, skin disease, all varieties of head-ache, catarrh, white swellings, tic doloreux, etc.; in all affections of the throat, loss of voice, etc. Toothache it promptly cures. Put a little in the tooth, on cotton, and rub a little over that affected tooth, on the cheek, and on the gum, etc. It is valuable in all spinal diseases, disposition to apoplexy, and nervousness. In neuralgia, rub it freely on the part, etc. It acts on all these by its control over the nervous system.[11]

So backward was medical science that Dr. Oliver Wendell Holmes felt justified in making this severe indictment of his fellow practitioners in 1860: "If the whole materia medica, as now used, could be sunk to the bottom of the sea, it would be all the better for mankind—and all the worse for the fishes."[12]

THE SAIRY GAMPS

By today's standards, most of the hospitals in the United States in the early 19th century were disgraceful. Dirty, unventilated, and contaminated by infections, they actually facilitated the spread of disease. Patients with discharging wounds filled the hospital wards and made the atmosphere so offensive

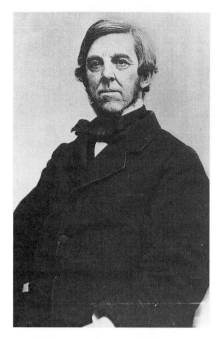

Oliver Wendell Holmes.

that the use of perfume was required. Nurses of the period adopted the use of snuff to make working conditions more tolerable. The same bed linen served several patients. Pain, hemorrhage, infections, and gangrene were rife in the wards.

Nursing was considered an inferior, undesirable occupation. During the previous century, religious attendants had been largely replaced by lay people employed without regard to their suitability. Often drawn from the criminal class and lacking a spirit of self-sacrifice, they exploited and abused the patients. Often the only lay nurses available were aged inmates or women who could obtain no other employment. Work was not subject to inspection or discipline. There was practically no nursing service at night except in cases of childbirth and impending death, at which times a "watcher" would be hired. Many of these nurses were widows with large families. Some drowned their grievances in alcohol. Others stooped to accepting bribes from patients and their relatives. Such nurses sometimes "aided" the dying by removing pillows and bedclothes and by performing other morbid activities designed to hasten the end.

In 1844 in England, Charles Dickens accurately portrayed this class of nurses in *Martin Chuzzlewit* through the characters of Sairy Gamp and Betsy Prig. In a later preface to the novel, he noted:

Mrs. Sarah Gamp is a representation of the hired attendant on the poor in sickness. The Hospitals of London are, in many respects, noble institutions; in others, very defective. I think it not the least among the instances of their mismanagement, that Mrs. Betsy Prig is a fair specimen of Hospital Nurse; and that the

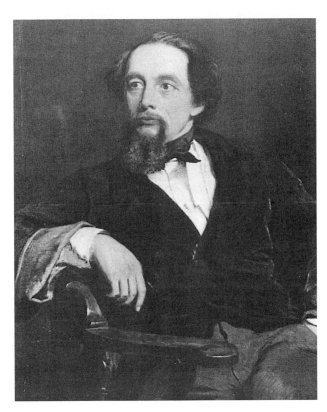

Charles Dickens.

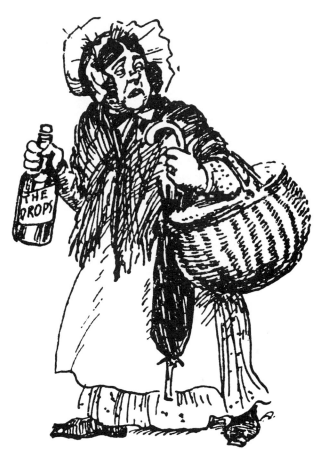

Mrs. Gamp epitomized the worst of untrained nurses.

> Hospitals, with their means and funds, should have left it to private humanity and enterprise, in the year Eighteen Hundred and Forty-nine, to enter on an attempt to improve that class of persons.[13]

Mrs. Gamp first appears in Chapter 19, when she is summoned by Mr. Pecksniff to prepare the body of Anthony Chuzzlewit for burial. After first awakening all the neighbors, Mr. Pecksniff finally rouses Mrs. Gamp, who consents to accompany him:

> Mrs. Gamp had a large bundle with her, a pair of patterns and a species of gig umbrella; the latter article in colour like a faded leaf, except where a circular path of a lively hue had been dexterously let in at the top. . . . She was a fat old woman, this Mrs. Gamp, with a husky voice, and a moist eye, which she had a remarkable power of turning up and showing the white of it. Having very little neck, it cost her some trouble to look over herself, if one may say so, to those to whom she talked. She wore a very rusty black gown, rather the worse for snuff, and a shawl and bonnet to correspond. In these dilapidated articles of dress she had, on principle, arrayed herself, time out of mind, on such occasions as the present; for this at once expressed a decent amount of veneration for the deceased, and invited the next of kin to present her with a fresher suit of weeds: an appeal so

> frequently successful, that the very fetch and ghost of Mrs. Gamp, bonnet and all, might be seen hanging up, any hour in the day, in at least a dozen of the second-hand clothes shops about Holborn. The face of Mrs. Gamp—the nose in particular—was somewhat red and swollen, and it was difficult to enjoy her society without becoming conscious of a smell of spirits. Like most persons who have attained to great eminence in their profession, she took to hers very kindly; insomuch, that setting aside her natural predilections as a woman, she went to a lying-in or a laying-out with equal zest and relish.[14]

An idea of the irresponsibility of the hospital nurses may be derived from the following extract describing an epidemic of cholera that occurred in the Philadelphia General Hospital during the spring of 1833:

> In the house the cases increased daily until a general panic took place. Nurses became clamorous for an increase in wages, which was granted. Those between terror and want of moral sense were seized with a kind of mad infatuation. They drank the stimulants provided

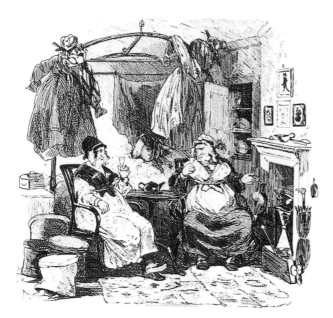

Sairy Gamp and Betsy Prig.

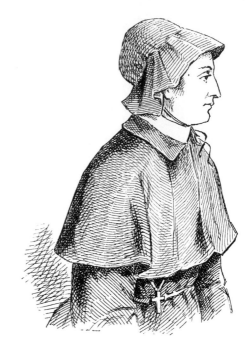

Elizabeth Bayley Seton.

for the sick, and in one ward where the pestilence raged in its most fearful forms, and where between the dead and the dying the sight was most appalling, these furies were seen lying drunk upon or fighting over the dead victims of the disease. In this state of disorder, application was made to Bishop Kendrick for Sisters of Charity. The request was granted, and these devoted ministers of mercy at once entered upon their mission of danger, restoring order and diffusing hope by the calm and self-possessed manner with which they moved among the diseased. These Sisters remained at their post until the 20th of May 1833.[15]

NURSING IN MODERN RELIGIOUS ORDERS

The Sisters of Charity had been founded in Paris in 1633 by St. Vincent de Paul, assisted by Mlle Louise Le Gras (Ste Louise de Marillac). Instead of taking perpetual vows, the Sisters took simple vows, which were renewed annually. They also took a fourth vow binding themselves to the care of the sick. In the United States, the Sisters of Charity began their charitable works under the direction of Elizabeth Bayley Seton. Mother Seton's first community, known as the Sisters of Charity of St. Joseph, was established at Emmitsburg, Maryland, in July 1809. Soon many orders and branches of orders in the Roman Catholic Church bore the name of Sisters of Charity. Some of them were also called "Gray Sisters" or "Gray Nuns," "Daughters of Charity," and "Sisters of St. Vincent de Paul."

Also deeply involved in nursing were the Sisters of Mercy, an order founded in Dublin in 1827 by Catherine McAuley, who later served as its mother superior. Besides their three primary vows, the Sisters took a fourth by promising to devote their lives to the service of the poor, the sick, and the ignorant—an obligation they zealously observed. The order was introduced into the United States in December 1843, when seven Sisters came from Carlow, Ireland, to establish a convent in Pittsburgh.

Several other Catholic orders were closely associated with nursing at this time. In 1822, the archbishop of Paris organized the Sisters of Bon Secours to care for the sick in their homes and for orphans in asylums. During the early 1840s, this order began its nursing activities in the United States. The goals of the Sisters of the Holy Cross—founded at Le Mans, France, in 1839—included the care of the sick in hospitals and orphanages. Their first American novitiate opened at Bertrand, Michigan, in 1844.

THE BIRTH OF MODERN NURSING

During the 19th century, deaconess orders, which had previously existed near the time of Christ, were revived by Protestant churches that felt the need for the assistance of women in conducting religious work.

The first modern order of deaconesses was established in 1836 by the German pastor Theodor Fliedner of Kaiserswerth, who needed an organized corps of nurses for his new infirmary. This experiment proved so successful that it was immediately copied by Lutheran organizations in other parts of Europe.

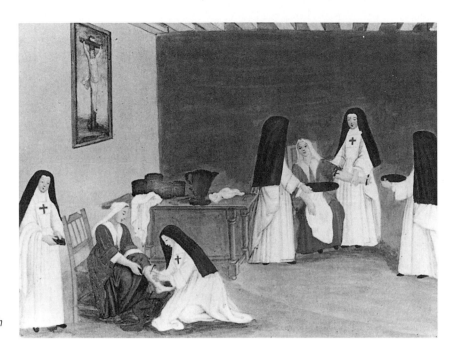

Sister nurses at work in the early 19th century.

As instituted by Pastor Fliedner, the Order of Deaconesses of the Rhenish Province of Westphalia comprised three classes of members: the first class devoted itself to the care of the sick poor and to the rescue of fallen women by the means of Magdalen homes; the second class served as teachers; and the third class, known as visitation deaconesses, assumed the responsibilities of regular parochial work.

The modern movement for nursing education began in the German town of Kaiserwerth. Here Pastor Fliedner and his devoted wife, Friederike, established a refuge for discharged prisoners. Aroused by the lack of facilities for the care of the sick and by physicians' bitter complaints "of the hireling service by day and night, of the drunkenness and immorality of the attendants" then available, they opened a small hospital with a training school for deaconesses in 1836. The first candidate, Gertrude Reichardt, was so disheartened when she saw the sparse facilities and poor equipment—"a shabby table, some brokenbacked chairs, wornout knives, two-pronged forks, worm-eaten beds and appliances to match"—that she almost returned home in despair. But soon a large bundle arrived containing a quantity of new bed linen, clothing, and ward fittings. She regarded this windfall as a providential sign and remained to become the first of the deaconesses dedicated to a new ideal of nursing. Thus, the efforts of the Fliedners resulted in the birth of modern nursing and prepared the way for Florence Nightingale.[16]

Eighteen years later, soon after the outbreak of the Crimean War—in which Britain, France, and Turkey fought against Russia for control of access to the Mediterranean from the Black Sea—ugly rumors of the neglect and mismanagement of casualties be-

gan to reach England. Reports dispatched by William Howard Russell, special correspondent to the *London Times*, and printed on October 9 and 12, 1854, revealed that the hospitals contained "neither surgeons, dressers, nurses, nor the commonest appliance of a workhouse sick ward." Later, after observing that the French were receiving nursing care from the Sisters of Charity, Russell demanded, "Why have we no Sisters of Charity?"

Regarding conditions in British hospitals, correspondent Russell wrote that "the commonest accessories of a hospital are wanting; there is not the least attention paid to decency or cleanliness; the stench is appalling; the fetid air can barely struggle out to taint the atmosphere, save through the chinks in the walls and roofs; and, for all I can observe, these men die without the slightest effort being made to save them." He added that "the sick appear to be tended by the sick, the dying by the dying."[17]

With the corridors and wards of the Barrack Hospital at Scutari paved with dirty broken stones, the damp, filthy building in a bad state of repair and infested with rats and vermin, sanitary conditions were appalling. No steps had been taken to clean the rooms, beds, and bedding, and all necessary equipment was lacking. Russell noted that "the manner in which the sick and wounded are treated is worthy only of the savage. . . . The hospitals have not the commonest appliances of a workhouse sick ward."[18]

The Duke of Newcastle, as secretary for war, was responsible for the administration of the army, and Sir Sidney Herbert, as secretary at war, was placed in charge of its finances. Even though grossly overworked, Newcastle quickly decided to send a commission to investigate Russell's allegations. Meanwhile Herbert, who for years had been interested in

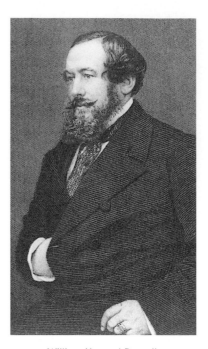

William Howard Russell.

FLORENCE NIGHTINGALE: PIONEER

Herbert's thoughts turned at once to Florence Nightingale. On Sunday, October 15, 1854, he wrote to Nightingale explaining the situation and the need for women nurses in the Crimea. He claimed that she was the only person in England capable of organizing and supervising such a plan. "Would you listen to the request to go and superintend the whole thing," he stated, "deriving your authority from the Government, your position would secure the respect and consideration of everyone."[19] With Nightingale's acceptance of this challenge, nursing took one of its longest steps forward.

Born in Florence, Italy, 34 years before, on May 13, 1820, Florence Nightingale had been named after the city of her birth. Her wealthy, influential English parents raised Nightingale in England, and, unlike the average English girl of the time, she received a thorough education. Governesses tutored Nightingale and her sister, Parthenope, the only other child of the family, and, as the girls grew older, their father took an active part in their education. As a young teen, Nightingale mastered the fundamentals of Greek and Latin; read Plato; studied history, mathematics, and philosophy; and wrote essays on subjects designated by her father. A shy, sensitive child, she was inclined to be pensive and somewhat morbid.

Soon after her 17th birthday, Nightingale returned to Italy. Later she took other trips with her parents or with family friends. During these travels, in addition to the usual itinerary of art, architecture, and nature study, she invariably took notes on the laws and social conditions of the lands she visited.

the care of the sick, took control of the situation. Russell had contrasted the deplorable medical and sanitary conditions of the British with those of the French, for whom 50 Sisters of Charity were providing admirable nursing care. Herbert saw no reason why Britain should not send a group of women nurses. He knew that there would be some opposition in Parliament, but he was determined to make the attempt.

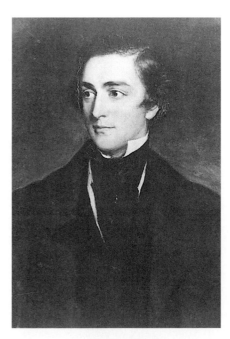

Sidney Herbert.

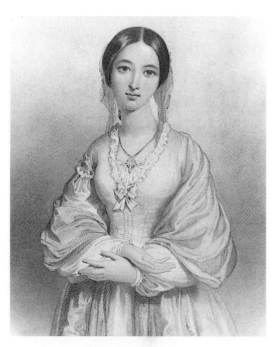

Florence Nightingale.

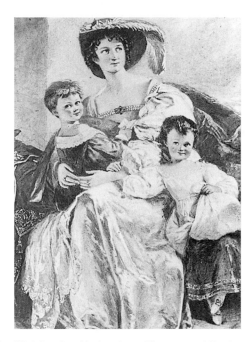

Mrs. Nightingale with daughters Florence and Parthenope.

Her sister, conversely, as an average girl of a prominent family, preferred social activities. On returning from their first continental trip, the girls were presented at court.

At an early age, Nightingale expressed to her parents a desire to enter the nursing field, but they were convinced that nursing was a profession suited only for women like Sairy Gamp. Although fully appreciating her parents' viewpoint, Nightingale determined that it would not be necessary for her to degrade herself to become a nurse. Moreover, she considered it unfair to condemn an occupation because of its existing poor reputation. Rather, she thought it better to correct the evils in nursing.

Nightingale's decision to train in an English hospital at the age of 25 years, 9 years before Herbert's summons, was met by the determined objections of her mother, who naturally expected her to marry wisely and assume her inherited place in society. Nightingale rejected matrimony, however, and took advantage of every opportunity to acquaint herself with nursing conditions.

In the autumn of 1849, Nightingale departed on a tour with family friends. They wintered in Egypt, where she spent time in Alexandria with the Sisters of Charity of St. Vincent de Paul. Spring 1850 found her in Athens, from where she set out, unaccompanied, for Kaiserswerth. Arriving in July 1850, she remained for 2 weeks and came away firmly resolved to return to train as a nurse, despite her family's objections.

The following year, with her ailing sister about to journey to the mineral springs of Carlsbad, Nightingale insisted on going to Kaiserswerth for nurses' training while her mother and Parthenope stayed at the resort. Permission was granted on the condition that no one outside the family learn of her destination. Nightingale reached the deaconess institution early in July 1851 and stayed 3 months.

Finally, after Nightingale returned from Germany and her family settled back home in England, provisions were made for her to enter her chosen profession. After arrangements had been made for Nightingale to go to France to work with several Catholic nursing sisters, her mother convinced her to postpone the trip. She did not reach Paris until 1853. Granted an official permit, she inspected hospitals and religious institutions and observed surgeons at their work. While in France, she negotiated for a position in England as superintendent of the Establishment for Gentlewomen During Illness, a charity hospital for governesses run by titled ladies. She assumed this position on her return to London, but friends soon persuaded her to leave the institution, for she was handicapped by an intolerant board of directors with little knowledge of good hospital management. Negotiations were underway for her appointment as the superintendent of nurses at King's College Hospital when the outbreak of the Crimean War presented her with a brilliant and unexpected opportunity for achievement.

At Herbert's insistence, the British government conferred on Nightingale the inspiring title, "Superintendent of the Female Nursing Establishment of the English General Hospitals in Turkey." This lofty title was a misnomer, for there was not yet any female nursing establishment to superintend, but a frantic recruiting drive in London soon remedied this deficiency. Two days after receipt of her orders, on October 21, 1854, the newly appointed superintendent set out for the Dardenelles with 38 self-proclaimed nurses of varied experience, including 24 nuns. The other 14 also claimed some nursing experience—which generally meant very little.

Florence Nightingale and her nursing force arrived at Scutari, a suburb of Constantinople on the Asiatic side of the Bosphorus, on November 4, 1854. Here the British military hospital had been established in a huge building called Selimah Kishler, which previously housed Turkish artillery. Renamed the "Barrack," this building had acquired an ignominious reputation. There were inadequate beds, no furniture, no eating utensils, no medical supplies, and no blankets. The latrines were clogged and the tubs standing in the passage were never emptied. Men lay naked on the floor in their own excrement. Later estimates held that three quarters of all the casualties suffered by the British army in the Crimean War resulted from diseases contracted in the hospital, such as dysentery, typhoid, and cholera. The Barrack Hospital had proved to be a death trap rather than a sanatorium. Moreover, it had been the subject of extremely unfavorable journalistic reports, much to the consternation of Dr. John Hall, chief of medical staff for the British Expeditionary Force.

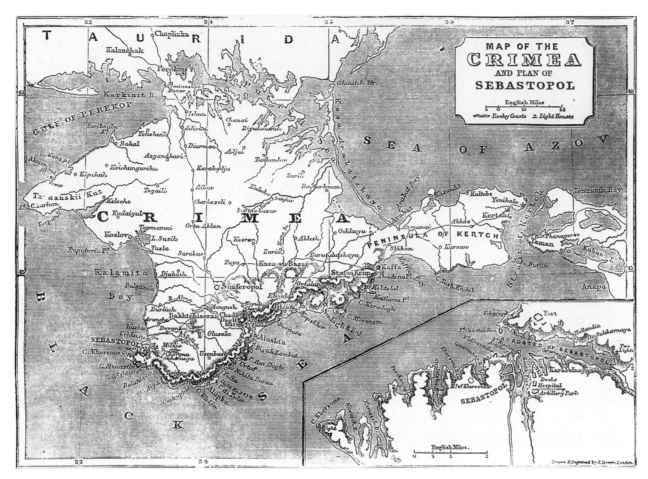

Map of Crimea.

Although some medical officers complained to each other about the ineptitude of the medical department and privately acknowledged the verity of William Howard Russell's exposés in the *Times* and the value of sending Nightingale and her nurses, most resented this outside interference and drew together into "a defensive phalanx" to justify and protect themselves. Most medical officers, like Hall, regarded Nightingale as an intruder who would undermine military authority. A powerful, mutual hatred soon developed between the two. When Hall was awarded the K.C.B. (Knight Commander of the Order of the Bath), Nightingale sarcastically referred to him as the "Knight of the Crimean Burial Grounds."

Because no accommodations had been arranged for Nightingale's group of 39 women, they crowded into six small rooms in one of the hospital's towers. Each room could hold only two comfortably. Meanwhile, the corresponding accommodations in the other tower were fully occupied by one major. The dirty rooms had no furniture, swarmed with vermin, and one even contained a long-neglected corpse. The Nightingale nurses wore gray tweed dresses, gray worsted jackets, plain white caps, short woolen cloaks, and brown scarves embroidered in red with the words "Scutari Hospital."

Designed to accommodate 1700 patients, the Barrack Hospital at Scutari had between 3000 and 4000 tightly packed into it when Nightingale arrived, with 4 miles of beds situated 16 inches apart. The mattresses on the bed, the tiles of the unglazed, unwashed floor, and even the plaster on the walls were soaked with liquid excrement. The building stood in "a sea of sewage." Lice, maggots, rats, and countless other forms of vermin crawled everywhere. Describing the conditions to Sidney Herbert, Nightingale wrote graphically that "the vermin might, if they had but unity of purpose, carry off the four miles of beds on their backs and march them into the War Office."[20]

Within 10 days of her arrival, Nightingale had set up a kitchen for special diets and had rented a house that she converted into a laundry. After she had hired soldiers' wives to do the washing, clean linen finally began to appear on the hospital wards. Unable to obtain any money from the authorities, Nightingale used the *Times* Relief Fund and even her own personal resources to purchase medical supplies, food, and hospital equipment for virtually an army. Once satisfied with the improvement in hospital

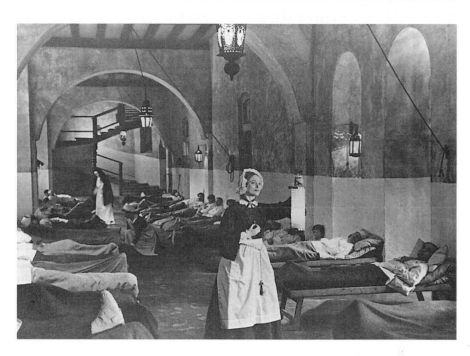

Depiction of Miss Nightingale in a Barrack Hospital ward.

conditions, she initiated social service work among the soldiers. This program of social welfare, however, earned her the criticism of the surgeons, who reproached her for "spoiling the brutes."[21]

In the small room where Nightingale sat at a plain wooden table and wrote requests, orders, letters, and reports, was a narrow bed, in which she seldom slept. In addition to her heavy administrative burden, she spent long hours nursing in the wards. Robert Robinson, a disabled 11-year-old drummer boy from the 68th Light Infantry, served as her personal attendant, delivering messages and carrying her lamp at night while she went among the crowds of wounded to help during an operation or sit by a dying man.

Nightingale often spent 8 hours at a time, sometimes on her knees, dressing wounds and comforting soldiers. At other times she stood for as long as 20 consecutive hours distributing stores, directing her staff, and assisting in operations. On one occasion, when she saw five soldiers laid aside as hopeless

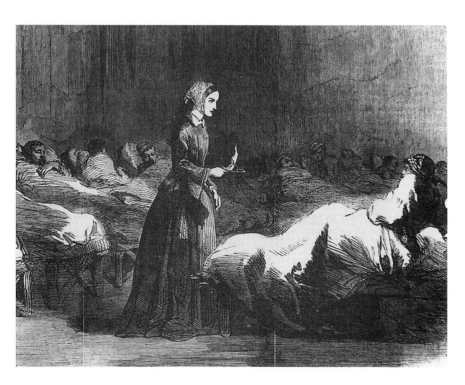

"The Lady with a Lamp." Florence Nightingale in the Barrack Hospital at Scutari.

cases, she asked permission to care for them. Next morning they were ready to be operated on. "Before she came," one soldier wrote home, "there was cussin' and swearin', but after that it was holy as a church." Another wrote, "What a comfort it was to see her pass even. She would speak to one and nod and smile to as many more, but she could not do it all, you know. We lay there by hundreds, but we could kiss her shadow as it fell, and lay our heads on the pillow again content." "She was all full of life and fun when she talked to us," said another, "especially if a man was a bit downhearted."[22]

Correspondent M.W. Macdonald of the *Times* filed a memorable report on Nightingale's work:

> Wherever there is disease in its most dangerous form, and the hand of the despoiler distressingly nigh, there is this incomparable woman [Florence Nightingale] sure to be seen; her benignant presence is an influence for good comfort, even amid the struggles of expiring nature. She is a "ministering angel," without any exaggeration, in these hospitals; and as her slender form glides quietly along each corridor, every poor fellow's face softens with gratitude at the sight of her. When all the medical officers have retired for the night, and silence and darkness have settled down upon those miles of prostrate sick, she may be observed alone, with a little lamp in her hand, making her solitary rounds.[23]

Victorian poet R.N. Cust immortalized Florence Nightingale for the British public in his poem "Scutari Hospital."

> *Moaning in agony,*
> *Writhing in pain,*
> *Fighting the dreadful fight*
> *Over again;*
> *Hearts yearning for home,*
> *Yearning in vain,*
> *Tears over manly cheeks*
> *Pouring like rain.*
> *Thus through the dreary day*
> *And dreary night*
> *Lie England's soldiers*
> *After the fight!*
> *Flitting like angels*
> *From bed to bed,*
> *Cooling the parched lips*
> *And aching head,*
> *Of the poor mangled limb*
> *Loosening the bands,*
> *Wiping the clammy brows*
> *With tender hands.*
> *Thus through the dreary night*
> *And dreary day*
> *To England's nurses*
> *Hours pass away!*

> *Many a blessing,*
> *Many a prayer,*
> *Burst from rough lips for*
> *Those angels there.*
> *England sends gladly*
> *Her mighty sons,*
> *With implements of war*
> *And battering guns.*
> *And England's daughters*
> *Proudly repair,*
> *In Liberty's battle,*
> *Perils to share![24]*

The difficulties Nightingale encountered and the prejudices she had to overcome were enormous. The revolutionary aspect of her work, which did more than just reorganize military hospitals and procure comfort for thousands of wounded soldiers, cannot be fully measured. As a result of the unprecedented introduction of women nurses into the British army, she succeeded in overcoming age-old prejudices and in elevating the status of all nurses. Probably for the first time in history, the overwhelming support of public opinion forced an antagonistic military hierarchy to accept a female administrator with extensive authority.

Six months later, in early May 1855, when conditions at the Barrack Hospital were reasonably satisfactory, Florence Nightingale journeyed across the Black Sea to the Crimea, where two British hospitals were located near the seaport of Balaclava. One, the General Hospital, had been established near the harbor on the arrival of the British in September 1854. The enormous numbers of sick from cholera, from wounds received at the battles of Balaclava (October 25, 1854) and Inkerman (November 5, 1854), and from the undernourishment and exposure during the winter of 1854–1855 had necessitated further accommodations, and a cluster of huts had been erected on the heights near the old Genoese Castle above Balaclava. This complex, which constituted the second hospital, was accordingly called the Castle Hospital.

Accompanying Nightingale to the Crimea was Alexis Soyer, chef at the Reform Club in London, whose task it was to supervise the army's diet. Because he had studied how to cook large quantities of food economically and at the same time serve delicious dishes, he rapidly trained the cooks in the hospital kitchens to prepare excellent meals made strictly with army rations. He invented a special cooking oven, the Soyer boiler, used long afterward, and the "Scutari teapot," which could brew tea for half a company of men.

After visiting the front and the hospitals, Nightingale contracted "Crimean fever" and was taken to the Castle Hospital, where she nearly died. Evacuated to Scutari, she narrowly avoided an underhanded effort by Dr. John Hall to ship her directly to England to eliminate her "interference" with medical staff

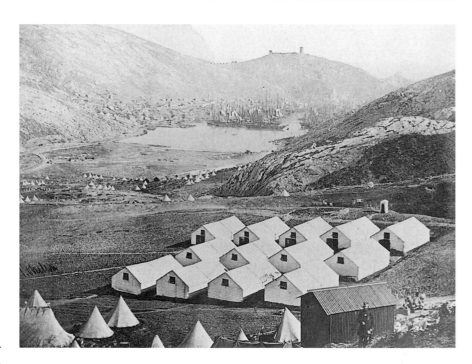

Castle Hospital above Balaclava.

affairs. Soldiers wept when news of her illness reached them, and all of England awaited the outcome in anxious suspense. Within a few weeks she had recovered and resumed her duties at Scutari, but the strain and responsibility of providing nursing care had undermined her health to such an extent that she would never again be able to work with her previous physical vigor.

By the end of the Crimean War, Florence Nightingale had supervised 125 nurses—a small number by later standards, but large when one considers the opposition of the army physicians. When she first arrived at the Barrack Hospital, its mortality rate stood at 60%; she left it at a fraction over 1%. The general improvement in all British military hospitals is perhaps best indicated by the overall drop in the mortality rate from 42% to 2.2%. Nightingale's immense courage and indomitable perseverance forced the military authorities to acknowledge that female nurses had a place in army hospitals. In recognition of her services, Queen Victoria presented her with a distinctive brooch bearing the inscription, "Blessed are the merciful."

After the Crimean War ended early in 1856, the hospitals closed one by one, and the nurses returned to England. Nightingale was among the last to leave in July 1856. On her return from the Crimea, she immediately began pursuing the two goals most vital to her: reform of army sanitary practices and the establishment of a school for nurses. The latter task was aided by the donation of more than $220,000 by the British public.

When the nurse training school began as an experiment at St. Thomas' Hospital in London in June of 1860, most London physicians opposed the proj-

ect. Of the 100 physicians asked, only 4 favored the school. Most replied that because nurses occupied much the same position as housemaids, they needed little instruction beyond poultice making, the enforcement of cleanliness, and attention to the patient's personal needs. Nightingale's ill health prevented her from taking charge of the program, but for years she acted as its chief adviser.

Besides establishing the training school, Nightingale worked to improve the health standards of the British army. She aimed to see the lessons taught by the Crimean War used to prepare for the future. To influence Parliament and the general staff of the British army, she wrote a study entitled *Notes on Matters Affecting the Health, Efficiency, and Hospital Administration of the British Army* (1858), which was respectfully received by Her Majesty's government. Her *Notes on Hospitals* (1858) was a seminal work, and her *Notes on Nursing* (1859) served for decades as the

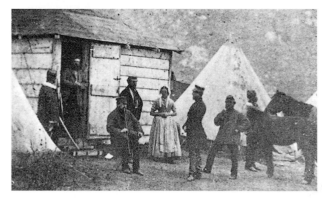

Nurse and soldiers outside hospital hut, Balaclava.

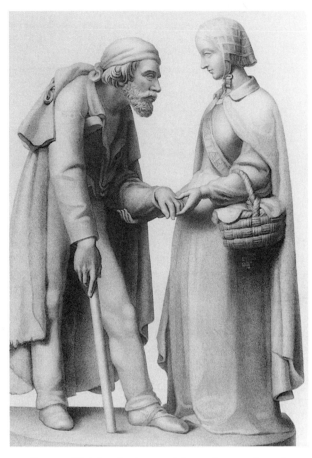

Florence Nightingale pioneered the modern nursing role.

standard text on nursing. On completion of these studies, she undertook the enormous project of investigating sanitary conditions in India.

Although the Crimean War caused untold suffering, it also led to one of the greatest humanitarian advances of history: modern military nursing, from which developed professional nursing in general. If it had not been for the horrible conditions in the British hospitals and camps at the beginning of this war, there would have been no nursing reform by Florence Nightingale. Possibly her indomitable spirit would have achieved its goal in some other way, but the frightful things that the "Lady with a Lamp" saw and the heroic things that she did reached the newspapers and gave her the backing of public opinion.

Across the Atlantic, Henry Wadsworth Longfellow paid popular tribute to the "Saint of the Crimea" with his poem "Santa Filomena":

> *Whene'er a noble deed is wrought,*
> *Whene'er is spoken a noble thought,*
> *Our hearts, in glad surprise,*
> *To higher levels rise.*
> *The tidal wave of deeper souls*
> *Into our inmost being rolls,*
> *And lifts us unawares*

> *Out of all meaner cares.*
> *Honour to those whose words or deeds*
> *Thus help us in our daily needs,*
> *And by their overflow*
> *Raise us from what is low!*
> *Thus thought I, as by night I read*
> *Of the great army of the dead,*
> *The trenches cold and damp,*
> *The starved and frozen camp—*
> *The wounded from the battle plain,*
> *In dreary hospitals of pain—*
> *The cheerless corridors,*
> *The cold and stony floors.*
> *Lo! in that house of misery,*
> *A lady with a lamp I see*
> *Pass through the glimmering gloom,*
> *And flit from room to room.*
> *And slow, as in a dream of bliss,*
> *The speechless sufferer turns to kiss*
> *Her shadow, as it falls*
> *Upon the darkening walls.*
> *As if a door in heaven should be,*
> *Opened, and then closed suddenly,*
> *The vision came and went—*
> *The light shone and was spent.*
> *On England's annals, through the long*
> *Hereafter of her speech and song,*
> *That light its rays shall cast*
> *From portals of the past.*
> *A lady with a lamp shall stand*
> *In the great history of the land,*
> *A noble type of good,*
> *Heroic womanhood.*
> *Nor even shall be wanting here*
> *The palm, the lily, and the spear,*
> *The symbols that of yore*
> *Saint Filomena bore.*[25]

REFERENCES

1. Edward Arber, ed., *Thomas Watson Poems* (Westminster: A. Constable & Co., 1895), p. 56.
2. Theodore G. Tappert and Helmut T. Lehmann, eds. and trans., *Luther's Works* (Philadelphia: Fortress Press, 1967), vol. 54, p. 296.
3. Quoted in W. S. Forbes, "Harvey and the Transit of Blood from the Arteries to the Veins," *Philadelphia Medical Times*, vol. 9 (March 1878):121–126.
4. Quoted in R. Dalton, "Hospitals: Their Origin and History," *Dublin Journal of Medical Science*, vol. 109 (January 1900): 17–27.
5. David Masson, ed., *The Poetical Works of John Milton* (New York: Macmillan Co., 1903), p. 255.
6. John Howard, *An Account of the Principal Lazarettos in Europe; with Various Papers Relative to the Plague; Together with Further Observations on Some Foreign Prisons and Hospitals; and Additional Remarks on the Present State of Those in Great Britain and Ireland* (Warrington: T. Cadell, 1789), pp. 1–259.
7. Board of Governors, New York Hospital, *Annual Report for Year 1803* (New York: The Hospital, 1804), p. 3.
8. Pennsylvania Hospital for the Insane, *Annual Report of the Physician-in-Chief and Superintendent to the Board of Managers for 1842* (Philadelphia: The Hospital, 1843), p. 6.
9. Dorothea Dix, *Memorial of D. L. Dix, Praying for a Grant of Land for the Relief and Support of the Indigent Curable and Incurable*

Insane in the United States (Washington, DC: Tippin & Streeper, 1848), pp. 1–21.

10. Samuel Sheldon Fitch, *Dr. S. S. Fitch's Health Almanac for 1854* (New York: S. S. Fitch & Co., 1854), p. 19.

11. Ibid., p. 20.

12. Oliver Wendell Holmes, *Currents and Counter-currents in Medical Science* (Boston: Ticknor & Fields, 1860), pp. 39–40.

13. Charles Dickens, *Martin Chuzzlewit* (New York: Macmillan Co., 1910), p. xxviii.

14. Ibid., pp. 312–313.

15. L. P. Bush, "Reminiscences of the Philadelphia Hospital and Remarks on Oldtime Doctors and Medicine," *Philadelphia General Hospital Reports,* vol. 1 (January 1890): 68–78.

16. M. Adelaide Nutting and Lavinia L. Dock, *A History of Nursing* (New York: G. P. Putnam's Sons, 1907), vol. 2, p. 15.

17. *London Times,* October 9 and 12, 1854.

18. Ibid., November 18, 1854.

19. Eliza F. Pollard, *Florence Nightingale* (London: S. W. Partridge Co., 1902), pp. 74–78.

20. Arthur Hamilton-Gordon Stanmore, *Sidney Herbert of Lea: A Memoir* (New York: E. P. Dutton & Co., 1906), vol. 1, pp. 393–394.

21. Alexis Soyer, *Soyer's Culinary Campaign* (London: G. Routledge & Co., 1857), p. 154.

22. Henry Tyrrell, *Pictorial History of the War with Russia 1854–1856* (London: W. & R. Chambers, 1856), p. 310.

23. *London Times,* November 20, 1854.

24. R. N. Cust, "Scutari Hospital," *Notes and Queries,* vol. 9 (August 25, 1908):337.

25. Henry Wadsworth Longfellow, "Santa Filomena," *Atlantic Monthly,* vol. 1 (November 1857):22–23.

UNTRAINED BUT UNDAUNTED

The Women Nurses of the Blue and the Gray

2

When the Civil War broke out in 1861, the concept of the trained nurse was still only being talked about. "It seems strange that what the aristocratic women of Great Britain have done with honor is a disgrace for their sisters on this side of the Atlantic to do," fretted a young Southern girl just after the war's outbreak.[1]

The alleged "disgrace" was the nursing of sick and wounded soldiers by women. For decades foreign visitors had remarked that American wives and mothers seemed to have been placed on a higher pedestal than had their European sisters. All agreed that American women excelled in modesty, humility, piety, and chastity, and American men generally concurred. Woman's place in society reflected her supposed physical delicacy: Smaller and weaker than man, she was believed mentally inferior as well. American men did acknowledge women's moral superiority. But that superiority would unquestionably be endangered if women were permitted to engage in such activities as nursing strange men on the battlefield. Yet unless someone undertook this tremendous task, thousands of sick and wounded would die of neglect.

The American Civil War lasted from April 1861 to April 1865 and was fought under conditions guaranteed to swell the casualty lists. Huge armies faced each other, firing as they advanced until one or the other gave ground. Combat, waged with rifled muskets and cannons, was often more dangerous than it would come to be in World Wars I and II. By the war's end, of 14 million free males, nearly 2 million were under arms—over 1 million in the blue of the North and over 900,000 in the gray of the South—a higher proportion than in any other American war. Either as battle casualties or as victims of disease, 618,000 men died in service—360,000 Union troops and 258,000 Confederate troops. Many died on the battlefield; the less seriously wounded faced the hazards of primitive sanitary conditions and a comparatively inept medical corps (Table 2-1).

A LESSON FROM ENGLAND

Florence Nightingale had been internationally celebrated for her tremendous contributions to the health of the British army in the Crimean War, and her methods had been called to the attention of America through the publication of her *Notes on Nursing: What It Is, and What It Is Not*; but the ambition of a few American women to engage in professional nursing service had been more than counterbalanced by opposition from the medical profession.

According to Nightingale, nurse training was necessary to

> teach not only what is to be done, but how to do it. The physician or surgeon orders what is to be done. Training has to teach the nurse how to do it to his order; and to teach, not only how to do it, but *why* such and such a thing is done, and not such and such another; as also to teach symptoms, and what symptoms indicate what of disease or change, and the "reason why" of such symptoms.
>
> Nearly all physicians' orders are conditional. Telling the nurse what to do is not enough and cannot be enough to perfect her—whatever her surroundings. The trained power of attending to one's own impressions made by one's own senses, so that these should *tell* the nurse how the patient is, is the *sine qua non* of being a nurse at all. The nurse's eye and ear must be trained—smell and touch are her two right hands—and her taste is sometimes as necessary to the nurse as her head. . . . Merely looking at the sick is not observing. To look is not always to see. It needs a high degree of training to look, so that looking shall tell the nurse aright, so that she may tell the medical officer aright what has happened in his absence.[2]

TABLE 2-1 Prevalence of Major Diseases in the Union Army During the Civil War*

CASES		DEATHS	
Disease	*Number*	*Disease*	*Number*
Diarrhea and dysentery	1,700,000	Diarrhea and dysentery	44,500
Malaria	1,300,000	Typhoid fever	34,800
Rheumatism	286,000	Pneumonia	20,000
Respiratory	283,000	Malaria	10,000
Typhoid fever	148,000	Smallpox	7,000
Syphilis and gonorrhea	80,000	Tuberculosis	7,000
Pneumonia	77,000	Measles	5,000
Measles	76,000	Meningitis	2,600
Jaundice	70,000	Scurvy	770
Scurvy	47,000	Rheumatism	710
Tuberculosis	29,000	Respiratory	500
Smallpox	19,000	Jaundice	400
Liver abscess	12,000	Yellow fever	400
Sunstroke	6,600	Liver abscess	300
Meningitis	4,000	Sunstroke	261
Insanity	2,600	Syphilis and gonorrhea	150
Yellow fever	1,300	Insanity	90

*United States War Department, Surgeon General's Office, *The Medical and Surgical History of the War of the Rebellion (1861–1865)* prepared in accordance with acts of Congress under the direction of the Surgeon General, Joseph K. Barnes, United States Army (Washington, D.C.: Government Printing Office, 1870–1888), three parts in six volumes.

Of significance to well-meaning amateur nurses was Nightingale's warning that

life or death may lie with the good observer. Without a trained power of observation, no nurse can be of any use in reporting to the medical attendant. The best one can hope for is that he will be clever enough not to mind her, as is so often the case. . . . It is most important to observe the symptoms of illness; it is, if possible, more important still to observe the symptoms of nursing; of what is the fault not of the illness but of the nursing. Observation tells *how* the patient is; reflection tells *what* is to be done; training tells *how* it is to be done. . . . Reflection needs training, as much as observation. The nurse is told by the medical attendant, "If such or such a change occurs, or if such or such symptoms appear, you are to do so and so, or to vary my treatment in such or such a manner." In no case is the physician or surgeon always there. The woman must have trained powers of observation and reflection, or she cannot obey. The patient's life is lost by her blunder . . . and people say, "The doctor is to blame"; or, worse still, they talk of it as if God were to blame—as if it were God's will. God's will is *not* that we should leave our nurses, in whose hands we must leave issues of life or death, without training to fulfill the responsibilities of such momentous issues.[3]

AMERICAN WOMEN ANSWER THE CALL

Almost before the echo of the first gun fired on Fort Sumter had died away, scores of Northern women were offering their services to the government. The president's call for 75,000 militia volunteers on April 14, 1861, was also answered by wives, sisters, and mothers. Within 3 weeks, 100 women had been selected, out of many hundreds of applicants, to take a special short course of training under physicians and surgeons in New York City. On June 10, 1861, Dorothea Lynde Dix, already well-known as a humanitarian on behalf of the mentally ill, was appointed by Secretary of War Simon Cameron to superintend the women nurses.

Her wide-ranging commission, dated April 23, 1861, theoretically gave her the power to organize hospitals for the care of all sick and wounded soldiers, to appoint nurses, and to "receive, control and disburse" special supplies donated by individuals or associations for distribution among the troops.[4] These were sweeping powers far in excess of those enjoyed by Florence Nightingale or, indeed, desired by Dix. Working as an individual, Dix had never had occasion to run an office force or to organize groups of workers for any sort of complicated program.

Even before Dix's appointment was made public, other agencies and individuals had already begun relief work. The medical department of the U.S. Army had begun organizing the hospitals, and the

U.S. Sanitary Commission had been authorized to channel supplies and comforts contributed by the home folks for the boys in the hospitals. Dix was left with the duty of organizing a corps of female nurses.

The eagerly awaited circular issued by Dix in 1862 stated that no woman younger than 35 need apply. All nurses were required to be plain-looking women, to wear simple brown or black dresses, and to eschew all bows, curls, jewelry, and especially hoop skirts. Good morals and common sense were the only other necessary qualifications. But plain-looking women older than 35 were not the only ones who burned with impatience to take an active part in the conflict in which their husbands and brothers were engaged. Many who were unable to meet Dix's requirements ignored them completely and nursed all through the war without official recognition or financial compensation; those who had been regularly appointed received $12 a month from the government.

In the North, the war quickly inspired a call for greater numbers of female nurses. On May 11, 1861, the *American Medical Times* warned, "We must not wait to learn by bitter experience what the Crimean War taught England and France; and we must now resolve that our intelligence shall anticipate and provide against all dangers not essentially fortuitous." An editorial pointed out that during the Crimean War female nursing in military hospitals had been put to a practical test and that the opinions of those who had witnessed its efficiency were worthy of consideration. Dr. E. A. Parkes, who had been in charge of the Renkioi Civil Military Hospital on the Dardanelles during the Crimean War, was cited as having testified, "I have a very high opinion of female nurses, if they have been trained and are proper nurses." The medical director of the British Civil Military Hospital at Smyrna, Turkey, was quoted as having said:

> They worked uncommonly well; out of 22 female nurses only one was removed for any misconduct. . . . Several of the ladies that we had did the work uncommonly well, and it would have been very difficult to have got a larger class of severe cases of fever attended to so well by night and day except by the agency of those ladies, who were thoroughly to be relied on, not only from their superior intelligence but also from their devotion to the work.[5]

CIRCULAR NO. 8.

Washington, *July* 24, 1862.

No candidate for service in the Women's Department for nursing in the Military Hospitals of the United States, will be received below the age of thirty-five years, nor above fifty.

Only women of strong health, not subjects of chronic d'sease, nor liable to sudden illnesses, need apply. The duties of the station make large and continued demands on strength.

Matronly persons of experience, good conduct, or superior education and serious disposition, will always have preference; habits of neatness, order, sobriety, and industry are prerequisites.

All applicants must present certificates of qualification and good character from at least two persons of trust, testifying to morality, integrity, seriousness, and capacity for care of the sick.

Obedience to rules of the service, and conformity to special regulations, will be required and enforced.

Compensation, as regulated by Act of Congress, forty cents a day and subsistence. Transportation furnished to and from the place of service.

Amount of luggage limited within small compass.

Dress plain (colors brown, grey, or black), and, while connected with the service, without ornaments of any sort.

No applicants accepted for less than three months' service; those for longer periods always have preference.

D. L. Dix.

Approved:

William A. Hammond,
Surgeon-General.

Dorothea Dix's circular on qualifications to become a nurse.

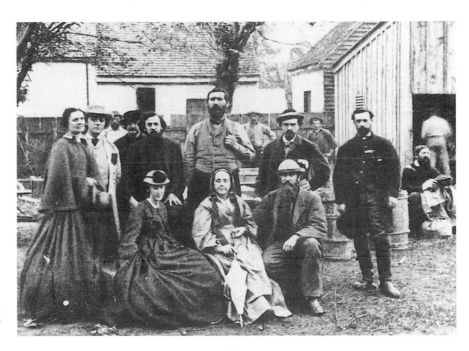

Nurses and officers of the U.S. Sanitary Commission at Fredericksburg, Virginia, in 1864.

Mary Livermore (1820–1905), a nurse in the U.S. Sanitary Commission and later a temperance and suffrage leader, asserted (rather naively) that the pain of men in battle was nothing next to the agony that women felt in sending their loved ones off to war "knowing full well the risks they run—this involves exquisite suffering, and calls for another kind of heroism." Livermore reasoned that the more highly cultivated and refined a volunteering lady was, the better a nurse she would make; such women were sure to submit to inconvenience and privation with much better grace than could those of the lower classes.[6]

WALT WHITMAN WRITES OF HOSPITAL NURSING

But it was a male nurse, Walt Whitman (1819–1892), who most poignantly captured the mood of nursing amid the carnage of battle. Journeying to Washington in December 1862 in search of a brother who had been wounded while serving with the Army of the Potomac in Virginia, Whitman found him to be safely recovered but saw enough misery to decide to devote himself to nursing wounded soldiers in the various hospitals of the city. He worked entirely on his own, going about the wards to talk with the soldiers or to read to them, bringing gifts of fruit, jelly, and candy and occasionally writing letters that they dictated for their families.

Several of Whitman's *Drum-Taps* poems reflect his hospital service. "The Wound-Dresser" provides an especially eloquent evocation of his experience among sick and dying soldiers:

Bearing the bandages, water and sponge,
Straight and swift to my wounded I go,
Where they lie on the ground after the battle brought in,
Where their priceless blood reddens the grass, the ground,
Or to the rows of the hospital tent, or under the roof'd hospital,
To the long rows of cots up and down each side I return,
To each and all one after another I draw near, not one do I miss,
An attendant follows holding a tray, he carries a refuse pail,

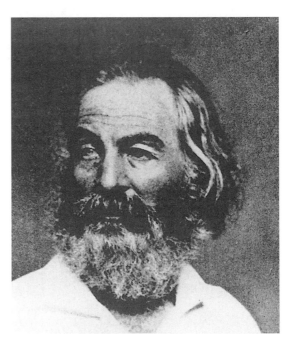

Walt Whitman. Photograph by Mathew Brady.

Soon to be fill'd with clotted rags and blood, emptied, and
*   fill'd again.*
I onward go, I stop,
With hinged knees and steady hand to dress wounds,
I am firm with each, the pangs are sharp yet unavoidable,
One turns to me his appealing eyes—poor boy! I never
*   knew you,*
Yet I think I could not refuse this moment to die for you, if
*   that would save you.*[7]

Although a few people approved and promoted the idea of women nursing in military hospitals, many others held that it was not the proper thing for a respectable woman to do. Even the liberal Whitman concluded, "It remains to be distinctly said that a few or no young ladies, under the irresistible conventions of society, answer the practical requirements of nurse for soldiers."[8] Physicians disliked the idea of women in the hospitals for other reasons. They charged that many of the women were opinionated, unreliable, and gossipy and that they showed favoritism. Military hospitals had traditional rules and regulations, and untrained, undisciplined women nurses did not fit in. Thus from the very beginning, some of the medical directors refused to accept the nurses Dorothea Dix had assigned to them or, when forced to allow them in, treated the nurses so badly that they soon took ill or quit in disgust.

The duties of the Civil War nurse who won admittance to the wards were extremely diverse. Many of the surgeons resented the presence of women nurses and, because they often came in without instruction in their proper duties, frequently assigned them to any housekeeping job that needed to be done, such as scrubbing wards or supervising laundry. Generally they would be called on for direct patient care only in moments of crisis, such as when a trainload of wounded troops arrived and hundreds had to be washed, fed, and put quickly to bed. Dix, on the other hand, expected the same women nurses to supervise the wards (including the male nurses), to dress wounds, and to administer medications.

HOSPITALS AND HOSPITAL ROUTINE

Large military hospitals were an obvious necessity throughout the war. Before this time, the largest military hospital had been the 41-bed facility at Fort Leavenworth, Kansas. Base hospitals, both Union and Confederate, were at first located in nearby hotels, churches, factories, warehouses, schools, academies, and private dwellings, such as the National Hotel, Georgetown College, and Odd Fellows Hall in Washington, DC, and the Tishomingo Hotel in Corinth, Mississippi. Unlikely places such as the Georgetown Prison in Washington, DC, the Capitol Rotunda, church pews, farmhouses, pigsties, and the Lee Mansion also housed federal casualties.

As casualties poured in from the great battles, additional wards sprang up around many of these buildings. In late 1861, assistant surgeon William A. Hammond, inspector of hospitals at Wheeling, West Virginia, recommended the construction of a pavilion-type hospital, based on the British experience in Crimea. The first such hospital was constructed at Parkersburg, West Virginia, in the spring of 1862 and consisted of an administrative building and two detached pavilions. Similar units at Grafton and Newkirk in the same state soon followed.

During and after 1862, hospital construction continued at a fast pace, although the practice of using existing nonhospital buildings as a core was to continue despite the growing recognition of the advantages of the pavilion plan. In November 1862, Dr. Hammond, who had been appointed surgeon general in April of that year, reported 151 military hospitals, with 58,715 patients, in operation throughout the North. Most of the hospitals built in early 1862 were comparatively small institutions. On May 1, 1862, construction commenced on what was to develop into the largest hospital north of the Mason-Dixon line.

Located in West Philadelphia, "removed from the close air and constant tumult of the crowded city," the new Satterlee Hospital was to have been completed in 40 days by terms of its contract. Seven wards were ready for occupancy on June 6, and in a few days they filled with patients. By October, all 28

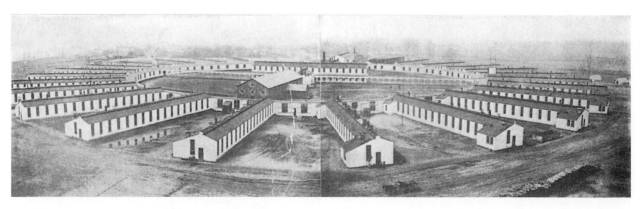

Rapidly constructed military hospitals had many pavilions.

wards, arranged in parallel rows of 14 each, were in operation, although eight large tents had already been added to house additional patients. Each of the wooden pavilion wards accommodated 70 patients. Eventually, the hospital added six additional pavilions to the east end of the structure and extended all on the south side as far as the site permitted. One hundred fifty hospital tents, accommodating 900 patients, were also set up. The hospital's official capacity as of 1865 was 3519 beds.

The most nearly complete military hospital, according to General Hammond, was the Mower General Hospital of Chestnut Hill, just within the city limits of Philadelphia. The entire facility consisted of 50 pavilions projecting from an interior circle 16 ft wide and 2400 ft long. The administration and service buildings were situated in the center of the site. With 3100 beds housed in wooden pavilions, it was actually larger than the neighboring Satterlee Hospital, whose greater bed capacity was due in part to an extensive use of tents. The North eventually had more than 200 military hospitals situated in most of the major cities, with 16 located in the Washington area alone.

Administrative surgeons instituted rigid rules concerning the work and behavior of nurses and patients. At Jarvis Army General Hospital in Baltimore, the edicts read as follows:

> The Nurses will be under the direct supervision of the Stewards and Chief Wardmaster. They will be held responsible for the proper administration of their wards, and they will take particular pains to carry out all orders emanating from the proper authority and pertaining to the welfare of the sick.
>
> The Patients will obey all lawful orders and instructions given them by the Nurses. They will be careful to be cleanly, and their conduct must be exemplary. All swearing, vulgar language, and indecent exposure are strictly prohibited, under penalty of severe punishment.
>
> The Wards must be thoroughly ventilated and cleaned once each day, and the beds must be arranged as often as they may require—care being taken to have things in proper condition at all times for inspection.
>
> The Nurses will guard against fires, and not use lights in their wards when not required, and they must report to the Surgeon in attendance on their Wards anything unusual occurring therein.
>
> If a patient needs medical or surgical attendance, the Nurse must at once see the Medical Officer of the Day, and request him to visit the person who is complaining. The interests of the afflicted require that the Nurses be mild and humane in waiting on their more unfortunate companions, and the Surgeon in Charge expects this of them.
>
> Should a patient not in sound mind be troublesome, the Nurses must bear with him;

> but if a patient, in his rational senses, conducts himself improperly, the Nurse will report the facts in the case to the Medical Officer of the Day.
>
> No lounging on beds or smoking in wards will be tolerated, and each bed, when not occupied, must be covered with clean bedding, which should be thoroughly changed at least once a week.
>
> The Female Nurses must be treated with the utmost respect and it must be remembered, a true soldier is always known by his good conduct.
>
> Convalescents must render every assistance to their companions who are disabled and assist in keeping their wards in proper police.
>
> Patients must take baths at regular intervals, and, when indicated by nature they must have their hair and beard cut, as there is no excuse for vermin in a well-regulated Hospital.
>
> The female Nurse will not be allowed in the wards after tatoo: and while all lady friends and relatives of Patients will be treated with proper courtesy and respect when visiting the Hospital, they will not be allowed in any of the wards after dark, except by special permission from the Surgeon in Charge.[9]

LOUISA MAY ALCOTT'S EXPERIENCES

A little book entitled *Hospital Sketches*, written by Louisa May Alcott (1832–1888), gives an idea of the nature of the work performed in Civil War hospitals by volunteer nurses. This slender volume—a little more

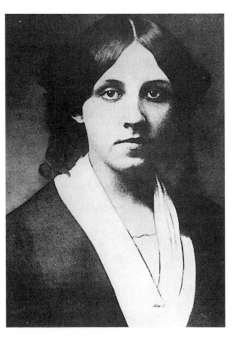

Louisa May Alcott.

than 100 pages—is written in a humorous, almost mock-heroic style, using the elegant circumlocutions, multisyllabic words, and formal syntax that marked fine writing in those times. In this case, the style relates to the structure of the book itself and to the author's philosophy of life and nursing. Humor is the key to both, despite the basic seriousness of the subject. The book is divided into six chapters: "Obtaining Supplies," "A Forward Movement," "A Day," "A Night," "Off Duty," and "A Postscript." The first chapter deals with her preparations for the trip and her oft-frustrated attempts to get the free railroad pass to Washington, DC, to which nurses were entitled. The second chapter is a spirited account of the actual trip, by trains and a boat, to "Hurly-burly House," her name for the makeshift army hospital hastily set up in an old Georgetown hotel.

The opening chapter implies much about the motivations, expectations, and attitudes then related to nursing. The narrator, calling herself Miss Tribulation Periwinkle, decides on her nursing career in an apparently offhand manner. The book opens starkly with her declaration, "I want something to do." She rejects in rapid succession various family members' suggestions to write a book, go back to teaching, get married, or become an actress. But when her brother (an invented character) says, "Go nurse the soldiers," she responds impulsively, "I will." A brief interview with an army nurse produces three results: "I felt that I could do the work, was offered a place, and accepted it." The expected position at Armory Hospital turns out to be filled, however, so Tribulation goes instead to "a much less desirable one at Hurly-burly House." And thus begins her career.[10]

The vague fervor that informed her choice, however, rapidly meets unforeseen realities, because nurses received no advance training. The third chapter,

"A Day," describes her first day on the job, but also serves as a microcosm of her entire time there. "What shall we have to do?" she asks as the casualties arrive all at once at the hospital—40 ambulances full. "Wash, dress, feed, warm and nurse them for the next three months" comes the prompt answer, with an immediate addition: "You won't probably find time to sit down all day, and may think yourself fortunate if you get to bed by midnight."

"Having a taste for 'ghastliness,'" says Nurse Periwinkle, "I had rather longed for the wounded to arrive." But when she sees the shattered, filthy collection of casualties and smells the vile odors that attend disease, infection, and death, she admits, "My ardor experienced a sudden chill, and I indulged in a most unpatriotic wish that I was safe at home again, with a quiet day before me." Furthermore, she is completely taken aback when asked for the first time to scrub the muddy soldiers: "If she had requested me to . . . dance a hornpipe on the stove funnel, I should have been less staggered; but to scrub some dozen lords of creation at a moment's notice was really—really–."[11]

Fortunately, she has determination and humor, and her first patient is an irrepressible Irishman who makes her laugh so hard that she "took heart and scrubbed away like any tidy parent on a Saturday night." In between anecdotes and descriptions of various patients, she tells of getting all the muddy soldiers washed, fed, and made comfortable in clean, warm beds. She makes rounds with the surgeons and learns how to dress wounds, groaning inwardly for the brave stoicism of these patients and beginning already to feel maternal toward them. It was "long past noon" before these basic nursing functions were completed, and, she says, "having got the bodies of my boys into something like order, the next task was to

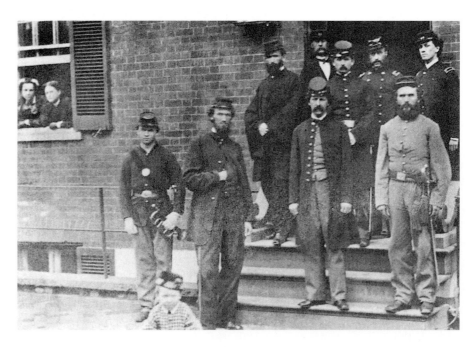

Nurses look out a window as soldiers pose at the Georgetown Hospital.

minister to their minds, by writing letters to the anxious souls at home; answering questions, reading papers, taking possession of money and valuables [for safekeeping]." Then it is all to do again as dinnertime arrives; she performs the evening duties: giving medicines, "washing fevered faces; smoothing tumbled beds; wetting wounds; singing lullabies; and [making] preparations for the night." By the time the chapter ends, Nurse Periwinkle seems to have been nursing for a long time, and only a second reading makes clear that just a single day has been described.

Likewise, the fourth chapter, "A Night," although ostensibly dealing with a single night of ward duty, in fact contains much more and marks Nurse Periwinkle's growth in skill, knowledge, and sympathy. Soon after her arrival she has been made superintendent of her ward, and her good instincts compensate for her lack of training. She anticipates modern practice by acting like a triage nurse. She separates her patients, according to the seriousness of their conditions, into three different rooms: her "duty room," "pleasure room," and "pathetic room." "One," she says, "I visited, armed with a dressing tray full of rollers, plasters, and pins; another, with books, flowers, games, and gossip; a third, with teapots, lullabies, consolation, and, sometimes, a shroud."[12]

There, where the sickest patients are, she keeps her watch as night nurse, making frequent checks also on the other rooms to make sure the watchman of the ward keeps the fires burning and the patients' wounds constantly wet. Some of what she sees as night nurse are funny, and this she describes with relish. But the main story in "A Night" is a sad one—the tale of the gentlest, most patient man in the ward, who, she learns with guilty surprise, is actually the most critically injured. She relates how she discovered that this stoic giant of a man actually longed to be comforted like a child and how she soothes him in his last days and eases his painful death. The arch humor that marks so much of the book is absent in this touching narration, and the tale shows Nurse Periwinkle at her finest moment, embodying the very spirit of nursing for all her lack of training.

The title of the fifth chapter, "Off Duty," is doubly apt, for it tells both of the narrator's hours off from nursing duties and of her final departure from duty. This chapter is most important for the revelations it makes about the awful conditions nurses had to endure in this hospital. Little provision is made for the nurses' comfort or health at "Hurly-burly House." The food is poor and limited in quantity; five of the window panes in her room are broken, letting in the cold winter air; furnishings are meager and uncomfortable; and rats haunt the closet and devour any food she might bring in to eke out the insufficient rations provided by the hospital.

The narrator describes these horrors with lighthearted humor and sarcasm, but clearly she feels the need to get away from such conditions. Whenever off duty, she leaves the hospital—taking brisk walks in the clean air, visiting monuments and museums—comparing Hurly-burly House with the efficient Armory hospital. She loses her appetite altogether, subsisting on small amounts of bread and water. Small wonder, then, that the long hours, the contact with desperately ill patients, the poor food, and the unsanitary conditions finally take their toll. By January, Nurse Periwinkle feels her strength giving out; although she resists urgings to go to bed and rest, she is finally forced to give in to the pain, exhaustion, and dizziness that overwhelm her. Doctors diagnose typhoid, and as her condition worsens, her father arrives to take her home, thus ending her brief nursing career.

The final chapter, "A Postscript," is just that—a section written after the original "Sketches" had appeared in print—and in it she answers readers' questions, makes suggestions for better hospital practices, discusses how nurses and families can most helpfully and sympathetically deal with death, tells readers what happened to some of the patients described in the sketches, and discusses the differences between nurses' and doctors' levels of sensitivity. She ends with a plea to provide hospitals for "the colored regiments," blacks apparently not having been allowed in the regular hospitals. Finally, she answers "the serious-minded party who objected to a tone of levity in some portions of the Sketches": "I can only say that it is a part of my religion to look well after the cheerfulness of life, and let the dismals shift for themselves; believing, with good Sir Thomas More, that it is wise to 'be merrie in God.'"[13]

MOTHER BICKERDYKE'S ADVENTURES

Another of the more famous untrained Civil War nurses was a little-educated but superbly shrewd Illinois woman in her 40s named Mary Ann Bickerdyke (1817–1901). She was soon called "Mother" Bickerdyke by the troops. When in 1861 she agreed to accompany medical supplies to Cairo, Illinois, she promised: "I'll go to Cairo, and I'll clean things up there. You don't have to worry about that, neither. Them generals and all ain't going to stop me. This is the Lord's work you're calling me to do."[14] Numerous stories were soon being told about "Mother's" exploits:

> Looking from his tent at midnight, an officer observed a faint light flitting hither and thither on the abandoned battlefield, and, after puzzling over it for some time, sent his servant to ascertain the cause. It was Mother Bickerdyke, with a lantern. Stooping down [among the dead] and turning their cold faces towards her, she scrutinized them searchingly, uneasy lest some might be left to die uncared for. She could not rest while she thought any were overlooked who were yet living.

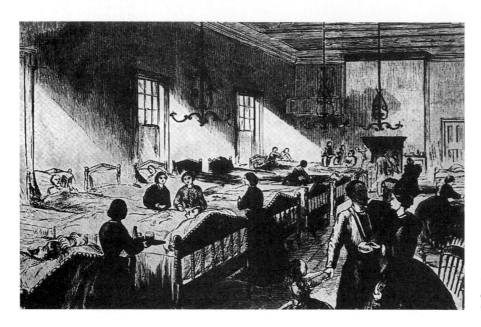

The scene of Alcott's nursing experience—the U.S. General Hospital at Georgetown in Washington, DC.

Observers recalled a hospital boat:

> Incessant cries of "Mother, Mother, Mother" rang through the boat, in every note of beseeching anguish. And to every man she turned with a heavenly tenderness, as if he were indeed her son. She moved about with a decisive air, and gave directions in such decided, clarion tones as to ensure prompt obedience.[15]

On one occasion a disrespectful Union officer snapped at Mrs. Bickerdyke: "Madam, you seem to combine in yourself a sick-diet kitchen and a medical staff. May I inquire under whose authority you are working?" Without pausing in her work, Mother answered: "I have received my authority from the Lord God Almighty. Have you anything that ranks higher than that?" This bold nurse was especially outraged when she saw lazy or corrupt medical officers, and the great efforts she made to secure their dismissals were often successful—although such action created much ill will among the physicians. Mrs. Bickerdyke wielded considerable power, largely because of her firm friendship with General Ulysses S. Grant and General William T. Sherman.[16]

Not all the women nurses of the North were as successful as Alcott and Mrs. Bickerdyke. Surgeons generally condemned them, although seldom citing any specific shortcomings. From their own accounts, the nurses did not always obey orders and sometimes substituted their own prescriptions for those of the physicians. Others fed men the food they wanted but were not supposed to have, while some lavished attention on favorite patients and were jealous of other nurses who had proved themselves more popular. A few took advantage of the weaknesses of the patients to reform them or to push on them a particular brand of religion.

JANE STUART WOOLSEY'S OBSERVATIONS

When Jane Woolsey set out for a Union hospital on a Virginia hill in sight of the nearly finished "wonderful white dome" of Washington, she cloaked herself "with an easy and cheerful-minded confidence in the unknown . . . which must," she added, "have been part of the spirit of the time." Indeed, her description of nursing during the Civil War manifests much of this "cheerful-minded" spirit; yet she writes also

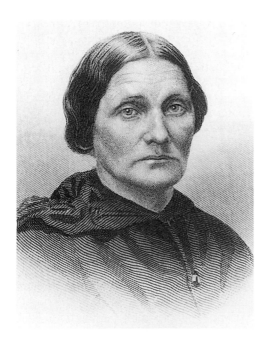

Mary Ann Bickerdyke.

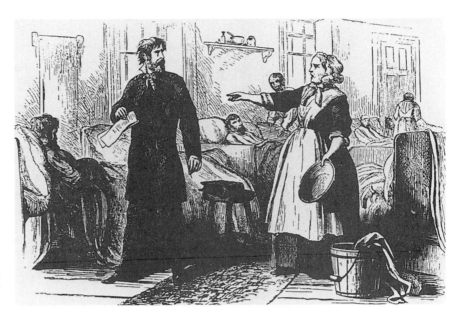

Mrs. Bickerdyke was outraged when confronted with lazy or corrupt medical officers.

with a sober air that seems to preserve her reminiscence in a pristine, objective state for the 20th-century reader. Because her account is thus balanced, it would seem a judicious indicator of the image of Union nursing during the Civil War.[17]

Woolsey began her service unlike many of her contemporaries. Whereas many nurses frequently battled to gain entrance to military hospitals, Jane and her sister "had been invited [to the hospital] by the officer in charge, as supervisors of the nursing and cooking department." Nor were their living conditions at the hospital as trying as many encountered:

> The officer in charge came out to meet them, and took them over to their lodgings in the parsonage, a few yards from the central offices. They were so fortunate as to be assigned to quarters in the house with the Chaplain and his family, and were shown into a large octagon-sided room, with bare, clean floor, two camp beds, with bed-sacks stuffed with straw, two little tables with regulation tin basins, and in the wide fireplace a huge black cylinder of sheet iron, giving out a dull roar, and growing red here and there in spots.[18]

If her hospital beginnings and personal lodgings differed from those of most nurses, Jane Woolsey's subsequent life as a Union nurse closely resembled that of her comrades. She expressed the same concern for an efficient professionalism that many other Union nurses observed, and her narrative praises the "division of labor and practice" that was becoming an integral part of hospital life behind the Union lines. To say that Union nursing was a model of orderly efficiency, however, would be an overstatement.

Woolsey's experience demonstrates that even in the best-run hospitals, "there never was any system" for selecting or training nurses on a widespread scale. Nurses were as likely to be wives of generals or destitute charwomen as to be reasonably qualified like herself. They were "volunteers paid or unpaid; soldiers' wives and sisters who had come to see their friends, and remained without any clear commission or duties; women sent by State agencies and aid societies; women assigned by the General Superintendent of Nurses"; or any woman who felt some reason to attach herself to a hospital. In short, although many urged and some tried to implement standards of selection and periods of training for nurses, the Union nursing corps nonetheless remained a motley group of women who shared little more than their lack of qualifications.[19]

Much of Woolsey's narrative thus provides us with a clear picture of opposing forces in Civil War nursing in the North. On the one hand, the sense of nursing as a profession with requisite standards existed at least among the elite of the nursing corps. On the other hand, all hospitals confronted an unending stream of women who, though little suited for their work, frequently out of necessity entered the ranks alongside more qualified personnel.

Such a dichotomy created in the incipient profession a tension that made the image of nursing during the Civil War somewhat ambiguous. Yet the very fact that nursing as a profession in America had its beginnings during this period of crisis did much to resolve that ambiguity. The lack of training on the part of many demonstrated, if nothing else, that training was imperative. It became increasingly evident as the war progressed that for the sick and wounded to survive, supplies and medical personnel had to be efficiently organized. Moreover, as competent women demonstrated their skill, they inspired a

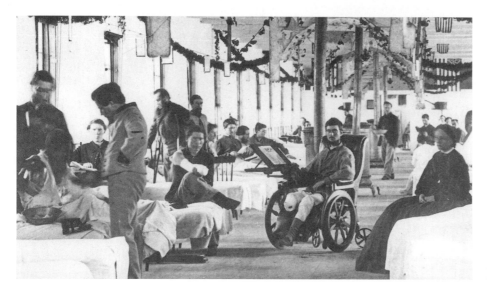

Nurse, patients, and physicians in a Union army hospital ward, 1864.

growing acceptance in the minds of surgeons and government officials and thus encouraged the participation of greater numbers of able women. There was, however, another ambiguity that circumstances did little to resolve: the question of what a nurse should be—a question that pervades the writings of even the women most qualified for nursing and most devoted to professionalism.

Clearly, nurses were not supposed to be machines. Just such an opprobrium was frequently registered, for example, against Catholic nuns who served in many Union hospitals. "The Roman Catholic system had features which commended it to medical officers of a certain cast of mind," Jane Woolsey wrote. They were particularly praised for their "order and discipline"—characteristics looked for in all nurses. Yet

more than anti-Catholic sentiment prompted Woolsey to add, "[T]aking the good, leaving the bad, and adapting the result to the uses of the country and the spirit of the time, we might have had an order of Protestant women better than the Romish 'sisterhoods,' by so much as heart and intelligence are better than machinery."[20]

Clearly, a traditional "womanly" character was just as important in a nurse, even to those women who led the fight for professionalization. Indeed, Woolsey describes many of the best nurses much as she does "Miss D-," who was "an excellent little creature, gentle-mannered, delicate, tremulous, full of intense and indignant patriotism." Miss D seems, if anything, the antithesis of "order and discipline." "She could not work by rule or method. She lost the

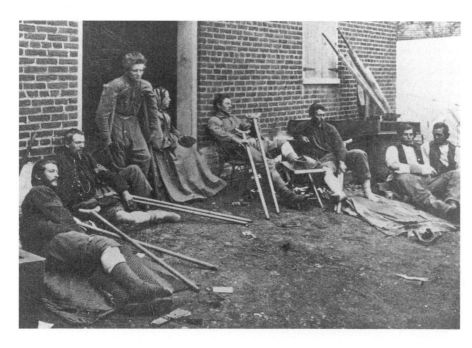

Wounded Union soldiers with nurse (in doorway) after the battle of Fredericksburg.

law in the exceptions. She took what she thought 'short-cuts,' and hand-to-mouth ways of doing what systematic effort would have accomplished in half the time." Moreover, Woolsey praises Miss D's ignorance of the chain of command so vital to an efficient organization. When Miss D, who "thought all military restriction atrocious," believed some injustice had been done, she "wanted 'to go and see Mr. Lincoln about it.'" Finally, what ensures Miss D's exaltation to the ranks of the gifted nurse is her "goodness and devotion."[21]

Woolsey's praise for the womanly virtues is not reserved for those nurses in less-responsible positions, but affects her perception of her own work. Although she sees her position much in terms of organizing supplies, keeping accounts, and supervising others, Woolsey feels as well the pull of more "traditional" duties:

> To these [supervisory] duties the Superintendent added in her own mind, among others, that of learning whether the permitted articles were cooked according to the taste and fancy of the individual, knowing well that A prefers salt and B sugar in the same kind of porridge, and disliking from her soul the tall-man-powders-short-men-pills system she observed elsewhere.[22]

A time that regarded women as the caretakers of virtue naturally emphasized the womanly virtues of nursing. A time when even minor bureaucratic barriers often posed immovable stumbling blocks just as naturally praised nurses for occasionally taking matters into their own hands. Woolsey's comment on the situation summed it up in a manner worthy of Dickens: "Sometimes it is a party of old gentlemen, in civil hats and tumbled, yellow dusters—a Board—for the Hospital is much infested with Boards out of which nothing is ever builded."

Yet one must remember that among leaders of the Union nursing corps, womanly virtues did not take precedence over the more professionally oriented qualities mentioned earlier. Along with her praise of Miss D, Woolsey includes another nurse who "possessed what many better educated women never attain—the ability to postpone the non-essential to the essential, and to distinguish clearly between them." Of herself, Woolsey says:

> Standing where she could see and sympathize with the "difficulties and scruples of authority," as well as with the needs and helplessness of suffering, the Superintendent eagerly availed herself of the privileges of her position. The diet system was from time to time altered and improved, until a set of tables, blanks, and orders was fixed on, so "fitly framed together" that the little department moved, without undue friction, fairly and smoothly to the end.[23]

In part, her duties included "little extra comforts" and as much sympathy "as she had time and inclination for," but overall, she said, "her serious business was to see that the women-nurses did their duty, and that the Special Diet was everything that it ought to be." For Woolsey, life in a Union hospital included the daily filing of forms and keeping of records that ensured at least some measure of organization, efficiency, and accountability.[24]

NURSING ON THE MISSISSIPPI

Another scene of nursing service took place on the muddy waters of the Mississippi, where the war saw the first use of a navy hospital ship. The steamer *Red Rover*, captured from the Confederates, was converted into a floating hospital to serve with the federal flotilla. The Western Sanitary Commission contributed $3500 to her conversion, and she was ready for service on June 10, 1862. The medical officer aboard made use of the services of Catholic nuns who had volunteered to nurse the wounded after the aborted first siege of Vicksburg in 1862. In effect, these Sisters of the Holy Cross were among the first navy nurses.

The description of the *Red Rover*, given by George D. Wise in the following excerpt from a letter to Flag Officer A. H. Foote, shows that no effort had been spared to provide excellent facilities for the care of the sick.

> I wish that you could see our hospital boat, the *Red Rover*, with all her comforts for the sick and disabled seamen. She is decided to be the most complete thing of her kind that ever floated, and is in every way a decided success. The Western Sanitary Commission gave us, in cost of articles, $3,500. The icebox of the steamer holds 300 tons. She has bathrooms, laundry, elevator for the sick from the lower to the upper deck, operating room, nine different water closets,

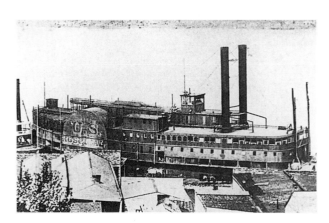

The Red Rover *near Vicksburg.*

gauze blinds to the windows to keep the cinders and smoke from annoying the sick, two separate kitchens for sick and well, a regular corps of nurses, and two water closets on every deck.[25]

NURSING IN THE SOUTH

In the Confederate states, the bulk of nursing duty fell into the rough hands of infantrymen detailed against their wishes to this type of duty. Many of these men were convalescent soldiers, selected more often because they were not strong enough for field duty than for any degree of aptitude or experience in caring for the sick. Moreover, as they grew well enough to be of any real help, they usually moved up to their line regiments. This gap in medical care was due to the South's slow recognition of the desirability of women as regular members of the medical department of the army. For the first 1½ years of the war, women had worked in the hospitals only as volunteers, and few of them had undergone any sort of training. Not until September 1862 did the Confederate Congress grant them official status.

In the Confederate states especially, widespread public prejudice militated against women serving in hospitals. An occupation involving such intimate contact with strange men was generally thought unfit for self-respecting women to pursue. There was no tolerance of young, unmarried women in these positions. "The simple truth is," wrote one Southern lady in withdrawing her application for a nursing position, "that my family is much opposed to my doing so, especially my brothers. . . . The boys have heard so much about ladies being in the hospitals that they cannot bear for me to go."[26]

Valor was exhibited by others not so easily discouraged, however. "I had never been inside of a hospital, and was wholly ignorant of what I should be called upon to do, but I knew that what one woman [Florence Nightingale] had done another could," wrote Kate Cumming (1828–1909) of Mobile of her decision to volunteer as a nurse. She later recorded:

> There is a good deal of trouble about the ladies in some of the hospitals of this department. Our friends here have advised us to go home, as they say it is not considered respectable to go into one. I must confess, from all I had heard and seen, for awhile I wavered about the propriety of it; but when I remembered the suffering I had witnessed, and the relief I had given, my mind was made up to go into one if allowed to do so.[27]

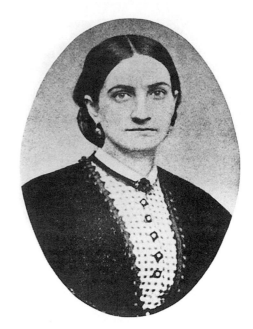

Kate Cumming.

The first entry in Kate Cumming's diary sets the stage of a straightforward Southern woman:

> *April 7, 1862.* I left Mobile by the Mobile and Ohio Railroad for Corinth, with Rev. Mr. Miller and a number of Mobile ladies. We are going for the purpose of taking care of the sick and wounded of the army.[28]

Indeed they were. For more than 300 pages, Kate Cumming chronicles the unflagging efforts of noble Southern women to care for their "boys." Although she does not hesitate to point out that many were oblivious of their duty—"I have said many a time that, if we [the Confederacy] did not succeed, the women of the South would be responsible"—she has mostly praise for the women who left their homes to serve as "matrons" in Confederate hospitals.[29]

Cumming's diary has much in common with Louisa May Alcott's *Hospital Sketches.* In the South as well as the North, many doctors resisted having any women in hospitals. Before Cumming even arrives at a hospital, she notes: "It seems that the surgeons entertain great prejudice against admitting ladies into the hospital in the capacity of nurses. The surgeon in charge, Dr. Caldwell, has carried this so far that he will not even allow the ladies of the place to visit his patients." But also, as in the North, the surgeons' ranks are divided. Another surgeon says of Dr. Caldwell's actions: "What can be expected from an old bachelor, who did not appreciate the ladies enough to marry one? He also said he did not think any hospital could get along without ladies. So we have one doctor on our side."[30]

Southern "matrons," at least from Cumming's account, endured even more social criticism than did their Northern sisters. Hospitals, known more for their filth and stench than for their ministrations to the sick and wounded, seemed hardly a fit place for a Southern belle. "The first thing we were told on our arrival [in Atlanta] was, that the citizens did not like the idea of the hospitals coming here." Hospital service, Cumming regrets, "is not respectable." Few of her pages, however, are given to musings about the position of nurses in society. In general, her main complaint against Southern society is directed toward those profiteers who charge hospitals exorbitant rates for food and supplies and toward those men and women in many towns who insist on living as if no war rages and refuse to supply either money or service to the soldiers. "I spent most of the day going around among the people, begging them for the loan of almost anything." A young man visited her "who was dressed in the extreme of fashion, with the addition of a few diamonds. . . . Foppish dress is bad taste in a man at any time; but if there is one time more than another when it is out of place, it is the present." Of course she also found many examples of community approval and of noble sacrifice: "A few weeks ago an article appeared in one of the papers of this place complimentary to the hospitals here. The editor said that, when the hospitals first came, there was great prejudice against them, on account of the sickness of which the people were afraid they might be the cause. But the reverse effect has been produced: All—rich and poor—sent something. One crowd of very poor-looking women brought some corn-bread and beans, which, I am certain, they could ill afford."[31]

The *social* situation of the Southern nurse, to this point, closely resembles that of her counterpart in the North. The professional situation, however, seems to differ. To begin with, female "nurses" are rarely, if ever, referred to by that title, which commonly denoted a male convalescent. (Southern nurses, called "matrons," will hereafter be called nurses for clarity.) Moreover, Southern nurses seemed even more than Northern nurses to be restricted to cooking, making bandages, and sewing, whereas Northern nurses spent more time comforting, washing faces, holding hands, and reading. This may have been due to the greater numbers of female nurses in the North—Southern nurses simply did not have time. As for doing the work of the surgeons, neither Northern nor Southern nurses engaged in much of that. Cumming, who entered service in April 1862, remarked on May 17, 1864: "Strange as it may seem, this was the first wound I had ever dressed. I had always had plenty of other work to do."[32]

Cumming also has described the menial position of nurses in the eyes of Southern doctors:

> Mrs. Dr. Pierce has sent a bottle of lotion for the use of the patients in cases of inflammation. As usual, the surgeons paid little or no attention to it, as it had been made by a lady. I found one of the patients suffering very much from a carbuncle. Dr. Wellford had been doing his best to get it ready for lancing. The head nurse said that Dr. Wellford told him to try any thing he pleased, as he was tired of trying things himself. I got him to try the lotion, and by next morning the carbuncle was ready for lancing. . . . This is a cause of triumph for us ladies.[33]

One never notices, as one frequently does in Alcott's *Hospital Sketches* or Woolsey's *Hospital Days*, a doctor asking a nurse's advice or a nurse volunteering advice to a doctor.

Cumming stayed with the hospital service of the army of Tennessee after the Battle of Shiloh and served with distinguished ability. Nursing in the Confederate army, often under primitive conditions, was exhausting and frustrating work. On November 13, 1864, then serving at a hospital in Atlanta, she noted in her diary:

> Our wounded are doing badly; gangrene in its worst form has broken out among them. Those whom we thought were almost well are now suffering severely. A wound which a few days ago was not the size of a silver dime is now eight or ten inches in diameter.
>
> The surgeons are doing all in their power to stop its progress. Nearly every man in the room where they were so full of jokes has taken it; there is very little laughing among them now. It is a most painful disease, and plays sad havoc with the men in every way. We cannot tempt them to eat, and we have very little sweet milk, and that is the cry with them all. Many a day I have felt as if I could walk any distance to get it for them.[34]

Of the work of such female nurses, Dr. S. H. Stout, medical director of Hospitals of the Army and Department of Tennessee, wrote:

> The gratitude of the soldiers was always manifest whenever these female nurses came into the wards. For they served them as amanuenses by writing letters to the families and friends of the disabled. They prayed for and with them when requested. They cooked appropriate and delicate food for them when needed. They wiped the sweat from the brows of the dying and closed the eyes of the dead. Often entrusted to send the last messages of the dying to their families and friends at home, these faithful matrons never failed to perform their promises.[35]

Conversely, Mary Boykin Chesnut (1823–1886), in *A Diary from Dixie*, reveals the reactions of a more typical woman of the Southern aristocracy, whose sentiments were later effectively mirrored in the experiences of Scarlett O'Hara in *Gone With the Wind*:

> August 19th, 1864. Began my regular attendance in the Wayside Hospital. Today we gave wounded men, as they stopped for an hour at the station, their breakfast. Those who are able to come to the table do so; the badly wounded remain in wards prepared for them where their wounds are dressed by nurses and surgeons, and we take bread and butter, beef, ham, hot coffee to them there. . . . They were awfully smashed-up objects of misery, wounded, maimed, diseased. I was really quite upset and came home ill. This kind of thing unnerves me quite. As I came into my room I stood there on the bare floor and made Ellen undress me and take every thread I had on and throw them all into a washtub out of doors. She had a bath ready for me, and a dressing-gown.[36]

EVALUATION OF CIVIL WAR NURSING

Close to 10,000 women served as nurses during the war. In the North, the 3214 nurses appointed by Dix and other officials held legal status as employees of the army and received salaries of 40 cents and one ration in kind each day. The several hundred Sisters of Charity or nuns of various orders constituted a second group of nurses. A third group consisted of those employed out of necessity over short periods to do the menial hospital chores. A fourth group consisted of black women employed under the General Orders of the War Department at a salary of $10 a month. The Federal Pension Office estimated the number of women serving in the third and fourth groups to be 4500. A fifth group included an unknown number of uncompensated volunteers. A sixth group consisted of women camp followers. The seventh and last group consisted of women employed by various relief organizations. Very few of these women had actual hospital experience or qualifications other than physical strength and willingness to serve. Probably at least 9000 women performed nursing duties of one kind or another in the North; fewer than 1000 did so in the South.

Jane Stuart Woolsey summarized her views of the women war nurses. These views, the result of observation and experience of a woman superintendent of nurses in military hospitals during the war, are probably a fair analysis of the true status and character of the Civil War nurses. "Was the system of women nurses in hospitals a failure?" she asked. Indeed, there had never been any system, she concluded; the experiment of a compact, general organization was

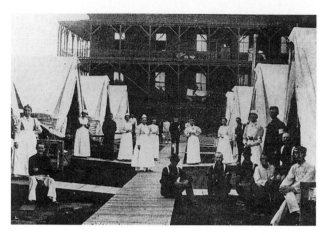

Several of 10,000 Civil War nurses at a hospital near Norfolk, VA.

never attempted. Hospital nurses were of "all sorts, and came from various sources of supply; volunteers, paid or unpaid; soldiers' wives and sisters who had come to see their friends, and remained without any clear commission or duties; women assigned by the General Superintendent of Nurses; sometimes, as in a case I knew of, the wife or daughter of a medical officer drawing the rations, but certainly not doing the work, of a 'laundress.'"[37]

These women were set adrift in a hospital—8 to 20 of them, slightly educated, for the most part, without training or discipline, without company organization or officers. They did their own "reporting" to the surgeons or to the general superintendent, which was very much "as if Private Robinson should 'report' to General Grant."[38]

Similarly, a first-hand investigation of the nursing system of the U.S. Sanitary Commission concluded:

> It is to be regretted that a more favorable account of the way in which the nurses have been received and treated in the hospitals cannot be given. They have not been placed, as they expected and were fitted to be, in the position of head nurses. On the contrary, with a very efficient force of male nurses, they have been called on to do every form of service, have been overtasked and worn down with menial and purely mechanical duties, additional to the more responsible offices and duties of nursing. They have encountered a certain amount of suspicion, jealousy and ill-treatment, which has rendered their situation very trying. . . . women nurses in military hospitals . . . are objects of continual evil speaking among coarse subordinates, are looked at with a doubtful eye by all but the most enlightened surgeons, and have a very uncertain, semi-legal position, with poor wages and little sympathy, except from the sick and wounded men they comfort and bless. Nothing but the most patriotic and humane motives could sustain women in this position.[39]

Although the nursing system was defective and the doctors did not approve of the women, certain parties to the experiment deemed it an unqualified success: the patients. The basis of the men's approval was rather sentimental and undiscriminating. As one of them replied when asked what he would have: "Anything just so it has a woman's finger on it."[40] Another recalled:

> Connected with our hospital was a lady who acted as matron. She frequently passed through the wards with some delicacy for the sick in her hands; this she gave to such as could take it; often the poor fellow had no stomach for anything, but the pleasure of receiving anything from the fair hands of a woman was too tempting to resist, and down it went, stomach or no stomach. Again she would pass from cot to cot, saying a kind word to each occupant, adjusting the blanket for this one, wiping the sweat from another's brow, and maybe writing to mother or wife for one too feeble to use a pen.[41]

In contrast, far too many women flooded Civil War hospitals as merely curious visitors and not to render any useful service. According to the account of one Indiana volunteer:

> The females . . . go gawking through the wards, peeping into every curtained couch, seldom exchanging a word with the occupant, but as they invariably "hunt" in couples giving vent to their pent up "pheelinks" in heart-rending outbursts of "Oh, my Savior," "Phoebe, do look here," "Only see what a horrid wound," "Goodness, gracious, how terrible war is," "My, my, my. Oh, let's go—I can't stand it any longer." And as they near the door, perhaps these dear creatures will wind up with an audible— "Heavens, what a smell. Worse than fried onions."[42]

A second class of women visitors frequented the hospitals generally in the company of "flashy youths got up in the latest style." These women were

> wasp-waisted, almond-eyed, cherry-lipped, finely-powdered damsels, carrying tiny baskets, containing an exquisitely embroidered handkerchief, highly perfumed, and a vial or two of restoratives (to be used in case of sudden indisposition). This batch of "sight seers," do-nothings, idlers, time-killers, fops, and butterflies skip through the hospital and like summer shadows, leave no trace behind.[43]

Although lacking a rigorous training for nursing, the more successful Civil War nurses had been driven by sentiment to enter hospital work. They saw nursing in a manner reminiscent of Longfellow, who had immortalized the work of Florence Nightingale in verse.

POSTWAR DEVELOPMENTS

After the war, several of the women who had been nurses helped lead the movement for the establishment of nurse training schools. Prominent among them were the Woolsey sisters—Abby, Jane, and Georgeanna. Abby (1828–1893) wrote one of the first books on the subject, *A Century of Nursing with Hints Toward the Organization of a Training School*, published in 1876. As directress of the Presbyterian Hospital in New York, Jane reorganized the nursing force, while Georgeanna (1833–1906) helped found the Connecticut Training School for Nurses in New Haven in June 1873.

About this time in England, Florence Nightingale was elaborating on what made a good training school for nurses:

> A year's practical and technical training in hospital wards, under trained head-nurses who themselves have been trained to train.
>
> The training of probationers should be as much a part of the duty of the head nurse ("sister") as directing the under-nurses or seeing to the patients.
>
> To tell the training, you require weekly records . . . kept by the head-nurses of the progress of each probationer (pupil) in her ward-work, and in the moral qualities necessary in her ward-work; a monthly record by the matron of the results of the weekly records; and a quarterly statement by her as to how each head-nurse has performed her duty to each probationer. The whole to be examined periodically by the governing body.
>
> Clinical lectures from the hospital professors . . . elementary instruction in chemistry . . . physiology . . . and general instruction on medical and surgical topics; examinations, written and oral, at least four of each in the year, all adapted to nurses; as also lectures and demonstrations with anatomical, chemical and other illustrations, adapted especially to nurses—all in the presence and under the care of the matron (Lady Superintendent) and mistress of probationers (Class-mistress and "Home"-sister); together with instruction from a medical instructor, one of the hospital professors and hospital medical staff, specially selected to teach the nurses.
>
> A good nurses' library of professional books, not for the probationers to skip and dip in at random, but to be made careful use of, under the medical instructor and class-mistress.

Classes for a competent mistress to drill the professorial teaching into the probationers' minds; the mistress of probationers to be above all a "home"-sister, capable of making the "home" a real home, and of training and disciplining the probationers there in all good—in moral qualities, customs, and habits, and manners, without which no woman can be a nurse, and in their duty and feeling to God as well as to their neighbor.

The authority and discipline over all the women of a trained lady-superintendent . . . who is herself the best nurse in the hospital, the example and leader of her nurses in all that she wishes her nurses to be. . . .

An organization not only to give this training systematically, and to test it by current tests and examinations, but also to give the probationers, by proper help in the wards, time to do their work as pupils as well as assistant-nurses, and above all to make it a real moral as well as nursing probation—for nursing is a probation as well as a mission.

Accommodation for sleeping, classes, and meals; arrangements for time and teaching and work; surroundings of a moral and religious, and hard-working and sober, yet cheerful tone and atmosphere, such as to make the training-school and hospital a "home" which no good young woman of any class need fear by entering to lose anything of health of body or mind; with moral and spiritual helps, and an elevating and motherly influence over all, such as to make the whole a place which will train really good women, who can withstand temptation and do real work, and neither be "romantic" nor "menial." For, make a hospital as good as you will, hospital-nurses require more such helps, and get less, than women either in their own homes or in domestic service.

Every hospital should have and be such a school for training nurses for itself and other institutions.[44]

Almost 3 decades later, Mary Livermore, one of the last of the famous untrained nurses of the Civil War, addressed the sixth annual convention of the Nurses' Associated Alumnae (later the American Nurses Association) on June 10, 1903, and declared: "I find all that is within me rising up in this presence in a semi-reverential attitude. A congregation of trained women nurses. Something that in my earlier days I never expected to see." She acknowledged a new profession that had grown in part from the seeds of the collective Civil War nursing experience.[45]

Whereas Mary Livermore and her associates had fought for "the right to tread so softly beside the

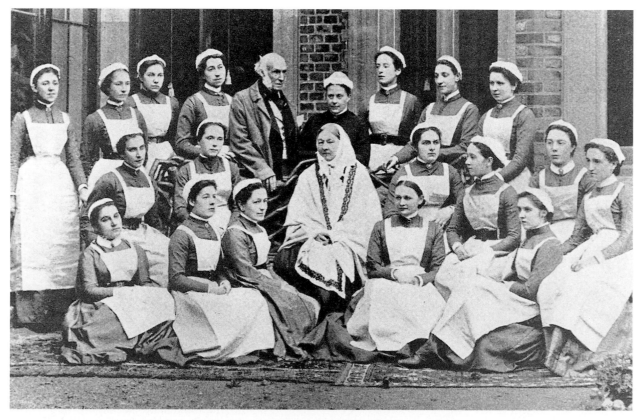

Florence Nightingale (seated, center), 1867, continued to provide direction to reforms in nursing.

couch of pain" and "to watch beside the dying in the still small hours of the night," the new generation of nurses being trained in scientific principles of patient care found that nursing demanded an abundance of strength, both of mind and body.[46] The romantic concept of the nurse as a guardian angel watching through the night and ceaselessly concerned with the patients ignored the reality of the woman with the scrub brush, the lady of soap and water, and the tireless cook of gruel and custard. But, no matter how beholders saw the wartime nurses and their work, the untrained Civil War nurses conferred on the women of the United States a great practical gift. Although most were amateurs, their humble efforts and the positive effects of their femininity on the sick and wounded troops made it legitimate for respectable women to enter the field of nursing and helped to create a new profession.

REFERENCES

1. Kate Cumming, *Journal of Hospital Life in the Confederate Army of Tennessee from the Battle of Shiloh to the End of the War: with Sketches of Life and Character and Brief Notices of Current Events During That Period* (Louisville: John P. Morton, 1866), p. 28.
2. Florence Nightingale, "Nurses, Training of," in Richard Quain, ed., *A Dictionary of Medicine* (New York: Appleton & Co., 1883), pp. 1038–1039.
3. Ibid., p. 1039.
4. L. P. Brockett and Mary C. Vaughan, *Woman's Work in the Civil War: A Record of Heroism, Patriotism, and Patience* (Philadelphia: Seigler, McCurdy, 1867), pp. 102–103.
5. *American Medical Times*, vol. 3 (July 13, 1861):25.
6. Mary A. Livermore, *My Story of the War: A Woman's Narrative of Four Years' Personal Experience as Nurse in the Union Army and in Relief Work at Home, in Hospitals, Camps, and at the Front During the War of the Rebellion. With Anecdotes, Pathetic Incidents, and Thrilling Reminiscences Portraying the Lights and Shadows of Hospital Life and the Sanitary Service of the War* (Hartford: A. D. Worthington, 1889), p. 110.
7. Walt Whitman, *The Works of Walt Whitman* (New York: Funk & Wagnalls, 1968), vol. 1, p. 285.
8. Mark Van Doren, *Walt Whitman* (New York: Viking Press, 1945), p. 557.
9. Rules for nurses and patients, Jarvis U.S.A. General Hospital, July 21, 1864 (placard), copy in Library of Congress, Washington, DC.
10. Louisa M. Alcott, *Hospital Sketches* (Boston: Roberts Brothers, 1885), pp. 3–10.
11. Ibid., pp. 26–39.
12. Ibid., pp. 40–59.
13. Ibid., pp. 80–96.
14. Nina Brown Baker, *Cyclone in Calico: The Story of Mary Ann Bickerdyke* (Boston: Little, Brown & Company, 1952), p. 11.
15. Florence Shaw Kellogg, *Mother Bickerdyke as I Knew Her* (Chicago: Unity Publishing Company, 1907), p. 30.
16. Margaret B. Davis, *The Woman Who Battled for the Boys in Blue—Mother Bickerdyke* (San Francisco: Pacific Press Publishing House, 1886), pp. 23–51.
17. Jane Stuart Woolsey, *Hospital Days* (New York: D. Van Nostrand, 1870), p. 45.
18. Ibid., pp. 45–49.
19. Ibid., pp. 29, 41.
20. Ibid., p. 43.
21. Ibid., p. 45.
22. Ibid., p. 35.
23. Ibid., pp. 16–17, 48.
24. Ibid., p. 16.
25. Louis H. Roddis, "The U.S. Hospital Ship *Red Rover* (1862–1865)," *Military Surgeon*, vol. 77 (August 1935):92.
26. Kate Cumming, *Gleanings from the Southland* (Birmingham: Roberts & Son, 1895), pp. 37–38.
27. Richard B. Harwell, ed., *Kate: The Journal of a Confederate Nurse* (Baton Rouge: Louisiana State University Press, 1959), p. 169.
28. Ibid., p. 9.
29. Ibid., p. 4.
30. Ibid., pp. 12–13.
31. Ibid., pp. 122, 136, 141, 207, 217.
32. Ibid., p. 198.
33. Ibid., p. 208.
34. Ibid., p. 169.
35. S. H. Stout, "Reminiscences of Medical Officers of the Confederate Army and Department of Tennessee," *St. Louis Medical and Surgical Journal*, vol. 64 (April 1893):228.
36. Mary Boykin Chesnut, *A Diary from Dixie*, ed. Ben Ames Williams (Boston: Houghton Mifflin Co., 1949), pp. 430–431.
37. Woolsey, op. cit., pp. 41–42.
38. Ibid., p. 42.
39. U.S. Sanitary Commission, *Report Concerning the Woman's Central Association of Relief at New York to the United States Sanitary Commission at Washington, October 12, 1861* (New York: The Commission, 1861), pp. 18–19.
40. Elvira J. Powers, *Hospital Pencilings* (Boston: Edward L. Mitchell, 1866), p. 172.
41. Charles B. Johnson, *Muskets and Medicine* (Philadelphia: F. A. Davis Co., 1917), p. 60.
42. "Prock's Letters from Camp, Battlefield, and Hospital," *Indiana Magazine of History*, vol. 34 (January 1938):96.
43. Ibid., pp. 96–97.
44. Nightingale, op. cit., pp. 1039–1041.
45. Mary A. Livermore, "Nurses in the Civil War," *Proceedings of the Sixth Annual Convention of the Nurses' Associated Alumnae of the United States, June 10, 11, and 12, 1903* (Philadelphia: J. B. Lippincott Co., 1903), pp. 1–6.
46. "Night Duty," *Trained Nurse and Hospital Review*, vol. 41 (October 1908):239.

3

THE FOUNDING OF EARLY SCHOOLS OF NURSING IN AMERICA

When the founding fathers in 1776 proclaimed that "all men are created equal," they did not see fit to include women. At the beginning of the 19th century, as legal wards of their husbands, wives had few legal rights over property or earnings. In practice, however, women fared better in America than in Europe because here men outnumbered women, and women were indispensable for running a farm household. But this demographic advantage did not immediately improve women's legal status nor did it open educational opportunity. Regarded as inferior to men, in mind as well as in body, women were declared unsuited for intellectual development. Instruction in painting, music, and embroidery seemed sufficient.

THE AMERICAN WOMAN'S PLACE

During the 19th century, common law and biblical tradition bound women to an inferior status. William Blackstone, the great British legal authority, had disposed of the independent rights of women by the simple common-law rule, "The husband and wife are one, and that one is the husband." In this state of wardship, the wife had no control over her property or her person. As a ward, she could not initiate a lawsuit by herself. If she ran away, her husband could forcibly reclaim and beat her as if she were a slave. If she resorted to divorce—where religious factors or complicated legal procedures permitted it—she might lose her home, children, and property. A drunken husband might sell his wife's clothing or require her employer—if she were employed—to turn over her earnings to him. A husband could even circumvent the complaints of a wife overly conscious of her human rights by committing her to an insane asylum.

Women were educated for marriage in a patriarchal society that revolved around their fathers and brothers and stressed property relationships rather than marital companionship. Despite the primacy placed on their reproductive functions, women were expected to know as little as possible about sex and to accept without complaint the double standard of morality.

The young lady of gentle background who wanted to step out of a strict family relationship to relieve the economic burden on her father or to seek an opportunity for self-development faced a real problem. Aside from teaching as a private governess or in the schoolroom and various types of handiwork such as dressmaking, millinery, and embroidery, few occupations were considered proper for a young woman to undertake. Mary Wollstonecraft passionately argued in the name of human dignity for justice to women. In her influential *Vindication of the Rights of Women* (1792), she urges that the trades and professions be opened to women according to their abilities, that women be educated in coeducational schools, and that society abolish the existing double standard of morality. Some of her ideas were popularized in the early 1800s by novelist Charles Brockden Brown and later by transcendentalist Margaret Fuller, whose *Women in the Nineteenth Century* (1845) makes a plea for the economic and intellectual emancipation of women.

American morality put women on a pedestal. The special function of women was to uphold virtue, serve as guardians of culture, and restrain the animal instincts of their mates. Men regarded their wives as creatures not only "purer and morally better" than themselves, but as "relatively impractical, emotional, unstable . . . incapable of facing facts or doing hard thinking." Man's arena was the factory and the marketplace, where aggressiveness and drive paid off. Women bore responsibility for maintaining a genteel atmosphere in the home, providing a refuge from the harsh workaday world ruled by force and power.

The sentimentality of the age produced an exaggerated chivalry and etiquette as confining to intellectually vigorous or sensitive women as the whalebone corsets and steel hoops that encased their bodies.

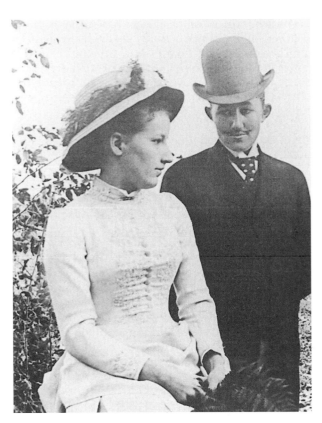

Extreme paternalism characterized 19th-century marital relations.

Popular Victorian literature in America idealized the fragile "lady" subject to self-induced faints, indifferent to exercise after marriage, languidly playing with her ringlets, idly moving her delicate fingers over the piano keys, and faithful to the minute ritual of etiquette books. Corseted tightly in gowns, these women decorated themselves with an assortment of laces, silks, trinkets, and rings, sat in parlors receiving visitors, changed ensembles several times a day, and patiently awaited their fathers' or husbands' return from the hectic business world.

Much of this routine was decidedly unhealthy. Dr. Robert L. Dickinson, a lecturer on obstetrics at the Long Island College Hospital, published a paper in the 1870s in the *New York Medical Journal* entitled, "The Corset: Questions of Pressure and Displacement." The results of his experiments and observations of corset pressure indicated that:

> The maximum pressure of the corset was 1.625 pounds to the square inch during inhalation, making the total estimated pressure 30 to 80 pounds.
> The capacity of expansion of the chest was restricted by one-fifth when the corset was on the body.
> The thoracic character of women's breathing was largely caused by wearing corsets.
> The abdominal wall was thinned and weakened by the pressure of stays; the liver suffered great direct pressure and was more frequently displaced than any other organ.
> The pelvic floor was bulged downwards, by tight-lacing, one-third of an inch.[1]

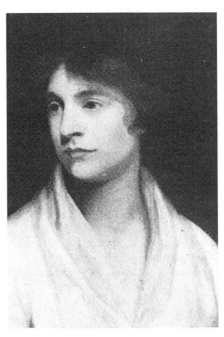

Mary Wollstonecraft.

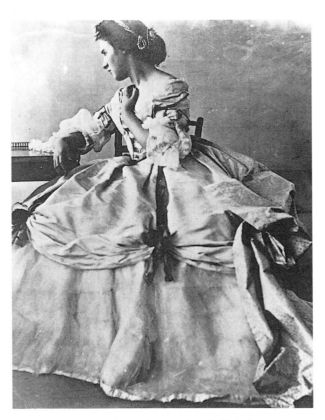

Victorians idealized the fragile "lady."

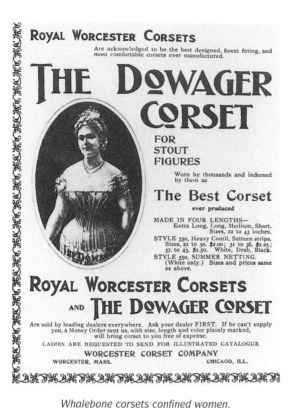

Whalebone corsets confined women.

One woman suffragist, Mary Livermore, challenged the doctrine that all men must support all women. She pointed out that such a view did not fit the facts. Many women with husbands were compelled to earn a living. Widows had to earn the livelihood for the entire family, she pointed out. The response to Horace Greeley's call "Go West, young man" had left an excess of women in the Eastern states without any opportunity to get married. Livermore noted that no girl should be considered well educated, no matter what her accomplishments, until she had learned a trade, business, vocation, or profession.

FIRST INSTRUCTION OF NURSES AND MIDWIVES

Intermittently throughout the first 70 years of the 19th century, physicians gave lectures to nurses and midwives at state hospitals in several large Eastern cities of the United States, but these activities could not be construed as formal courses of instruction. Just before the turn of the century, Dr. Valentine Seaman, an attending physician at New York Hospital, had conceived and initiated the first comprehensive course of instruction for nurses on the North American continent. This achievement was commemorated in an inscription placed below his portrait in the original hospital building: "In 1798 he organized in the New York Hospital the first regular training school for

nurses, from which other schools have since been established and extended their blessings throughout the Community."[2] In connection with the maternity department of New York Hospital, Seaman, far ahead of his time, had organized a course of 24 nursing lectures, including outlines of anatomy, physiology, and child care. The three concluding lectures were published in 1800 as *The Midwives Monitor, and Mothers Mirror, Being Three Concluding Lectures of a Course of Instruction of Midwifery; Containing Directions for Pregnant Women; and Roles for the Management of Natural Births, and for Early Discovering When the Aid of a Physician is Necessary and Cautions for Nurses, Respecting Both the Mother and Child. To Which is Prefixed, a Syllabus of Lectures on that Subject.*

The practice of obstetrics by male physicians had been practically unknown in the British colonies of North America. Early public disapproval of this practice was indicated in 1646 when a man was arrested and heavily fined for practicing as a midwife in Massachusetts. But in 1752, when Dr. James Lloyd returned to Boston after having studied in London and announced himself as a physician and male midwife, he introduced a new vogue. Twenty years later, a female midwife moving from Boston to Salem felt compelled to announce in an advertisement that her reason for relocating was that male midwives were too numerous in Boston. The practice of obstetrics by male physicians became so common that the male designation of "man midwife" had disappeared by 1800.

Another training course for nurses was organized by liberal Quaker physician Joseph Warrington, who in 1828 established the Philadelphia Lying-in Charity. Warrington, a graduate of the University of Pennsylvania, was obstetric physician to the Philadelphia Dispensary for the Medical Relief of the Poor, founded in 1786. While working in this capacity, he became aware of the urgent need for trained midwives who would deliver, without fee, the babies of poor women in their homes. On May 7, 1832, he formed an additional institution, incorporated as the Philadelphia Lying-in Charity for Attending Indigent Females in Their Own Homes.

Warrington began to train nurses in midwifery during classes with his medical students. Later, he expanded the training program to include experience in medical and surgical nursing. In 1839, Warrington wrote *The Nurses' Guide, Containing a Series of Instructions to Females Who Wish to Engage in the Important Business of Nursing Mother and Child in the Lying-in Chamber.* Faced with a shortage of applicants, Warrington, in 1854, wrote a six-page pamphlet entitled *An Appeal for the Supply of a Greater Number of Intelligent Women to Become Trained as Nurses for the Sick.*

In Boston, Dr. Samuel Gregory helped to start a second school for nurse-midwives in 1846. Gregory published a number of pamphlets urging more courses and better instruction in this field. One of his addresses was entitled *Man Midwifery Exposed and*

Corrected; or the Employment of Men to Attend Women in Childbirth, shown to be a Modern Innovation, Unnecessary, Unnatural and Injurious to the Physical Welfare of the Community and Pernicious in its Influences on Professional and Public Morality. Gregory wanted to make it possible for aspiring female midwives to acquire some scientific knowledge as a basis for their practice. In that era, midwives acquired their skill primarily through trial and error.

Gregory also wrote a pamphlet published in February 1846 titled *Licentiousness, Its Cause and Effects.* It stated that "There is demanded now, as formerly, a supply of female accoucheurs [midwives]; also a class of female physicians, qualified at least to attend to the peculiar complaints of their own sex."[3] Gregory cited the success of Mme. Lachapelle and Mme. Boivin of Paris, who were so skilled in saving the lives of mothers and babies that the mortality among patients confined in Paris was much less than that in Boston. Midwives in the United States needed instruction in anatomy and physiology, especially in the physiology of pregnancy and parturition.

ELIZABETH BLACKWELL OPENS MEDICINE TO WOMEN

Before the Civil War, females were generally admitted on an equal basis to elementary and secondary schools, but the doors of most colleges were closed to them. A few private colleges for women had been founded, but only three schools admitted women to study with men. An application for admission to attend medical lectures at Harvard was made as early as 1847 by Harriet K. Hunt. It was refused, but, without benefit of a medical degree, she gained some success both as a practitioner of hydropathy and as a lecturer on temperance, phrenology, the evils of tobacco, and sex hygiene.

The first woman to study medicine in America—and in modern times the first anywhere—was Elizabeth Blackwell. Born in England in 1821, she immigrated to the United States with her parents, who eventually settled in Cincinnati in 1832. On completion of her education, Elizabeth and her younger sister Emily engaged in school teaching. The remarks of a friend dying slowly of cancer, whom she was nursing, first inspired Blackwell to seek a medical education. "Why don't you study medicine?" the patient asked. "It would have been so much less harassing for me to have been taken care of by a woman than by a man." Blackwell found it impossible, however, to secure the opportunity to pursue a regular medical education.[4]

In 1845, Blackwell met Dr. Joseph Warrington, who did not believe in the existence of any mental or physical deficiency that should disqualify a woman from studying medicine. Warrington suggested that she wear men's clothing, as Dr. Mary Edwards Walker later did, because he thought that a woman would be less conspicuous in trousers. Blackwell, however, refused to disguise herself. Warrington tried to help her gain admission to one of the Philadelphia medical schools. She followed up her applications with personal appeals to faculty members, but although many of them were impressed by her poise, personality, and preparation, she was turned down by every medical school in Philadelphia and New York and also by Harvard, Yale, and Bowdoin. Disheartened but still determined, she began studying anatomy in the private school of Dr. Joseph M. Allen and applied to several rural medical schools.

Elizabeth Blackwell applied for admission to 12 different medical colleges and was rejected by all of them. Finally, in October 1847, the faculty of the Geneva Medical School of Western New York decided to refer the decision on her pending application to the all-male student body. The circumstances surrounding this incident were later recalled by Dr. Stephen Smith, an eyewitness to the proceedings:

> Being located in the country, the class of students was largely made up of the sons of farmers, tradesmen, and mechanics. A common saying among the people of that vicinity was that a boy who proved to be unfit for anything else must become a doctor. And the "royal road" to a medical degree was made remarkably easy at that time. The full term of study was three years and the fee was reduced to a minimum.
>
> Under these circumstances the class contained a large element of rude and uncouth country youths whose love of "fun" far exceeded their love of learning. During the interval of lectures every form of athletic sport might be

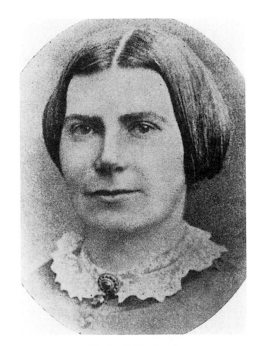

Elizabeth Blackwell.

witnessed with occasional "fisticuff" exercises which elicited ear-splitting shouts of the spectators. Nor did the excitement cease with the commencement of the lecture, but often continued through it to the great annoyance of those students who were attentive and studious. The rowdyism of the class may be realized when it is stated that the residents in the vicinity endeavored to have the college declared and treated as a public nuisance.

One morning early in the session, the Dean of the Faculty, an elderly, courtly, nervous gentleman, entered the classroom with a letter in his hand. He stated, with trembling voice, that the Faculty had received a very important communication from an eminent physician of Philadelphia and he had been requested to lay the letter before the class and ask its serious and thoughtful consideration of the request which the writer made.

A profound silence fell upon the class-room as he proceeded. The writer stated that he had a lady medical student who had attended a course of lectures in a college in Cincinnati; that he wished to have her attend one of the Eastern city colleges and graduate, but that everyone had refused her admittance; that he thought that a country college like Geneva might not object to her entrance; that if refused admission, she would be compelled to go to Edinburgh, Scotland to graduate. The Dean remarked that the request was so unusual, and so vitally interested the members of the class, that the Faculty decided to submit the question of admission of a woman student to its judgment, and had determined that, if there was one negative vote, the faculty would deny the request.

It was subsequently learned that the Faculty was unanimously opposed to the admission of a woman to the class, but did not care to take the responsibility of opposing the request of the eminent Philadelphia physician. Believing that the class would quite unanimously reject the proposal, the Faculty determined to place their denial upon the action of the students. To make the action of the class certainly negative they decided that a single vote against the request would enable the Faculty to refuse admission.

But the Faculty did not understand the tone and temper of the class. For a minute or two, after the departure of the Dean, there was a pause, then the ludicrousness of the situation seemed to seize the entire class, and a perfect babble of talk, laughter, and catcalls followed. Congratulations upon the new source of excitement were everywhere heard, and a demand was made for a class meeting to take action on the Faculty's communication.

A meeting was accordingly called for the evening, and a more uproarious scene can scarcely be imagined. Fulsome speeches were made in favor of admitting women to all the rights and privileges of the profession, which were cheered to the echo. At length the question was put to vote, and the whole class arose and voted "Aye" with waving of handkerchiefs, throwing up hats, and all manner of vocal demonstrations.

When the tumult had subsided, the chairman called for the negative votes, in a perfectly perfunctory way, when a faint "Nay" was heard in a remote corner of the room. At that instant, the class arose as one man and rushed to the corner from which the voice proceeded. Amid screams of "cuff him," "crack his skull," "throw him down stairs," a young man was dragged to the platform screaming, "Aye, aye! I vote 'aye.'" A unanimous vote in favor of the woman student had thus been obtained by the class, and the Faculty was notified of the result.[5]

Initially ostracized by the townspeople of Geneva and by the faculty—both groups regarded her as immoral or "queer"—Blackwell gradually won acceptance through her diligence and enthusiasm for her studies. During her 1848 summer vacation she gained admittance to the wards of Philadelphia General Hospital, where she pursued clinical study and helped combat an epidemic of typhus that had broken out among the patients. This experience inspired her to write her M.D. thesis on the subject of typhus and the importance of sanitary measures in combating disease. On January 23, 1849, Elizabeth Blackwell graduated at the head of her class.

Immediately after graduation she went to Europe and spent 2 years in several hospitals of London and Paris. Perplexed male authorities first suggested, as Warrington had done, that she dress as a man, but they finally admitted her in her usual attire. She studied at La Maternité, the famous school of midwifery in Paris, where life was "infernal." It seemed that the female midwifery students were "pretty generally the mistresses of the teachers." While passing through England in April 1851, she visited Florence Nightingale. One afternoon during the visit, Blackwell openly admired the facade of Embley Estate, where she was staying. "Do you know what I always think when I look at that row of windows?" asked Nightingale. "I think how I should turn it into a hospital and just where I should place the beds."[6]

After studying privately with the demonstrator of anatomy at Cincinnati Medical College, Emily Blackwell applied for admission to the medical college at Geneva in 1851 but was refused. The faculty agreed that the presence of Elizabeth Blackwell had resulted in a positive effect on the conduct and attainments of the other students, but they would not

PHYSICIANS IN MUSLIN.

CONTEMPORARY states that an English lady has just completed her medical studies at Paris, and obtained a diploma to practise as a physician; so that she has now become DR. EMILY. The surname of the lady is immaterial, and, moreover, it may he hoped, will speedily be exchanged for another; since if to be cherished in sickness is a important object in marriage, a wife who in her own person combines the physician with the nurse must be a treasure indeed. The difficulty, not to say impossibility, of getting the ordinary nurse to act in concert with the rational and honest physician is too well known to all who have experienced the blessings of a nursery, and have ever paid any attention to its affairs as well as paying its expenses. A consort, uniting the two characters in her single and at the same time her married person, would insure reasonable conduct, and expenditure to match, in that department of the household. She would also maintain, without DAFFY or MRS. JOHNSON, comparative quiet in that same region whence although it is mostly situated at the top of the house, continually proceed the very same kind of noises with those described by the poet as first saluting the ears of the Trojan hero upon the threshold of another and a lower place.

A medical wife, moreover, would not need, on her own account, that enormous amount of cherishing in sickness which some ladies require, and which, though in itself a duty which is also a pleasure to gentlemen of independent property, is yet somewhat of an embarrassment for men whose duty it is to attend, at the same time, to the business whereby they have to support themselves and their families. She would save her husband all the cost of those continual doctors who beset the house of that man who has an ignorant hypochondriacal wife, continually in want, not of medicine, but of medical consolation and condolence.

She would likewise, through her sanitary knowledge— her learning in the laws of health —be enabled to dispense with much of that travelling and change of scene, which, whilst they are gratifying to the inclinations of so many, are suitable to the circumstances of so few. She, although in a station of some gentility, would manage to exist without those sumptuous indulgences, for the want of which it is wonderful that almost all women of the working classes do not perish.

The above considerations cause us to rejoice in the embellishment of the Faculty by the fair sex. DR. EMILY has a sister, DR. ELIZABETH, who preceded her in walking the Parisian hospitals, and who is now practising at New York. May we venture to hope that they will prove ornaments to the fee-male sex? We shall be glad to see the gold-handled parasol extensively sported in Old England too; and trust that a clause will be introduced into MR. HEADLAM's Medical Bill, providing every facility for British ladies desirous of following the praiseworthy example which has been set them by these two daughters of Æsculapius.

THE EAST WIND!

LAST week, when the east wind was at its sharpest, a nursery maid, walking with her charge in the Regent's Park, had a remarkably fine baby cut into twins!

The Blackwells' pursuit of a medical education stirred social controversy.

consider her admission as a precedent and feared that if they opened their doors to women in general, they would become unpopular, thereby decreasing their enrollment. After Emily's applications had been rejected by several other medical schools, Rush Medical College in Chicago admitted her as a student for the first year of the program but, after censure by the State Medical Society of Illinois, refused to allow her to proceed with the second year. Finally, the Medical Department of Western Reserve University in Cleveland accepted her application, and she graduated in 1854.

In the meantime, concern over the Blackwells' difficulties had induced a group of Quakers to aid in establishing a full medical course for women in Philadelphia. The Quakers' initiative laid the foundation for the Woman's Medical College of Pennsylvania, which opened in March 1850 and graduated its first eight female physicians on December 31, 1851. They possessed only a theoretical knowledge of medicine, however, because the college could not gain access to clinical facilities. Although male physicians could not prevent women from studying medicine, they were unwilling to introduce them, as they did their male students, into the houses of even their poorest patients for fear that they might lose their clientele by making themselves odious as reformers.

THE NEED FOR TRAINED NURSES IS RECOGNIZED

In 1849, the Massachusetts Legislature appointed a state sanitary commission to propose plans for promoting public health. The commission recommended in its report early in 1850 "that institutions be formed to educate and qualify females to be nurses of the sick." To this end, the education of nurses was one of the purposes included in the 1850 charter of the New England Female Medical College. The college's annual catalogs urged aspiring nurses to attend the medical college lectures. A few women were given bedside training in nursing during the 3 years in which the medical college operated a hospital. A desire to establish a more complete course of instruction for nurses was mentioned in the manuscript records of the trustees, who at one time contemplated applying to the state legislature for funds with which to found a school for nurses.[7]

FOUNDING OF THE FIRST HOSPITALS FOR WOMEN

After her return from Europe, Elizabeth Blackwell settled in New York in 1851. The few patients who availed themselves of her counsel did not nearly constitute a "practice." In fact, not one female physician in any city could yet support herself entirely from the results of her medical studies. No respectable family in a good neighborhood would rent rooms to a "female physician"—a term then used by the notorious New York City abortionist Ann Trow Lohman. Even friends refused to help. Blackwell was forced to buy a house to obtain the privilege of publicly offering her services as a regularly educated physician.

The editor of the *Buffalo Medical Journal* later speculated, "If I were to plan with malicious hate the greatest curse I could conceive for women, if I would estrange them from the protection of women and make them as far as possible loathsome and disgusting to men, I would favor the so-called reform which proposes to make doctors of them."[8] The

Medical and Surgical Reporter declared "The opposition of medical men arises because this movement outrages all their enlightened estimate of what a woman should be. It shocks their refined appreciation of woman to see her assume to follow a profession with repulsive details at every step, after the disgusting preliminaries have been passed."[9] It was asserted that much of a man's more delicate feeling and refined sensibility had to be subdued before he could study medicine. In women, therefore, such delicate feeling and sensibility would be entirely destroyed. Nowhere were women who sought entrance to medical schools met by legitimate objections. Their requests were seen simply as an affront to the profession and an instance of women's obsession to intrude into affairs outside their proper sphere.

By the mid-1850s, Philadelphia and Boston had medical schools for women, but the level of instruction was inadequate and in no way comparable to the training given to men. Blackwell saw a definite need for a medical school to give women proper training and for a hospital to provide female physicians with clinical experience. By speaking frequently before various civic organizations, she eventually obtained financial support from an influential group of New York women. In 1853, Elizabeth Blackwell established a small dispensary in a New York tenement district. Four years later she expanded this facility into the New York Infirmary for Women and Children, with herself and Drs. Emily Blackwell and Marie E. Zakrzewska as administrative physicians. The first of its kind in the world, this institution offered care to the poor as a dispensary and soon opened a lying-in ward with 12 beds.

After the opening of the New York Infirmary for Women and Children on May 12, 1857, Zakrzewska wrote, "We kept true to our promise to begin at once a system for training nurses although the time specified for that purpose was only six months."[10] The school began with two nurses, one of whom remained for several years to become invaluable as a head nurse. Zakrzewska was evidently not satisfied with the success of this first system, however, because 8 months later she said:

> We . . . began to make more positive plans for the education and training of nurses. The first women who presented themselves . . . were unwilling to give a longer time than four months. During this time they received no compensation except their keeping and one weekly lesson from me on the different branches of nursing.[11]

At that time, the New York Infirmary was the only place in New York, other than the debauched and dissolute wards of Bellevue and Blackwell's Island, where an unwed pregnant girl could find refuge. When the Civil War broke out, Blackwell tried to obtain a post with the Union army, but she was refused. In May 1861 she converted Bellevue Hospital into a training center for nurses, in which an intensive 4-week course prepared about 100 women for service in military hospitals.

Meanwhile, in March 1861, the Woman's Hospital of Philadelphia was founded as an adjunct to the Woman's Medical College of Pennsylvania. Dr. Ann Preston, a member of the first graduating class of the college, was the leading force behind the establishment of this hospital, the purpose of which was to treat women's and children's diseases and to provide obstetric care, clinical instruction, and "practical training of nurses." About 1 year later, Preston instituted a 6-month training course for nurses and wrote a pamphlet entitled *Nursing the Sick and the Training of Nurses*, in which she described the ideal nurse as having "maternal tenderness, common sense, and a training in 'the greatness of little things.'" She noted that the nurse had to have "the patience of hope [and] the faith of love. The good nurse is an artist!" Nurse training accordingly became part of hospital routine, and although initially the hospital awarded no formal diploma, it was soon able "to send out capable nurses into private families."[12] The first known graduate was Harriet Neuton Phillips, who completed her training in 1869 and immediately assumed the position of head nurse at the hospital at a salary of $4 per week.

NURSING SERVICE PERSONNEL WOEFULLY INADEQUATE

During the 1860s, the nursing service at most hospitals was haphazard and disorganized. Although some women developed an aptitude for nursing and achieved positive results in caring for the sick, most nurses at that time were uneducated and often morally unfit to assume responsibility for patient care. This was especially true in large city hospitals, which often recruited nurses from among the poor who had sought shelter in almshouses.

At Bellevue Hospital in New York, former inmates of the workhouse on Blackwell's Island, known as "ten-day women," staffed the wards. Arrested for public drunkenness or disorderly conduct and sentenced to 10 days in the workhouse, they were paroled as soon as they had recovered sufficiently to be of service, provided that they agreed to undertake nursing in the Bellevue wards. One of these so-called nurses was enlisted for every 20 patients, a proportion that increased in times of severe epidemic.

The Philadelphia General Hospital employed so few nurses that it could not adequately care for the patients. Sometimes the nurses' inability to read directions on medicine bottles resulted in unexpected disasters and even in loss of life. Little more could be expected of these nurses, however, when one examined the conditions under which they were forced to live. In 1866, the hospital's warden, Dr. T.N. McLaughlin, wrote:

> While we have some excellent nurses, some that cannot be improved upon, the majority are not what we desire. With a few exceptions we have been obliged to utilize the convalescent patients, who have had no training, and from their previous habits and vocations do not possess the requirements to make good nurses. They are illiterate and have never been accustomed to any refinement, and that feeling of sympathy which is so essential is entirely wanting. They are . . . compelled to sleep in small, overcrowded and ill-ventilated rooms adjoining the wards, and in some instances in the wards. Four or five persons are often crowded into one room that is only of sufficient size to accommodate one, where they inhale the impure atmosphere of the hospital and are annoyed by the cries and moans of the suffering.[13]

Most of the better American hospitals used the services of Catholic sisters and Protestant deaconesses. St. Luke's Hospital in New York, for example, had been staffed since its foundation in 1853 by a Protestant order of nurses, and a similar order provided care in the Syracuse Hospital. Although these nursing sisters were far superior to the women otherwise hired, they were still untrained, and their best intentions were no substitute for adequate knowledge of medical procedures.

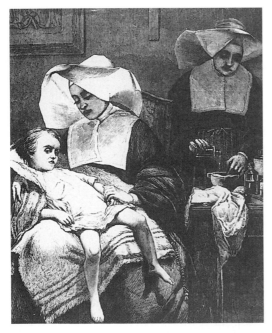

In American hospitals of the 1850s, religious orders provided exemplary nursing service.

PHYSICIANS EXPRESS A NEED FOR TRAINED NURSES

At the 1868 meeting of the American Medical Association (AMA), the AMA president, Dr. Samuel D. Gross, advocated the training of nurses:

> I am not aware that the education of nurses has received any attention from this body; a circumstance the more surprising when we consider the great importance of the subject. It seems to me to be just as necessary to have well trained, well instructed nurses as to have intelligent and skillful physicians. I have long been of the opinion that there ought to be in all the principal towns and cities of the Union institutions for the education of men and women whose duty it is to take care of the sick and to carry out the injunctions of the medical attendant. There is hardly one nurse, of either sex, in twenty who has a perfect appreciation of the requirements of the sick room, or who is capable of affording the aid and comfort so necessary to a patient when oppressed by disease or injury. It does not matter what may be the skill of the medical practitioner, how assiduous or faithful he may be in the discharge of his functions as guardian of health and life, his efforts can be of comparatively little avail unless they are seconded by an intelligent and devoted nurse. Myriads of human beings perish annually in the so called civilized world for the want of good nursing.[14]

The following year, Gross presented a committee report that called attention to the absence of organized efforts to upgrade nursing care. This report emphasized the importance of nursing care and concluded that nursing should be of universal interest because of its effect on every class of society and its importance as a complement to the services of physicians everywhere. Gross also recounted the history of nurse training efforts in other countries and referred to the large number of women in the United States who were potential candidates for such training. In conclusion, he suggested that schools of nursing be attached to hospitals, that instruction be provided by the medical staff and by the resident physician of each hospital, and that nursing schools be formed under the aegis of county medical societies throughout the nation.

POPULAR AGITATION FOR NURSE TRAINING

For years, Sarah Josepha Hale of Philadelphia edited the popular women's magazine *Godey's Lady Book*, which had a monthly circulation of more than 150,000. Although *Godey's* offered mainly fashion plates and

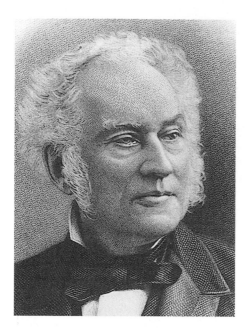

Dr. Samuel D. Gross.

sentimental tales, Hale encouraged middle-class women to learn to enjoy their leisure time without inhibition by discarding their tight corsets and engaging in activities such as swimming, horseback riding, sponsoring and patronizing public playgrounds, and enjoying the family "picnic"—a term she popularized. More importantly, she influenced the generations before and after the Civil War to create greater social and educational opportunities for women. In the spring of 1871, Hale made a plea for "lady nurses":

> Much has been lately said of the benefits that would follow if the calling of [the] sick nurse were elevated to a profession which an educated lady might adopt without a sense of derogation. . . . There can be no doubt that the duties of a sick nurse, to be properly performed, require an education and training little, if at all, inferior to those possessed by members of the medical profession. To leave these duties to untaught and ill-trained persons is as great a mistake as it was to allow the office of surgeon to be held by one whose proper calling was that of a mechanic of the humblest class. . . . Every medical college should have a course of study and training especially adapted for ladies who desire to qualify themselves for the profession of nurse; and those who had gone through the course, and passed the requisite examination, should receive a degree and diploma, which would at once establish their position in society. The "graduate nurse" would in general estimation be as much above the ordinary nurse of the present day as the professional surgeon of our times is above the barber-surgeon of the last century.

> When once the value of the "graduate nurses" became known, there is no doubt that the demand for them would be very great. Every village of a thousand inhabitants would, with the country about it, give occupation for two or three, at least. In any case of severe and protracted illness, their services would be called for as a matter of course, when the circumstances of the family allowed it. . . .
>
> There would be the further advantage that the nurse would not be an ignorant and unrefined person, with whom association would be unpleasant, but an educated lady, who would form an acceptable addition to the family circle during a period of anxiety and trouble—one who could give useful counsel on many subjects besides those of the sick chamber, and who would know how to economize not only her own health and strength, but the health and strength of the household. . . . In short, whenever such a profession is once established, it will soon be deemed as useful and respectable as any other.[15]

"Training-Schools for Nurses," an unsigned eight-page essay in the December 1874 issue of *Fraser's Magazine*, called for hospital-based training schools and homes for nurses. The author argues that (1) there is a great need for nurses all over the world, (2) this need can be met only by training schools, (3) such schools would provide not only proper training but also services and protections for both nurses and patients, and (4) "the welfare of such training schools is worthy of the attention and liberality of the intelligent and benevolent" (that is, a fit subject for charitable contribution).[16]

The author suggests numerous reasons for the shortage of nurses, all of which could be remedied by the institution of training schools or homes. Nursing has been found variously repulsive, overly laborious (so taxing, in fact, that the average nursing career lasted no more than 10 years), and miserably paid. Others have decided against a career in nursing because of the prospectless future awaiting the frequently incapacitated or superannuated nurse. Moreover, the work style of the average private nurse places her, when out of an assignment, at the mercy of boarding-house keepers who often require extra payment for the privilege, necessary for the private nurse, of surrendering lodgings at short notice.

By elevating nursing to the dignity of a profession, by providing enough hands to divide the labor, by making remuneration more secure, and by offering a year-round home for active and retired nurses, the hospital training school would serve not only to attract women into nursing, but also to enhance the quality of nursing care. Such a school, contrary to the opinion of many, is decidedly appropriate for the benevolence of charity:

> Is it not a charity in the first place to see that the sick and suffering, whether rich or poor, are as well taken care of as the science and knowledge of the day will admit? Is it not a charity to furnish one way more for good, well-disposed women to earn their living honourable and usefully, when so many of them are now helpless and discouraged?[17]

These latter concerns reflect fairly accurately the general tone of this article. The author of the essay writes thoughtfully and with compassion of the concerns of the working nurse. Yet the quality that most often appears here in association with good nurses and nursing is *discipline*. "The greatest trial to many who would be nurses," writes the author, "is the necessity of implicit obedience to the orders of superiors." Though the writer admits that these orders are "often arbitrary and peremptory," it is nevertheless not for the nurse to question them; her place is "to do what she is told, and never complain or disobey." He writes further that it is the quality of "implicit obedience to authority which proves the sincerity of purpose and abnegation of self essential in a good nurse."[18]

Although the author clearly recognizes the importance of good nursing care, he conveys a limited respect not only for the professional standing of nursing but also for the character of women in general. He defines nursing as "merely the care of the sick" and a nurse as "a useful assistant when one is ill; a kind of servant under the doctor's orders." He adds that general opinion has altered of late, moving toward a definition of nursing as "an art, and the well-being of the nurse a public question." Although the writer proves his endorsement of the latter development, the viewing of nursing as an "art" rests uncomfortably on him; in another place he sets the word in italics and feels compelled to note that it is "Miss Nightingale" who so defines it. Women in general seem here to be melting, helpless creatures who can survive the more indelicate aspects of hospital life—and, for that matter, tolerate each other without "jealousy and quarrels"—only through "great system and discipline."[19]

The following year, Dr. J. P. Chesney of New Market, Missouri, declared:

> As a nurse a woman's physical capabilities are incomparably superior to those of a man. . . . Who ever heard of a woman succumbing to the toils and exhausting vigils incident to nursing those in whom she was interested? Her eye is never closed, her ear is never deaf, her feet are never weary while the necessities of the sick have a claim upon her. The morning's dews or the gloom of midnight deter her not from her humane ministrations; not one like her can smooth the painful couch, make sweet the bitter draught, or

calm the aching heart; no one so ready to gratify the childish caprices or soothe the distempered imagination when "thick coming fancies" oppress the troubled brain. In fact, it would appear that there is a strange compatibility between women and the chamber of the sick; their benevolence relieving it of many of its terrors, while in its solemn precincts they learn, and teach, those lessons of humility and self-sacrifice.[20]

At about the same time, Dr. Horatio Storer, in his pamphlet *Nurses and Nursing*, clearly described the organization of nursing schools as they would exist in the following decade: "There must, sooner or later, be established, in connection with all large hospitals, scholarships, as it were, for nurses, corresponding somewhat to those already provided for ambitious medical students, who, for six months or a year, receive the appointment of resident or house physician."[21] Storer believed that many capable women would gladly offer their services for room and board only, in exchange for the privilege of caring for patients and for a certificate indicating the faithful completion of hospital training.

BIRTH OF THE FIRST TRAINING SCHOOL FOR NURSES

The associate of the Blackwells, Dr. Marie Zakrzewska (or "Dr. Zak," as she was called), also exerted a profound influence on nursing. Born in Berlin in 1829, she demonstrated at an early age a keen interest in medicine. In 1851 she graduated from the school for midwives at the Charité Hospital in Berlin, where she obtained the appointment of chief midwife and

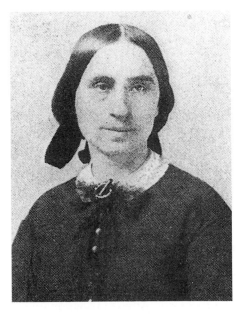

Dr. Marie Zakrzewska.

Nurse Training School of the Woman's Hospital.

———

This paper is to be filled out in applicant's own hand writing.

What is your Name?

What is your Age?

State whether you are Married or Single?

What your present Occupation?

What is your state of Health?

Can you Read and Write?

What References can you give?

You will be required to remain under instruction for twelve months, the first month of which is probationary. The Hospital furnishes you with Board and Lodging, and has your Laundry work done. After the month of probation, for the first five months, the pay is..................dollars per month. For the last six months of training the pay is.........................dollars per month.

You will be required to sign the following agreement, should the month of probation be satisfactory to both parties.

"*I promise to remain for one year under instruction in the Training School of the Woman's Hospital, and to observe faithfully all Rules of the School.*"

The month of probation is included in the year's instruction.

Upon passing a satisfactory examination at the close of the year of training, a certificate will be given you, and your name is recorded on the books of the Hospital, to which Physicians and others, desiring Nurses, are privileged to apply.

Application form used by the first American nurse training school.

professor in the following year. The knowledge and experience that she gained from this position increased her desire to practice medicine. Because German medical schools refused to accept her, however, she decided to immigrate to the United States, where she expected to find a more tolerant attitude toward women wishing to study medicine. In May 1854, she was introduced to Dr. Elizabeth Blackwell, who advised her to learn English and secured her admission to the medical department of Western Reserve University. Two years later, in March 1856, she received her M.D. degree.

After working with the Drs. Blackwell for 2 years at the New York Infirmary, Zakrzewska in 1859 accepted an appointment from the New England Female Medical College of Boston as professor of obstetrics and resident physician of a proposed woman's hospital. After a dispute with the college's administrators, she succeeded in founding her own institution, the New England Hospital for Women and Children, which opened July 1, 1862. Its act of incorporation expressly stated the training of nurses as one of its fundamental purposes. In connection with the nurse training course, the board of directors proudly announced, "We offer peculiar advantages for training nurses for their important duties, under the superintendence of a physician."[22] Students were required to attend the course for 6 months. After a probationary period of 1 month, they were granted a small wage, board, and laundry service. Despite these incentives, few women were willing to invest the required 6 months' time.

Because Zakrzewska experienced difficulty in attracting qualified female physicians for the new hospital, she began the practice of employing one female premedical student in the wards each year to give her practical experience and to induce her to return to the hospital on completion of her medical studies. In 1867, Susan Dimock, a Southern girl aged 18 years, came to the hospital for such preparation. Acting on the advice of Zakrzewska and Dr. Lucy Sewall, both of whom recognized her outstanding potential, she applied successfully to the medical school of the University of Zurich.

Four years later, in 1871, Dimock graduated with high honors—the sixth woman to obtain a medical degree from Zurich between 1867 and 1872. The topic of her dissertation, written in German, was "The Different Forms of Puerperal Fever." After graduation she spent 6 months in Vienna and 3 months in Paris for further study and observation in hospitals. In July 1872, she returned to the United States to assume the post of resident physician at the New England Hospital for Women and Children. Dr. Dimock's 3-year appointment provided her with an annual salary of $300, board, an office in the hospital, and the privilege of a private practice. As a result of her superb training in Europe, she brought with her the most recent diagnostic methods, the correct

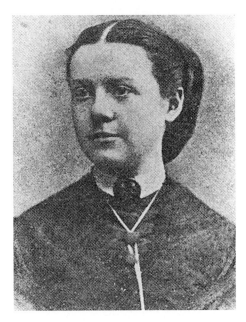

Susan Dimock.

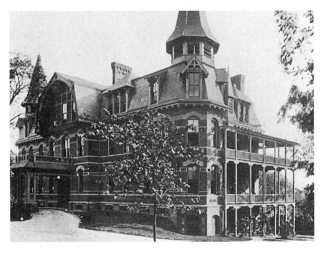

New England Hospital for Women and Children.

procedure for taking medical history, and the latest surgical techniques.

Immediately after completion of a new hospital building in July 1872, the New England Hospital nursing course was expanded into the "first general training school for nurses in America." Organized and equipped to give full general training along modern, practical lines, it employed a staff of physician-instructors in all medical branches and offered a hospital service program that included medicine, surgery, and obstetrics. The school's administration announced in its 1872 report:

> In order more fully to carry out our purpose of fitting women thoroughly for the profession of nursing, we have made the following arrangements. Young women of suitable acquirements and character will be admitted to

the hospital as school nurses for one year. This year will be divided into four periods: three months will be given respectively to the practical study of nursing in the medical, surgical, and maternity wards, and [of] night nursing. Here the pupil will aid the head nurse in all the care and work of the ward under the direction of the attending and resident physicians and medical students. In order to enable women entirely dependent upon their work for support to obtain a thorough training, the nurses will be paid for their work from one to four dollars per week after the first fortnight, according to the actual value of their services to the hospital. A course of lectures will be given to nurses at the hospital by physicians connected with the institution, beginning January 21st. Other nurses desirous of attending these lectures may obtain permits from our physicians. Certificates will be given to such nurses as have satisfactorily passed a year in practical training in the hospital.

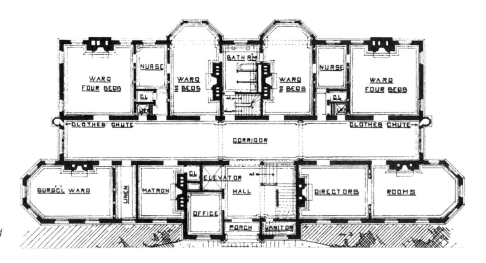

Street-level floor plan, New England Hospital for Women and Children.

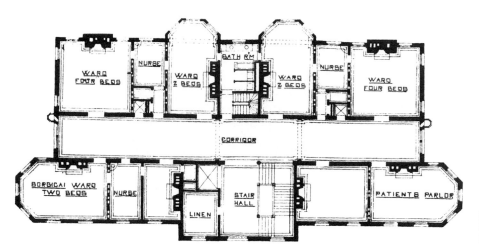

Second-level floor plan, New England Hospital for Women and Children.

The report continued:

> As long as we were in the old hospital, with space so inadequate to our needs, we were able to carry out only partially our plans for training nurses, but finding the demand so constant for those we have already trained, and the need of good nurses so great in the community, we have now determined to use our increased facilities to the utmost, and each year to send out a small band of trained nurses.[23]

While in Europe, Dimock had visited Florence Nightingale, from whom she had learned something about the essentials of a legitimate training school. Nightingale had stressed the organization of the nursing staff along authoritarian lines. Just as the superintendent regarded the probationers as her children, the head nurses, who were responsible for training both the probationers and student nurses, were supposed to consider their charges as students rather than as servants. In addition, physicians were to lecture once a week on pertinent medical and surgical topics.

Based on these guidelines, the first American nurse training school to offer a graded course in scientific nursing began, with five probationers, on September 1, 1872. The students worked from 5:30 a.m. to 9:00 p.m. and slept in rooms placed near the ward so that they could be quickly awakened for emergencies during the night. In return for their 1 year of service, they received 12 lectures given by several women physicians on medical, surgical, and obstetric nursing.

On October 1, 1873, the first diploma was awarded to 32-year-old Linda Richards—America's first professionally trained nurse. It must be remembered, however, that the New England Training School was not located in a general hospital, that the training course was short, and that the lectures were comparatively meager. Dimock's untimely death in 1875 aboard the steamship *Schiller*, which sank en route to England, cut short a promising career, but not before she had organized a definite curriculum and working plan for the school.

ESTABLISHMENT OF THE FIRST NIGHTINGALE SCHOOL

Even as Linda Richards was graduating, three more nurse training schools were opening in New York, New Haven, and Boston. The New York Training School, attached to the Bellevue Hospital, was the first in the United States to be modeled after Florence Nightingale's school at the famous St. Thomas' Hospital in London.

In 1872, the prominent New York socialite Louisa Schuyler, a descendant of Alexander Hamilton and Revolutionary War major-general Philip Schuyler,

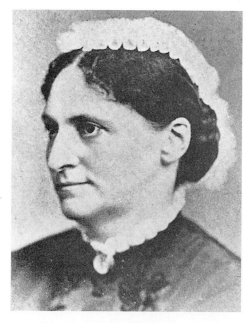

Linda Richards.

convened a group of society ladies in her home. Organized as the State Charities Aid Association of New York, these citizens regularly visited the various charitable institutions of the city and took note of needed reforms. One committee of the association was assigned to visit Bellevue Hospital. Including such prominent women as Mrs. Joseph Hobson, Mrs. William H. Osborn, Julia Gould, and the Misses E. and B. Van Rensselaer, the committee followed a route from the Schuyler home to Bellevue Hospital that was described as "the fashionable promenade of the city."

At Bellevue, the visitors found 900 patients, most of them in terrible distress and in need of a great deal more nursing care. Many had to sleep on the floor, without blankets or pillows, because the only extra bedding was the unwashed blankets of recently deceased patients. There were no night nurses and only three night watchmen for hundreds of patients. These watchmen sometimes drugged patients with morphine to keep them quiet and to counteract the stimulants that they had taken during the day. In the kitchen, tea and soup were frequently made in the same boiler. Moreover, the coffee was nauseating and the beef dry and hard. "Special diets" generally existed in name only. Moreover, much of the food was confiscated on its way up from the kitchen by the "ten-day" women who had been committed to the workhouse on Blackwell's Island for drunkenness and disorderly conduct and had subsequently been transferred to Bellevue Hospital as "nurses."

Official statistics drew a dismal picture. In 1871, about 15 of every 100 patients had died on the premises. Of 1102 hospital deaths, 69 were attributed to infections acquired from within the wards. The risk involved in delivering a baby at Bellevue was high: 33 of 376 mothers (9%) died of puerperal fever. Surgery was even more dangerous. The 18 months beginning in January 1872 saw 58 amputations, 28 of which ended in deaths because of shock, hospital gangrene, exhaustion, or tetanus. Amazingly, even relatively simple operations proved fatal: three of five hand amputations, five of seven arm removals, and four of eight foot amputations. The committee recalled the words of Florence Nightingale, who had insisted, "The most delicate test of sanitary conditions in hospitals is afforded by the progress and termination of surgical cases after operation, together with the complications which they present."[24]

In view of these gloomy statistics, the committee concluded that to delay a massive reform of Bellevue Hospital would be "simply criminal." The members were convinced that the hospital could not function effectively until the nursing service had been completely reorganized. Inspired by the success of similar projects begun in England by Florence Nightingale, they boldly attacked the problem but received little encouragement from the medical profession. One distinguished physician stated: "I do not believe in the success of a training-school for nurses at Bellevue. The patients are of a class so difficult to deal with, and the service is so laborious, that the conscientious, intelligent woman you are looking for will lose heart and hope long before the two years of training are over." A clergyman well acquainted with the hospital echoed this opinion and thought it "not a proper place for ladies to visit."[25]

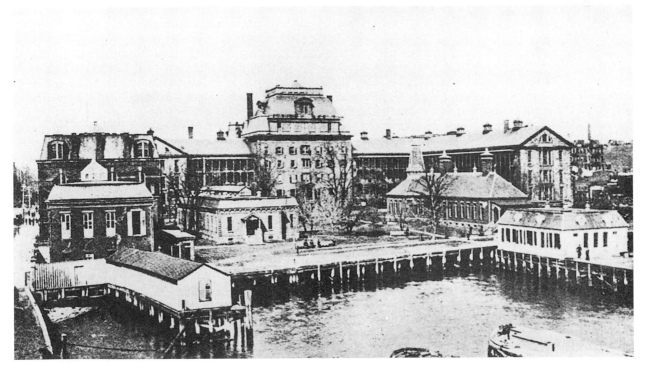

Bellevue Hospital in the 1870s.

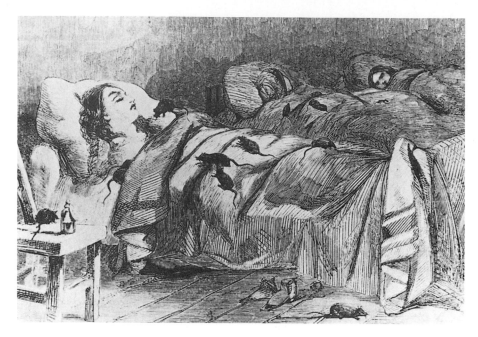

Appalling conditions at Bellevue Hospital.

To organize a nurse training school in the most effective manner, the committee dispatched Gill Wylie, a young resident physician, to London, where he observed the methods of the training school that Florence Nightingale had established at St. Thomas' Hospital. Returning with a favorable impression of this school, Wylie strongly recommended that the one at Bellevue Hospital be similarly organized, even though he realized that some features of the British system would be unsuitable. He even suggested that the governing board of Bellevue invite the school at St. Thomas' Hospital to send some of its nurses to New York to assist in the establishment of an American counterpart.

This recommendation was referred to a committee consisting of Drs. James R. Wood, Alonzo Clark, and Stephen Smith. Only Smith favored the complete implementation of Wylie's proposals. By contrast, Wood and Clark maintained that women who had received medical training would automatically consider themselves capable of practicing medicine and would immediately go out into the country to do so. Given the laxity of state laws regulating medical practice at that time, in theory a trained nurse might practice as a physician without legal interference. To alleviate fears of local physicians, the exact limits of the nurses' duties were carefully defined.

Fully aware of the controversial nature of this plan, Schuyler's group raised more than $23,000 to establish the nurse training school and rented a house near the hospital for the nurses to live in. Finding a person capable of taking charge of the new school, however, proved to be an arduous task. "Sister Helen" Bowden of the Sisterhood of All Saints finally agreed to fill this position.

Recruiting enough qualified students for the school, which opened on May 24, 1873, was difficult, because strict admission requirements deterred many who might otherwise have come. These requirements included a solid previous education, strong constitution and freedom from physical defects (including those of eyesight and hearing), and excellent references. The recruiting effort for the first class was far from satisfactory, as only 29 of 73 applicants from states as far away as California were considered worthy of acceptance. In addition, 10 admittants were dismissed for various reasons within the first 9 months.

The story of the gradual replacement of the old order was later recounted by Smith: "The school soon proved so efficient that it was not long before the old nurses were entirely supplanted."[26] These displaced women left in a foul disposition, however, venting their wrath on Bellevue authorities with coarse expletives and throwing stones at the new student nurses.

Until this experiment succeeded or failed, the students were given charge of only the women's wards at Bellevue. Even though conditions in the men's wards were far worse than in the women's, authorities gave no serious thought to asking "lady nurses" to care for male patients. When Smith, who had found the student nurses so successful with his female patients, proposed sending them into his male wards, he encountered tremendous opposition from the medical board. Opponents argued that the male patients of Bellevue were "nothing but a raft of bums from Five Points and the Bowery, and to send women nurses among them would be an outrage."[27] Undaunted, Smith sent one of the students to work on the male wards. She proved successful, and within a week additional students improved conditions to a level comparable with those in the female wards. This improvement seemed so remarkable to Wood, who at

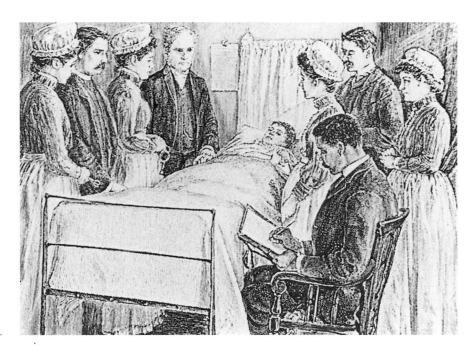

Student nurses being trained.

first particularly opposed the new idea, that he soon asked that nurses be assigned to his male wards.

The course of training consisted of dressing wounds; applying fomentations; making beds; and positioning, bathing, and caring for helpless patients. Moreover, the nursing students learned to prepare and apply bandages, make rollers, and line splints. They also learned how to cook for and serve food to patients. Instruction stressed the best methods of securing fresh air and of warming and ventilating the sickroom. Exemplary deportment, patience, perseverance, and obedience were expected as a matter of course throughout the training program.

Although the program lasted 2 years, the trainees received instruction for the first year only. During this time, they attended lectures by experienced physicians and were considered to be under the supervision of the superintendent of the school. These first-year students received $10 per month after a probationary period of 1 month. During the second year, the salary of the students, who now simply provided service without receiving additional instruction, increased slightly. Not until each student had satisfactorily completed the entire 2-year program did she receive her coveted, ornate diploma.

THE CONNECTICUT TRAINING SCHOOL FOR NURSES AT NEW HAVEN STATE HOSPITAL

Meanwhile, the New Haven State Hospital was also starting a nurse training school based on the Nightingale plan. On May 21, 1873, the founding committee for what was to become the Connecticut Training School for Nurses held its first formal meeting to appoint a superintendent of nursing. This was not an easy task, given the small pool of experienced nurses from hospitals that had conducted nursing courses. After many inquiries and visits, the committee selected Miss Bayard, superintendent of the recently upgraded Training School for Nurses of the Woman's Hospital of Philadelphia. Of 21 student applicants, 6 were finally selected, but 2 of these failed to appear because of illness when the course of instruction began on October 6, 1873.

The four student nurses and their superintendent immediately found themselves faced with demanding duties. Ten typhoid patients occupied the north ward of the hospital. The founding committee's journal relates:

> Our nurses for the first five weeks did very hard work. The fever cases were severe, some of the patients entirely delirious, throwing themselves out of bed, or getting up and dragging their sheets and blankets out into the entry. . . . The four nurses in turn sat up night after night and did duty during the day in the other wards or diet kitchen, where the special diet for thirty [patients] was cooked and distributed to all parts of the hospital by the nurse who cooked it.[28]

One of the first problems that had to be resolved was the elimination of the students' trailing skirts and superfluous jewelry, which did not constitute proper nursing attire. Dr. Francis Bacon later recalled: "I remember one morning I was met by the head nurse with the despairing question, 'What *shall* I do with Miss ——? She appeared at breakfast with all her long hair curled down her back.'" Bacon suggested the use of large caps and soon no one needed

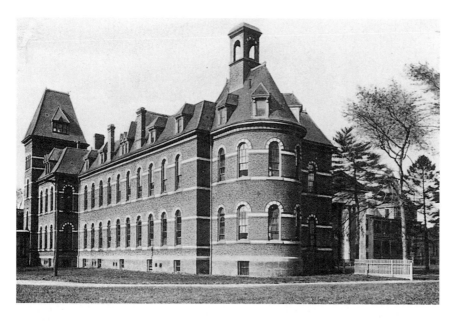

New Haven (CT) State Hospital.

to be told that elaborate hairstyles were out of place in a sickroom. He further related that when the hospital surgeons were assured of the provision of good nursing care to combat the danger of "hospital disease," they began to undertake surgery never before attempted in the hospital.[29]

On March 26, 1874, 6 months after the school opened, the hospital committee, which had ordered an evaluation of the performance of the student nurses, concluded, "In regard to the work undertaken by the school in the care of the sick and disabled, we find for it many general commendations. The physicians and surgeons report a decided improvement in the nursing, and speak strongly of the good already accomplished." By the end of the first year, nearly 100 applications for admission to the school were on file, but most of the young women withdrew their names after learning of the large amount of work required.[30]

By the end of the second year of operation, the Connecticut Training School for Nurses was able to supply trained graduates for the field of private-duty

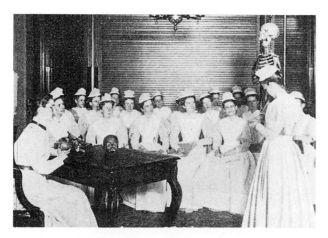

Nursing fundamentals class.

nursing; by the fourth year it began to graduate candidates for jobs as superintendents of nursing in other hospitals; and by the sixth year the school faculty had published a handbook of nursing.

THE BOSTON TRAINING SCHOOL FOR NURSES

In November 1873, the third American school of nursing modeled after the Nightingale system began operation in Boston as the Boston Training School for Nurses at Massachusetts General Hospital. The *Report of the United States Commissioner of Education for 1873* contains the following description of this school, which was

giving a systematic training to women who wish to become nurses. With a small and manageable number for a beginning, an influential body of ladies and gentlemen has made arrangements with the trustees of the Massachusetts General Hospital for exercise of the pupils in their wards. Lodging and boarding at a house near the hospital, these pupils are to receive instruction there in the theoretic part of their profession and in the preparation of diet for the sick, and for a year will practice in the wards under the direction of the hospital-physicians. During that year they will receive $10 a month for clothing and personal expenses. At the expiration of the year they will become full nurses and receive as such a salary sufficient for their support, but must remain another year for further practice and instruction. This full term of two years completed, they will, if approved, receive diplomas certifying their knowledge of nursing, their physical ability, and good character.[31]

The first superintendent, Mrs. Billings, a former nurse with the Union army during the Civil War, was succeeded 3 months later, in January 1874, by Mary Phinney von Olnhausen, a German baroness who had also served as a volunteer nurse with the Union army and later with the German army during the Franco-Prussian War. Only one of the staff physicians at Massachusetts General supported the establishment of the nurse training school. Because the others refused to cooperate in providing instruction for the student nurses, female physicians from the New England Hospital for Women and Children helped to give the weekly lectures. In November 1874, Linda Richards became superintendent of nurses at an annual salary of $600 and continued in this capacity for the next 2½ years.

Throughout the next decade, Linda Richards enjoyed phenomenal success in organizing training schools for nurses. Richards, who had served as night superintendent at Bellevue Hospital during its first year (1873), not only supervised the early development of the Boston Training School for Nurses at Massachusetts General Hospital but also organized or reorganized five other important schools in subsequent years, including the new school at Boston City Hospital in 1878. It is significant that these early "Nightingale" training schools for nurses, each affiliated with a general hospital, enjoyed semi-autonomous status. Soon, however, this trend toward autonomy reversed as nursing "schools" tended to become the nursing service departments of their respective hospitals. Because these early schools lacked substantial endowments and permanent independent budgets, they depended totally on private donations and the good will of hospital authorities for their funding.

THE NURSE TRAINING SCHOOL EXPERIENCE IN THE LATE 1870s

If you had been one of the student pioneers in one of the early nurse training schools more than a century ago, your experience as a probationer would have conformed to the following general pattern. At the time of your entrance to the school you would have been between the ages of 25 and 35 years. Before your admission, you would have completed an application form in which you would have stated your marital status (single or widowed—married women were not accepted), present occupation, height, weight, education, and state of health (in particular, whether your sight and hearing were perfect). Any physical defect, especially pulmonary, would have disqualified you. Two persons would already have submitted character references.

Once granted admission, you immediately entered the hospital. You did not arrive as part of a group of students, because students were not usually received in classes but were admitted as needed. One of the older trainees showed you to your room, actually a 6- to 8-ft-high stall containing three separate beds. These stalls were erected under the dome of what had once been the operating theater of the hospital and had later been converted into the servants' quarters. The room received no heat and little light, only that which filtered through the painted white glass of the dome, seemingly 100 ft above the room. There was no privacy because the servants who came up to their rooms at all hours of the day and night chatted, scolded each other, and told stories. Except for the beds, which were in fairly good condition, the rooms were sparsely furnished. Your roommates might not be at all congenial, for they too were undergoing much emotional strain.

Later, at dinnertime, you were taken to another part of the hospital for your first of many institutional meals. You found the food of poor quality, because the cook, despite all her years of service, seemed to hate nurses in training and regarded you as an intruder with no rights. You soon discovered that many of the student nurses spent nearly all their monthly wages on additional food. Later, when you had mustered up enough courage to complain about the fare, you found that your complaints actually jeopardized your future in the school.

After dinner you received a notebook and pencil with instructions to proceed to an operating theater to hear your first lecture. Because you had just arrived at the school, you were not too tired that first evening, but you found the lecturing physician

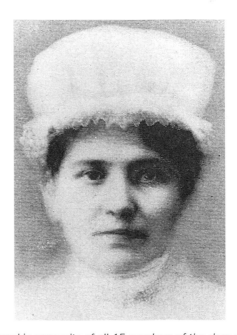

Photographic composite of all 15 members of the class of 1886 of the McLean Asylum Training School for Nurses, Waverly, MA. Negatives of 15 individual portraits were overlaid to make this composite.

exhausted from his long day at work. The next week, however, when you attended the second lecture, you too were tired and unable to follow much of his presentation.

After class that first night, you noticed no place where you could really socialize with the other students. Soon you sensed a cliquishness: As a new student occupying one of the stalls in the oldest part of the hospital, you were looked down on by the more advanced students, who enjoyed the privilege of occupying the rooms adjacent to the superintendent's quarters. You also encountered ingratiating types who curried favor with the superintendent by offering her dainties, making her a cup of tea, or sewing a seam for her.

Early the next morning, you put on one of the wash dresses from home and at 6:30 a.m. began your probationer's duties on the hospital wards. As you entered the ward, you were introduced to the head nurse. At first you were asked to do only simple work, like arranging the linen closet and folding clothes. Later you were given more arduous tasks, such as sweeping and cleaning, polishing the floors and furniture, and washing and ironing. You were surprised that you had to beg for the materials with which to do this drudgery. In folding the linen you were told to do the sheets, the towels, the pillowslips, and then the washcloths, in that order. You also learned that all the sheets had to be folded to exactly the same size and that the folded items were to be placed in neat, separate piles in the linen cupboard. The appearance of this closet was a major source of pride for the nurses.

Before coming to the school, you had considered yourself particularly well suited for nursing, and, having read Florence Nightingale's *Notes on Nursing,* you had become somewhat informed about nursing duties. As the first clinical day progressed, however, you discovered that you were not required to know *anything.* In fact, the head nurse preferred to work with raw material, so to speak, who had no preconceptions about nursing. What *was* required was receptiveness, intelligence, and, above all, an energetic nature. If you did have any prior knowledge or opinions of nursing, it was wise to keep them to yourself! On the wards you adhered to principles of order and decorum that absolutely subordinated the nurses to the physicians.

As the afternoon wore on, you found yourself looking at the clock and waiting for 8:00 p.m. to come so that you could go off duty. The hospital atmosphere, a combination of strange sights and sounds and the smell of drugs and other unavoidable odors most perceptible to the uninitiated, had managed to produce in you a mild case of first-day shock. You were unable to sleep that night, and by the end of the week you found yourself crying in bed with pain in your feet and legs. You kept these little ailments to yourself, however, because you were anxious to satisfy your superiors and perform your duties as directed. By the end of the first week, you were grateful for the half-day off. Although you worked only 6 hours that day, you were so exhausted that you spent your free time resting indoors instead of leaving the hospital for recreation.

With the second week came greater responsibility. You were given charge of 10 to 15 patients. The head or senior nurse went around the ward with you for the first time and demonstrated how to make beds, change soiled linen, move an invalid from one bed to another, cover a patient and avoid fatiguing her while sitting her up to have her bed made, and

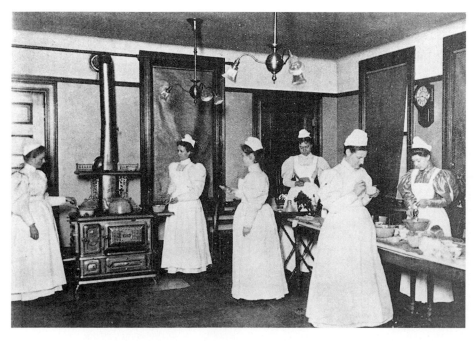

Cooking patient meals in a ward kitchen.

get a patient in and out of bed. You also learned the importance of having patients make their own beds when able. The latter part of the day was spent in waiting on your patients and keeping your side of the ward in order at all times. The first month was a probationary period, during which you had to master a host of difficult techniques and procedures. Instruction was given by visiting and resident physicians; by surgeons; and by the superintendent, assistant superintendent, and head nurses (themselves students). Demonstrations took place occasionally, with examinations administered at regular intervals.

To your great satisfaction you finally passed through the probationary period and became a junior nurse. Having shown yourself qualified, you were required to sign the following agreement: "I hereby agree to remain for two years in the Training-School for Nurses as a pupil nurse and to obey the rules of the school and hospital." Board, lodging, and laundry were furnished, and a monthly stipend of $7 provided for clothes, textbooks, and incidental expenses. This stipend, you were told, represented an allowance rather than wages.

For 3 more months you engaged in the same work that you had done as a probationer, and then you went on night duty. You were beginning to feel somewhat independent by this time, although you had not yet acted completely alone because there was always an experienced nurse on the top floor from whom you could seek help in case of emergency. Because you had probably never before remained awake the entire night, you found your first night duty rather exciting and anxious. You kept alert until about 2:00 a.m., when the effort to stay

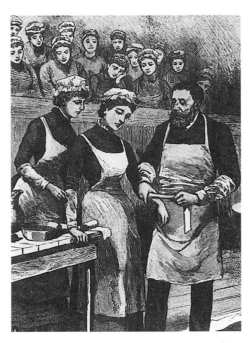

Nurse training school class receiving instruction in bandaging.

awake began to grow painful. With the aid of an antiquated lantern that cast large shadows and a tiny ray of light, you peered about the large ward. Sometimes the miserable little lamp went out while the wick spit and sputtered. To your dismay, you found that patients had a way of dying during the night despite your utmost efforts to keep them alive until dawn. It required considerable nerve on your part to "lay out" a dead patient in the small hours of the morning. Something uncanny hung in the air that first night in the silent, gloomy wards, but you got used to it after a time. Because your night duty lasted 14 hours, you began to feel completely exhausted about 5:00 a.m. You braced yourself, however, and summoned up a last spurt of energy to get through the early day's work until 8:00 a.m., when you collapsed, without breakfast, into bed.

Your nurse's training divided into several "services." You spent so many months in each of the different branches—medical; surgical; maternity; gynecologic; eye, skin, and throat; and pediatric—unless needed by another service. Then you found that the training school's rotation plan was quickly overlooked. About 6 months of your training period was devoted to night duty, spread out over 2 years. During the day, each of the 30-bed wards of the hospital had four nurses: two juniors, one senior, and a head nurse, who were also responsible for the "special cases" in adjacent private rooms.

When you became a senior nurse at the beginning of the second year, your duties changed somewhat and you now felt more important. You no longer had to attend evening lectures or take bothersome quizzes, and your monthly allowance increased to $12. You took charge of the linen

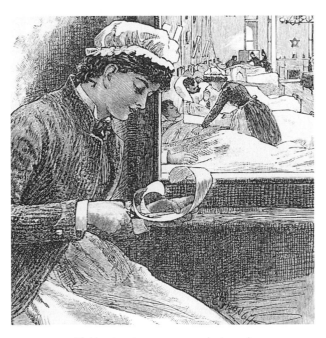

Making bandages on a surgical ward.

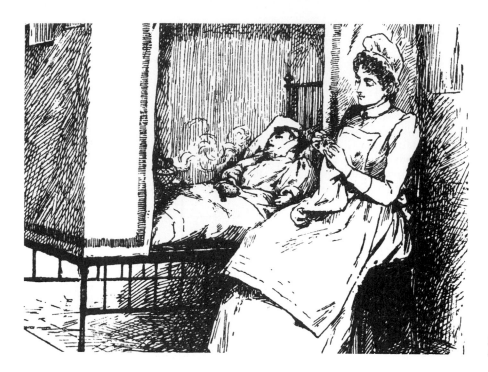

Night duty—an exciting but anxious experience.

closets, assisted in serving food and dispensing medicine, and carried out orders for various patients' treatments. The prescription list for patients carried 30 names, and some patients received as many as five or six different medicines. After sufficient practice and with the assistance of another nurse, you were able to dispense all medications within 40 minutes.

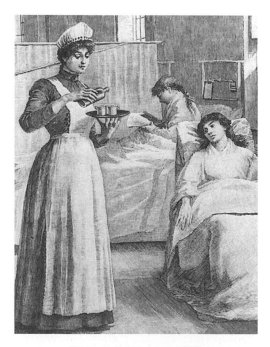

Giving medicines, circa 1888.

When elevated to the position of head nurse, you were given charge of an entire ward. You assumed responsibility for the condition of this ward, for the care of its patients, and for the instruction of less-experienced student nurses—in fact, for whatever was done or not done on the ward. Dealing with the various personalities of the physicians who relied on you to carry out their orders faithfully required mature judgment and tact. After receiving the notes of the night nurse and seeing that all the work was proceeding smoothly, you went around with a notebook in hand and examined the condition of each patient. You questioned the patient, listened to what he or she had to say, and made your own observations. In this way you became acquainted with all your patients and were able to report every important detail to the attending physicians.

Each week, as you proceeded with your training, you gained confidence in yourself while others gained confidence in you. You found no time for dreaming, and amidst sickness and death you invariably acquired a matter-of-fact disposition. Except for an annual 2-week vacation and the half day off every other week, you devoted 7 days a week to nursing. After you had made up any sick days that you had been granted during your 2 years of training, a board of physicians gave you a final examination, and, after passing it, you received a fancy diploma signed by the examining board and by a committee of the training school board of directors. Because your name was now listed on the school rolls, a patient or physician needing a nurse could summon you. At last you were ready to begin a career in private-duty nursing in the homes of patients.

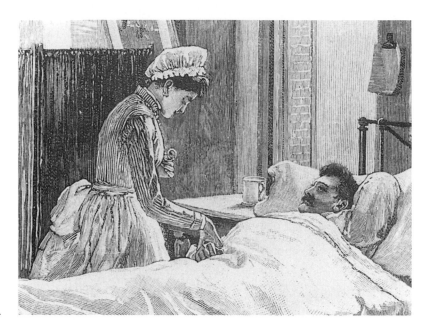

Taking a patient's pulse, circa 1888.

UNIFORMS AND CAPS

The new graduate always proudly wore her school cap and uniform on her private-duty nursing assignments. The practice of wearing uniform and cap, important symbols of nursing, grew out of its military and religious heritage, which had always placed high value on the wearing of uniforms. Until the 1850s, the religious orders had been the dominant factor in the evolution of nursing service. After this time, Florence Nightingale's military nursing experience during the Crimean War exerted a powerful influence on the subsequent development of professional symbols.

The New York Training School for Nurses at Bellevue Hospital was the first school to adopt a standard uniform for student nurses. After the school had been operating for about a year, the board of directors decided that the students should wear a gingham apron in the morning and a white one in the afternoon, in addition to the required dark woolen dresses and variously shaped white caps. For reasons of economy as well as neatness, the school committee concluded in 1876 that the adoption of a standard uniform, which would have the same psychological effect on nurses as on a company of military recruits, was necessary and advantageous.

The most well-bred woman of the first Bellevue class was Euphemia Van Rensselaer of New York, whose aristocratic relatives held high positions in business and government. After her father, Union army Brigadier General Henry B. Van Rensselaer, died of typhoid fever during the Civil War, she resolved to

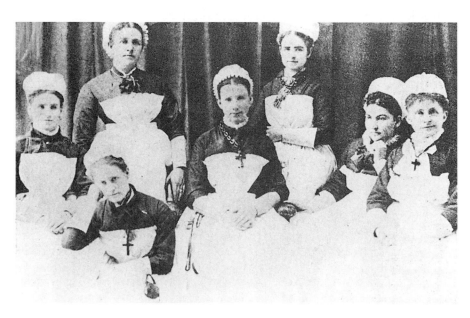

Graduating class, Bellevue Hospital, mid-1870s.

become a trained nurse. In describing Euphemia's return from the New York Training School, a relative, Mrs. John King Van Rensselaer, wrote: "When she returned to her family's home, she entered the basement, took off her verminous clothes, and then stood on a sheet while her old nurse cleansed her body and combed her hair. Only after this purification would she permit the rest of the household to greet her."

Euphemia Van Rensselaer introduced the uniform, apron, and cap of the Bellevue Training School for Nurses. At first the students had opposed the wearing of uniforms, which were commonly worn by servants at that time. Certain members of the school committee decided to grant Euphemia 2 days' leave of absence to have a uniform made for herself. When she returned to the hospital in her new attire, the other students saw how attractive she looked in her tailored uniform and became eager to adopt it as standard dress. The new outfit consisted of a long gray dress for winter and a calico version for summer, both with white apron and cap and brown linen cuffs covering the sleeves from the wrist to the elbow. In 1880, the gray dress for winter was replaced by an easily laundered dress that could be worn throughout the year.

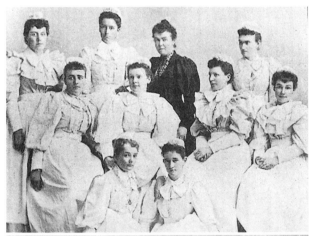

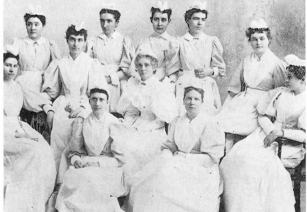

Graduation pictures, circa 1880, show elaborate uniforms.

Not until the 1890s was a regulation uniform generally established as a distinguishing mark of each nurse training school. The use of stripes and checks on student nursing uniforms derived from the old calico summer attire. The bib and apron, also worn in early European nurse training schools, were similar to those worn by gentlewomen while performing their household duties.

During this period, nurses generally wore a waist and skirt of white material, adjustable white cuffs, a stiff white collar, a white cap, and sometimes a cape of blue or red. Emphasis on an hourglass female silhouette required a high neckline, full bosom, wasp waist, leg-of-mutton sleeves, and bell-shaped skirt. To achieve the desired effect, a tightly laced, boned, long corset was essential. The predominant view was that "a nurse is a gentlewoman and as such should show her individuality in her style of dress." Femininity and gracious manners and behavior marked the lady nurse. The ankles were not to be seen, and nurses wore long dust-raising skirts in the interest of modesty.

Uniforms enforced social distinctions within the hospital as well as outside in private-duty nursing homes. A proper nurse's uniform assured the wealthy that a trained nurse remain distinguishable from a lowly domestic. An editorial in the February 1890 *Trained Nurse* ridiculed "the nurse who believes in a rattling starched domestic uniform to be worn at all times, in all seasons, and under all circumstances, and in which she cannot be told from the cook, laundress or second-girl, without a square, front view." It was recommended that the ideal uniform for day nursing consist of "a plain tea-gown, a round skirt and surplice waist, or any other not too elaborate house-dress. Other handy things to have, are a large apron, as long as the dress, and sleeve protectors, made of fast black sateen, which is found at the lining counter; to put on when giving baths, etc."[32] Local dressmakers rather than retail stores or uniform companies furnished most uniforms.

Rounding out the proper attire for the well-dressed nurse was the cap and nursing "badge," or "pins," as they later became known. The nurse's cap was originally designed to cover the long hair fashionable during the late 19th century. In the 1880s, most caps were made of lace-trimmed organdy; they were large, almost circular, and meant to be worn directly on the top of the head. The 1890s caps tended to become smaller, more elongated, and lower in the back, and they began to be worn further back on the nurse's head. Each school developed its own distinctive cap, and the black bands on some caps indicated a student's rank. The mandatory use of a standard cap style was first introduced at Massachusetts General Hospital in 1878, along with a regulation uniform.

The first Nightingale School of Nursing in the United States, at Bellevue Hospital, also created the first school badge or pin, which was presented to the class of 1880. It contained a crane in the center to signify the nurse's vigilance, an inner circular

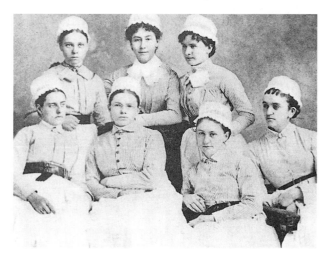

Uniforms were often made by local dressmakers.

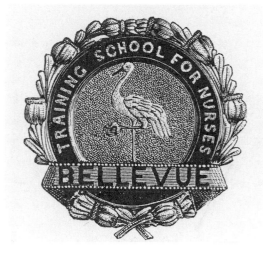

The first school of nursing badge of pin in the United States.

field of blue to connote constancy, and an outer circle of poppy capsules to symbolize mercy and the relief of suffering. The school of nursing pin was always worn very prominently on the uniform and proved to be a lasting symbol of considerable pride for the wearer.

Nurses continued to wear their school caps, uniforms, and school pins after graduation, whether as private-duty nurses or superintendents. Physicians and patients, therefore, began to recognize the various caps and uniforms and to associate them with the reputations of the various training schools. The distinctive uniform and pin began to symbolize the nurse's

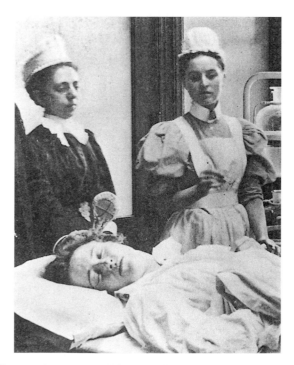

The nurse's cap was originally designed to cover the long hair styles of the late 19th century.

pride in the high standards of the training school from which she had graduated.

Because intent centered on the creation of the image of a refined "lady nurse," these early nurses' uniforms were neither practical nor hygienic. The uniforms reproduced Edwardian fashions in their characteristic features: charming frills and laces, long implacable corsets, long full skirts covering the ankles, layers of starched petticoats, tight bodices, stiff cuffs, and high choking collars. Although this style fostered an impressively romantic portrait of a woman in white, a nurse taking care of a patient with an infection could not be on duty more than a half hour without getting her sleeves contaminated. Although elaborate cuffs and sleeves were carriers of infection, nurses who rolled them up were severely criticized, because their "unladylike" appearance suggested the image of a laundress or scrubwoman.

Despite the disadvantages of these confining uniforms, however, they had a pronounced effect on the public. In a popular account of the nursing students at St. Luke's Hospital in New York, a reporter for *Munsey's Magazine* raved that their appearance was "all that the most inveterate reader of sentimental war stories could desire."[33] The nurses of St. Luke's wore a neat uniform of blue-and-white striped gingham. Their bibbed white aprons, neckbands of stiff linen, and crisply erect and airily poised little caps of sheer white mull conjured up an image of exquisite orderliness believed capable of inspiring hope in the hearts of their patients. The reporter for *Munsey's* thought "it would be impossible to conceive of anything so manifestly out of place as disease daring to persist near them." Every ward had a head nurse who could easily be recognized by the black velvet band on her cap.

Despite its limitations, the early nurse's uniform conveyed considerable authority and was greatly admired by the public. Popular support for the early

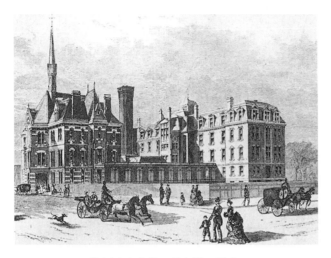

Saint Luke's Hospital, New York.

nurse's uniform appeared as early as 1886 in an editorial in the earliest nursing journal, *The Nightingale*, which noted that the nurse's uniform had captured the hearts of the late-19th-century public, as the "uniform presents the necessary lights and shadows." To the public, the nurse "is like a figure in a kaleidoscope. She is here, but the whence and whither of

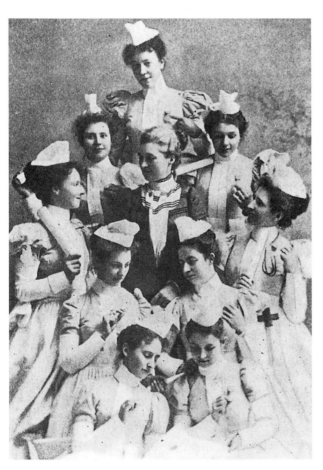

The nurse's uniform became a status symbol.

her destiny are unknown." The editor further commented that "every nurse has listened to the remark, 'How did you happen to do it?' People do not wonder why a woman becomes a teacher, but they require something romantic about the reason why she becomes a nurse."[34] The uniform helped supply this romantic image. In 1905, Oldfield wrote:

> The adoption of a pretty and distinctive uniform, worn in public, was the real starting point of the modern professional nurse. . . . The uniform gave a status, an attractive status, to those thousands of young women who wanted occupation and status, or status without much occupation.[35]

The origins of professional nursing in the United States can be attributed to the desire of respectable women for a broader occupational role, to the pioneering efforts of the first female physicians, to humanitarian sentiments among certain liberal physicians and magazine editors, and to the financial support of various civic and philanthropic groups in New York, New Haven, and Boston. In the beginning, the training schools engaged in a desperate struggle to prove their worth to society in the face of constant criticism from the medical profession. Their success in convincing the public of their usefulness enabled them to impart a higher degree of professionalism to their graduates.

REFERENCES

1. Robert L. Dickinson, "The Corset: Questions of Pressure and Displacement," *New York Medical Journal*, vol. 46 (November 5, 1887):507–516.
2. M. Adelaide Nutting and Lavinia L. Dock, *A History of Nursing* (New York: G. P. Putnam's Sons, 1907), vol. 2, p. 339.
3. Samuel Gregory, *Licentiousness, Its Causes and Effects* (Boston: G. Gregory, 1857), p. 6.
4. Elizabeth Blackwell, *Pioneer Work in Opening the Medical Profession to Women: Autobiographical Sketches* (New York: Longmans, Green & Co., 1895), p. 23.
5. Stephen Smith, "In Memory of Dr. Elizabeth Blackwell and Dr. Emily Blackwell," *Bulletin of the New York Academy of Medicine*, vol. 25 (January 1911):3–7.
6. Rachel Baker, *The First Woman Doctor: The Story of Elizabeth Blackwell, M.D.* (New York: Julian Messner, Inc., 1944), pp. 161–175.
7. Commonwealth of Massachusetts, *Report of a General Plan for the Promotion of Public and Personal Health, Devised, Prepared, and Recommended by the Commissioners Appointed Under a Resolve of the Legislature of Massachusetts Relating to a Sanitary Survey of the State* (Boston: Dutton & Wentworth, 1850).
8. "Editorial," *Buffalo Medical Journal*, vol. 24 (July 1869):191.
9. "Women as Physicians," *Medical and Surgical Reporter*, vol. 44 (May 1881):354–356.
10. Agnes C. Vietor, *A Woman's Quest: The Life of Marie E. Zakrzewska, M.D.* (New York: Appleton & Co., 1924), p. 360.
11. Ibid., p. 361.
12. Ann Preston, *Nursing the Sick and the Training of Nurses* (Philadelphia: King & Baird, 1863), pp. 1–14.
13. Philadelphia General Hospital, *Annual Report of the Philadelphia General Hospital for 1866* (Philadelphia: The Hospital, 1866), p. 7.

14. "Report of the Committee on the Training of Nurses," *Transactions of the American Medical Association*, vol. 20 (1869):161.
15. Sarah J. Hale, "Lady Nurses," *Godey's Lady's Book*, vol. 92 (March 1871):188–189.
16. "Training Schools for Nurses," *Fraser's Magazine*, vol. 10 (December 1974):706.
17. Ibid., p. 713.
18. Ibid., pp. 709–710.
19. Ibid., pp. 706–710.
20. J. P. Chesney, "Woman as a Physician," *Richmond and Louisville Medical Journal*, vol. 11 (January 1871):1–15.
21. Horatio Storer, *Nurses and Nursing* (Boston: Lee & Shepard, 1868), p. 10.
22. New England Hospital for Women and Children, *Annual Report of the Officers to the Society and Friends, 1862–1863* (Boston: The Hospital, 1863), p. 3.
23. New England Hospital for Women and Children, *Annual Report of the Officers to the Society and Friends, 1871–1872* (Boston: The Hospital, 1872), p. 5.
24. New York State Charities Aid Association, *Report of the Committee on Hospitals, Dec. 23, 1872, on the Training School for Nurses to Be Attached to Bellevue Hospital* (New York: The Association, 1873), pp. 11–16.
25. Ibid., pp. 16–17.
26. *New York Evening Sun*, March 11, 1911.
27. Ibid.
28. Francis Bacon, "Founding of the Connecticut Training School for Nurses," *Trained Nurse*, vol. 15 (October 1895):187.
29. Ibid., pp. 188–189.
30. Ibid., p. 189.
31. U.S. Commissioner of Education, *Annual Report of the U.S. Commissioner of Education for 1873* (Washington, DC: Government Printing Office, 1874), p. 60.
32. "Editorial," *Trained Nurse*, vol. 5 (February 1890):22.
33. K. Hoffman, "St. Luke's, N.Y.: Model Hospital," *Munsey's Magazine*, vol. 22 (January 1900):487–496.
34. Sarah Post, "Editorial," *The Nightingale: A Paper in the Interests of the Methodical Nursing of the Sick*, vol. 1 (September 4, 1886):40.
35. J. Oldfield, "The Nurse of the Future," *The Westminister Review*, vol. 164 (December 1905):655–656.

THE RISE OF SCIENTIFIC MEDICINE AND ITS IMPACT ON NURSING

4

Physicians of the centennial year 1876 did their best to control the prevailing diseases, but the profession was still hampered by ignorance and superstition inherited from the past. In a sober essay written in 1876, Professor Edward H. Clarke of Harvard reviewed what he regarded as the major scientific accomplishment of medicine in the preceding 50 years, which consisted of studies proving that patients with typhoid and typhus fever could recover without medical intervention and often did better untreated than when they received the bizarre herbs, heavy metals, and fomentations popular at that time. Delirium tremens, a disorder long believed to be fatal in all cases unless subjected to constant and aggressive medical intervention, was observed to subside more readily in patients left untreated, with a substantially improved rate of survival.

The erroneous Hippocratic concept of the "epidemic constitution of the atmosphere" still clouded the medical profession's thinking. Even as late as 1882, the superintendent of health of Providence, Rhode Island, reported that he had known of one situation in his city where nearly all the residents of a large house had developed typhoid fever due to the decomposition of a large quantity of potatoes stored in the basement. Medical literature still contained references to the "zymotic" (fermentative) diseases— a term applied to specific infections such as Asiatic cholera, smallpox, typhus, diphtheria, dysentery, typhoid, whooping cough, and syphilis.

YELLOW FEVER EPIDEMICS

In the summer of 1878, one of these scourges—yellow fever—reappeared in New Orleans. The *New York Times* of July 24, 1878, noted the outbreak and told of four deaths occurring in 48 hours. Before the end of the month, the newspaper announced that other cities along the Mississippi had become alarmed and were establishing a rigid quarantine on vessels and travelers from New Orleans. Despite this precaution, the disease spread rapidly upriver, causing serious outbreaks in eight states. Hysteria permeated the entire South.

The epidemic hit Memphis hardest. More than half its population fled. Of the 20,000 who remained, more than 17,000 developed yellow fever within 3 months, and 5000 of those people died. Many who ran away carried the seeds of yellow fever with them and set off new outbreaks in other parts of the country. Even physicians and nurses who stayed to care for the sick fell ill: In one group of 39 volunteer helpers, 32 developed yellow fever and 12 of them died. The cost of this great epidemic in money, suffering, and lives was enormous. New Orleans, Vicksburg (Mississippi), and Memphis bore the brunt of the outbreak, but hundreds of other communities suffered. Commerce practically stopped in the Lower Mississippi Valley, and the economic loss rose into the millions of dollars. No one knew what caused yellow fever or how it spread, and therefore no one knew how to cure or prevent it.

Speculation about the cause of the disease filled the medical journals along with heated controversy about its prevention and treatment. Because Americans had been so thoroughly frightened by the epidemic, Congress appointed a special commission to investigate the causes and existing remedies of yellow fever. The commission failed. Americans of the 1870s would remain exposed to yellow fever and a host of other diseases of unknown cause.

LAG IN MEDICAL KNOWLEDGE

Because of the comparatively primitive state of medical knowledge and practice in the 1880s, it is doubtful that the medical profession exerted any significant net influence on the morbidity or mortality of infants and young children of the time. Records of vital statistics for the large cities of America show

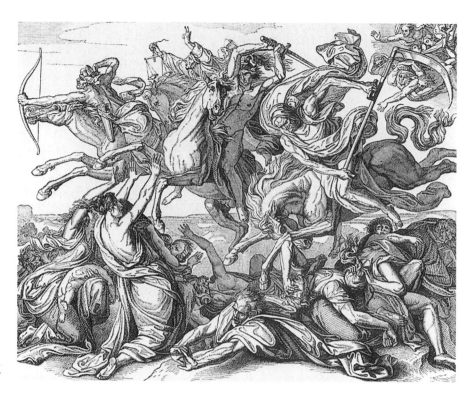

The erroneous concept of the "epidemic constitution of the atmosphere."

similar patterns of astonishingly high mortality rates among the very young.

Reliable official lists of live births and of burials indicate that the infant mortality rate (number of deaths occurring during the first year of life per 1000 live births) varied between 250 and 500. The highest rates were among artificially fed babies confined to foundling homes, with between 75% and 95% of such babies dying within their first year. Some metropolitan records show that more than half the total deaths from all causes in the average community occurred among children younger than

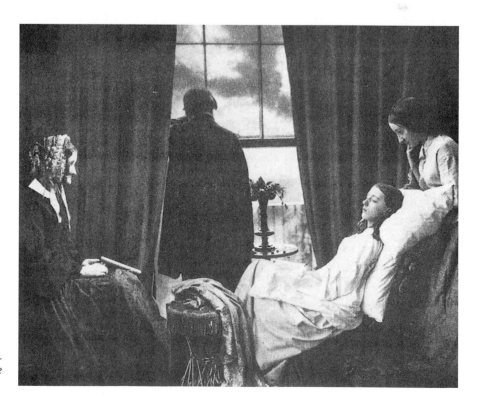

Extremely high infant and child mortality rates lowered the average life expectancy.

5 years of age. Three fourths of the total occurred among children younger than age 12 years. These high mortality rates of the late 19th century accounted in large measure for the average life span's remaining at 35 to 38 years. Although adequate records are not available, one can assume that the morbidity rates of the time were also extremely high. Enteric disorders, malnutrition, and the common respiratory and contagious diseases constituted the major causes of death.

In the pharmaceutical field during the 1870s, coal tar products were displacing calomel and whiskey as the panacea for febrile illnesses. Serious abuses occurred. Antipyrine, which came first, was used to such an extent during earlier epidemics of influenza in this country that it often produced serious, if not fatal, results. Acetanilid, which followed, became a favorite popular remedy for headaches and probably did more harm than antipyrine. The salicylates, introduced for rheumatism and long thought to be specific for that affliction, came to be used for all possible aches and pains. A series of coal tar hypnotics, each introduced with the definite assurance that it had all the advantages and none of the disadvantages

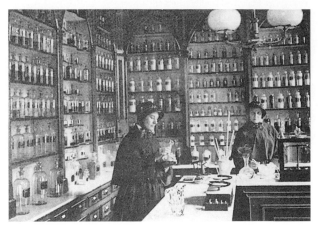

Coal tar products were the drugs of choice in the late 19th century.

of opium, proved in succession to have serious, lasting side effects that rendered them unsafe when used over long periods. By the 1890s, the 10 most important drugs in medical practice were (1) ether, (2) morphine, (3) digitalis, (4) diphtheria antitoxin,

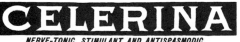
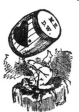
Most patent medicine remedies for disease were worthless.

(5) smallpox vaccine, (6) iron, (7) quinine, (8) iodine, (9) alcohol, and (10) mercury.

A few physicians perceptive enough to realize the inadequacy of their American training went to Europe to complete their education. There they found a different world—a world of laboratories and carefully controlled experiments. They learned to use the microscope to distinguish between normal and abnormal tissue and to identify the conditions that accompanied certain diseases. Pathology and physiology, barely recognized in American medical schools, were well advanced abroad. Bacteriology—the science destined to revolutionize medicine more than any other—was in a stage of vigorous youth. European scientists turned to projects relating to the cause and prevention of disease, and American graduate students crossed the Atlantic to learn the new techniques and to bring "modern medicine" back to their schools and hospitals.

FOUNDERS OF BACTERIOLOGY AND ANTISEPSIS

During the last quarter of the 19th century, an almost unbelievable advance in medicine stemmed from an unusual number of medical discoveries resulting from the development of scientific methods in the approach to problems of medicine. The growth of work in the basic sciences and the use of the experimental process in seeking answers greatly accelerated understanding in bacteriology and pathology and laid the groundwork for developments in biochemistry, physiology, and pharmacology.

The effects of nitrous oxide and ether on the nerves had been tried on people at fairgrounds long before it occurred to anyone to use these drugs in surgery. American dentists first took advantage of their anesthetic properties. In 1845, Horace Wells demonstrated the use of nitrous oxide but failed to convince a medical audience that his method was efficacious. His assistant, W. T. G. Morton, with the advice of the chemist Charles T. Jackson, had recourse to ether; but the first surgical operation with ether—the ablation of a tumor of the neck by J. Collins Warren—took place at the Massachusetts General Hospital in Boston on October 16, 1846, and was successful. The method spread quickly in Europe, but chloroform soon came to be preferred to ether. Pure chloroform had been available since 1834. In 1847, the Scottish obstetrician James Y. Simpson used it during deliveries, with excellent results.

With anesthetics, the surgeon could take his time, allowing more drastic operations than had been possible before. Advances in abdominal surgery followed, but many fatal infections also occurred. In simple surgeries, more than 30% of the patients died. The draining of incisions and the use of hemostatic forces, which began around 1860, were merely helpful expedients. Oliver Wendell Holmes, of

THE

New England Druggist

A monthly publication devoted to the interests of the Wholesale and Retail Druggists of New England, New York and the British Provinces.

BOSTON, MAY, 1890.

FORMULAS.

WHOOPING COUGH.

FORMULA NO. 1.

Sulph. Zinc.....................10 grains.
Pulv Myrrh,.....................1½ drams.
Confect. Rosarum q s
Make twenty pills. Dose—one pill.

FORMULA NO. 2.

Ext. of Belladonna, ...2 grains.
Aqua, ...2 ounces.

Mix. Dose—five or six drops four times a day.

FORMULA NO. 3.

Chloral hydrate, ...1 dram.
Simple syrup, ...4 ounces.

Mix. Dose.—Teaspoonful, according to severity.

FORMULA NO. 4.

Acid. Nit. Dil., ...,12 drams.
Tinct. Card. Comp., ...3 drams.
Simple syrup ....3½ ounces.
Aqua, ...1 ounce.

Mix. Dose.—Teaspoonful every hour, or second hour, with soda gargle immediately after administering.

PNEUMONIA.

Ammonia muriatis, ...3 drams
Antim. et Pot. tartrat, ...2 grains
Sulph. morphia, ...3   "
Syrup glycyrrhizae, ...4 ounces

Mix.

Dose. Teaspoonful every two hours.

Hydrag. chlor. mitis, ...6 grains
Ipecac pulveris, ...6   "
Opii pulveris,...........................3   "
Sacchar. alb.,...........................30 "

Mix.

Make six powders. Dose. One powder every four hours, alternately with the preceding prescription. At the same time cover the chest with emollient poultices. At the end of twenty-four hours omit the powders, and if the bowels have not been moved, give a mild laxative. If the symptoms are not favorably modified in three or four days, a blister is placed on the side of the chest most affected.

Recommended formulas for whooping cough in 1890.

Boston, who had observed that physicians and midwives were themselves responsible for puerperal infections because of a lack of sanitary precautions, wrote a devastatingly accurate description of puerperal fever in 1843. It was ignored.

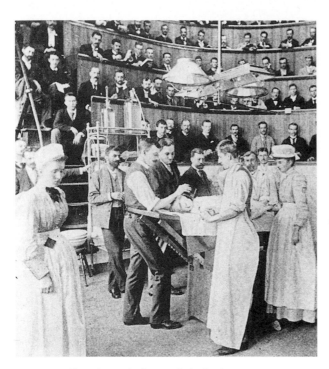

Use of anesthetics revolutionized surgery.

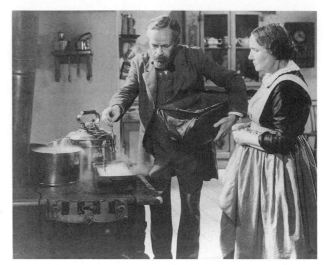

Louis Pasteur proved that bacteria are living microorganisms.

Working in a Viennese obstetric unit in 1847, Ignaz Philipp Semmelweis noted a much higher incidence of puerperal fever in the ward where physicians or students examined pregnant women than in the room where midwives tended the women. Semmelweis became convinced that the physicians and students, who went directly from the postmortem room to the obstetric clinic, communicated some highly pathogenic substances. On the basis of his autopsies, he went as far as to claim that puerperal infection was identical with the fever of the seriously wounded. He therefore stipulated that his physicians sterilize their hands in a solution of chlorine before examinations. His book, *The Aetiology, Concept and Prophylaxis of Childbirth Fever*, gave the world theories and methods of treatment that had been validated when he reduced the death rate in the maternity wards by more than 90% between 1846 and 1848 through the simple expedient of cleanliness. Semmelweis, in advocating antisepsis, pointed the way to elimination of maternal mortality, but his ideas were ridiculed in America and in Europe for a long time afterward. Eventually, he lost his sanity and died in an asylum.

Later, the French chemist Louis Pasteur demonstrated the scientific basis for Semmelweis's theory when he proved that bacteria were living microorganisms. From Pasteur's chemical studies of the optical power of tartaric acid, he was led to study the biology of fermentation. By September 1857, he had reached a notable conclusion, which he communicated to his friend, the natural philosopher J. B. Biot: "It should then be admitted," he wrote, "that all fermentation is an activity related to the vital

processes . . . to the organization of globules, and of myodermic plants." This idea received a hostile reception from certain scientists of the time, notably the German chemist Liebig, who regarded fermentation as a purely chemical phenomenon independent of any living organism. After studying the ferment responsible for the putrefaction of wine, Pasteur began to wrestle with the general problem of infection. That the bacilli found in fermented or putrefied substances were the cause and not the result of the process had yet to be proved.[1]

Perhaps Pasteur's religious convictions inspired him to oppose the materialist hypothesis of spontaneous generation. In any case, he proceeded to conduct experiments that demonstrated decisively that if a solution of putrescible substances is boiled, it can only be infected thereafter by contact with the air. If the air is filtered or passed through a tube with an upward-pointing convexity, the solution will remain sterile. Pasteur's *Mémoire sur les corpuscules organisés qui existent dans l'atmosphére* (Memoir on the organized bodies existing in the air) dates from 1861. Two years later he perfected the procedure that bears his name: pasteurization.

Lord Lister (1827–1912), 20 years after Semmelweis's failure, finally achieved success against germs. From his youth he had been interested in the problem of inflammation. After reading Pasteur's writings, he concluded that if the air carries dangerous germs, the area around the operating table should be disinfected. Noting that carbolic acid used with open fractures removed the danger of suppuration, he conceived the idea of spraying the operating area with vaporized carbolic acid.

Under antisepsis, infected wounds were opened widely and antiseptics used freely in them in the hope of killing the infectious agents. Unfortunately, the earlier antiseptics were extremely toxic and often killed tissue cells to a greater extent than the bacteria

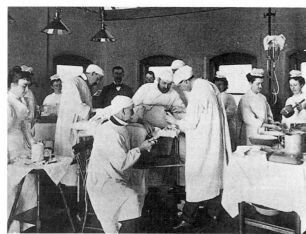

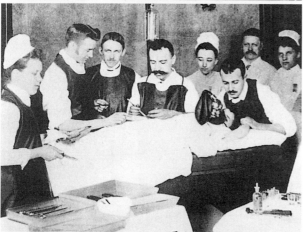

Surgery in the 1880s.

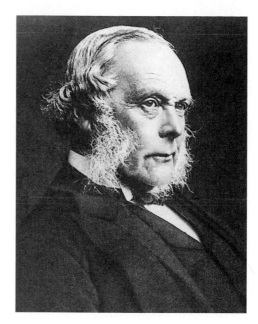

Joseph Lister.

present. The better surgeons used drainage tubes to flush the wound surfaces thoroughly with antiseptic solution at regular intervals. Gradually, fewer and fewer badly infected wounds occurred. Skepticism persisted, however, in Pasteur's own country and elsewhere. As late as 1886, Dr. Morris Longstreth of Philadelphia published a serious 16-page dissertation, "Against the Germ Theory of Disease," in the *Therapeutic Gazette.*

As a result of antiseptic techniques, puerperal sepsis was no longer "childbed fever," but streptococcal septicemia. To understand the effect of the antiseptic principle in extending the scope of surgery, one must remember that in the days before listerism, the mortality rate for amputation ran around 40% to 60% as a result of infection and secondary hemorrhage.

Despite Lister's theories, laudable as they were, it was soon realized that the air itself was not the most dangerous element in infection. The major risk came from the surgeon's hands, his instruments, his clothes, and the dressings he used. At that period, physicians still gave little thought to cleanliness. Operations usually took place in tiny, badly lit rooms, and the surgeon commonly kept in a closet an old, unwashed frock coat that he used repeatedly during surgical procedures.

Gradually, it became clear that paying meticulous attention to sterility during surgery—sterility of hands, clothes, instruments, and dressings—produced results far more effective than spraying the operating chamber with Lister's disagreeable carbolic acid vapor. Thus the practice of asepsis—now universally adopted—came to replace the older antiseptic method. Originally, every item used in surgery was boiled, but under the influence of Pasteur and others, various types of sterilizers were developed, some capable of raising the temperature up to and beyond 130°C.

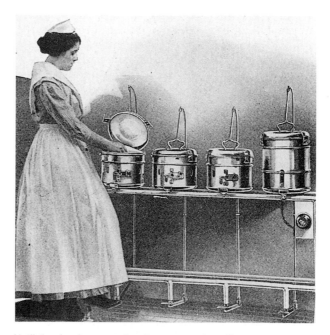

Until the development of various types of sterilizers, every instrument used in surgery was boiled.

In 1891, William Halsted of Baltimore introduced the use of rubber gloves—initially, it must be admitted, to protect the skin of the hands of his scrub nurse. Physicians later generally adopted the face mask. These developments aided significantly in the continued development of hospitals because the ability to limit infections soon became a necessary preliminary to gaining the public's confidence.

The first nurse anesthetists chosen by the surgeons with whom they were to work were considered as especially qualified for this type of duty. The nurse was expected to devote her entire attention to the conduct of the anesthesia—as opposed to the intern, whose interest would naturally be divided between the anesthesia and the surgical procedure. By the time the intern had become proficient in administering anesthesia, his term of service usually ended; in contrast, the nurse would stay on indefinitely and become increasingly valuable.

Administering ether in the late 1890s was not easy for the nurse. Patients commonly came to the operating room expressing greater repugnance and fear toward the anesthesia than toward the actual operation. Little innovation had been made in the administration of ether since its inception. A so-called ether cone was fashioned from a folded newspaper or butcher's straw cuff, covered snugly with a folded towel, and fastened tightly at the top by safety pins; its inside was stuffed with fluffed gauze. An indefinite amount of ether, ranging from a dram or two to an ounce or two according to the judgment of the nurse anesthetist, was poured into the gauze and the cone applied near to or in contact with the patient's face. Then, as now, followed the constant admonition to "take a deep breath."

Often the ether vapor was so strong that one or two deep breaths would nearly choke the patient, but prevailing practice expected this; the only thing to do was to rush the patient through the agony as quickly as possible. So, the more the patient choked and struggled for air, the more the ether was pushed and force applied to keep him sufficiently still. Inhalation of ether vapor at first stimulated the mucous glands: the stronger the vapor, the greater the stimulation. With luck, the anesthetist might accidentally allow the patient to return to a lighter ether-tension stage, and coughing and vomiting might clear out the frothy mucus; thus the anesthesia maintenance stage would be much improved. But all too often the anesthesia was kept at too deep a level; the mucus remained in the air passages (more or less obstructing them and causing a subcyanosis due to poor respiratory exchange); and irritation of the bronchial epithelium led to prolonged postoperative nausea and vomiting, aggravated by swallowing ether-laden mucus. Under these conditions—although anesthesia had been accomplished, the operation performed, the patient (usually) still alive—the horror of "taking ether" could not easily be forgotten.

The advent of antiseptic surgery necessitated a re-arrangement of operating rooms in all hospitals. The early hospitals performed operations in connection with the surgical wards, but the necessities of medical teaching soon rendered it essential that amphitheaters be built to permit medical and nursing students to view clinics and surgical operations. No special effort was made in these amphitheaters to guard against the possibility of infection from the surroundings of the patient or from those who came in contact with him or her. Usually brought in under the influence of an anesthetic, the patient was operated on before the students, with subsequent dressings made on the ward or in some adjoining room. The advent of antiseptic surgery and the altered conditions of surgical work required the provision of new operating rooms.

Antiseptic surgery and anesthesia increased the demand for hospitals. Anesthesia could be more

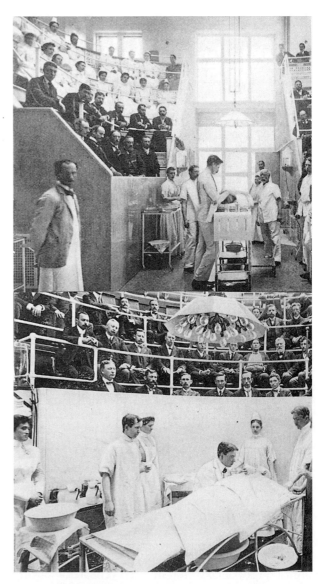

Surgery in hospital amphitheaters in the 1890s.

ETHER INHALERS.

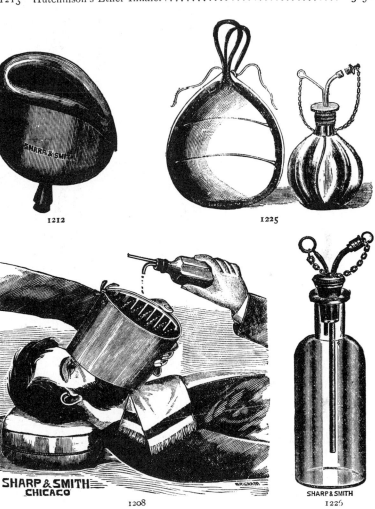

1212   1225

SHARP & SMITH
CHICAGO   1208

SHARP & SMITH
1226

Various devices for the administration of ether in the 1880s.

conveniently administered in a hospital than in a home, and the operating-room equipment for antiseptic surgery and administration of anesthesia demanded a highly specialized department furnished with technical equipment seldom found outside a hospital. Thus the developing complexities of the operating room began to make the hospital a necessity.

The development of blood transfusion also had great effect on the craft of surgery. It appears that transfusion was first practiced as early as 1867, but the modern period began in 1901, when it became possible to describe the four blood groups, thus making compatible blood transfusions possible and opening the way for the development of blood banks and for the method of supportive therapy that

has become basic to much of the success of modern surgical treatment.

IMPROVED DIAGNOSTIC INSTRUMENTS

One of the most striking developments in the medical practice of the era came with the introduction of the thermometer. It seems almost impossible now to understand why physicians were so slow to accept this indispensable diagnostic aid. Not until the 1880s was the thermometer generally used by city physicians in the United States, and it was nearly 1890 before it was generally used in country practice. Older physicians made all sorts of objections to its use, asked why a physician should bother to carry

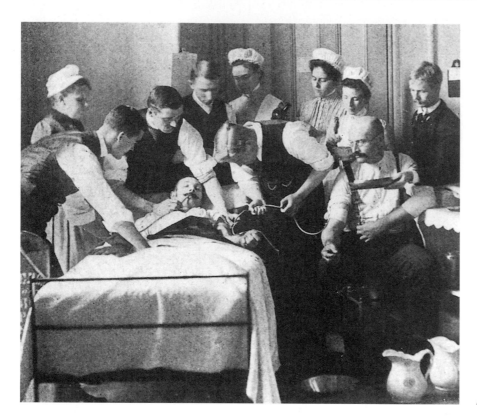

A blood transfusion in 1888.

such a toy around with him, and fretted over the possibility of delirious patients injuring themselves with broken thermometers. The introduction of the thermometer literally revolutionized the study and treatment of various illnesses.

Other instruments were equally important. Dr. George Elliott of New York gave a new stimulus to therapeutics when he brought the hypodermic syringe with him from Edinburgh in 1860. Because of professional conservatism and the fear that the hypodermic might readily lead to drug abuse, it did not become a common instrument in the hands of physicians for more than 20 years. The double stethoscope (an American modification of the basic instrument that had been around since 1816) added to the knowledge of diseases of the chest as well as of the condition of the fetus at any given time. In addition, that long-used instrument, the microscope, soon came into much greater use.

The invention of precision instruments during this period contributed to more accurate diagnoses. Among these were the ophthalmoscope and laryngoscope, developed before 1860; the gastroscope, sphygmomanometer, and cystoscope, developed before 1883; and the bronchoscope, developed in 1898. Thomas Edison's invention of the incandescent light made the visual instruments even more useful. High-frequency oscillating currents were introduced by Jacques-Arsène d'Arsonval in the late 1880s and later used in diathermy. In 1893, Niels Finsen introduced light therapy for the treatment of

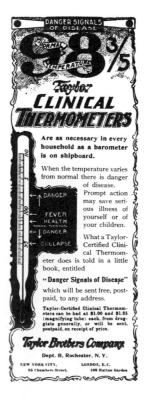

New clinical thermometers, 1888.

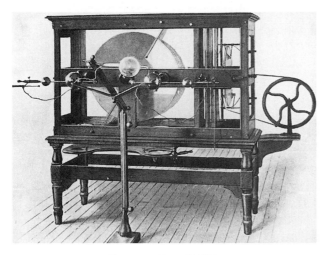

X-ray machine of 1898.

skin diseases, and in 1896 he published the results of his work on the use of ultraviolet rays.

Perhaps no diagnostic method caused a greater revolution in medical practice and diagnosis than the discovery of the X-ray by Wilhelm Konrad Roentgen in 1895. The rapid application of this discovery to clinical medicine brought much information concerning the previously invisible organs of living patients. Correlation of the findings of photographic films or fluoroscopic screens with those at operations and postmortem examinations quickly demonstrated the tremendous usefulness of this method of diagnosis and rapidly established radiology as a separate medical specialty. The introduction of radiopaque substances into the gastrointestinal tract and bronchial tree and the selective

excretion of radiopaque dyes by the liver into the gallbladder and by the kidneys into the urinary tract revolutionized the diagnostic capabilities of physicians in these fields. Introduction of air and occasionally of other contrast media into the cerebrospinal fluid spaces, into serous-lined cavities (peritoneum, pleura, pericardium, and joints), and, at times, into the retroperitoneal space offered more limited, but at times equally important, diagnostic aid.

The early hospital X-ray services were limited chiefly to the examination of bony structures. The equipment was crude and its operation hazardous to both patient and roentgenologist. Nevertheless, the X-ray increased confidence in medical diagnosis and brought hundreds of additional patients to the hospital for treatment. Moreover, the first use of the X-ray marked the beginning of medical care requiring equipment so elaborate that the average practitioner could not afford to install it. The great cost of these machines encouraged the founding of more community hospitals, in which local physicians could use such apparatuses jointly.

PATHOLOGY, MICROBIOLOGY, MEDICAL ENTOMOLOGY, AND IMMUNOLOGY

Modern pathology in this country found its inspiration in the German and Austrian universities of the mid-19th century. Autopsy was used extensively in the study of disease, and most of the great advances in gross descriptive pathology had already been made. Much of the knowledge thus gained had been transferred to clinical practice, particularly in surgery. Probably the greatest pathologist of the day was Rudolf Virchow, director of the Pathological Institute of the University of Berlin. By the mid-1870s, he had already completed the creative work that left such an imprint on medicine. He had instituted the first modern journal in pathology, *Archiv fur Pathologische Anatomie und Physiologie*. The new concepts of disease put forth in his book *Die Cellularpathologie* (1858) stemmed from the use of the microscope in the study of diseased tissues. Virchow furthered experimental inquiry into the nature of pathologic phenomena and the application to pathology of advances in physiology.

From the standpoint of future developments in pathology in America, the influence of one of Virchow's pupils, Julius Cohnheim, was most important. Cohnheim's laboratory, in Breslau, Prussia, actively emphasized the experimental approach to pathology. His experiments on inflammation furnished the basis for current conceptions of this fundamental process. It was in Cohnheim's laboratory that William Henry Welch, often referred to as the dean of modern American medicine and as America's great pioneer pathologist, did his first experimental work. Welch published *On the Pathology of Lung Edema* in 1878. The

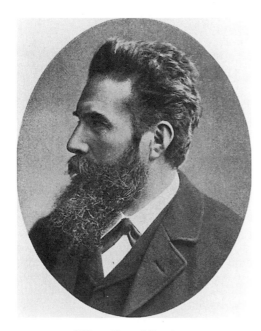

Wilhem Konrad Roentgen.

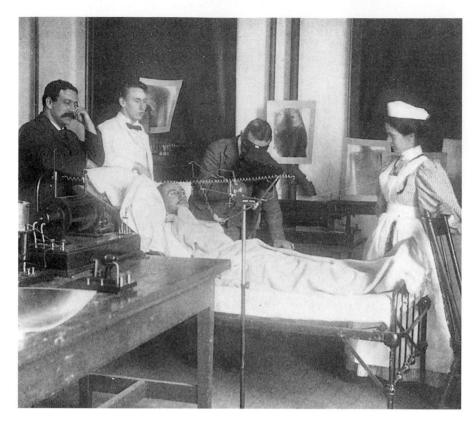

X-ray machine in use at the Philadelphia Polyclinic.

dynamic concept of disease that Welch had studied in Breslau influenced future developments in this country, not only in pathology but in medical education and general medical thought as well.

In contrast to Europe, opportunities in America for investigations in pathology remained limited.

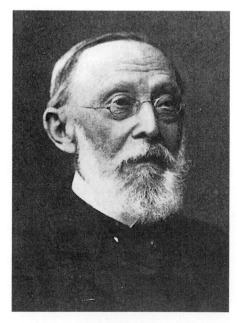

Rudolf Virchow.

Before the 1890s, neither medical schools nor hospitals had pathology laboratories in the modern sense, and few, if any, medical men devoted full time to pathology. The well-known pathologists of the day, such as Samuel D. Gross in Philadelphia and Francis A. Delafield in New York, were primarily clinicians who gave special attention to pathology. Despite many limitations, some Americans made basic contributions to pathology. In 1885, Francis A. Delafield and Theophile M. Prudden published the first modern textbook of pathology in this country.

Along with the identification of microbes—a great forward stride in the art of diagnosis—came the discovery of new serums and vaccines revolutionizing medical treatment and public hygiene. The basic rules governing bacteriologic research were formulated by Robert Koch (1843–1910). According to Koch, (1) the infectious agent of a given disease must be shown to be present in every case of that disease, (2) it must be absent from all other diseases, (3) we should be able to isolate it, (4) we should be able to cultivate it, (5) an animal inoculated with it must contract that same disease, and (6) we should be able to trace the agent again in the organism of the inoculated animal. In Koch's time these rules could not be applied to diseases caused by viruses because the infectious agents of many diseases—so-called filterable viruses—could pass through the filters that effectively retained bacteria.

Bacteriologists and their associates in pathology and medical microbiology stimulated widespread

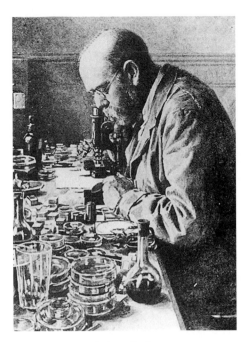

Robert Koch.

investigations. By 1890, the causes of the following diseases had been isolated: European relapsing fever (*Borrelia recurrentis,* by Otto Obermeier, 1873), leprosy (*Mycobacterium leprae,* by G. Armauer Hansen, 1874), anthrax (*Bacillus anthracis,* by Robert Koch, 1876), gonorrhea (*Neisseria gonorrhoeae,* by Albert Neisser, 1879), typhoid fever (*E. typhosa,* by Karl Eberth, 1880), malaria (*Plasmodium malariae,* by Charles Laveran, 1880), lobar pneumonia (*Diplococcus pneumoniae,* by Louis Pasteur and George Sternberg, 1880), tuberculosis (*Mycobacterium tuberculosis,* by Robert Koch, 1882), diphtheria (*Corynebacterium diphtheriae,* by Theodor Klebs, 1883), tetanus (*Clostridium tetani,* by Arthur Nicolaier, 1884), cholera (*Vibrio cholerae,* by Robert Koch, 1884), bacillus coli infection (*Escherichia coli,* by Theodor Escherich, 1886), and Malta fever (*Brucella melitensis,* by David Bruce, 1887).

During this era of discoveries, the foundation was laid for another new science: medical entomology. In 1877, Patrick Manson in Hong Kong showed that mosquitoes could carry the microfilaria of *Wuchereria bancrofti,* and in 1881 Carlos Finlay in Cuba believed that he had succeeded in transmitting yellow fever through *Stegomyia* mosquitoes. Eight years later, Theobald Smith described the transmission of Texas cattle fever by ticks. Such a rich harvest of new scientific facts intensified interest in research as the medical revolution continued to gain momentum.

The last 7 years of the century witnessed a surge in experimental activity and the discovery of still more organisms. These included the influenza bacillus (*Haemophilus influenzae,* by Richard Pfeiffer, 1892), *Clostridium welchii* (*Clostridium perfringens,* by William H. Welch and George H. Nuttall, 1892), and the

bacillus of plague (*Yersinia pestis,* by Alexandre Yersin and Shibasacuro Kitasato, 1894). In 1894, David Bruce began his work on anemia in Africa, which led to the incrimination of tsetse flies as vectors of trypanosomiasis. The same year, Patrick Manson suggested to Ronald Ross that the parasites of malaria might develop in the body of the mosquito and be transmitted between people in this way. In 1895, Ross went to India to test Manson's theory, and by 1897 he had shown that *Anopheles* mosquitoes could transmit human malaria. In 1898, Kiyoshi Shiga of Japan discovered the dysentery bacillus that bears his name.

Immunology developed almost hand in hand with bacteriology. In 1881, Louis Pasteur inoculated 25 sheep with weakened anthrax bacteria and left the same number unvaccinated. Later, he gave all 50 a virulent form of the disease. The unvaccinated animals died, whereas the treated sheep remained well. With the establishment of the principle that the injection of a mild form of disease bacteria will cause the formation of antibodies that will prevent the inoculated person from getting the virulent form of the disease, the science of immunology began in earnest. In 1890, Emil von Behring discovered the possibility of passive immunization against tetanus and diphtheria, which led to the concept of antitoxins. Prevention of smallpox by vaccination had long since been introduced by Edward Jenner, to be followed by efforts to establish immunity against typhoid, rabies, whooping cough, typhus, and cholera.

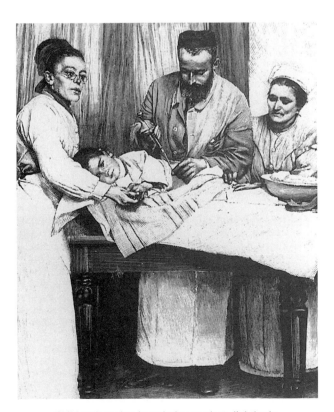

Child undergoing inoculation against diphtheria.

GYNECOLOGY AND OBSTETRICS

Modern gynecology is a product almost entirely of the 19th century. Of his book *The Principles and Practices of Gynecology* (1879), Thomas Addis Emmet wrote, "It was published, unfortunately, just before the full development or adoption of the aseptic treatment as applied to abdominal surgery."[2] In other words, the principles and application of the aseptic techniques, prerequisite to successful operative gynecology, were just beginning to gain acceptance. Peritonitis was but poorly understood until 1880, when T. Gaillard Thomas clearly identified so-called cellulitis as peritonitis.

With the general use of antiseptic and aseptic techniques, operative gynecology, along with abdominal surgery, had its real beginning, and the next few decades saw reports of countless new operative procedures. The first conditions addressed were those most urgent, such as ruptured ectopic pregnancy. The progenitor of surgery in ectopic pregnancy was the great British gynecologist Lawson Tait, who first operated for this condition in 1883. Rapid progress followed: By 1891, Friedrich Schauta demonstrated that prompt surgery in ectopic pregnancy had reduced the mortality rate from 86.9% to 5.7%. With the advent of modern blood transfusion, the mortality rate fell still lower.

Hysterectomy had its beginning in the epic struggle with myomata, an affliction characterized by fibrous muscular tumors. Throughout the greater part of the 19th century, myoma victims took vast quantities of ergot (rye plant derivative) in the futile hope that blood loss from these tumors could thus be stemmed. Although a few abdominal hysterectomies had been performed in the first half of the century,

the mortality rate was extremely high because of hemorrhage and sepsis from the thick pedicle. In 1889, a general surgeon, Lewis A. Stimson, first suggested and practiced the systematic ligation of the ovarian and uterine arterial trunks as the cardinal principle of hysterectomy. This transformed the operation, which has since gained many refinements in technique. Likewise, the whole field of female urology developed as the result of the invention of the air cystoscope by Howard A. Kelly in 1894. Surpassing these developments in operative gynecology in basic importance, if not in practical use, was the vast array of advances made in knowledge of ovarian function, the menstrual cycle, and gynecologic pathology.

In the 1870s, childbearing was a hazardous undertaking, and any substantial deviation from the normal physiologic processes meant death. Throughout the greater part of the 19th century, cesarean section was the most fatal of surgical procedures. In Great Britain and Ireland in 1865, the maternal mortality rate from the operation had mounted to the appalling figure of 85%. In Paris, during the 90 years ending in 1876, not a single successful cesarean section had been performed. As late as 1887, Robert P. Harris reported in the *American Journal of Medical Science* that cesarean section was actually more successful when performed by the patient herself. He collected 9 such cases from the literature, with 5 recoveries, and contrasted them with 12 cesarean sections performed with only 1 recovery, in New York City during the same period. Considering such results, it is not surprising that many obstetricians of the 19th century doubted the wisdom of ever resorting to cesarean section and predicted that the operation would shortly become obsolete.

The turning point in the evolution of cesarean section was the appearance in 1882 of a monograph by Max Sanger, 28-year-old assistant to Karl Crede in the University Clinic at Leipzig. This monograph recommended the routine use of carefully placed uterine sutures in cesarean section. Within a few years, uterine suture was generally recognized as an indispensable step in cesarean section, and forthwith the modern operation came into being.

PEDIATRICS

Largely as a result of the unprecedented application of the scientific method to the study of clinical problems in the laboratory as well as in the clinic, pediatrics finally emerged as a fledgling branch of scientific medicine during the waning decades of the century and proved itself to be a discipline less fettered by accumulated misinformation and more willing to adopt new concepts than were other long-established clinical specialties. In this atmosphere, the American Pediatric Society was founded in 1888. During the same year, Harvard University organized

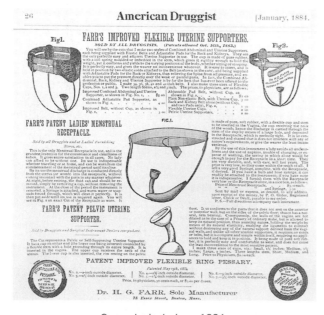

Gynecologic devices, 1884.

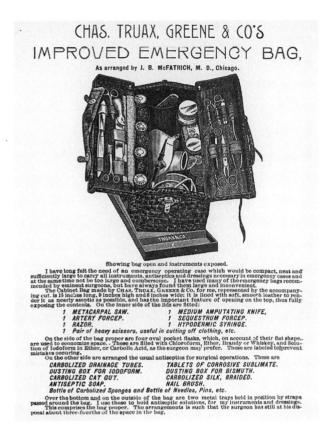

CHAS. TRUAX, GREENE & CO'S
IMPROVED EMERGENCY BAG,

As arranged by J. B. McFATRICH, M. D., Chicago.

Showing bag open and instruments exposed.

I have long felt the need of an emergency operating case which would be compact, neat and sufficiently large to carry all instruments, antiseptics and dressings necessary in emergency cases and at the same time not be too large and cumbersome. I have used many of the emergency bags recommended by eminent surgeons, but have always found them large and inconvenient.
The Cabinet Bag made by CHAS. TRUAX, GREENE & Co. for me, represented by the accompanying cut, is 15 inches long, 9 inches high and 8 inches wide; it is lined with soft, smooth leather to render it as nearly aseptic as possible, and has the important feature of opening on the top, thus fully exposing the contents. On the inner side of the lids are fitted:

1 METACARPAL SAW.	1 MEDIUM AMPUTATING KNIFE.
1 ARTERY FORCEP.	1 SEQUESTRUM FORCEP.
1 RAZOR.	1 HYPODERMIC SYRINGE.
1 Pair of heavy scissors, useful in cutting off clothing, etc.	

On the side of the bag proper are four oval pocket flasks, which, on account of their flat shape, are used to economize space. These are filled with Chloroform, Ether, Brandy or Whiskey, and Solution of Iodoform in Ether, or Carbolic Acid, as the surgeon may prefer. These are labeled to prevent mistakes occurring.
On the other side are arranged the usual antiseptics for surgical operations. These are

CARBOLIZED DRAINAGE TUBES.	TABLETS OF CORROSIVE SUBLIMATE.
DUSTING BOX FOR IODOFORM.	DUSTING BOX FOR BISMUTH.
CARBOLIZED CAT GUT.	CARBOLIZED SILK, BRAIDED.
ANTISEPTIC SOAP.	NAIL BRUSH.
Bottle of Carbolized Sponges and Bottle of Needles, Pins, etc.	

Over the bottom and on the outside of the bag are two metal trays held in position by straps passed around the bag. I use these to hold antiseptic solutions, for my instruments and dressings. This comprises the bag proper. The arrangements is such that the surgeon has still at his disposal about three-fourths of the space in the bag.

Contents of a physician's emergency bag, late 1890s.

the first independent university department of pediatrics for formal teaching of the subject.

The most spectacular reduction in the previously high mortality among children resulted from the discovery of the relationship between the contamination of water and food supplies, including milk, and the occurrence of enteric or diarrheal diseases. Since then, in no other major health care area has cooperation among private practitioners, public health officials, and voluntary lay organizations accomplished so much as it accomplished in eliminating food and water contamination throughout communities.

Of the many advances made in the medical care of infants and young children, the most important pertained to malnutrition. All physicians admitted the unsatisfactory results of artificial feeding of newborn infants, especially premature infants. A major portion of every pediatrician's practice until 1900 concerned the problems of artificial feeding and the search for a formula that might be substituted for human milk.

"Wet nursing" registries and human milk stations organized in the large population centers were woefully inadequate, even under the best conditions. Unmodified raw milk from other animal sources proved to "upset digestion," whereas highly diluted cow's milk formulas failed to produce acceptable weight gains. Thus elaborate milk modifications were devised, with sick infants frequently shifted from one formula to another without benefit. Acute infection

often ensued. Many babies had severe vomiting and diarrhea with attendant dehydration, exhaustion, and acidosis. Without adequate replacement of water and electrolytes lost in the course of such illness, mortality among these babies was extremely high.

The entire picture changed with the advent of greatly improved sanitation and the practice of boiling cow's milk formulas. Artificially fed babies began to thrive, and the mortality rates rapidly decreased to one fourth their former levels as the serious dangers of infection, exhaustion, and vitamin deficiencies declined. No longer were such disease entities as hypoproteinemic edema, scurvy, rickets, rachitic tetany, vitamin A deficiency, beriberi, pellagra, ariboflavinosis, and iron-deficiency anemia inevitable in the child population.

AMERICA'S FIRST CENTER OF MODERN MEDICINE

The great developments in medicine during this period occurred principally in the university medical centers of Germany, Austria, France, and England. Just before the turn of the century, scientific methods in medicine came from the European countries to the United States; at the same time, a full-fledged university medical school was introduced here. In 1873 in Baltimore, Johns Hopkins, bachelor merchant and financier, had willed his great fortune to found a hospital and a university within which a medical school was to be organized. While the university was getting underway, the trustees sought to build the hospital. Members of this board depended greatly on John Shaw Billings, whom they had chosen as their official adviser. Billings was a military physician and librarian attached to the army surgeon general's office who had acquired wide hospital experience during the Civil War. Billings designed the Johns Hopkins Hospital buildings and assisted in preparing plans for hospital management and for integration of the hospital with the proposed medical school. He included plans for a school of nursing and for various supporting services, such as pharmacies.

On May 7, 1889, the doors of the Johns Hopkins Hospital and nursing school formally opened, followed several years later by the medical school. Significantly, all faculty members who would be chosen for the Johns Hopkins University Medical School over the next few years would be comparatively young. The first to be named was William H. Welch, as pathologist, in 1884. Then 34 years of age, Welch went on to serve the university in various capacities for 50 years and became the most influential of the faculty members. Welch at once began to organize postgraduate courses in bacteriology and pathology for practicing physicians, using hospital facilities for teaching, because there was, as yet, no medical school. Much of the responsibility for selection of the rest of the medical school faculty fell to Welch.

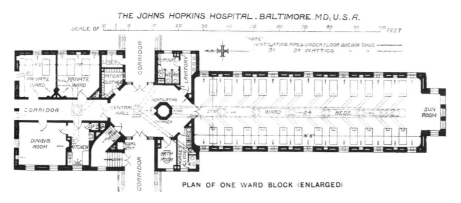

THE JOHNS HOPKINS HOSPITAL . BALTIMORE . MD; U.S.A.

PLAN OF ONE WARD BLOCK (ENLARGED)

Typical ward at Johns Hopkins Hospital, 1890s.

Next to come, in 1888, was Canadian-born William Osler, called from his post at the University of Pennsylvania to become physician-in-chief at the hospital and professor of the theory and practice of medicine at the university. Osler devoted much of his time to organizing the clinical staff. Organized on the unit system, with a graded resident staff, as in German universities, the new medical school used teaching methods similar to those used in Great Britain and France. The teaching program included instruction of small groups of students who served on the wards as clinical clerks and surgical dressers and in practical work in clinical laboratories, amphitheater clinics, and outpatient clinics.

A New York surgeon, William S. Halsted, working temporarily in Welch's laboratory, became acting surgeon to the hospital, and Howard A. Kelly moved from the University of Pennsylvania to become staff gynecologist and obstetrician. As a team, these men remade the face of American medical education. Bedside teaching and observation correlated with data obtained at the autopsy table and in the laboratory revolutionized medical education, medical practice, and medicine as a whole.

HOSPITAL USAGE CLIMBS

General hospitals were slow to develop, and not until around 1900 did the use of hospitals for the care of all types of illness and all types of patients become widely accepted. By then the advances in medical science and the development of surgical X-ray and laboratory facilities in hospitals, coupled with the decrease in the size of houses (especially in the urban areas), the increase in families living in apartments, and the tendency to rely more and more on agencies outside the home, made it increasingly difficult to care for the ill at home, particularly in serious cases.

The original hospitals kept few medical records. During the early part of the century, most had but a register of admissions and discharges that contained a summary of the age, nationality, and condition of each patient, with a statement of the name of the disease and the condition at discharge. With advances in medical science, however, and with an increase in the size of the medical staffs of hospitals, a system of casebooks grew in which were recorded the history of the patient, the course of his or her disease, a description of the operation performed (if any), and the condition of the patient on discharge from the hospital. Routine notes on cases were made daily by clinical clerks appointed for that purpose. Generally bulky volumes, the casebooks could not be conveniently handled and carried to the wards, so notes could not be easily made at bedside. Thus a modification of this system was adopted in all hospitals whereby notes were made at

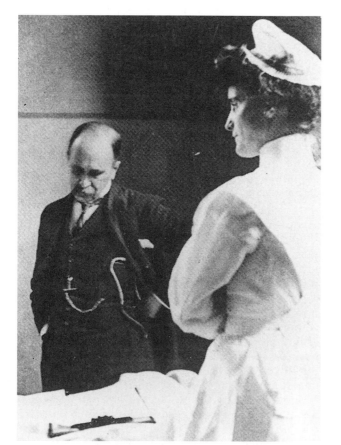

William Osler on rounds with nurse.

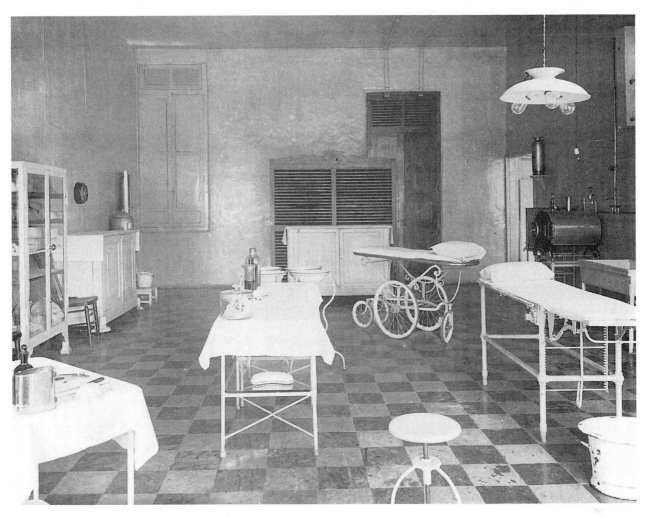

Fully equipped hospital operating room, 1900.

the bedside on loose sheets of paper and afterward collected, collated with charts, photographs, and graphic representations, and finally bound.

Every history of a patient's disease contained a full account of his or her condition before admission to the hospital. Inherited tendencies to disease were carefully noted along with previous illness, lifestyle, occupation, place of residence, exposure to unhealthful surroundings, and known addiction to alcohol or drugs. The state of the patient on admission was carefully described, and daily notes of his or her signs and symptoms followed, together with the findings in the clinical and bacteriologic laboratories. Surgical operations were accurately described, and records made of the pathologic changes in the tissue or tumor removed, along with any information obtained by the microscope. The termination of the disease was made a matter of similar record, and in the event of death a full protocol of the autopsy findings was added. Such histories were permanently bound and indexed for future reference. Cross-references kept on index cards allowed the diseases to be grouped and all the clinical material of the hospital

used for the description and further study of disease. In many hospitals, this work took place under the charge of a paid registrar, who devoted his whole time to the preparation of casebooks and histories.

During the last quarter of the 19th century, great strides in the science of medicine and in the improvement of hospitals led to the attainment of better health. A baby born in 1875 had a life expectancy of 40 years. Although in 1900 a child could be expected to live 47 years, much remained to be done. In 1900 in the United States, the principal causes of death were (1) tuberculosis, (2) pneumonia, (3) diarrhea and enteritis, (4) heart disease, and (5) diseases of infancy and congenital malformations.

The developments that revolutionized medicine in the last quarter of the 19th century probably yielded more progress toward the amelioration of human suffering than all the fumbling efforts of the preceding 1000 years. The implications of this revolution for nurses and nursing were great. As physicians embraced the tenets of this new medicine, with its concomitant reliance on laboratory work, advanced surgery, and clinical diagnosis, many areas of

TABLE 4-1 Reports of 12 Hospitals in a Large American City, 1990

HOSPITAL	INPATIENTS	OUTPATIENTS	TOTAL PATIENTS	TOTAL RUNNING EXPENSES	COST PER HOSPITAL
A	1,854	8,197	10,051	$187,079.37	$10.65
B	1,894	11,810	13,704	105,635.16	7.71
C	3,850	12,559	16,409	83,410.06	5.08
D	901	11,423	12,334	53,787.05	4.36
E	3,026	34,100	37,126	125,939.43	3.39
F	4,079	30,860	34,939	116,790.30	3.34
G	4,654	15,374	20,328	64,053.22	3.15
H	973	14,608	15,851	34,717.45	2.23
I	1,266	24,011	25,217	53,392.86	2.12
J	745	23,666	24,411	45,813.40	1.87
K	2,052	18,614	20,666	37,781.17	1.83
L	1,898	34,281	36,179	63,378.79	1.75

their former domain—particularly those related to the so-called art of medicine—became the province of the nurse. As a result, the practice of nursing was markedly altered. The nurse not only stepped into the vacuum created by the physician's move into the world of scientific medicine but also began to participate in the more complicated medical and surgical procedures that were required for modern treatment. Most importantly, she faced new nursing care problems and unforeseen complications that came with the new methods of treatment. The result was a rapid increase in the number of hospitals. All the nation's general hospitals in 1880 contained approximately 85,000 beds; in 1890, approximately 150,000; and in 1900, approximately 250,000. The ratio of one hospital bed to 817 people in 1872 had by 1900 become one bed to 304 people.

Sources of hospital revenue also began to change. Separate facilities for the private patients of staff physicians were added to the standard ward facilities. Patients began to pay an increasing proportion of the rising costs of hospital care. In accordance with the theory that the wealthy patients should be charged enough to provide funds for hospital care of the poor, the patients in the private rooms became not merely "pay patients" but often "overpay patients." However, despite the growth in income from patients, financing in voluntary hospitals still relied on deficit funding. The chief duty of the board of trustees in the early decades of the current century was to furnish or obtain philanthropic funds to make up the inevitable deficits. In 1900, the average cost per patient per day for all hospitals was estimated to be $2.00, with total annual expenditures for hospital care estimated at $120 million. Payroll expenditures, including administration salaries, were estimated to be less than one fourth of total expense. The figures in Table 4-1 reveal stark differences in per capita cost among various hospitals.[3]

The turn of the century saw a tendency to organize hospitals for specific diseases. Special hospitals emerged for skin diseases; eye, ear, nose, and throat diseases; cancer; tuberculosis; fever; and diseases of the digestive tract. It was soon realized, however, that the hospital organized to treat only one type of disease was too limited in service, and the emphasis veered from hospitals organized for specific diseases to hospitals organized for certain age, sex, or occupational groups. Hospitals were built for maternity, orthopedic, isolation, industrial, incurable, convalescent, chronic, pediatric, and cancer patients. With the addition of active surgical and medical clinics, sanatoriums for convalescents, for patients with nervous and mental disorders, and for victims of drug addiction became hospitals.

REFERENCES

1. James Bryant Conant, *Pasteur's Study of Fermentation* (Cambridge, MA: Harvard University Press, 1952), p. 56.
2. Thomas Addis Emmet, "Personal Reminiscences Associated with the Progress of Gynecology," *American Gynecological and Obstetrical Journal*, vol. 18 (May–June 1900):301–324.
3. "Some Hospital Statistics," *National Hospital Record*, vol. 5 (May 1902):13.

5

THE NOT-SO-GAY EIGHTIES AND NINETIES IN NURSE TRAINING SCHOOLS

The growth of nurse training schools had to await the acceleration of the general hospital movement in the United States. It was only when the concept of the community hospital became attractive to every major town and city throughout the country that these institutions began to acquire respectability, multiply, and elicit a much broader clientele. Let us examine just what the status of the hospital was as the nation moved into the 1880s and what conditions brought on the realization that trained nurses would be socially and economically useful in caring for the increasing hospital population.

HOSPITALS OF THE LATE 19TH CENTURY

In the early 1880s, only a few hundred hospitals existed in the United States. Most medical care was provided in patients' homes and physicians' offices. As primarily charitable institutions, hospitals provided care for indigent patients who had nowhere else to go. The image of the hospital was that of an almshouse, a place for the poor and needy. The hospital was not a place for the living, but a place to go to die. Patient wards were like flophouses, where patients were removed from society. With the expansion of the influence of Florence Nightingale, the image of the hospital as a place to die slowly transformed into the image of a place with skilled nursing care that "would do no harm to the patient." Nursing hospitals that would do no harm soon developed into major providers of quality health care and rapidly spread across the nation.

The first complete census of hospitals in the United States was published in 1873, when the report of a survey of 178 institutions by the United States Bureau of Education appeared in *Transactions of the American Medical Association*. This report showed that 146,472 patients had been admitted to hospitals in 1872, that there were 35,604 beds, that 46 hospitals had between 100 and 200 beds and

38 had between 200 and 400 beds, and that 18 had more than 400 beds.[1]

Fifteen of the hospitals were supported by cities, 4 by counties, 7 by religious bodies, and 67 "by patients and other sources." Because several of the institutions established before that time were not named in this early survey, the statistics probably do not include all existing hospital facilities, but they represent enough to establish a fair basis for comparison with the present.

The Civil War did much to develop the hospitals of America, and certain features of hospital service were derived from the U.S. Army medical department. The most important of these was ambulance service, originated in New York City in 1868. In 1869, Dr. E. B. Dalton, who had served in the U.S. Army as a medical officer and had had considerable experience in the transportation of sick and wounded soldiers, divided New York City into districts to respond better to all calls for emergencies, accidents, and transfer of the sick from their homes to the various hospitals of the city.

Under his direction, ambulances with medicines, instruments, and other articles were built for the speedy and comfortable transportation of the sick and the wounded. Arrangements were also made to have the vehicles accompanied by experienced surgeons who could give attention to the patients on the way to the hospital. Dr. Emily Dunning successfully challenged the conventions of male medicine in New York's Gouveneur Hospital in 1890 by becoming the first female ambulance surgeon. To prevent delay in the run between home and hospital, ambulances were given the right of way by an order of the police department.

The showcase of hospital architecture of the 1880s was the new 100-bed Presbyterian Hospital in New York City, which opened its nurse training school in 1892. The hospital complex had been designed by Richard Hunt, at that time New York's most distinguished architect. The complex consisted of two

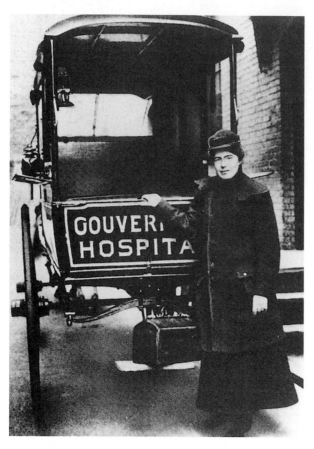

Emily Dunning, America's first female ambulance surgeon.

The plan of the hospital building was simple. The first floor was devoted mainly to rooms for private patients. These rooms were of fair size and comfortably furnished; the charge for them was $30 to $50 a week. The surgical operating rooms, located on the third and fourth floors, were considered among the best of their day, although they were paneled with wood, less sanitary than tile. They received excellent outside light and were conveniently equipped. The three upper floors were each divided equally into two wards of 12 beds. The ceilings were high, and the many windows of the wards were large enough to secure excellent ventilation. The walls were hard-finished and the floors were made of pitch pine to withstand heavy scrubbing. There were no passenger elevators: A staircase ran up through the center of the building.

PROLIFERATION OF NURSING SCHOOLS

To the planners of hospitals, it was doubtful whether a successful hospital could be developed without an affiliated training school for nurses. This was not simply because the training school had proved to be the most economic means of providing nursing care, but because it was supposedly impossible to create the desired home atmosphere if graduates from various schools were employed. Each graduate nurse from outside would come with habits firmly fixed and with her own hospital traditions and ideas of service.

Consequently, after the founding of the first four schools of nursing in 1872 and 1873, other hospitals opened schools of their own, and by 1880 there were 15 schools, 323 students, and 157 graduates in the United States. Twenty years later, these figures had soared to 432 schools, 11,164 students, and 3546 graduates. Irene Sutliffe, superintendent of the Long Island College Hospital Training School for Nurses, and Isabel Hampton, superintendent of the Johns Hopkins Training School for Nurses, warned against the premature organization of schools of nursing, but this warning was not

major buildings, one for administration and the other for the hospital wards. Between them were a small structure that included the kitchen, laundry, and heating plants; another smaller one, the mortuary; and one for the ambulance. The hospital property comprised the block bounded by Manhattan's 70th and 71st streets and Madison and Park avenues. The administration and hospital buildings sat on the property lines of their respective streets and were connected by two long covered corridors, the tops of which served as roof gardens.

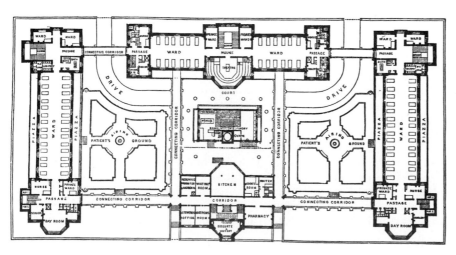

First-level floor plan of Presbyterian hospital.

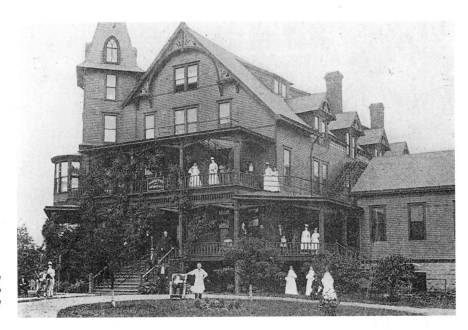

Most hospitals wanted a training school for nurses in order to develop their own economical student nursing force.

heeded. New York State alone was responsible for the organization of 25 schools before 1890 and by 1902 had added 54 more of varying quality. By 1902, four states accounted for 230 of the 492 existing schools.[2]

NURSE TRAINING SCHOOLS, PUBLIC SCHOOLS, AND HIGHER EDUCATION

If the nation's cultural level could be gauged by the status of the public school, then the latter part of the century showed a significant advance in American culture. The 7 million pupils enrolled in the public schools in 1870 increased to 15.5 million in 1900; the 300 public high schools of 1860 increased to more than 6000, while the 12 state normal schools of 1860 increased to 175. At the end of the century, there were almost 500 colleges—about double the number in 1860. Illiteracy declined from 17% in 1880 to less than 11% in 1900. By the end of the 1870s, most of the state universities had opened their gates to women. In the meantime, women's colleges on a par with the best schools for men had been founded: Vassar, opened in 1865 and supported by a rich brewer from Poughkeepsie; Mount Holyoke, transformed from a girls' seminary into a college; Smith, founded in 1871 through the vision of a country minister and the wealth of a village spinster; and Wellesley, created in 1875 through the largess of a Boston lawyer. Women's colleges were added to the great universities: Barnard at Columbia in 1889 and Radcliffe at Harvard in 1894. More significant was that secondary schools as well as elementary schools were being taught largely by women by this time.

Compared with other professional schools or with colleges of the time, nurse training schools, despite their 7-day week, had an unprecedentedly long year. In most schools, the academic year ran 50 weeks, with no Christmas, Easter, or Thanksgiving holidays and rarely a whole free Sunday. The annual vacation period generally lasted 2 weeks, and although some schools allowed 3 weeks or even a month, others gave but 10 days of vacation annually. All schools required the student to make up to the hospital every day or half-day lost through illness or absence. The 50 weeks of the training school year contrasted with the 32 or 36 weeks of the academic year in the college or professional school.

Several months before entering a hospital training school, one prospective student nurse came across some stanzas entitled "Woman's Rights," one of which particularly impressed her:

> *The right to tread so softly beside the couch of pain,*
> *To smooth with gentle fingers the tangled locks again,*
> *To watch beside the dying in the still small hours of night,*
> *And breathe a consecrating prayer as the spirit takes its*
> *flight.[3]*

This privilege to practice those "dearest rights of her sex" meant, in fact, the right to train and work under incredibly rigorous conditions, but that did not seem to discourage the young woman or a host of other new applicants.

TRAINING SCHOOL APPLICANTS

The enormous number of applications received each year by the more famous training schools made it possible for them to attract students of a much higher caliber than formerly had been the case. The approximate number of applicants to the following training

Touro Infirmary

NEW ORLEANS, LA.

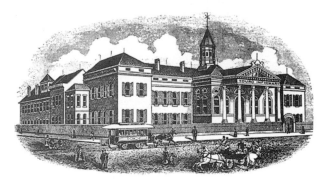

A MEDICAL STAFF OF THE MOST EMINENT PHYSICIANS AND SURGEONS OF OUR CITY,

A Corps of Experienced Nurses, and the tender care bestowed upon the sick entrusted to us, are sure guarantees for those who desire to avail themselves of its advantages.

Situated in the most beautiful portion of the City, its surroundings are most pleasant to the eye, whilst the rooms well furnished, high and airy, give every comfort desired, equal to any modern hotel.

ST. JOSEPH'S HOSPITAL

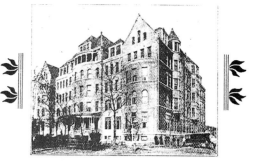

Is located west of Lincoln Park, on Garfield Avenue, between Halsted and Burling Streets. It is conducted by Sisters of Charity, who, after the usual examination have obtained diplomas in their profession, and in connection with it is a model Training School for Nurses, under the special patronage of Prof. N. Senn, M. D., Surgeon in Charge, to whose watchful care it is deeply indebted for the efficiency of its pupils.

Almost every hospital started a school of nursing.

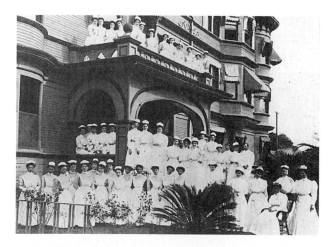

Nursing schools grew much larger in the 1890s.

schools in 1905 substantiated their well-deserved reputations:[4]

Bellevue Hospital, New York	2000
Johns Hopkins Hospital, Baltimore	1400
St. Luke's Hospital, New York	1200
Presbyterian Hospital, New York	1100
New York Hospital, New York	1000
Illinois Training School, Chicago	1000
Boston City Hospital, Boston	1000
Massachusetts General Hospital, Boston	1000
Carney Hospital, Boston	900
Margaret Fahnestock Training School, New York	800
Lakeside Hospital, Cleveland	800

On the other end of the continuum were several hundred assorted schools that barely managed to attract enough students to allow the maintenance of even a skeleton student nursing staff. The enormous increase in the number of hospitals and sanatoriums throughout the country and the consequent unrestricted development of training schools as a part of their working organizations led to a large demand for students trained essentially for utilitarian purposes. In the face of an inadequate student supply, training schools sacrificed standards to meet the current institutional staffing needs. Evidence accumulated as to the inferiority of many candidates. A school that could state honestly that it had 100 quality applicants annually was fortunate. The average large school of the time admitted a class of about 30 to 35 students each year.

STUDENT CHARACTERISTICS

What were the students like? Nightingale standards dictated "good education; good character; good background; good health." Naturally, "good" meant what each hospital labeled as such. Eight years of prior schooling was an accepted educational standard, but often the required amount of preparatory education varied. Requirements concerning health and background differed as well. Although the minimum age varied, the students were typically older than young women enrolled in trade schools or colleges. Competition from other fields open to women soon put pressure on schools of nursing to take younger students to prevent them from drifting into other lines of work, and consequently the minimum age requirement of 25 years was decreased to 21 years or younger.

Of course, one of the prevailing characteristics of nurse training school students was that all were female. American nursing, based on Nightingale ideals, had no place for men except where physical strength was needed, and men attendants were used only in the care of alcoholics, insane and violent patients, and men with genitourinary diseases. In 1888,

The Lakeside Hospital Training School for Nurses

offers a three-year course of training to young women from twenty to thirty years of age. Requirements, good health, good moral character and a high school education.

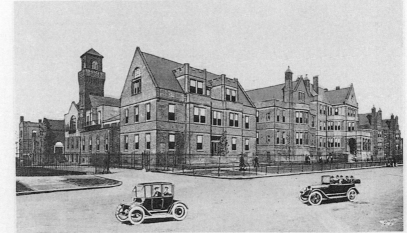

For further information, address
LAURA FELL WHITE, Superintendent, Lakeside Hospital.
4147 Lake Avenue, CHICAGO.

One of the 492 schools of nursing in 1902.

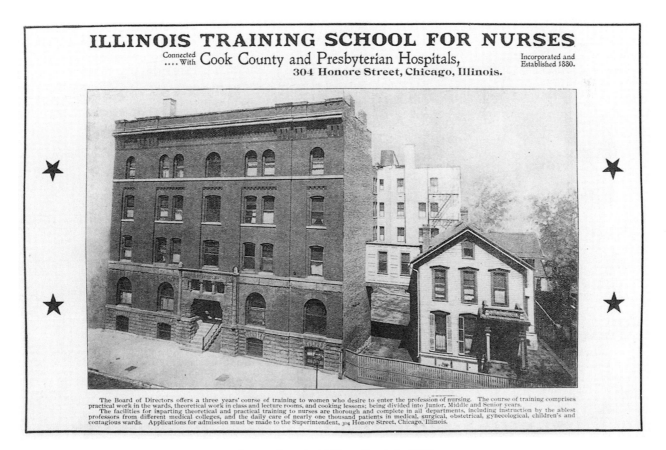

ILLINOIS TRAINING SCHOOL FOR NURSES

Connected ....With Cook County and Presbyterian Hospitals,
304 Honore Street, Chicago, Illinois.

Incorporated and Established 1880.

The Board of Directors offers a three years' course of training to women who desire to enter the profession of nursing. The course of training comprises practical work in the wards, theoretical work in class and lecture rooms, and cooking lessons; being divided into Junior, Middle and Senior years.
The facilities for imparting theoretical and practical training to nurses are thorough and complete in all departments, including instruction by the ablest professors from different medical colleges, and the daily care of nearly one thousand patients in medical, surgical, obstetrical, gynecological, children's and contagious wards. Applications for admission must be made to the Superintendent, 304 Honore Street, Chicago, Illinois.

The Illinois Training School for Nurses attracted approximately 1000 applicants in 1905.

Sanitarium Training-School for Nurses.

Regular Terms Begin Nov. 1. Students Received at Any Time.

This School has now been in operation for five years, with constantly increasing patronage and success.

Course of Instruction:

The course of instruction comprises two series of lectures, recitations and practical instruction, continuing through two years.

Methods of Instruction:

The instruction is both theoretical and practical. Several lectures and recitations are given each week. Each student is required to become familiar with the subjects taught, by actual practice. The following are among the leading topics taught: *Anatomy; Physiology; Elementary Chemistry. Nature and Causes of Disease; Language of Disease. Principles of Cure; Management of Common Diseases; Dressing of Simple Wounds and Injuries; General and Individual Hygiene. Ventilation, Disinfection; Air and Water Contamination; General Nursing. Surgical Nursing; Monthly Nursing; Bandaging, Hydrotherapy — theoretical and practical; Application of Electricity — Faradic, Galvanic, Static, and the care and management of batteries; Diet for the Sick; Massage, Swedish Movements; Calisthenics; What to Do in Emergencies.*

Qualifications:

The requirements for admission are good health, a good moral character, a fair education, and natural ability adapted to the profession. Students are not received under nineteen years of age, nor over forty.

Special Advantages:

The advantages offered by this school are in many respects superior to those offered by any other, not excepting the older schools in the large cities.

TERMS. — Students pay board and tuition in labor the first year; wages are paid the second year.

For Circulars giving full information, address, **SANITARIUM, Battle Creek, Mich.**

This school took in new students at any time.

however, the training of male nurses for general patient care became a possibility with the establishment of the Mills School of Nursing at Bellevue Hospital. A course comparable with that offered to the female students was developed, but this action was not widely emulated.

The first black nursing school graduate was Mary E. P. Mahoney. She attended the New England Hospital for Women and Children, completing her course of study in 16 months on August 1, 1879. The first separate school to educate black nurses was founded in 1886 at Spelman Seminary in Atlanta, and two other similar institutions—Hampton Institute in Virginia and Providence Hospital in Chicago—opened their doors in 1891. Tuskegee Institute in Alabama started a school of nursing in 1892. As the 20th century

approached, the number of black students enrolled in schools of nursing—primarily in separate schools, but also in integrated ones—slowly increased.

STRICT DISCIPLINE

During the Middle Ages, nursing had been a function of religious orders, and the monastic ideals of asceticism, self-abnegation, and obedience to authority had survived as ideals deemed appropriate to nursing. In addition, a military influence on nursing education was evident because the first hospital training schools had been built on the English model, which had closely followed Florence Nightingale's reorganization of the army medical service in the Crimea.

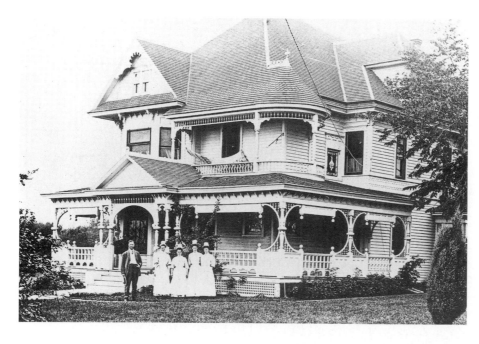

Hospitals with as few as 10 to 20 beds also established nurse training schools.

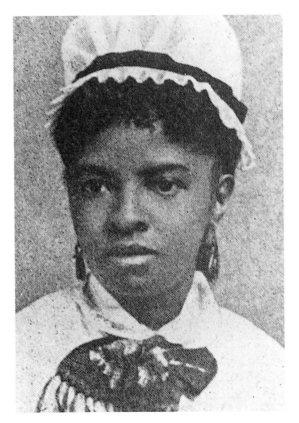

Mary E. P. Mahoney, first black graduate nurse.

Monastic and military traditions heavily influenced not only the actual workings of the schools of nursing but also the public's conception of them. The nurse in training was expected to yield to her superiors obedience characteristic of a good soldier and actions governed by the dedication to duty derived from religious devotion. Hospital administrators shared these expectations. A leading hospital administration manual of the era warned: "Most of the women who enter the training school are only half-made women. They are but half-bridled in their moral and mental as well as their physical makeup."[5] The superintendents of the training schools took it as their duty to mold the young women along proper lines; to teach them good morals, truthfulness, conscientiousness, devotion to duty, and unselfishness; and to teach them to think less of themselves and of their pleasures and comforts and more of the happiness and comfort of others.

Any nurse probationer who in her early days showed a tendency to shirk distasteful tasks was declared unfit. Perhaps the most difficult problem came when a young woman, who had proved promising and worthwhile during her probation and had been subsequently advanced, unexpectedly developed undesirable qualities. She might have grumbled at extra-duty assignments or she might have regarded some rules as having been made to be broken, or perhaps she had developed a too-familiar attitude while dealing with men or her records were untrustworthy or she could not get along "sweetly" in all places she was assigned to or she talked too much and openly criticized the physicians and head nurses. After having ignored a word of warning, such a borderline student would quickly be dismissed as a "troublemaker."

That strict discipline for student nurses was the order of the day was evidenced by one of the major questions at an early hospital association meeting: "Who has a successful method of disciplining pupils?" The participants had found it generally most

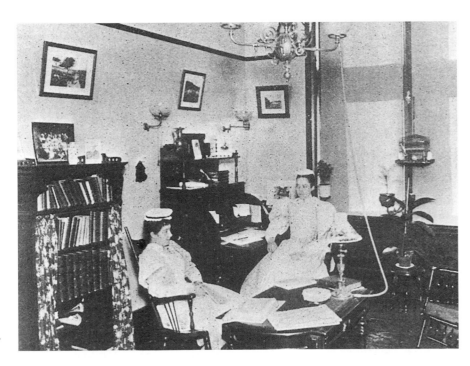

Superintendent of nurses' quarters, 1895.

RULES FOR NURSES IN TRAINING

I.
Application for admission to the school must be made to the Resident Physician of the Hospital. The Physician shall select intelligent women only, who can read and write, of good character and habits, for which testimonial is required. Applicants must be between 21 and 45 years of age.

II.
A record shall be kept by the Resident Physician of the names of nurse-students; their time of entering and leaving the school; their standing as graduates; and, when practicable, of their engagements as nurses, with name and address of physicians under whom they are employed.

III.
Nurses shall be under training twelve months, one month of which is probationary. They must sign a written agreement to remain under instruction for one year.

IV.
Their duties shall not only be within the Hospital, but they shall serve in the out-clinic as the Resident Physician may require. The last six months of their training shall be spent in the ward assigned by the Philadelphia Hopsital to the Woman's Hospital Training School.

V.
After the month of probation, for five months the instruction and a small compensation are considered a fair equivalent for their services. For the last six months of training they receive increased pay.

VI.
The right is reserved by the Resident Physician and Nurse Committee to discharge a student for misconduct or inefficiency.

VII.
The Resident Physician is empowered to invite any one or more of the graduated nurses to assist her in emergency, when the Hospital needs may require. But no nurse, upon leaving the Hospital shall be privileged to return for residence, except as invited by the Physician, nor to retain any right before accorded to her, except that of leaving her address and record of engagements.

VIII.
Nurses, while on duty, shall wear cotton dresses without crinoline and without trains, and soft shoes without heels. The dresses shall be changed at least once in two weeks. White aprons must be worn. The utmost simplicity is enjoined both in outer and under-clothing; as no ruffled, tucked, or flounced skirts, nor trimmed garments are allowed to be sent to the hospital laundry. The number of garments shall not exceed eighteen per week.

IX.
Nurses in training are instructed to change the bed-linen in the medical wards twice weekly; in surgical cases every two days, unless directions to the contrary are given. In the lying-in wards, bed-linen and clothing to be changed daily. Each confinement patient shall be washed three times daily, unless special directions are given. No sponges allowed to be used in the lying-in wards. The babies shall be washed after the morning visit, their mouths carefully washed after each nursing.

X.
The temperature of each patient must be measured, and the pulse and respiration counted and carefully noted twice daily.

XI.
The nurses shall see that each ward is thoroughly ventilated; the temperature shall be maintained at 65° Fahrenheit, unless special directions to the contrary are given.

XII.
Soiled clothing shall be removed immediately from the wards. Bed-pans, syringes, &c., to be carefully washed and disinfected after use.

XIII.
Exact information with respect to the appearance, amount and frequency of discharges is expected of the nurse.

XIV.
Each nurse is required to be present at the morning visit in her ward. In the evening visit she will accompany the Physician through all the wards and receive bed-side instruction.

XV.
No nurse shall leave her ward at any time without providing a substitute upon whom any patient therein or the attending Physician may call.

XVI.
Each nurse is required to serve on night-duty one week in every six. During this time the day is entirely at her disposal for rest and recreation.

XVII.
The night-nurse shall see that the wards be kept perfectly quiet between 9 P. M. and 6 A. M.

XVIII.
Medicines in each ward are to be administered by the nurse, and kept in a locked closet of which she holds the keys.

XIX.
Nurses shall roll the bandages to be used in their wards.

XX.
All unnecessary exposure of a patient is to be avoided in washing and dressing.

XXI.
The temperature and duration of a bath will be ordered by the physician. Mean duration of a general bath, five minutes; of a hip bath, twenty minutes. No bath to be given within two hours of a meal.

XXII.
Nurses are required to be present at the nurse-lectures, unless detailed for special duty at the time.

XXIII.
Each nurse shall serve the prescribed length of time in the diet-kitchen, where she shall prepare all gruels, beef-teas, eggnogs, etc.

XXIV.
The nurses shall see that visitors bring no food to the patients.

XXV.
The nurse shall not permit a lying-in woman to sit up in bed, or leave her bed, without the full sanction of the physician.

XXVI.
A strict watch of the patient and her every symptom shall be kept by the nurse and reported to the resident physican. A written record in special cases is required.

XXVII.
Gentleness and kindness to all patients is strictly enjoined upon the nurses. No personal remarks or criticism will be permitted, no forebodings expressed, nor comparison with other cases.

XXVIII.
Nurses shall in no instance be permitted to receive money from the patients.

Rules for student nurses at Women's Hospital Training School, Philadelphia, 1881.

satisfactory to give erring student nurses extra hours of duty and maintained that discipline in the nursing school either made or broke a student's character. The superintendent of nurses decided whether a troublesome student was incorrigible or incapable of nursing. Those who went through the full nursing school course were expected to emerge from the experience with strong characters, disciplined wills, and a capacity for self-sacrifice.

Other authoritarian characteristics prevailed. The dining room had separate tables for head nurses, seniors, juniors, and probationers. A student who entered a hospital was expected to readily accept that she would have no time for social activities and that she would be able to visit her friends at home only once or twice a year. Even then, it was recommended that friends allow her to rest when she was visiting them.

These rigid rules of conduct were difficult for young ladies of the era to tolerate. One student secretly complained:

> Rules are necessary, of course, but surely we are subject to rather many. I have hitherto submitted meekly to every rule, but there are times when they chafe. Of late I have sometimes found myself longing to yield to the voice of an inward tempter that bids me defy red tape and regulations when it can be done without interfering with my duty to the patients. There are so many rules, such battalions of regulations, such miles and miles of red tape that to me seem totally unnecessary—the existence of some of them is a positive insult to the manners and discretion of the nurses. The idea of it being made compulsory for us to ask the lady superintendent's permission every time we want to go out on the street, even though we are off duty. It isn't as if we were very young girls.

> When a girl is fitted for a hospital nurse she is fitted to regulate her own conduct without the aid of a thousand rules. I think that when the rules of this training school were framed it was surely done upon the principle of making life as trying as it possibly could be made for the nurses. I fancy that the board must have sat down and made out a list of everything it seemed likely that young women would care to do for innocent pleasure and then passed a sweeping motion to the effect that they weren't to be allowed to do any of them.[6]

Schools tolerated no student misconduct. They generally excluded married and older women because, as one superintendent put it, "We see so few women past 30 who begin the career of a trained nurse, and who fall in with the life successfully, that we are constrained almost to take the broad ground that women over 30 are unfit for admission to a training school." She added that "of course it goes without saying that married women—divorced or separated from their husbands, with perhaps divorce in the background—are not proper probationers for a training school." Such women were "self-centered; their interests are elsewhere; in their own minds at least they have been abused, and they are unable to devote themselves to others to the exclusion of their personal affairs."[7]

The systematic hospital socialization of student nurses may best be understood as a concern with authority and self-control. Supervised by a trusted "director of nurses" and surrounded by a tight wall of security, the school intended to raise a plentiful supply of women nurses—respectful, obedient, cheerful, submissive, hard-working, loyal, passive, and religious. As workers on massive hospital wards, student nurses buried the Victorian stereotype of the woman-as-lady under a mountain of reality. Indeed it was

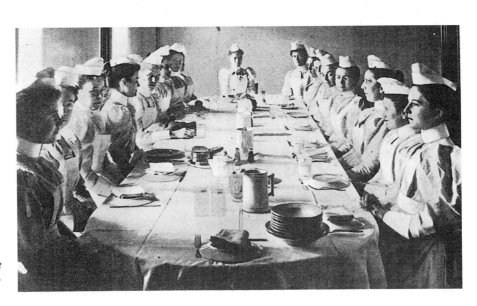

Dinner at eight: student nurses at the Jefferson Medical College Hospital, Philadelphia, 1898.

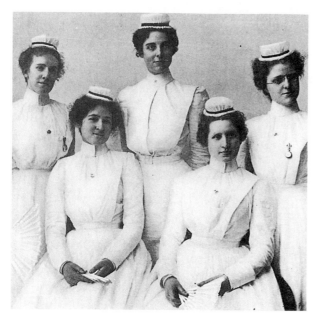

Total dedication to nursing was a requirement.

difficult to argue that young women as a sex must be weak, timid, incompetent, fragile vessels of spirituality when thousands of them were exposed daily to a ritual of long hours, disease, death, human misery, and suffering.

THE FLORENCE NIGHTINGALE PLEDGE

Early in 1893, Lystra E. Gretter, superintendent of nursing at the Farrand Training School for Nurses at Harper Hospital in Detroit, became convinced that the fledgling nursing profession needed a code of ethics to guide the graduates in their work. Amid the trappings of surrounding Victorian America, Gretter led a small committee of nurses to compose the "Florence Nightingale Pledge." A document with marked similarities to the Hippocratic oath and reflecting the idealism of the era, the pledge was first administered to the graduating class of Farrand Training School on April 25, 1893, as follows:

> I solemnly pledge myself before God, and in the presence of this assembly: to pass my life in purity and to practice my profession faithfully. I will abstain from whatever is deleterious and mischievous, and will not take or knowingly administer any harmful drug. I will do all in my power to maintain and elevate the standard of my profession and will hold in confidence all personal matters committed to my keeping and all family affairs coming to my knowledge in the practice of my calling. With loyalty will I endeavor to aid the physician in his work and devote myself to the welfare of those committed to my care.[8]

TEACHERS AND TEXTBOOKS

Who taught the students? Records of the early schools reveal that in the 1880s and 1890s physicians imparted nursing theory, whereas the superintendent and her assistants taught nursing practice. A few of the physician lecturers had some knowledge of educational methods, but most of them merely repeated to tired students notes that they themselves had taken in medical school classes. Sometimes even this poor formal instruction had to be modified when the pressure of ward work kept either the students or the teachers away and the class had to be canceled.

Lack of teaching materials and textbooks also posed a serious problem (Table 5-1). The leading schools developed their own instructional manuals of nursing arts, such as the *Hand-Book of Nursing for Family and General Use*, written by a committee of physicians and nurses connected with the Connecticut Training School at the New Haven Hospital and published by Lippincott in 1878. The committee thought it important to give a summary of hospital nursing directions to each student nurse as well as to any graduate nurse who might be hired from another school. Written simply to be easily understood, it was comprehensive enough to provide aid in the ordinary duties of the nurse.

The New Haven manual was soon introduced for textbook use in other training schools. During the next 2 years, similar nursing manuals were published elsewhere. In 1885, Clark Weeks Shaw wrote *A Textbook of Nursing for the Use of Training Schools, Families and Private Students*. The title reveals that the level of presentation and content were designed for use by both nurses and the general public. The first substantial nursing care text, Isabel Hampton's *Nursing: Its Principles and Practice for Hospital and Private Use*, appeared in 1893 and was widely used in schools for the next 20 years.

The first anatomy book for nurses was written in 1893 by Diana Kimber of the Charity Hospital School for Nurses in New York. Lavinia Dock, an 1886 Bellevue Hospital graduate, wrote *The Textbook on Materia Medica for Nurses* in 1890. Five different journals for nurses were published before 1901. The first, the *Nightingale*, appeared in 1886 and was edited by a Bellevue graduate who was also a female physician. It died from lack of support in 1891. A second periodical, the *Trained Nurse and Hospital Review*, began business in August 1888 and continued to appear monthly for more than 70 years. Two other journals, the *Nursing Record* and the *Nursing World*, appeared for several years during the Gay Nineties before folding. In 1899, under the leadership of Mary E. P. Davis, a stock company was formed with about 550 cash subscriptions, and a new journal, the *American Journal of Nursing*, managed entirely by nurses, made its debut in October 1900 and continues to the present.

TABLE 5-1	Results of a Survey of Hospital Superintendents Associated With Five Major Schools of Nursing in 1883				
CHARACTERISTICS	NEW YORK TRAINING SCHOOL AT BELLEVUE HOSPITAL	CONNECTICUT TRAINING SCHOOL AT NEW HAVEN STATE HOSPITAL	TRAINING SCHOOL AT MASSACHUSETTS GENERAL HOSPITAL	TRAINING SCHOOL OF THE NEW YORK HOSPITAL	BOSTON CITY HOSPITAL TRAINING SCHOOL
Year organized	1873	1873	1873	1877	1878
Admission requirements	Aged 25–35, sound health, good moral character, and a knowledge of arithmetic, reading, penmanship, and English dictation	Aged 22–40, good health and character, and common school education	Aged 25–35, preferred, must be in sound health, and must present on application a certificate from some responsible person as to their good character	Aged 25–35, sound health, perfect senses, good moral character, and good common school education	Aged 21–35, preferred, good health and character
Salary paid pupils	$9 a month for the 1st year, $15 a month for the 2nd year	$170 for the term of 18 months (average of $9.44 a month)	$10 a month for the 1st year, $14 a month for the 2nd year	$10, $13, $16 a month for the 1st, 2nd, and 3rd 6 months, respectively; graduates, $25 a month	$10 a month for the 1st year, $14 a month for the 2nd year; graduate head nurses, $20–$30 a month
Text books used (by number)*	1, 4, and 7	4 and 6	2 and 3	4, 6, 7, and 8	3, 5, 7, 10 and 11
No. of nurses excluding superintendent	50	22	53	36	61
Average no. of patients	260	112	170	140	286
Average patients assigned per nurse	5	5	3	4	5
Does hospital bear all expenses of school?	Salaries and washing partly	Board, lodging, and washing	Board, lodging and washing, and part salaries	Entire	Entire expense
Yearly average of training school salaries paid by hospital	$6,722.00		$8,527.33	$5,700.00	$8,820.00
Does the superintendent of the hospital think the training school valuable to the hospital?	"Certainly I do."	"I do."	"No Hospital of any size is complete without one."	"In all its developments and departments good and always good."	"Yes"
Does he know of any as a good and cheaper plan?	"No."	"Not that I know of."	"Any other system inferior in every respect."	"No."	"The cheapest and best."
Course length	1 year	18 months	2 years	18 months	2 years

Source: W.B. Platt, "Table of Statistics of Several Training Schools for Nurses," *Medical News,* vol. 47 (June, 1885):444. *(1) Bartholow, Robert. *A Practical Treatise on Material Medica Therapeutics.* New York: D. Appleton, 1876; (2) Cutter, Calvin. *Second Book on Analytic Anatomy, Physiology and Hygiene.* Philadelphia: Lippincott, 1875; (3) Domville, Edward J. *A Manual for Hospital Nurses and Others Engaged in Attending on the Sick.* London: J & A Churchill, 1872; (4) Draper, John W. *Human Physiology.* New York: Harper, 1870; (5) Lees, Florence. *Handbook for Hospital Sisters* (ed. by H. W. Acland). London: W. Isbister & Co., 1874; (6) New Haven State Hospital, Connecticut Training School for Nurses. *Hand-Book of Nursing for Family and General Use.* Philadelphia: Lippincott, 1878; (7) New York Training School for Nurses Attached to Bellevue Hospital. *Manual of Nursing.* New York: The Hospital, 1878; (8) Nightingale, Florence. *Notes on Nursing: What It Is and What It Is Not.* New York: Appleton, 1860; (9) Smith, William R. *Lectures on Nursing.* London: J & A Churchill, 1875; (10) Williams, Rachel, and Alice Fisher. *Hints for Hospital Nurses.* Edinburgh: Maclachlan and Stewart, 1877; (11) Woolsey, Abby H. *Handbook for Hospital Visitors.* New York: G. P. Putnam's Sons, 1877.

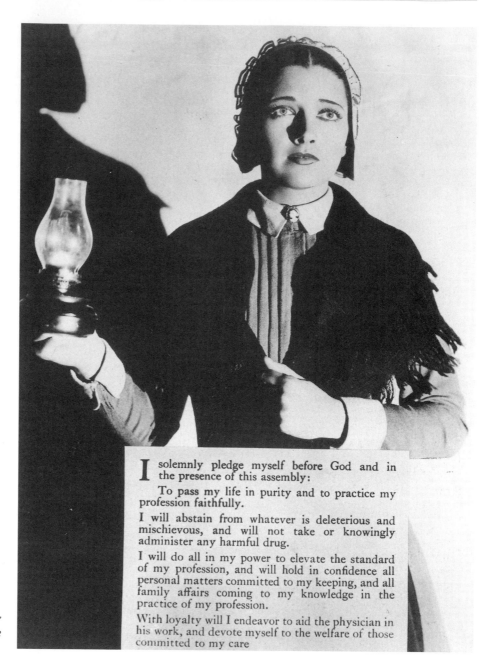

I solemnly pledge myself before God and in the presence of this assembly:

To pass my life in purity and to practice my profession faithfully.

I will abstain from whatever is deleterious and mischievous, and will not take or knowingly administer any harmful drug.

I will do all in my power to elevate the standard of my profession, and will hold in confidence all personal matters committed to my keeping, and all family affairs coming to my knowledge in the practice of my profession.

With loyalty will I endeavor to aid the physician in his work, and devote myself to the welfare of those committed to my care

"The Florence Nightingale Pledge" reflected the ethical ideals of the Victorian era.

THEORY PORTION OF NURSE TRAINING

Although the theory portion of nurse training had been expanded somewhat since the late 1870s, when it had constituted less than 1% of the entire time spent in school, in the 1890s it still accounted for only about 2% of the total required hours. The other 98% to 99% was devoted to practice. Curricula of early days contained some anatomy and physiology, materia medica, and lectures on "special diseases."

In 1884–1885, at one of the better institutions of the time, the Farrand Training School for Nurses at Harper Hospital in Detroit, the students had two annual series of lectures, which constituted the total theory content of the 24-month course. The distribu-

tion and time devoted to the various subjects included anatomy (4 hours), physiology (4 hours), surgical emergencies (4 hours), medical emergencies (4 hours), dietetics (2 hours), and hygiene (2 hours). All lectures, including those on nursing, were given by physicians from 8:00 p.m. to 9:00 p.m. between October and March. For the remainder of the year, students provided service without the benefit of formal classes.

Final examination questions at Evansville Sanitarium Training School in Evansville, Indiana, for the class of 1899 reveal the state of nursing theory of that time (Box 5-1).[9]

Let us look at the work of an outstanding student in one of the schools of nursing with a large

---

| BOX 5-1 | FINAL EXAMINATION QUESTIONS |

SURGERY

How would you prepare for a celiotomy or a laparotomy at a patient's house?

How would you prepare for adjustment of a fracture of the forearm, and what would you do before the doctor came if he were long delayed? What is a simple fracture? A compound fracture? A comminuted fracture? A multiple fracture?

What means can you give for stopping hemorrhage?

What instruments should be prepared by curettage with repair of laceration of cervix and perineum?

What are the following operations: Ventral fixation? Alexander's operation? Vaginal puncture? Colpoperineoplasty? Colectomy? Hysterectomy? Paracentesis? Cholecystectomy? Nephrectomy? Gastroenterotomy?

MEDICINE

What is the temperature and pulse range in an average case of typhoid fever? What is a high temperature in this fever?

What is a relapse?

OBSTETRICS

If you were alone with a woman when she gives birth to a child, what would you do?

What does fever following delivery indicate?

What is puerperal eclampsia? What would you do for a case of it before the doctor came?

With what would you feed the baby until the milk appeared? When does the milk appear? Is its advent accompanied by fever?

Give the stages of labor.

What is Crede's method?

PHYSIOLOGY AND HYGIENE

Give the difference between excretion and secretion.

Give systemic circulation; pulmonary circulation.

How would you ventilate a sickroom which had only one window and one door? What is natural ventilation? What is ventilation by extraction? Name three important rules in regard to ventilation.

How would you take care of the flush closets, stationary basins, and old dressings?

Give a thirty-line treatise on digestion.

ANATOMY

How many vertebrae are there? Name the divisions.

Name the bones of the head; of the face; of the leg.

Give the divisions of the alimentary canal. Of the region of the chest. Locate the heart, the liver, the spleen, and the kidneys.

Name five arteries; five nerves.

What kind of nerves are the fifth and seventh cranial nerves?

BACTERIOLOGY

Name five pyogenic germs which cause disease. How are they killed? What are the requirements for their growth?

What is asepsis? What is antisepsis?

MATERIA MEDICA AND THERAPEUTICS

What is the dose of sulphate of atropia? Of sulfate of strychnia? Of hyoscine hydrobromate?

What would you do for a patient who had taken an overdose of opium, or morphine?

What are poisons generally? What is a special antidote for carbolic acid poisoning?

In strychnine mixture with grs. II to 3VI of water, how much strychnine will be given to 3I dose?

How much morphia would you give to a child two years old? Four years old? Seven years old? How much strychnine sulphate to a child three years old? Eight years old? Twelve years old? Give the standard rule by which the dose for children is reduced.

CHEMISTRY

Give the meaning in reaction of urine, or acid, alkaline, and neutral. Give test for albumin and sugar and the normal specific gravity of urine.

How would you obtain a specimen of urine for examination? How is it often contaminated?

Write about one hundred words of general urinalysis.

How do you make saturated solution of boric acid? Normal salt solution? Ten percent solution of nitrate of silver? How do you make bichloride solution 1-2000, 1-5000, 1-10,000?

Credit: U.S. Commissioner of Education, "Final Examination Questions of the Evansville Sanitarium Training School of Nurses," Annual Report of the U.S. Commissioner of Education for 1903 (Washington, DC: Government Printing Office, 1904), pp. 2231—2233.

---

component of theory. In November 1890, *Trained Nurse* announced the offer of "a prize of $10 cash for an essay upon the following subject: Give full particulars, with Notes, as to Temperature, Dietary, etc., of a Typhoid Fever Case, nursed by the Competitor herself, and describing, if possible, the Case from its commencement to its termination. Temperature and Diet-Charts, etc., should accompany Essay, if possible." Ambitious nurses eager to test their writing ability and knowledge of clinical nursing flooded the journal's office with material. The winner was Mary Adelaide Nutting, a student at Johns Hopkins School of Nursing. Her "Notes of a Typhoid Fever Case" appeared in the March 1891

issue and documented the expert bedside observations she had made.

In her record of the initial day of nursing care, Nutting noted:

> In order to follow satisfactorily the development of this case, it will be necessary to have some definite idea of the patient's surroundings and conditions previous to admission to the Hospital.
>
> The case had been reported to the Superintendent of the Hospital on December 18th, 1890, and a member of the staff was promptly sent out to investigate. In a locality amidst surroundings which were wretched in the

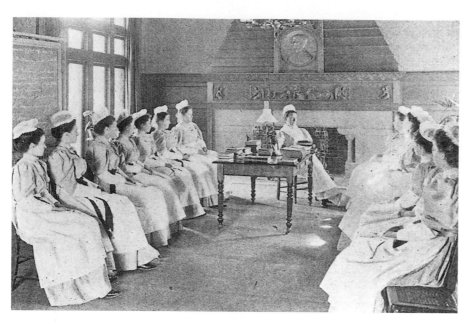

Class in session at the Henry W. Bishop Memorial Training School for Nurses, Pittsfield, MA, 1895.

extreme, and in quarters where poverty and filth held undisputed sway, this is what he found. On a sofa in the corner of a small room which was almost destitute of furniture, yet evidently served for kitchen, bedroom and living-room generally, the patient, a young man about twenty-one years of age, was discovered, lying in his clothes.

The room was already occupied by a woman and three small children, and the stench which pervaded the atmosphere was sickening to a degree, almost unendurable. The distress of abject poverty and accumulations of filth were visible everywhere. It was quite impossible to obtain accurate information concerning the first days and date of the patient's illness, but, from what could be gathered, it was now the

beginning of the fourth week. For this length of time the poor creature had been lying in his clothes and was now in a state of neglect which beggars description. The first point to attract the attention was his mouth, in which not only the tongue but the lips and teeth and even the roof of the mouth were so covered with a thick, dry, dark, almost black crust that their original form and color were almost entirely lost. The cheeks and nose had a very peculiar dusky flush, and between the partially closed eyelids, the white of the eye only was visible. He was in a state of low muttering delirium and displayed a marked subsultus. His abdomen was found to be greatly distended, tense and tympantic, and it was discovered that involuntary movements of the

NURSING:
ITS PRINCIPLES AND PRACTICE.

By ISABEL ADAMS HAMPTON,

Graduate of the New York Training School for Nurses attached to Bellevue Hospital; Superintendent of Nurses and Principal of the Training School for Nurses, Johns Hopkins Hospital, Baltimore, Md.; Late Superintendent of Nurses, Illinois Training School for Nurses, Chicago, Ill.

In one very handsome 12mo. volume of 484 pages, profusely illustrated.

Price, Cloth, $2.00 net.

This entirely new work on the important subject of nursing is at once comprehensive and systematic. It is written in a clear, accurate, and readable style, suitable alike to the student and the lay reader. Such a work has long been a desiderata with those intrusted with the management of hospitals and the instruction of nurses in training schools. It is also of especial value to the graduated nurse who desires to acquire a practical working knowledge of the care of the sick and the hygiene of the sick-room.

The first substantial nursing-care textbook.

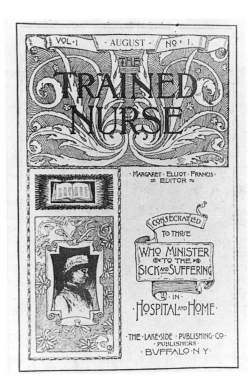

The first important nursing journal.

THE AMERICAN JOURNAL OF NURSING

PUBLISHED MONTHLY BY
J. B. LIPPINCOTT COMPANY
624 CHESTNUT STREET,   PHILADELPHIA, PENNA.
FOR THE
ASSOCIATED ALUMNAE OF TRAINED NURSES OF THE UNITED STATES

SUBSCRIPTION PRICE, $2.00 A YEAR   SINGLE COPY, 20 CENTS

The oldest active professional nursing journal.

COURSE OF LECTURES 1884-5.

FARRAND TRAINING SCHOOL FOR NURSES.

ANATOMY,	Oct. 29, Nov. 12, Nov. 26, Dec. 10.
	DR. CARRIER.
PHYSIOLOGY,	Nov. 1, Nov. 14, Nov. 28, Dec. 12.
	DR. GILBERT.
SURGICAL EMERGENCIES,	November 15, November 19.
	DR. BOOK.
SURGICAL EMERGENCIES,	December 3, December 17.
	DR. WALKER.
MEDICAL EMERGENCIES,	November 17, November 20.
	DR. ANDREWS.
MEDICAL EMERGENCIES,	December 6, December 20.
	DR. CLELAND.
DIETETICS,	December 24, January 7.
	DR. FLINTERMANN.
HYGIENE,	December 27, January 10.
	DR. RUSSEL.
OBSTETRIC NURSING,	December 31, January 14.
	DR. DAVENDORF.
OBSTETRIC NURSING,	January 28, February. 28.
	DR. ANDREWS.
SICK ROOM NURSING,	January 3, January 17.
	DR. SHURLEY.
SICK ROOM NURSING.	January 31, February 14.
	DR. LYSTER.
GYNÆOCOLOGICAL NURSING,	January 21, February 4.
	DR. CARSTENS.
GYNÆOCOLOGICAL NURSING,	February 18, March 4.
	DR. LONGYEAR.
SURGICAL SICK ROOM NURSING,	January 24, February 7.
	DR. McGRAW.
SURGICAL SICK ROOM NURSING,	February 21, March 7.
	DR. MACLEAN.
NURSING CHILDREN,	March 14, January 21.
	DR. DOUGLASS.
NURSING CHILDREN,	March 18, February 25.
	DR. CLELAND.
EYE AND EAR,	February 25, March 11.
	DR. CONNOR.
NERVOUS DISEASES,	March 25, March 28.
	DR. EMERSON.

LECTURES FROM 8 TO 9 P. M.

Course of lectures for the 1884–1885 session at the Farrand Training School for Nurses, Detroit.

bowels had been going on for some days, with the passage, also involuntary, of large quantities of urine. His pulse was irregular, intermittent and compressible, the respiration rapid and feeble, and it was questionable if he could live to reach the hospital. By exercise, however, of the very greatest care, they succeeded in removing him, and he was brought to the ward on the evening of December 18th at nine o'clock.

After admission his temperature was 102.5°, pulse 108, and very dicrotic, and respiration 42. An hour later the temperature rose to 103.6° and he was then given a tub bath, 70°F. of fifteen minutes duration, which brought it down to 98.6°. It was quite evident, however, that the temperature was not the great difficulty to overcome; the grave trouble lay in the extreme weakness of the heart, in which there was almost no impulse, the heart sounds indistinct, and the pulse thready and fluttering. Free stimulation

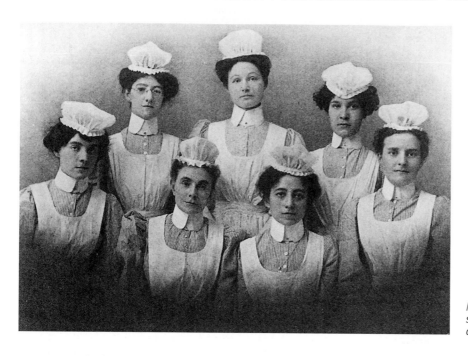

Nursing students formed close relationships while enduring rigorous work demands.

was at once resorted to, brandy being administered in half ounce doses every two hours, and for a further cardiac stimulus was given 01. Terebinth M.*v* every three hours, for three doses. At 4 A.M. his temperature rose to 103.8° and he was given a second bath bringing it down to 99.8°; at this time his respiration had become 44, shallow and quivering, his pulse 124, still compressible and intermittent, and the cheeks showed a steadily deepening purplish flush. The lips and tongue were so dry, and the scabs so adherent, that it was with difficulty they

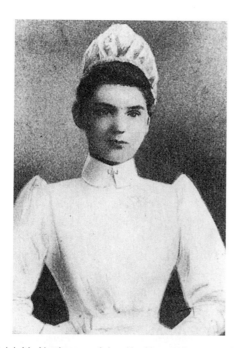

Mary Adelaide Nutting as a Johns Hopkins student nurse in 1891.

could be removed, and then only with forceps and after repeated softening applications of glycerine and Boracic Acid Solution. With the utmost care that could be used they would bleed with every small portion that was removed and it was thought advisable to do only a very little at a time and vaseline was applied liberally after each attack.

Owing to his extreme weakness and prostration no attempt was made to give him the thorough cleansing bath he needed, but he was merely sponged off with tepid water, softened with Aromatic Spirits of Ammonia. At this point, 10 A.M., the application of Turpentine stupes to the abdomen was begun, applying them just as hot as could be borne, and changing every fifteen minutes when possible. For nourishment he had albumen, the whites of two eggs, every two hours, well beated, strained, diluted with cold water one-third, flavored a little with about two drachms of whisky and served with crushed ice. This he took easily, and never seemed to grow tired of. At 10 A.M. he was ordered Tr. Digitalis M.*xv* to be given every three hours, but this was discontinued after five doses (*M.lxxv*) had been given. At 10:39 the temperature had risen to 104.4°, and the bath which was given reduced it to 98°, and him to a condition which looked very much like collapse, for in addition to the subsultus, there was much tremor, coldness and blueness of the extremities, continuing for more than an hour, a feeble and fluttering pulse, a rapid and shallow respiration. He was able, however, to take both stimulant and nourishment very well, and drank water whenever it was brought him, most eagerly, this was generally done every hour, at regular intervals between nourishments. At 3 P.M. a bath was again due, the temperature being 103.6°, pulse 132, respiration 32, and the result was a reduction of temperature to 101.6°, pulse 132, respiration 44. At 10 P.M. it had risen again to 104, pulse 140, respiration 40, and was reduced to 98.2°, pulse 130, respiration 36, by a bath of seventeen minutes duration at 70°F. His condition after this was very much as described before, only with each feature more marked, and on this occasion, it was fully an hour and a half before the tremor ceased to be visible, while the pulse was extremely thready and fluttering, ranging from 132 to 140 and dropping a beat frequently. Later he became somnolent and remained in that state during the rest of the night. Although his temperature was 102.8°, above bathing point (which had been fixed at 102.5°), and remained there without moving for six hours, no baths were given, but he was roused every hour for stimulant and nourishment which came alternately, and the fomentations were steadily kept up. On the morning of the second day the tympanites was if anything increased, and as there had been about nineteen movements within twenty-four hours, it will be seen that the diarrhoea was not materially diminished. The movements were of course still involuntary as was also the passage of a really enormous quantity of urine. Later in the morning at 10 A.M. the baths were started once more, and the temperature from 102.8° was brought down to 99°, the effect after being that of the previous day. It was at this period that the pulmonary trouble began to be apparent, and dullness was noted at the left base, the exact cause of which was doubtful. A hypodermic puncture was made for diagnostic purposes, and a small syringe full of bloody pus was withdrawn. Aspiration was decided upon for the following day, and the diagnosis of pneumonia was made. Here I may say that upon aspirating the next day much to the surprise of everybody no fluid was found.[10]

PHYSICIANS ATTACK THEORY FOR NURSES

From the beginning, physicians vigorously debated the proper mix of theory and practice in the education of the nurse. According to an 1875 paper by Dr. Samuel Howard, a professor of the theory and practice of medicine in Montreal, the new profession of nursing should require

> a liberal preliminary education at least equal to that now required of the medical student, assigning, however, a first place to natural

science and a lower one to the classics. And, second, a professional education extending over three full years, and embracing the following scheme of subjects: anatomy, physiology, chemistry, materia medica, pharmacy, dietetics, hygiene, and clinical instruction in nursing the sick and wounded, in dressing wounds, and applying splints, etc., for which education they would, of course, receive pay as medical students do.[11]

Howard thought that nurses trained along these lines should receive a diploma, after an extensive examination, entitling them to practice nursing among the general public and to charge fees in rates proportionate to physicians. Such nurses would then not only be the helpmates of physicians but would also complement the work of the entire medical profession.

Such liberal ideas, however, were generally unwelcome. An opposing view voiced in a leading international medical journal warned of the dangers that would follow if such a course were to be pursued:

> The principal argument in favour of the medical education of nurses is the necessity for their knowing the reason why in reference to all the details of management and treatment which fall under their cognisance. . . . To attempt to give nurses instruction as to the reason why . . . would be, in the majority of instances, to inflict a heavy task upon them and to lift them more or less out of their proper sphere, possibly at the risk of withdrawing them from due attention to their less intellectual but equally useful functions. To give them more than an insight into it is to demand for them complete education as medical practitioners and to transform them from nurses into doctors—a consummation assuredly not to be desired. . . . There are fashions in opinion as well as in dress, and there are enthusiasts in practical as well as in theoretical matters; and it is from time to time needful to show the folly or distortions of fashion and to put the curb upon such enthusiasm.[12]

Twenty-five years later, the opinion of most physicians had not changed. During the early 1900s a Boston surgeon lecturing to a class of nurses surprised them by saying that, if he had to choose, he would prefer a nurse who knew a few ways of dressing hair to one well grounded in anatomy and physiology. Physicians repeatedly attacked attempts to increase the theoretical portion of nurse training. One claimed that if asked to state the function of the trained nurse, he would answer as follows: first, to care for the bodily needs of the patient; second, to carry out the orders of the physician; and, third, to record

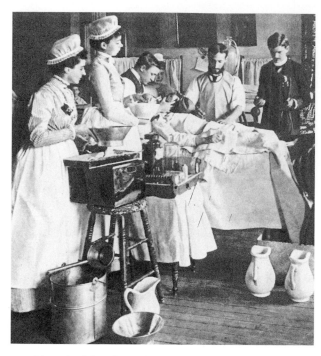

Most physicians favored practice-based nurse training.

the "vital phenomena" of the patient. The entire scope of nursing practice should fall under one of these headings.

Yet in many proposed nurse training courses, alarmed physicians discovered such topics as mineral food and mineral waters; the amount of salt found in the body and its necessity in food; food value in heat, energy, and tissue building; and the uses of calcium, sodium, phosphorus, magnesium, iron, sulfur, and potassium in the body. Dismayed physicians saw that, under the heading of practical work, nursing students received laboratory instruction in pipe analysis where they applied the flame test for sodium, potassium, calcium, and strontium. Another lesson focused on sucrose, glucose, levulose, and lactose, comparing sources, preparations, composition, properties, and digestion. The pages of course outlines in such innovative curricula revealed lessons in chemistry and physiology that, according to some physicians of the day, had absolutely nothing to do with nursing the sick.

Physicians quickly pointed out that if such "foolishness" continued, society would have a nurse with knowledge that would not be of the slightest use to her patient; at least 2 years of her time would have been wasted in the acquisition of theory that had no bearing on her work. Why should the nurse, they fumed, be taught urinalysis or the use of the microscope? Such objections as these kept the theory portion of nurse training at a rudimentary level, and some curricula embraced less controversial content, such as how to make cranberry jelly, bake apples, and prepare peanut brittle.

The *Medical Record* of February 29, 1896, carried an article, "The Monstrous Regiment of Nurses," complaining of

> a tendency of the trained nurse to interfere excessively in the conduct of medical and surgical cases. They hint . . . that doctors' prescriptions and treatment might be a little amended. They make suggestions of their own as to diagnosis and prognosis. They elevate themselves in a measure to the order of the medical practitioner himself. Their smattering of knowledge of anatomy and physiology leads them to suggest to their patients diseases which never could, by any possibility, have entered the heads of the patients themselves. To a person with a stomach ache they talk "peritonitis" and "appendicitis," and to a person with eczema they talk about "lupus" and "scleroderma."[13]

The *Western Medical Journal* in March 1900 commented:

> These ladies claim that the medical and nursing professions are entirely distinct, and that a doctor cannot possibly understand nurses or nursing. This proposition is so absurd that it is difficult to realize how an intelligent woman can believe it.
> It is physicians who lecture in the training schools, and one of the cardinal principles of nursing ethics is, that the nurse must always be subordinate to the doctor, the nursing being part of his treatment. She is trained to be his (or her) assistant—an instrument to an end, and is employed for the purpose of carrying out the doctor's orders. In private practice or in hospital practice, no nurse could succeed who worked on the principle that nursing was a separate profession which should be quite independent of medical direction.[14]

Physicians also interfered with the distribution of experience. If assisted by a student whose work he liked, a physician frequently used his influence to keep her on his service far beyond the stipulated length of time.

Soon after schools of nursing came into being, some began to send students out as special private-duty nurses and confiscated the money that the students earned. This development sprang from the premise that training in a hospital did not automatically qualify a nurse to work in the home—the major kind of employment available after graduation. Thus, to overcome this deficiency, hospitals sent their students into the community to nurse in homes, supposedly under school supervision. A lucrative system of exploitation resulted. A student might be kept on and on with a chronic or convalescent patient for reasons

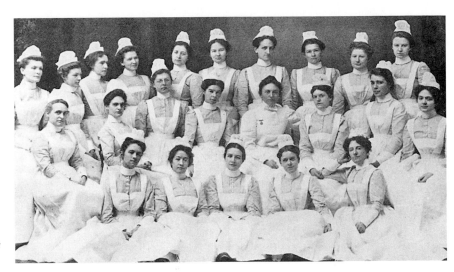

Medicine debated the independence of the nursing profession in 1900.

such as "The patient doesn't want to give her up," "The family can't pay a graduate," or, more openly, "The hospital wants the money" long after any teaching value remained in the experience. Even in shorter cases, supervision often proved inadequate, with the patient left to the care of a partially trained student, who in the meantime missed the theory background and more balanced clinical experience she needed and deserved.

Even in the early 1900s, the complaints that nurses were overtrained continued. For example, a meeting of the Academy of Medicine in New York City on the evening of March 29, 1906, assembled an audience of physicians and nurses for a symposium on the training of nurses. With one exception, the speakers voiced the opinion that nurses of the day were overtrained, with too much theory and too little practice. Some of the public seemed to agree with the physicians on the matter. Indeed, an editorial that appeared in the *New York Evening Sun* of March 3, 1906, maintained:

> Nurses nowadays are instructed in a great variety of topics, and it is a question whether the smattering of knowledge they acquire is not often more mischievous than useful. Some of them are too apt to think that their position entitles them to censure the work of the doctor and to carry out his orders or not as they see fit. Thus we have known of one who persuaded her patient that his surgeon was incompetent in having failed to remove some catgut sutures from a wound at the proper time; another, in a public hospital, who ignored the house physician's prescription of a narcotic in the case of a boy on the ground that "it was a shame to expose him to the danger of acquiring a drug habit." What we want in nurses is less theory and more practice. The place of the nurse is an honorable one, and every candid physician is glad to acknowledge

> that the successful issue in many cases, such as pneumonia and so on, depends at least as much on her services as on his. But to stuff her head with scraps of knowledge about a number of subjects which do not concern her duties at all would surely be foolish. A thoroughly trained nurse is indispensable. An overtrained and "learned" nurse is apt to be a nuisance.[15]

Dr. W. Gilman Thompson made similar charges in a paper entitled "The Overtrained Nurse" in the April 28, 1908, issue of the *New York Medical Journal.* The editor noted that this paper "was read with huge enjoyment by physicians generally," as Thompson lashed out in measured prose:

> Nursing is not, strictly speaking, a profession. A profession implies professed attainments in special knowledge as distinguished from mere skill; nursing is an honorable calling, nothing further, implying proficiency in certain more or less mechanical duties; it is not primarily designed to contribute to the sum of human knowledge or the advancement of science. The great and principal duty of a nurse is to make a patient comfortable in bed, something not always attained by the most bookish of nurses. Any intelligent, not necessarily educated woman can in a short time acquire the skill to carry out with implicit obedience the physician's directions.[16]

THE PRACTICE COMPONENT

The better schools of nursing attempted to give varied experience on all hospital nursing services, but if the hospital's need for personnel on a certain unit was acute, students would be assigned there regardless of their educational needs.

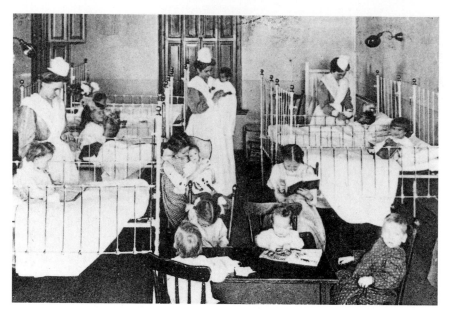

The better schools attempted to provide a balanced program of clinical experience.

Income derived from this practice was supposed to go into the training school budget, but hospitals were supporting the schools, and the money for nursing service inevitably found its way into the hospital coffers. This encouraged several unethical 10- and 20-bed hospitals to recruit students from kitchens and restaurants, pay them $5 to $10 a month, and then, as soon as the students put on uniforms, send them on special cases—for which the hospital received at least $21 per week. Physician stockholders of such proprietary hospitals might profit greatly by encouraging such practices. Progressive nurses of the day saw clearly that nurse training schools could be exploited as important subsidiaries to dividend-paying businesses.

Even at better schools, "specialing" was common. At the Illinois Training School for Nurses in Chicago, the students brought in more than $2000 annually from such work. The school proudly mentioned this amount as income in its annual reports and occasionally expressed regret that the press of work at the hospital had prevented more students from being available to answer the many calls for private-duty assignments.

A PROBATIONER'S LIFE

Much of the work required of the probationer was decidedly not nursing. Instead of being taught to care for the sick intelligently, in many hospitals the probationer was made to do the work of a chambermaid or scullion. She dusted, scrubbed, and washed dishes. Training for probationers of the 1890s usually meant working 14 hours a day, 7 days a week. It meant each student being under continuous surveillance, with the superintendent at her heels, ready to pounce on her for the slightest mistake.

One can visualize the rigorous probationary period by hypothesizing the case of Miss X in 1895. The hospital Miss X entered required a probationary period of 6 weeks. She felt glad that her own probation would be no longer than 42 days. She often wondered if the school really meant to keep her as she scrubbed floors, cleaned windows, polished furniture, cleaned out patients' rooms and wards, and scoured tubs and copper cookers used in rheumatic cases. Probationers in her hospital, called "probies" for short, spent most of their time cleaning. "Well, if

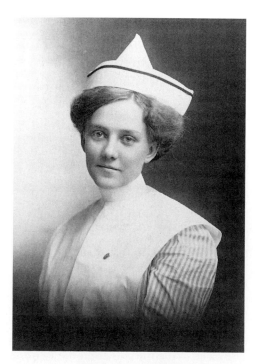

Miss X, class of 1895.

I'd ever had any idea that being a trained nurse was like this!" she moaned to a fellow student one day as they polished the "coppers." While she did not finish the sentence, it could easily be filled in: If she had known, she would have stayed home.

Several women who entered with Miss X did drop out during the 6 weeks. The school characterized them as the type who had been attracted to nursing only for romantic reasons. They had pictured themselves in glossy white linen stooping to soothe the brow of a sick (but handsome) young man. Now they found themselves in blue chambray, bent over a kitchen floor, where sentiment could not even nudge them.

Miss X's experience reflected not only her own school. The attrition rate among students was astonishingly high. For example, the Farrand Training School at Harper Hospital in Detroit received about 100 applications in response to advertisements for admission to the January 1884 class and selected 16 of these applicants as probationers. Of this number, the school soon rejected 12 probationers as not meeting the required standard of clinical performance, advanced a mere 4 students to the status of "pupil nurse," and eventually graduated the same 4, for an attrition rate of 75%.

After the probationary period, the work of the students continued to be strenuous. Nursing demanded muscle and endurance. A student could generally count on being on her feet the whole time she spent on the wards, which contributed to the prevalence of the complaint known among student nurses as flat feet. In hospitals, a law of etiquette held that the nurse should never sit down while on the ward, even if she had the opportunity.

The intensity of the work varied greatly in different hospitals and depended much on whether they were situated in busy urban centers or in quiet towns. In big-city general hospitals, where patients were seriously ill and required much attention, student nurses were more effectively used, and the greater part of the manual labor in the ward might be performed by ward maids and orderlies. In smaller rural hospitals or infirmaries, where the patients had mostly chronic illnesses, the proportion of students to patients was low, and all the time not spent giving nursing care was filled with scrubbing, sewing, washing bandages, and even cleaning windows. Thus the work of the nurse seemed to adjust itself to the circumstances at hand and essentially comprised whatever needed to be done.

LONG HOURS AND 7-DAY WORK WEEKS

Extremely long hours of service for student nurses continued to be the accepted pattern, with no improvement in this regard over the earlier practices in schools of nursing during the 1870s. In most hospitals, the students on day duty arose at 5:30 a.m. to the sound of a loud bell, then dressed, made their beds, and cooked breakfast for themselves. At 6:45 a.m., another bell sent the students scurrying to the parlor to join their fellow nurses in a hymn, a Bible reading, and a prayer. They arrived on the wards at 7:00 a.m. and worked until 8:00 or 9:00 p.m. with about 75 minutes off for meals. In the large general city hospitals, students typically had 2 hours off duty between sleep and work each day. Lectures for the students were held between 8:00 and 9:00 p.m. or

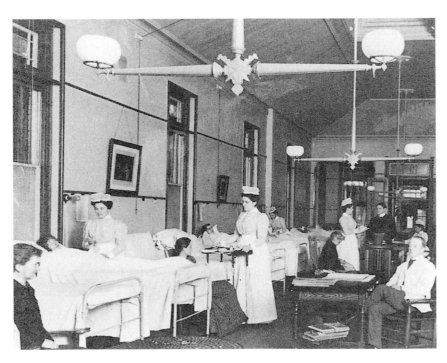

Manual labor around the hospital awaited students at the completion of nursing tasks.

later. Compulsory attendance at evening prayers often deprived students of an extra hour's rest in bed. Night duty hours were even longer, and most hospitals required a night duty of 12 hours per day, 7 days a week, for a total of 84 hours.

A brief study made in 1895 of the hours of work at 111 schools throughout the country showed that in about two thirds of these training schools, students were on duty for 10 hours or more daily. The hours of night duty were found to be 12 hours in 70% of the schools, and in the remaining hospitals they exceeded that number and ranged from 13 to 13.5 hours. In no instance were the night duty hours found to be less than 12 hours daily. This first study of the working hours of students concluded that the hours were universally excessive and that such requirements were injurious to students' health and to the welfare of the patients and the hospital.

A young woman who worked 10 to 12 hours a day was in no mental condition to profit by class instruction offered during the evenings. A common schedule of required hours per week in the 1890s follows:

Monday	9 hr work, 1 hr class
Tuesday	10 hr work, 1 hr class
Wednesday	5 hr day duty, 5 hr night duty
Thursday	12 hr night duty
Friday	11 hr night duty, 1 hr class
Saturday	7 hr night duty, 5 hr private duty ("specialing")
Sunday	15 hr private duty in two shifts
Total	82 hr

In 1896, a bill introduced into the Massachusetts state legislature aimed to limit the working hours of student nurses in private or public hospitals to 12 hours out of 24 and to supply them with sleeping apartments separate from those of the patients. Nurse administrators strongly opposed the bill. Maria P. Brown, superintendent of the Boston Training School for Nurses, attached to the Massachusetts General Hospital, said it was impossible to regulate the work and daily lives of student nurses by such arbitrary laws, and only those who were familiar with the needs, variations, and emergencies of the work could realize how impractical such rules would be. She claimed that a hospital was not like a workshop, which could have definite hours of work as a part of its operation. In the student nurse's life, she insisted, every day brought new demands, in that each patient constituted an individual requirement that called for some new and extra effort on the part of the nurse.

The rules governing the nurses at the Massachusetts General Hospital resembled those at other institutions, Brown explained. Although to the superficial observer the hours seemed wearisome, they were, she pointed out, arranged with tact and consideration for the nurses' welfare. The day nurses were on duty 13 hours, minus 1 hour for relaxation and mealtime. They also found relief in turning from one kind of work to another—from the classroom to the ward and back to the lecture room. Students had an afternoon off every week and a part of every Sunday.

Of course, as Brown noted, emergency calls were likely at any time, which might prolong the ordinary hours. A day nurse might be called on to do extra night duty in the case of a bad accident or other emergency, but the superintendent usually tried to select a nurse who had been given the afternoon off that day or a nurse especially strong and well fitted to bear the extra strain.

Although such extra calls came many times within some weeks, at other times they did not occur for long periods. When they did come, however, they had to be met, and it was thought that no regulations should hamper the hospital in carrying out its responsibilities to the patients. Brown acknowledged that some smaller schools might need a degree of restraint in their practices, but, in her view, any state law would prove more of a hindrance than a help to nurses in their work. The main thing, she pointed out, was to have efficient graduate nurses in command of the schools and then to entrust to their judgment and discretion the direction and control of the students. The superintendent's rules would generally be found more efficient and practical than a direct and definite law passed by the legislature.

Despite such objections to outside regulation, the long hours in schools of nursing were clearly out of step with the times. Federal statistics show that the average hours per work week in all industrial establishments averaged 58.4 in 1890, 58.1 in 1895, 57.3 in 1900, and 55.7 in 1905. To expect 70 to 90 hours of work from a student nurse for a period of 2 or 3 years approached a form of slavery.

EXCESSIVE ILLNESS AMONG STUDENTS

It quickly became apparent that illness among student nurses greatly exceeded illness among other young working women. A nurse of 8 years' standing declared, "Doctor, there must be something wrong in the system which takes young women who are sound and healthy at the commencement of their training and graduates them three years later mostly wrecks." One student nurse poignantly testified:

> I certainly cannot stand this much longer. I fainted last night for the first time in my life. Miss Gray said I must have eaten something that didn't agree with me and seemed to feel very much injured by my thoughtless action. She was greatly relieved when she found that I soon recovered sufficiently to continue my duty. I could stand the loss of sleep at night all right if I did not have to work so extremely hard. I think it a shame to have so few nurses on duty at night, when the work is the most trying. It oughtn't to

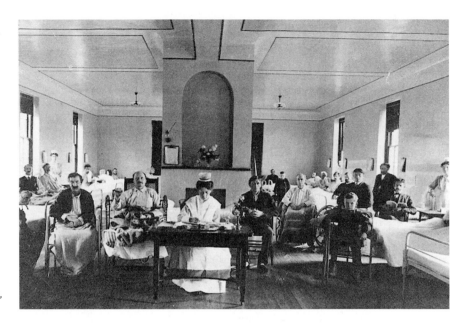

Students staffed most hospital wards, including the head nurse role.

be necessary to break down one's health in order to become a graduate nurse, but that is what it amounts to.[17]

One investigator succeeded in obtaining from seven of the large hospitals of New York City data concerning the number of days of illness that kept student nurses from duty. His findings, ranging from slightly less than 2 days to nearly 22 days, were as follows:

Hospital A—Average number of patients, 173; number of nurses in training school, 41, being a little over 4 patients per nurse. Each nurse in this hospital average 19/10 days' illness of sufficient severity to keep her in her room. This was the best record of any of the seven hospitals.

Hospital B—Average number of patients, 178; student nurses, 99, being not quite 2 patients for a nurse. In this hospital, the average illness per annum per nurse, 41/3 days.

Hospital C—Average number of patients, 110; student nurses, 51, a little over 2 patients for a nurse; average illness per annum per nurse, 6 days.

Hospital D—Average number of patients, 189; student nurses, 47; patients per nurse, 4; average illness per annum per nurse, 11 days.

Hospital E—Average number of patients, 130; student nurses, 56; average patients per nurse, 2 1/3; average illness, 117/8 days per annum per nurse.

Hospital F—Average number of patients, 268; student nurses, 22; average patients per nurse, 12.5; average illness per annum per nurse, 21 days. In this training school, more than 50 percent of the nurses were afflicted with flat and painful feet, and there was a high incidence of acute digestive disturbances (50 cases of 2 to 3 attacks each).

Hospital G—Average number of patients, 105; student nurses, 28; average patients per nurse, 33/4; average illness per annum per nurse, 117/8 days.[18]

It is illuminating to apply to other lines of work the system that had become characteristic of nurse training. One might speculate on the outcome of the growing stenographic field if every business or industry needing 10 or more stenographers had said, "We will have a stenographic school; we will have the president's secretary do the teaching (that will cost us nothing); the vice-president's and treasurer's secretaries will help (also without expense to us); we will keep our pupils 3 years and after the first 6 months expect them to work 7 days a week, including some nights; we will give them room, board, and laundry; at the end of 3 years we will have a little celebration, perhaps in a church, and give each one a cheap gold pin; we will then take in a new group of students to do our work; we will recommend our graduates to people who need stenographers; of course, we will have no need to employ our own graduates, unless we can't get enough student stenographers."

AN ADDED YEAR OF HARD LABOR

Although the course of nurse training up to the early 1890s generally lasted 2 years, it soon expanded to 3 years. Ten or more hours a day in addition to class work and study might be endured for a period of 2 years, but the same hours extended to 3 years placed an even more serious strain on the student's physical resources. Isabel Hampton, superintendent of the Johns Hopkins Training School for Nurses, repeatedly pointed out the dangers of adopting the 3-year course requirement unless shorter hours came with it. She insisted that superintendents of nurses should maintain their 2-year courses unless they were prepared to limit practice to 8 hours a day. In an 1895 paper on this subject, Hampton warned:

> I am sure that many of you have had some qualms of conscience at the way in which we are sometimes forced, I might almost say, to drive our pupil nurses through a two years' course. I assure you that I have had myself many anxious moments for the future of certain of my pupils as regards their health. It is well known that a combination of physical and mental labor is more exhausting than simple manual or simple mental occupation. It is true that for a time such a strain can be borne without producing any permanent injurious effects, and it is possible in most cases for women to stand the strain imposed upon them for two years, although I am afraid that not all of them come out of the trial unscathed. If, however, this high pressure is to be kept up for three years, I am sure that the health of the nurses will suffer. A woman who works physically over eight hours a day is in no mental condition to profit to any extent by class instruction or lectures. I maintain, therefore, that the three years' course must not be considered at all unless the hours of practical work are shortened, but if the two changes can be made together, then the preservation of the health of the nurse and the extension of her education and training will be insured. This again will result in an increase in her competency and consequently will be productive of greater benefits to the patients who come under her care during her training, and after she has graduated.[19]

FOUNDING OF THE FIRST NURSES' ASSOCIATIONS

The advance of the United States as a nation achieved vivid dramatization in a great spectacle, the World's Fair and Columbian Exposition, held in Chicago from May to October 1893 to celebrate the 400th anniversary of Columbus' arrival in the New World. The outstanding American architects, painters, and sculptors of the time joined in fashioning the gleaming and ornate "White City" that rose from the bogs and dunes along Lake Michigan. By the time the exposition closed its gates, it had attracted more than 27 million visitors. Planned as a miniature of the ideal metropolis, the World's Fair boasted fine macadam roads, an excellent sanitation

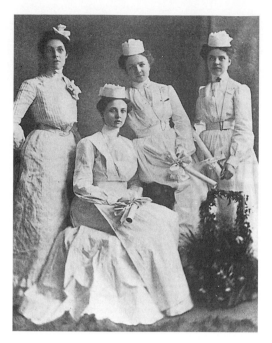

Graduating class of the City Hospital, Memphis, 1902.

and water supply, underground telephone and telegraph wires, and ample hospital facilities. Its great dynamo showed that electricity was destined to displace steam as the prime mover of modern industrial civilization. The Chicago World's Fair symbolized a new stage in the development of an urban industrial society. It also marked the coming of age of nursing as a profession.

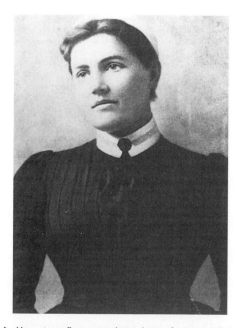

Isabel A. Hampton, first superintendent of nurses of the Johns Hopkins Training School for Nurses.

The exposition grounds provided the meeting place for various congresses and conferences, including, among many others, an international congress of charities, correction, and philanthropy, with a section devoted to hospital care of the sick, to the training of nurses, to dispensary work, and to first aid to the injured as well as a subsection on nursing. The chairman of this subsection was Isabel Hampton.

The nurses' meetings were held in the Hall of Columbus from June 15 to June 17, 1893. Attended by nurses from throughout the United States and Canada, the event marked the first time that nurses had met as a united body. Isabel Hampton read a paper, "Educational Standards for Nurses." Florence Nightingale, although not present, sent an address that was delivered before a large crowd. She wrote, in part: "Nursing proper can be taught only by the patient's bedside and in the sick room or ward. Neither can it be taught by books, though these are valuable accessories if used as such; otherwise what is in the book stays in the book."

"What is training?" she asked. "Training is to teach the nurse to help the patient to live. Nursing the sick is an art, and an art requiring an organized, practical, and scientific training, for nursing is the skilled servant of medicine, surgery and hygiene." Nightingale observed that a good nurse of 20 years before had not had to do one twentieth of the work required by her physician or surgeon in 1893. The physician prescribed "for supplying the vital force, but the nurse supplies it," she concluded.

Lavinia L. Dock spoke on the relation of training schools to hospitals. She said that the training school idea did not originate within the hospital but had been grafted to it by the efforts of a few inspired women outside, who had seen the terrible needs of the sick, who knew the inadequacy of the care they received, and who bravely knocked at the hospital doors.[20]

This meeting saw the birth of the first national nursing organization, the American Society of Superintendents of Training Schools of Nursing. This body had as its objectives "(1) to promote fellowship of members, (2) to establish and maintain a universal standard of training, (3) to further the best interests of the nursing profession." Forty-four superintendents attended the first official meeting of the new society in January 1894.

The need remained for a national association of trained nurses. Isabel Hampton noted that the first alumnae association of nurses in the United States had been formed in 1889 by the graduates of the Bellevue Hospital Training School and that the next had been formed in 1890 at the Illinois Training School. By 1893, there were 21 such associations or clubs organized and in active operation and 10 in process of organization, all with the objective of advancing the interests of trained nurses and their role in society.

Three years later, in 1896, Hampton's dream of one great official organization of trained nurses became a reality at the third annual meeting of the American Society of Superintendents of Training Schools. A committee prepared a constitution and bylaws for the proposed national organization and met with delegates from various alumnae associations to establish this association. The following year, the constitution and bylaws prepared by the group were accepted, and the national nursing body completed its organization as the Nurses' Associated Alumnae of the United States and Canada.

Yet another group, the American Hospital Association (AHA)—an international charitable and educational association of hospitals and hospital people—was organized first as the Association of Hospital Superintendents in 1899 with a membership of nine people. Its purpose was to "establish and maintain high standards of hospital service, to promote the efficient care of the sick, and to assist through its membership in the control and prevention of disease." Many nurses holding positions as hospital administrators played passive roles in the earlier years of the AHA, and this passivity cast a negative influence over nurse training standards.[21]

The 1880s and 1890s saw schools of nursing established by the hundreds in all parts of the nation as the financial advantages of the training system were fully exploited. This was a corollary to the rapid proliferation of general hospitals, and the two movements developed hand in hand. The initial skirmishes fought between physicians and nurses over the amount of theory instruction that students should be exposed to provided a prelude to a long-standing controversy. Giving focus to such matters, the professional nursing and hospital associations organized and began to exert influence on the direction of nursing education and practice.

REFERENCES

1. "Statistics of Hospitals in the United States, 1872–73. Derived from Replies to Inquiries by the U.S. Bureau of Education," *Transactions of the American Medical Association*, vol. 14 (1873):314–333.
2. U.S. Commissioner of Education, *Report of the U.S. Commissioner of Education for 1902* (Washington, DC: Government Printing Office, 1903), pp. 2043–2061.
3. "Night Duty," *Trained Nurse and Hospital Review*, vol. 41 (October 1908):239–240.
4. U.S. Commissioner of Education, *Annual Report of the U.S. Commissioner of Education for 1906* (Washington, DC: Government Printing Office, 1907), p. 177.
5. A. J. Ochsner and M. J. Sturm, *The Organization, Construction, and Management of Hospitals* (Chicago: Cleveland Press, 1907), pp. 92–95.
6. "The Journal of a Pupil Nurse," *Trained Nurse and Hospital Review*, vol. 40 (May 1908):314.
7. "Training Schools," *Transactions of the American Hospital Association*, vol. 13 (October 1911):397–399.
8. Agnes G. Deans and Anne L. Austin, *The History of the Farrand*

Training School for Nurses (Detroit: Alumnae Association of the Farrand Training School for Nurses, 1936), p. 58.

9. U.S. Commissioner of Education, "Final Examination Questions of the Evansville Sanitarium Training School for Nurses," *Annual Report of the U.S. Commissioner of Education for 1903* (Washington, DC: Government Printing Office, 1904), pp. 2231–2233.

10. M. Adelaide Nutting, "Notes of a Typhoid Fever Case," *Trained Nurse*, vol. 6 (March 1891):121.

11. Samuel Howard, *The New Profession of Nursing* (Montreal: Privately printed, 1875), p. 3.

12. "Nurses and Nursing," *British and Foreign Medico-Chirurgical Review*, vol. 57 (April 1876):283–301.

13. "The Monstrous Regiment of Nurses," *Medical Record*, vol. 48 (February 29, 1896):3.

14. "The Trained Nurse and the Doctor," *Western Medical Journal*, vol. 12 (March 1900):110.

15. *New York Evening Sun*, March 3, 1906.

16. W. Gilman Thompson, "The Over-Trained Nurse," *New York Medical Journal*, vol. 83 (April 28, 1906):845–849.

17. Ibid., vol. 40 (May 1908):311–314.

18. A. T. Bristow, "Is the Present System of Training Fair to the Pupil Nurse?" *American Journal of Nursing*, vol. 7 (March 1907):447–455.

19. Isabel A. Hampton, "Three Years Course of Training in Connection with the Eight-hour System," *Transactions of the American Society of Superintendents of Training Schools for Nurses*, vol. 2 (1895):36.

20. J. S. Billings and H. M. Hurd, eds., "Hospitals, Dispensaries, and Nursing," *International Congress of Charities, Correction, and Philanthropy, Sec. III* (Baltimore: Johns Hopkins Press, 1894), pp. 86–98.

21. American Hospital Association, "Constitution and By-laws," *Transactions of the American Hospital Association*, vol. 25 (October–November 1923):605–606.

6

GASLIGHT AND SHADOW

The Practice of Nursing at the Turn of the Century

No large laboring or wage-earning class had developed in the United States before the Civil War. Although growing industries and other economic activities employed increasing millions of people, most of the population was occupied in agriculture: As late as 1860, about 60% of the gainfully employed were farmers. But the rise of large-scale industry and big business between 1870 and 1900 added millions of wage earners to the labor force.

One of the most important developments of the post–Civil War era was the rapid growth of cities. So swift was the transition that within a single generation the United States changed from a predominantly rural nation to one that was predominantly urban. In 1860, communities with populations of 2500 or more accounted for less than 21% of the total population; by 1900 this figure had grown to 39.9%.

Increasing urbanism facilitated the rapid growth of hospitals after the Civil War. Towns and cities sprouted up all across the United States. Cities, with their concentrated populations, new wealth, and numerous poor, offered a magnificent challenge to churches, religious orders, and enterprising physicians to found general hospitals. These groups looked for the sure thing, for opportunities to minimize costs and maximize services. Hospital administrators who could keep the books in the black and transfer a healthy surplus to the building fund became important and powerful figures.

WOMEN IN THE LABOR FORCE

The movement for increased rights for women was part of the Industrial Revolution and its consequent process of urbanization, and women advanced on various fronts during the 1880s and 1890s. A basic factor was the rapid increase in the number of jobs for women, amounting to a form of female emancipation. Even the conservative South dropped its severe restrictions on remarriage after divorce. In 1882, New

York courts allowed married women greater rights of property ownership and declared that wives could sue their husbands for damages incurred as the result of brutality. Gradually, most of the states conceded to wives their rights to own and to control their personal property, to retain their earnings, to sue, and to make contracts.

More employment alternatives for women opened up in the urban-industrialized society of the late 19th century. Many career-minded ladies of the middle class still believed that elementary school teaching represented the chief form of employment for women, however. Philo Remington had started to mass-manufacture the typewriter, an invention that would open a new form of livelihood for women, and new jobs emerged for women as clerks and salespeople in the department stores and other merchandising establishments that had come into existence since the Civil War. Uneducated working women had been accepted long before into the first factories born of the Industrial Revolution, but now, for the first time, middle-class women in large numbers were moving from the home to industry and business. The number of female breadwinners rose from 2,500,000 in 1880 to 4,500,000 in 1890.

OPPORTUNITIES FOR GRADUATE NURSES

Nursing did not fare well compared with many other lines of work that were opening up for women. After graduation from a school of nursing, a nurse had two main career options: she could work in a home as a private-duty nurse or in a hospital as a superintendent or head nurse. Opportunities for hospital work were few for trained nurses. Even at the very best schools, few if any graduates were retained each year to fill the limited number of vacancies that occurred in the relatively permanent staffs of head nurses; as the size of the classes

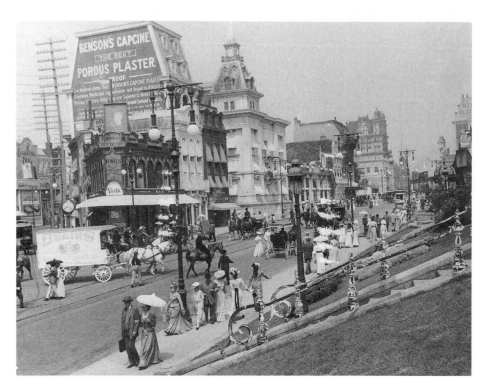

Cities grew rapidly in the post–Civil War era.

grew, the head nurse positions usually went to students rather than graduate nurses. At the Massachusetts General Hospital, the first class graduated in 1875 with only three nurses. The second class had 11 graduates; the third class, 5; the fourth class, 20; and the fifth class, 6. The Boston City Hospital Training School had a similar history, graduating its first class in 1880 and averaging 18 graduates annually until 1887.

It is interesting to note what had become of the 300 graduates from these two schools by 1887:[1,2]

Remaining in the parent hospital	24
In other institutions	30
In district nursing	8
Total in institutional and public work	62
Private-duty nursing	170
Total continuing in nursing	232
Married	37
Died	10
Studied medicine	1
Unknown as to abode and occupation	20
Total out of nursing	68

At the same time, trained nurses were beginning to make inroads against the women and men working as nurses without the benefit of formal training, traditional until the advent and growth of nursing schools: Figures at the Registry for Nurses in Boston showed 245 graduate female nurses on the roll, as opposed to 408 nongraduate female nurses and 84 nongraduate male nurses. Untrained nurses, however, would still dominate nursing service for several more decades.

THE HOSPITAL ROUTE

As the schools produced more nurses, new graduates began to migrate to other sections of the country without nursing schools. Emily L. Loveridge, a graduate of Bellevue Training School for Nurses, went west in 1890 to establish the first school of nursing in the Northwest at the Good Samaritan Hospital in Portland, Oregon. Her reminiscences vividly portray the challenges of those early nursing pioneers:

> Coming to Oregon forty years ago to establish the first training school for nurses in the Northwest, I found myself one of three graduate nurses in a city of 70,000 people and entering a hospital of less than fifty beds. The Good Samaritan Hospital was a two-story frame building in those days, situated six blocks from the end of a street car line. The place looked small after the rambling buildings of Bellevue. I had plenty of courage but needed it. For six long months I was very homesick for the East.
>
> In addition to being superintendent of nurses, I was the floor nurse and operating room supervisor, and in my leisure moments did any necessary work—sewing, cleaning, painting, etc.—that was to be done. We all worked and no one grumbled, not even at the end of a perfect day of twelve to sixteen hours of labor, for there were no hours off, and sometimes no afternoons off, in our schedule.
>
> Our school of nursing, known at that time as the training school, started with five nurses,

ST. LUKE'S HOSPITAL

1420-1434 INDIANA AVENUE, CHICAGO, ILLS.

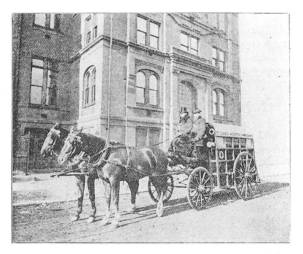

The Hospital is for the treatment of acute, curable, and non-contagious diseases. Sufferers from chronic or incurable diseases cannot be permanently provided for.

St. Luke's is centrally located and our private ambulance will meet patients at the train at any hour of the day or night. Special facilities for operative work. The Medical Board is made up of the most prominent practitioners of the city. We have a large number of private rooms from $12.00 to $30.00 per week. Address,

The **Good Samaritan Hospital**

Corner 6th and Lock Sts., Cincinnati, O.

Under the Efficient Management of the Sisters of Charity.

The private department comprises forty well ventilated, neat, attractive and comfortable rooms, a number being elegantly furnished and calculated to please the most fastidious; two operating rooms, large, well lighted, models of convenience and cleanliness, and up-to-date in every particular. The prestige, incidental to an existence of thirty years, together with the assiduous care and efficient nursing administered by the sisters, insures to its patrons the most proficient surgical and medical attendance.

The ward service is complete in every particular; the occupants receive a degree of privacy unknown in other institutions, the best of medical skill and the kindest nursing. The portals of the institution have ever been open to those afflicted and in need, irrespective of creed, condition or color, and during the years of its existence the accommodations have never been commensurate with the desire to care for the unfortunate.

Twice weekly, clinics are held by the most renowned talent the city possesses, in a commodious, well heated, well lighted amphitheatre, capable of seating two hundred and fifty people. Here patients, suffering with every variety of disease and injury, who are financially unable to engage the best medical attention are treated in the most scientific and effectual manner, and students of medicine are given an opportunity to see, examine and witness the treatment of all cases. For detailed information address

SISTER SEBASTIAN, SISTER SUPERIOR.

City hospitals at the turn of the century were becoming more substantial enterprises.

three of whom were on the hospital force at the time the school opened. All classes were held in the evenings.

Our first operating room had a double window at the end and single one at the side. Mrs. Wakeman conducted the first operation after my arrival, and my Bellevue training of even that period received a shock. She described an operation she witnessed in another hospital, where she was impressed with the convenient place used for the threaded surgical needles. They were stuck in the window shade! Our needles were run in a piece of bandage and boiled with the other instruments, or "carbolized."

The cold water used was boiled by the night nurse. Each kettle had to boil for fifteen minutes and was then emptied into a large covered granite can. The hot water was boiled in the diet kitchen and was carried in large porcelain pitchers covered with bichloride towels.

The field of operation was vigorously scrubbed and rinsed and washed in bichloride. We never felt that the patient's skin was properly cleansed until it was red from the scrubbing. After this the field was covered with towels soaked overnight in a 1/1000 bichloride solution and wrung as dry as possible. Every surgeon irrigated, using a rubber bag which had previously been sterilized by boiling. Not only the field of operation but all of the assistants at the operation were irrigated at the same time, and clothing and shoes had to be changed after a morning in the operating room.

At each operation one nurse was assigned as official brow wiper, for at that time the surgeons and assistants did not wear face masks. A few of the surgeons objected, preferring to let beads of perspiration fall when and where they would. One surgeon dropped his eye glasses into an abdominal cavity, but we irrigated more than usual and the wound healed by first intention.

Catgut was cut into yard lengths, wound on pieces of glass rods, put into glass jars, covered with alcohol, and boiled in water bath for four successive boilings at three day intervals. Preparing catgut was rather nervous work and there were several explosions during the time catgut was prepared in this manner.

When we bought our first operating gloves, only the surgeon operating wore them, then they were used by his assistant, and soon everyone used rubber gloves during an operation.

I recall the first abdominal operation performed. It took days to gather enough supplies and prepare them. . . . All went well during the operation until the ligature slipped from the pedicle and the patient died of internal hemorrhage. All of us were heartbroken.

Sunday was our busy day for operations. It was the only day that the doctors did not schedule for office hours—and there was no golf!

Our first ward beds had straw ticks, washed and refilled with straw during the interim between the discharge of one patient and the admission of another.

For ordinary heat we used stone jugs, bricks, and quart bottles, all in flannel covers. A few selected rubber bags were kept for abdominal application.

We had a diet kitchen in which each nurse in training served her allotted time. Here were made the softdiets, broths, etc. We sorted our milk in pans in the milk room. Some of these were skimmed for the cream and the thin milk was used for cooking.

In those days people frequently refused to come to the hospital—they were afraid of them—so the hospital went to the patient for operative work. All of the necessary paraphernalia was carried from the hospital. The kitchen table was frequently used as the operating table, and bedroom stands and marble top tables with the marble turned upside down were used for instrument and sponge tables. The operating room nurse usually went out a couple of hours previous to the operation and scrubbed everything. The tables were covered with bichloride towels and hot water was kept in pans and kettles on the stove. Occasionally members of the family helped. It was better to keep them occupied and away from interfering with our surgical supplies.[3]

Loveridge found that Good Samaritan Hospital's management could function with relative simplicity. The annual report for 1891–1892 contained the following statistics regarding the services rendered:

Patients under treatment, May 31, 1891	73
Admitted during the year 1891–1892	907
Total	980
Died in hospital, 65; discharged, 846	911
Remaining under treatment, June 1, 1892	69
Total	980
Of this number, 234 were free or charity patients and 746 were paying patients.	
Number of days of care given charity patients	4793
Number of days of care given paying patients	23,551
Total number of days of care	28,344

The report also included a classification of diseases treated, a note about the hospital's nurse training school, and a tabulation of patients according to religious belief.

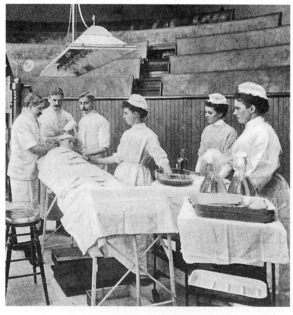

Hospital surgery in the late 1890s.

HOUSEKEEPING TASKS

The practice of nursing at the turn of the century included many housekeeping tasks. The nurse of this time had to maintain an appropriate sickroom environment—room temperature, humidity, and ventilation—as well as prepare, cook, and serve food to patients. Every ward had its own kitchen. Scrubbing, cleaning, polishing, controlling insects, oiling furniture, washing clothes, folding linen, making bandages and rollers, and other similar duties were in the domain of the nurse, who spent many, many hours on these lower level duties.

The following job description of a hospital nurse during the 1880s vividly underscores just how arduous, task-oriented, and regimented nursing was:

> In addition to caring for your 50 patients each bedside nurse will follow these regulations:
>
> Daily sweep and mop the floors of your ward, dust the patients' furniture and window sills.
>
> Maintain an even temperature in your ward by bringing in a scuttle of coal for the day's business.
>
> Light is important to observe the patient's condition. Therefore, each day fill the kerosene lamps, clean chimneys and trim wicks. Wash the windows once a week.
>
> The nurse's notes are important in aiding the physician's work. Make your pens carefully. You may whittle nibs to your individual taste.
>
> Each nurse on day duty will report to duty every day at 7 A.M. and leave at 8 P.M., except on the Sabbath, on which day you will be off from 12 noon to 2 P.M.
>
> Graduate nurses in good standing with the director of nurses will be given an evening off each week for courting purposes, or two evenings a week if they go to church regularly.
>
> Each nurse should lay aside from each pay day a goodly sum of her earnings for her benefits during her declining years so that she will not be a burden. For example, if you earn $30 a month you should set aside $15.
>
> Any nurse who smokes, uses liquor in any form, gets her hair done at a beauty shop, or frequents dance halls will give the director of nurses good reason to suspect her worth, intentions, and integrity.
>
> The nurse who performs her labors and serves her patients and doctors faithfully and without fault for a period of five years will be given an increase by the hospital administration of five cents a day, providing there are no hospital debts that are outstanding.[4]

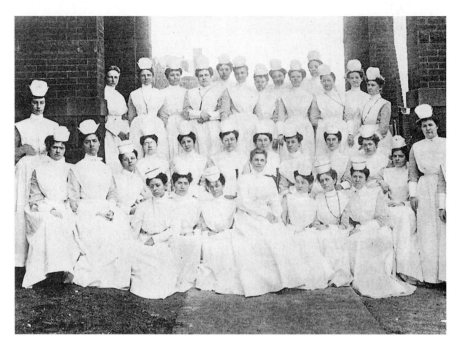

Nurses in good standing received an evening off each week, City Hospital, Cleveland, 1904.

In 1894, one nurse described the scrubbing duties in the ward lavatory as follows:

> The nurses scrub a board about 2½ ft. long and 2 ft. wide, which usually lies on the tub, and is called a poultice-board. . . . It is always kept spotlessly white, and instead of feeling it a humiliation, one soon learns to take pride—and a great deal of pride, too, let me tell you—in seeing how white one can keep it. . . . One of the first things a nurse learns is that she must leave everything thoroughly "aseptic." . . . You see, now, why it is that nurses do this part of the work instead of maids, who do not understand the importance of these things.[5]

NURSING CARE RESPONSIBILITIES

Besides these housekeeping tasks, the practice of nursing included making beds; giving baths; preventing and dressing bedsores; applying "friction to the body and extremities"; giving enemas; inserting catheters; bandaging; dressing blisters, burns, sores, and wounds; and observing secretions, expectorations, pulse, skin, appetite, body temperature, consciousness, respirations, sleep, condition of wounds, skin eruptions, elimination, and the effect of diet, stimulants, and medications. Administering medications and treatments as ordered by the physician was another major responsibility of the nurse.

The degree of autonomy that the nurse could exercise in completing these tasks varied. In the early 1870s at the Woman's Hospital in Philadelphia, the temperature and the duration of the bath were ordered by the physician primarily because baths constituted a means of therapy. The "half-bath," for example, given in a long tub filled with 6 inches of cold or temperate water so that it covered only the legs and thighs, treated selected cases of typhoid fever. One nurse, wetting her hands repeatedly with the bath water, rapidly rubbed the patient's shoulders, back, and chest while another nurse vigorously massaged the lower extremities and thighs. The patient splashed water on his or her own face. This procedure lasted 3 to 4 minutes and was repeated every 6 to 8 hours. Other types of baths included the hot-air bath, the sheet bath, the gelatin bath, the reducing or graduated bath, the vapor bath, the mud bath, the narcotic bath, the sand bath, the mustard bath, and the sea bath.

Catheterization of male patients by female nurses provoked considerable controversy in the late 1890s. The director of nurses at St. Luke's Hospital in New York, Mrs. L. W. Quintard, read a paper on the subject at the Superintendents' Convention in 1896. She expressed grave concern about the practice of using male orderlies to catheterize, bathe, and dress wounds or blisters in the pelvic region of male patients, because the men hired as orderlies in these hospitals tended to be careless and ignorant. Private-duty nurses had no one to delegate such care to, and because most nurses did private nursing at one time or another, she believed they should learn the procedure on "children and unconscious patients." Quintard's suggestions were liberal for the Victorian times:

> Is it wise to allow nurses to give a full massage or rubbing to male patients? When convalescence is once established such treatment should not be given by a male attendant. . . . In caring for the very sick we must, as far as possible, forget both sex and self. In their weakness men appeal

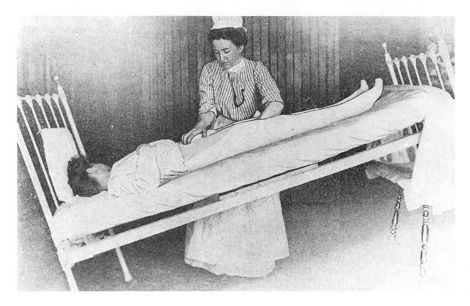

Concern arose in the 1890s as to the propriety of female nurses attending to certain nursing procedures for male patients.

to us as little children, and the motherliness inherent in every true woman's nature responds to their cry for help, and we give them what they need without any regard to our relation, except as patient and nurse.[6]

LEECHING

Among the more frequently administered treatments were applications of leeches, cups, poultices, counterirritants, and blisters. Leeches were used at that time to treat a wide variety of ailments, including meningitis and conjunctivitis (leech from the temples), otitis (leech from the mastoid area), and orchitis (leech from the perineum). Inflammations or engorgements were often treated by applying leeches to the affected area. Nurses were warned never to apply leeches near the eyelids or the scrotum.

In administering this treatment, the nurse first washed and dried the part of the body to which the leeches would be applied. She dried the leeches in the folds of a soft towel and then held them in place with a wine glass or the top of a pillbox. They were never applied over a large vein. If they delayed taking hold, the nurse pricked her finger and put a drop of blood on the spot or a drop of sugar water or milk. If applying the leech to the mouth area of the person, the nurse put it in a test tube or small bottle held to the spot. The leech would usually continue to draw blood until fully engorged, then drop off. Each leech consumed about one teaspoon of blood. If the nurse wanted to remove the leech before it dropped off, she put a drop of water or some salt on its head to induce it to cease feeding. Conversely, if the bleeding had been insufficient, the application of warmth to the wound, particularly with a poultice, served to continue the bleeding and increase the depletion.

The number of leeches used varied with the patients' circumstances and the variety of leech. Embarrassing accidents sometimes happened owing to the migratory tendencies of the leeches, and caution was taken not to apply them too near a bodily orifice and to count every leech as applied and later removed. If a leech was swallowed, salt water or port wine was given and followed, if necessary, by an emetic. If the leech entered the rectum, the salt water was given in an enema. A leech could be used more than once, because it could be forced to disgorge the blood it had swallowed by drawing it, tail first, between the fingers, thus emptying it by pressure. After detachment, the leech was placed in clean water and left for later use.

NURSING PROCEDURES ASSOCIATED WITH THE USE OF COUNTERIRRITANTS

Counterirritants were agents used to irritate the surface of one part of the body in an attempt to relieve disease in another part of the body. They were indicated for inflammation, congestion, and the absorption of "inflammatory products." They were also used for pain relief and as a stimulant in acute depression and narcotic overdose.

Dispute arose during the 1890s over why this treatment was effective. One theory that gained acceptance held that a counterirritant drew the blood supply away from the diseased part of the body. Another scientific explanation suggested that the irritation of peripheral nerves changed their molecular structure. This change was then communicated to the nerves in the affected organ. The choice of sites for application of counterirritants frequently reflected the theory to which the practitioner subscribed. Milder forms of counterirritants, such as heat or friction, tended to be used more frequently and closer to the affected part of the body. Vigorous forms, such as blistering, were used more judiciously and farther away from the affected area. Counterirritants fell into four categories: rubefacients, vesicants, pustulants, and cauterants.

Rubefacients were agents that reddened the skin without destroying its integrity. The most common procedure used in the 1890s to achieve the rubefacient effect was dry cupping, a treatment commonly performed by the nurse. This therapeutic procedure involved the application of a cup to the body's surface by means of a vacuum. This vacuum created local vascular congestion. The cup was made of rubber, glass, china, or metal. The objective was to establish a vacuum in one of these vessels, and this demanded elaborate procedures requiring considerable manual dexterity as the nurse burned paper in the cup and applied it to the patient's skin at the precise moment the paper was ready to extinguish. As the cup cooled, a vacuum formed and local circulation increased. The nurse was admonished not to burn or bruise the skin.

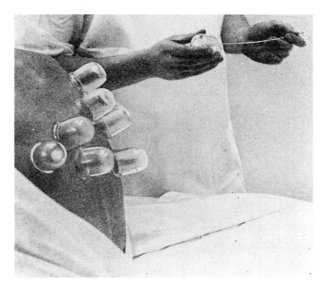

Male nurse cupping the back of a patient, circa 1900.

CUPPING INSTRUMENTS.

FIG.			
3000	8–blade Scarificators..	$3	00
*3001	10 " plain Scarificators.............................	3	00
*3002	10 " reverse "	3	75
*3003	12 " plain "	.3	50
*3004	12 " reverse "	4	50
*3005	Cupping Case complete.................................	5	50
3006	Plain Glass Cupping Cups.....................per doz.	1	00
*3007	" " " " with Rubber Bulb.............each.		50
3008	All Rubber Cupping Cups		75
3009	Cupping Cup Caps.....................................		60
3010	" Pump, metal, nickel plated......	1	85
3011	" " " with Stop Cock............	3	00
3012	Stop Cocks for Cupping Cups..........................		60

Sharp & Smith.

3001-3003   3002-3004

3005
This case contains : Three Glass Cups, mounted ; three Stop-cocks, and fine nickel plated Pump. In morocco case, velvet lined.

3007

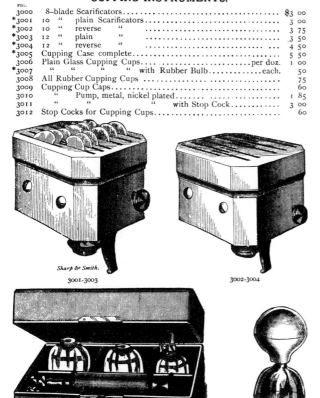

Cupping instruments used in the 1890s.

Widely used in a variety of cases, cupping was believed to temporarily relieve congested organs and tissues of surplus blood, thus affording relief to the patient during medical crises. As a rule, dyspnea due to cardiac disease and the pain and cough of acute pulmonary and pleural diseases were believed to be temporarily relieved by dry cups applied to the chest and back. Acute inflammation and congestion of the kidneys were treated with a large number of dry cups applied over the lumbar region, whereas intracranial congestion and inflammations were improved by cups applied to the nape of the neck or over the mastoid region.

A variation of dry cupping, more akin to the use of leeches than counterirritants, was "wet cupping." The skin was cupped, the cup removed, and a prick made in the reddened area. Another cup was reapplied in the same area to suction out blood, creating a wet cup. This was an alternative to the various methods of bloodletting and should not be confused with the use of "dry cupping" as a counterirritant.

Poultices were also used extensively as rubefacients to allay pain and inflammation. They were moist substances applied externally in such a consistency that they adhered to the surface of the skin without spreading to adjacent areas and without becoming so thick that they stuck to the skin.

Poultices were made from a variety of substances. Quite popular were linseed or flaxseed poultices, a mixture of linseed and boiling water gradually mixed by constant stirring until the correct consistency was achieved. Bread poultices were made from pulverized stale bread and hot water or hot milk, the latter being referred to as the "bread-and-milk" poultice. The disadvantages of bread poultices were that they cooled and dried quickly, crumbled, and became sour, whereas linseed had oily mucilaginous characteristics.

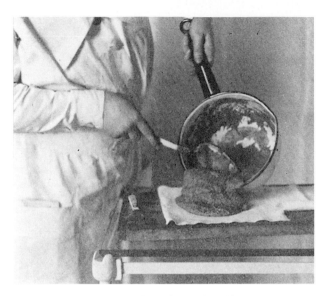

Nurse preparing a flaxseed poultice.

Indian-meal poultices prepared from Indian corn meal were believed to retain their heat longer than linseed poultices. Bran had the advantage of lightness. Powdered charcoal was added to flaxseed to treat "offensive ulcers." Similarly, warm yeast was smeared on the surface of bread poultices and placed near the fire to rise. An "iodide-of-starch" poultice, used to clean sloughing ulcers, was made with starch, boiling water, and liquor iodide. To eliminate "gaseous emanations from unhealthy sores," a chlorine poultice was applied. Poultices were also prepared with oatmeal, slippery elm, mashed potatoes, carrots boiled and mashed, starch, and wheat. Various medicines, such as opium, were added to the poultices for rapid pain relief.

The chief use of poultices was to relieve congestion and inflammation of internal organs, such as the lungs in cases of bronchitis, pleurisy, or pericarditis. Similarly, acute abdominal, lumbago, intestinal, and hepatic "inflammations," and even peritonitis, were believed to be alleviated with this treatment.

When the nurse applied the poultice, she followed a number of important steps. Because it was believed that pain extended beyond the inflamed part, she made a poultice large enough to cover the surrounding surface. She spread the substance from ½ to 1 inch thick on a heavy piece of cotton, making the edges as thick as the middle so that the poultice would not dry too rapidly and be painful. She then covered the surface of the poultice with a very thin gauze of muslin, mosquito net, or lace so that it would not stick to the surface and could later be removed in one piece. In applying it to the chest, the nurse was cautioned to avoid covering the nipples. The cloth on which the poultice was spread had to be large enough to double up around the four sides and up over the edges of the poultice to prevent it from oozing out. The nurse prepared everything beforehand and had

the patient's clothing unfastened before she brought the poultice to the bed. She applied it immediately, as hot as the patient could stand. She covered it with oiled silk or rubber sheeting and then with flannel to keep it warm for as long as possible. It was changed before it became cold, usually every 2 hours. During the poultice change, the nurse was careful to keep the skin covered at all times, thus preventing rapid loss of body heat. She changed the poultices promptly, because if left too long, they dried and adhered to the skin. A sleeveless poultice jacket, made out of two layers of muslin sewed together at the edges, was devised to hold the poultice in its proper location.

Fomentations, or stupes, were warmed liquids applied to the surface of the body with absorbent material, usually a cloth. Sometimes an irritant, such as oil of turpentine, was added. The reasons for applying the fomentations were the same as for poultices, both treatments offering heat and moisture. But a fomentation lasted only a few minutes, compared with 2 hours for a poultice. Colic was treated with fomentations, because a prompt, short action was required.

Another favorite rubefacient treatment was the mustard plaster. To apply a mustard plaster, the nurse mixed ground mustard with boiling water into a thin paste, spread it on heavy paper or cloth, covered it with gauze or very thin cloth, and applied it to the patient's skin. It was removed after the skin became reddened. If a slower, milder, and continuous burning process was desired, she made a thick paste of Indian meal or flour and stirred in a tablespoon or more of ground mustard. This was applied and kept in place with a bandage. Mustard plasters treated a variety of clinical problems. They were said to relieve pain when placed over an area of soreness. Colds and bronchitis responded remarkably well to mustard plasters applied over the entire lateral surface of the affected lung or lungs. Diarrhea was treated with a plaster applied to the abdomen, nausea with one over the stomach, and migraine with one over the hepatic region.

Vesicants, agents that produced blisters, were used as a more vigorous form of counterirritant. The nurse was cautioned not to blister the skin's surface larger than a silver dollar. A number of small blisters seemed to be most effective. The agent used to blister the skin was most commonly Cantharis, which could be used in ointment or oil, applied to paper, or dissolved in collodion. To apply a blister, the nurse first washed and dried the location and then applied the blister agent to the area, holding it in place with strips of adhesive plaster or bandage. The time required for the blister to rise varied among patients. The nurse would examine it in 3 hours, then hourly, to determine when the blister appeared. The plaster came off easily when the blister had risen. She then snipped the puffed skin in several places with sharp-pointed scissors. The nurse gently wiped away the fluid that ran out, spread an ointment over the area,

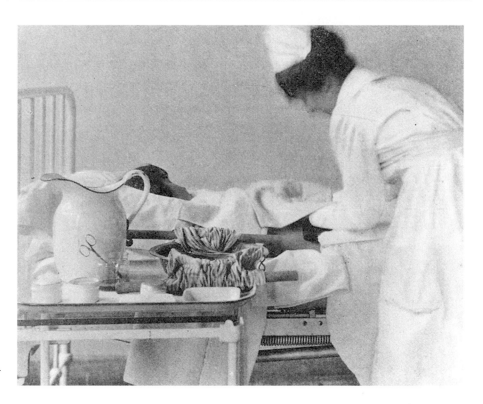

Applying turpentine stupes to a female patient.

and applied a soft lint bandage. Examples of specific diseases and the location of the blistering are spinal meningitis (blister on nape of neck); headache due to intracranial lesions (blister over mastoid process); persistent nausea, gastric ulcer, colic (blister on abdomen); and neuralgia (blister over affected nerve exiting from osseous canal).

Nurses administered the remaining two categories of counterirritants, pustulants and cauterants, less frequently. Pustulants caused a pus-containing lesion on the skin, due to the use of agents such as croton oil or silver nitrate, or, more likely, to the introduction of bacteria through poor technique. The result of this kind of counterirritant was quite painful and difficult to heal. Cauterants were agents that burned and destroyed tissue. They were believed to achieve a more powerful therapeutic effect than blistering, but without the pain of pustules. In this procedure, the nurse passed white-hot metal over the skin but stopped short of actually searing the tissue, because this was not necessary to achieve the counterirritant effect.

ORGANIZATION OF NURSING SERVICE

The method of dividing up the day's work varied among hospitals according to the number of nurses, students, orderlies, and ward maids available and to the patient load. A pattern of functional nursing service was practiced, with the following division of work a typical one. The "temperature nurse" took temperatures and charted them, gave out medicines and kept the medicine closet in order, made out and gave to the head nurse the list of medicines for replenishment each day, served the meals and special nourishments to the patients, and took responsibility for the kitchen. In many hospitals, this nurse also cooked the meals. The "right-side nurse" cared for the patients on the right side of the ward (exclusive of administering medicines, taking temperatures, and serving meals). This nurse bathed and ambulated these patients, made their beds, gave skin care, and maintained everything in good order on her side of the ward. She kept every bed in line and was responsible for the orderliness of the linen closet and for folding the fresh linen. The "left-side nurse" had the same duties as the nurse on the right side but was responsible for the bathroom and lavatory instead of the linen closet. A fourth nurse took care of the special patients in the small private or semiprivate rooms off the ward and was responsible for taking care of the dressing carriage and preparing patients for surgery.

The probationers assisted in making beds, dusting, carbolizing the beds, cleaning mackintoshes, itemizing soiled clothes for the laundry lists, putting away new patients' clothes, and giving out meals. The ward maid, when available, assisted in the preparation of meals; washed dishes; scrubbed the stairs, woodwork, floors, closets, and lavatories; and cleaned the refrigerator, stove, and fireplaces. The orderly was usually hired for the male wards only, and there he was expected to ambulate and bathe the men as well as collect and wash urinals and sputum cups, give enemas, catheterize the patients, and assist in heavy lifting.

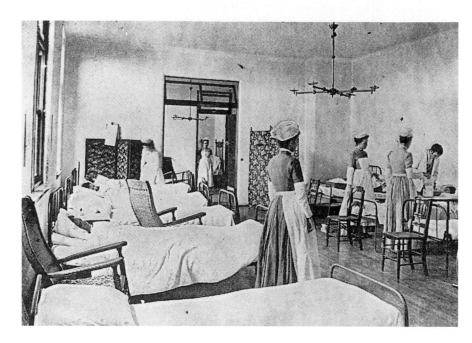

Functional nursing service was practiced at the turn of the century.

The head nurse, generally a senior nursing student, was held responsible for everything pertaining to her ward, including furniture, medicine chest, and linen. She was to make the rounds of the patients with the physicians during their visits, take down their orders, and see that those orders were faithfully carried out.

CARE OF THE SURGICAL PATIENT

As the number of surgical operations increased, the student nurses took on new responsibilities. In the operating room of the 1890s, the student nurse had to make sure that everything connected with the operation was antiseptic. She prepared the room and scrubbed the floors, walls, and other surfaces with antiseptic solution. The surgical dressings were boiled, soaked, and wrapped in antiseptic towels or kept in large glass jars until needed. The nurse also set up the room with everything the surgeon might possibly need, such as hot water bottles, stimulants, clean towels, soft rags, lint, basins, pails, hot and cold water, ice, pins, needles, silk, scissors, petroleum jelly, soap, oil silk, sponges, bran, sticking plaster, carbolized water, a rubber blanket, a pillow, and a sheet to cover the patient.

The nurse also assumed preoperative preparation. She bathed the patient, braided the hair for women, and dressed the patient in loose-fitting clothing. A pint of beef tea, or its equivalent in beef juice, was given 4 hours before the operation along with an enema (especially if the surgery was to be in the region of the rectum or bladder).

After arranging the patient on the operating table, the student nurse had to be prepared for any emergency that might arise. She might help the physician to give the anesthetic, or in some cases she would administer it herself. Generally there were three nurses present at a surgical procedure of any importance: the head nurse and two others. The head nurse kept her eye on the surgeon and stood in a place where she could readily hand him hot towels, sponges, bowls of solution, or anything else he needed. The second nurse maintained the supply of hot towels, solutions, sponges, and hot and cold water, while the third nurse helped the person who was etherizing the patient. She also carried buckets of water, filled empty pitchers, and wrung out sponges.

PHYSICIAN DOMINANCE

Wherever she worked, one of the first rules the student nurse had to remember was that the physician was always her director. She was told over and over that every good nurse was "wise as a serpent," quick to understand and obey whatever orders might be given, and "harmless as a dove" in remaining oblivious to any function of greater importance than that which the physician gave her to perform. According to medical dogma of the 1890s, few professions marked the scope of duties more rigidly than nursing. Medicine, theology, art, music, law—all had unknown depths, and the student who drank at any one of these wells of knowledge could profit by the old quotation, "Drink deep, or taste not." Only to the student nurse did the mandate apply, "Thus far shalt thou come, but no farther." Any nursing student who did not heed this advice was assured that she would fail miserably.

Illustrative of the childlike respect accorded 1890s physicians was a descriptive poem written by

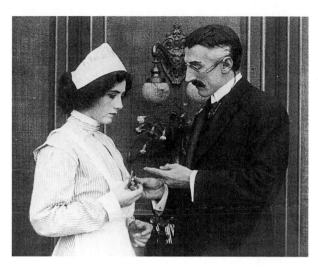

Nurses learned to obey physician authority without question.

a nurse of the era, entitled "When Doctor's on the Floor":

> *Nurses moving quietly,*
> *Voices hushed in awe,*
> *All things silent waiting,*
> *Obedient to the law*
> *That we have heard so often,*
> *But I'll repeat once more:*
> *"All things must be in order*
> *When Doctor's on the floor."*
>
> *Soon a startled murmur*
> *Bursts upon the throng:*
> *"Here's the Head Nurse for the rounds!"*
> *They'll be made ere long!*
> *And now when long we've waited,*
> *As many a time before,*
> *The rounds at last will soon be made,*
> *The Doctor's on the floor.*
>
> *Quick I write a temperature*
> *Just as quick the spread,*
> *Which hangs across a chair-back*
> *I put on baby's bed.*
> *With my apron, quick I wipe*
> *The dust from off the door*
> *Everything must be in state*
> *For Doctor's on the floor.*
>
> *Nurses get their sleeves on,*
> *And straighten up their caps;*
> *They gaze at spots on aprons,*
> *Which may be seen, perhaps.*
> *The patients lie in silence,*
> *The babies cry no more;*
> *They seem to know by instinct*
> *That Doctor's on the floor.*
>
> *We nurses drop our quarrels*
> *And other little sins;*
> *And when a breast is bandaged*

> *We share our safety-pins.*
> *To wipe up water that in haste*
> *Is spilt from door to door,*
> *Down goes a nurse upon her knees,*
> *When Doctor's on the floor.*
>
> *If you pass the class-room*
> *On any lecture night,*
> *You can hear the merry voices*
> *Each one talks with all her might.*
> *But what a sudden silence comes*
> *If you approach the door,*
> *And stop to whisper softly*
> *That Doctor's on the floor.*⁷

This attitude derived chiefly from the dependence of nursing on the medical profession, in many respects nursing's progenitor. Yet nursing was supposedly a profession in itself. According to Victorian sentiments, the cultured, educated, and "womanly" woman intuitively discovered and appreciated her limitations and did not venture beyond them. Once the student or graduate nurse overstepped the boundary of her prerogative, she was labeled a menace to society. Her intelligence, experience, and knowledge were inconsequential if she forgot the limitations of her training. The nurse was to read no medical books: if she had wished to be a physician, she should have gone to medical school, and then the field of medicine would have legitimately been open to her.

Physicians contended that any nurse who read medical books and journals overburdened her brain with useless knowledge that, in any case, she would probably not remember much longer than overnight. Such a nurse was apt to disgrace herself by daring to use obscure medical terms that only exposed her real ignorance and would quickly bring down the censure of the superintendent, the disgust of the physician, and the scorn of her patients.

In most situations, physicians found the use of medical terms by a nurse to be objectionable. If a physician asked a nurse, "Has this man had a nosebleed?" and she brashly answered, "Yes, doctor, he had quite an attack of epistaxis last evening," she would be scorned and probably accused behind her back of keeping "soiled medicine bottles in her ward closets" or of having "patients with long fingernails." Nursing textbooks stressed that physicians objected to the pedantic nurse. They would far rather have an ignorant "good, old-time Sairy Gamp," whom they could command and perhaps swear at a little and who would carry out their orders to the letter, out of ignorance. This pattern of interpersonal relations extended into the social level, where interaction between the nursing and medical staffs was strictly prohibited. The reasons given were many and amusing. Some schools reported that it was for "disciplinary reasons," others said "professional," and several naively explained that "the nurses would lose respect for the doctors."

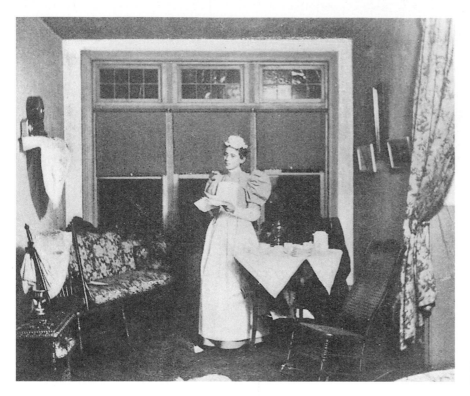

The nurse was expected never to step beyond the bounds of her training.

THE WORLD OF THE PRIVATE-DUTY NURSE

Private-duty nursing took place in the patient's home, and the graduate nurse who undertook such a job was frequently expected to work 24 hours a day for as long as needed. The nurse's time was considered the property of anyone who employed her. She was ordinarily called into a private family when everyone was worn out and needed immediate relief from home nursing. For this reason the nurse did not expect to begin a case with an easy first night, even though she might arrive exhausted from a long carriage ride. The family was usually very anxious, and the nurse had to move quickly to shoulder the patient-care burden that they were too weary to carry a moment longer.

Entering the patient's room for the first time, she might give a pleasant look or a bow because her first objective was to get acquainted with the patient and discern his or her needs. She did not sit where the patient could see her, and, although she was not to

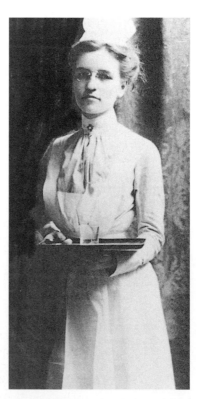

The private-duty nurse and her time were considered the property of the family she served.

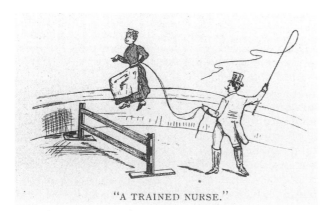

"A TRAINED NURSE."

A medical student's conception of a "trained nurse," 1895.

appear to be watching the patient, she would observe him or her constantly. The private-duty nurse was to avoid whispered conversations and walking on tiptoe because such behavior caused the patient to strain to hear. She was to use a low, distinct tone when conversation was necessary and walk with light step. She was to avoid sitting on the bed, rattling newspapers, turning book pages, creaking a rocking chair, sewing, or clicking knitting needles. Neither was she to turn the gas lights up bright to improve the light for knitting or reading, because the gas burners were said to consume a large amount of the air needed by the patient.

The "good" nurse moved quietly, promptly putting things in their places. She anticipated the patient's wants and tried not to question the patient about his or her needs. If the patient was delirious, she was not to contradict him or her. The nurse listened attentively when the patient spoke, trying never to ask him or her to repeat. She never spoke to the patient from a distance or while standing behind him or her. She shut doors quickly and softly and oiled the hinges if rusty.

The private-duty nurse of the 1890s had learned in her training school that a pleasant personal appearance would go far toward inspiring confidence. Therefore, she developed habits of extreme neatness in dress, always having clean handkerchiefs, collars, and stockings; spotless sleeves and aprons; starched caps;

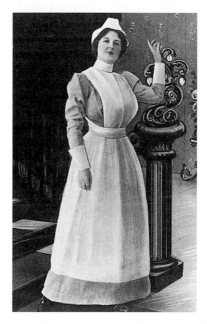

A pleasant appearance went far in inspiring confidence.

and a simple arrangement of the hair. Trailing skirts, flounces, hoop petticoats, frizzed or loose hair, rings, and all other jewelry were considered out of place in a sickroom. For her night use, the nurse was to have warm slippers and a close-fitting dressing gown.

Recommended private-duty nurse's basic outfit, obstetrical outfit, and operation outfit from the B. S. Cooban Nurse's Directory, Chicago.

NURSE'S OUTFIT.

Hot Water Bag ....
Irrigating Bag ....
Rectal Tube ....
Ice Cap ....
Oil Muslin ....
Hypodermic Syringe ....
Syringe for saline injections ....
Thermometer for baths ....
Fever Thermometer ....
Hypodermic Tablets:
    Nitroglycerin 1/100 ....
    Morphine Sulphate ¼ ....
    Morphine ¼ and Atropine 1/150 ....
    Strychnine Sulph. 1/60 ....
    Digitalin 1/100 ....
    Codeine ¼ ....
Glass Douche Point ....
Glass Catheter ....

OBSTETRICAL OUTFIT.

1 qt. Alcohol ....
1 pt. Witch Hazel ....
1 oz. Fld. Ext. Ergot ....
1 oz. Aromatic Spts. Ammonia ....
2 oz. Whisky ....
25 yds. Gauze ....
1 lb. Cotton ....
2 oz. Green Soap ....
2 sml. Bottles Vaselin ....
1 Breast Pump ....
1 Nipple Protector ....
1 Hot Water Bag ....
1 Hard Rubber Syringe ....
1 lb. Boracic Acid ....
1 Soft Catheter No. 8. ....
1 yd. of 1½ yd. Rubber Sheeting ....
1 Porcelain Douche Pan ....
1 Glass Catheter ....
1   "   Douche Point ....
¼ lb. Epsom Salt ....
8 oz. Pure Olive Oil ....
1 oz. Chloroform ....
1 Hand Brush ....
1 Box Mennen's Borated Talcum ....
2 oz. Carbolic Acid ....
5 yds. Iodoform Gauze ....
5   "   Corros. Sub. G., 1 to 2000 ....

OPERATION OUTFIT.

1 lb. Cotton ....
5 yds. Gauze ....
1 glass Catheter ....
8 oz. Olive Oil ....
1 oz. Formaldehyde ....
2 oz. Carbolic Acid ....
2 lbs. Boric Acid ....
1 Small Bottle Seiler's Tablets ....
1 Cake Bichloride Soap ....
1 Bottle Bichloride Tablets ....
1 yd. Adhesive Plaster ....
1 qt. Alcohol ....
2—5c Bottles Vaselin ....
1 pt. Witch Hazel ....
1 yd. Iodoform Gauze ....
½ lb. Ether ....
½ lb. Chloroform ....
2 dr. Aristol ....
1 oz. Iodoform Powder ....
¼ gr. Codeine Tablets ....
2 doz. Aloin, Strych., and Bellad. Pills ....
2 oz. Aromatic Spts. Ammonia ....
1 oz. Tr. Opium ....
4 oz. Epsom Salt ....
100 1 gr. Acetanilide Tablets ....
2 oz. Borolyptol ....
1 oz. Ergot ....
2 oz. Whisky ....
4 oz. Peroxide of Hydrogen ....
2 Cheap Hand Brushes ....
1 Glass Douche Point ....
1 Medicine Dropper ....
½ lb. Green Soap ....
1 Box Mennen's Borated Talcum Powder ....
1 oz. Collodion ....
2 Hand Brushes ....

The nurse was careful to maintain her freshness with a daily bath. She accomplished this with a basin and towel by wringing out a rough cloth in soap and water and rubbing herself briskly from head to foot. She kept her nails scrupulously clean but never cleaned or pared her nails in front of the patient. She made a point not to use a toothpick or to arrange hairpins in public.

Because the private-duty nurse literally moved in with the household, relationships with the family became important. If she was there for any length of time, she soon became a part of the inner family circle as interests hovered around the sickroom and private matters were openly discussed. According to the thinking of the day, the family had the right to expect a cheerful, helping disposition from the private-duty nurse at all times. Although she carried out the physician's orders and did what was essential for the patient, she was to readily accept suggestions from members of the family. She was to remember that she was responsible to the family as well as to the physician whose orders she followed.

Private-duty nursing was strenuous work with low pay, often requiring weeks of continuous service. If the patient was dangerously ill, the nurse sat up all night and sometimes for more than a month had only 2 to 6 hours' sleep, snatched during daylight.

The average private-duty engagement lasted 3 weeks. The first 10 days of each case usually meant 2 hours of sleep out of 24, and the next 10 days might allow 6 hours of sleep per night. When the patient reached the convalescent stage, the nurse slept on a couch close by. If her patient was sleepless, the nurse was to stay awake to keep the patient comfortable. During the day, if the patient was not seriously ill, the nurse was expected to assist the family in sewing and other household chores.

There was not 1 hour of the long day and night that the private-duty nurse could call her own except the time when she took her daily walk. Even that had to suit the convenience of everyone in the family. If no arrangements had been made with the family for the nurse to get some fresh air, she usually stated her case pleasantly and asked for relief—but she was never to show an unwillingness to attend to her patient, and she was never to let anyone see her tired or upset. After a case had been completed, the private-duty nurse generally went home with a trunkful of soiled clothes, thoroughly exhausted.

ECONOMICS OF PRIVATE-DUTY NURSING

In 1888, the Department of Labor investigated the weekly wages paid to women in 22 large cities. It found that average weekly wages varied from a high of $6.91 in San Francisco to a low of $3.93 in Richmond, whereas most women averaged from $4.00 to $6.00 a week. A government report noted that this was hardly enough to buy the necessities of life. Such inadequate wages, said the report, "must inevitably lead in many cases to the adoption of a life of immorality, and in fact there is no doubt that the low rate of wages paid to women is one of the frequent causes of prostitution."[8]

In 1890, private-duty nursing was proclaimed one of the very best fields for women:

> Trained nurses receive good pay in comparison with that of the ordinary employments of women, ranging from ten dollars per week upward to twenty, thirty, or even forty dollars, according to the difficulty of the case. While these prices are by no means higher than should reward a nurse who has given years in preparation for her profession and who works faithfully in it, they are yet burdensome to many families. A surgeon will sometimes refuse to take a case unless he can have the skilled nursing that he believes essential to success, and yet the pay of the nurse will take all the earnings of the father, on which the family rely for support.[9]

However, the public did not generally know that a private-duty nurse was overworked for some months yet idle for others. Consequently, an excellent nurse was very fortunate if she could gross $600 a year. Like all other independent practitioners in business for themselves, nurses found that sometimes they could not collect their fees. Instead, when the time came for settling the account, the family would offer food, old clothing, and trinkets along with whatever small portion of her fee they might deem sufficient pay.

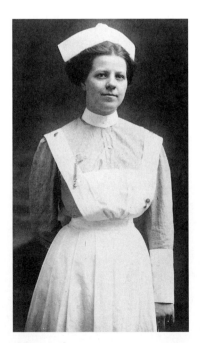

Private-duty nursing was considered one of the best fields of employment for women in the 1890s.

Despite difficulties in fee collection, some physicians charged that graduates of nurse training schools were overpaid. Dr. A. W. Catlin of Brooklyn, in December 1894, publicly stated that the need for intelligent aid in the sickroom was apparent and that trained nurses were needed rather than ignorant Sairy Gamps. Yet the system of having trained nurses for private duty was fast becoming undesirable because of its exclusiveness. The private-duty nurse was more and more of a luxury, he warned, and would soon be far beyond the means of the average family. He charged that schools of nursing taught students that on graduation they should not take patients for less than $3 a day, and many schools stood firm on $25 a week as their unalterable fee. The wealthy could easily afford nurses along with many other comforts, whereas people of moderate income had to deny themselves this service and, because of this denial, take additional risks on their lives.

Catlin's remarks outraged several private-duty nurses, who quickly refuted his charges in a series of letters to the *Brooklyn Eagle*. One commented that among the first principles she had been taught in training was loyalty to the physician, and she wondered why there should not be some loyalty given to the nurse by the physician. She had also been taught that by devoting 2 years of hard work to a hospital, she would be given a diploma and then enter a profession that would enable her to make a living. Even the strongest nurses had to take a rest between patients, she noted, and it was often necessary to wait many weeks for calls—which brought the average nurse's income down to the price of unskilled labor. Private-duty nurses were deprived of pleasures of every kind and spent their time in the sickroom, night and day for weeks and even months, without rest, giving their very lives for their patients. Could anyone think that it would be right to alter their charges so as to deny them regular prices, she asked, when all physicians in good standing were entitled to their standard fees?

Another nurse could not see why Catlin was so desirous of reducing a nurse's pay, although she knew some physicians preferred to have inexpensive nurses attending their patients to enable patients to pay the physicians' larger fees. Physicians knew, she continued, that where a good trained nurse was employed to care for a patient, it was unnecessary for the physician to make as many calls as otherwise would be required. Catlin, she thought, was no doubt getting at least $3 for one 15- or 20-minute house call, and yet he wanted a nurse to settle for $2 for working a 24-hour day for the same patient. She deplored the fact that any man would attempt to thwart a woman who was only trying to earn a decent living: "What right has Dr. Catlin to set salaries? No more right than the nurses have to say that his house calls are only worth 50 cents a visit." Catlin, she pointed out, wanted to know who would join hands with him in building a home where he and several other medical men could teach 30 or 40 women to work cheaply as untrained nurses. Why not build a home for cheap physicians, this nurse retorted, assuring the newspaper readers that trained nurses would be willing to teach aspiring cheap physicians free of charge. What a beautiful memorial that would be for future generations, she speculated: a home where anyone could secure a physician for 50 cents a call. Trained nurses could then easily charge $30 a week.[10]

Not surprisingly, a nurse's practice began to wane soon after she reached age 40. Physicians and families favored younger nurses. At one of the large training schools in New York, where many wealthy families requested names of graduates for private-duty assignments, three fourths of the requests were for nurses in their 20s. Private-duty nurses with 10 or 20 years' experience behind them frequently lacked the physical vitality required for long night vigils and the hard work connected with demanding assignments. Although private-duty nursing by trained nurses was still a young field, an increasing problem was how to provide for nurses older than age 50. Occasionally, unmarried nurses achieved long careers by obtaining permanent positions in wealthy families, where they had duty no more arduous than in superintending other nurses under them. In one instance, a trained nurse who had been sent from New York to Europe found that her sole work was to make sure that the daughter of a millionaire never went out in damp weather without overshoes.

Such nurses found the very wealthy of this era burdened with more money than they had time to use. They often spent it competitively to impress and surpass one another. They spent millions on huge mansions. Their parties, especially their masked balls, were spectacular functions to which the elite came by the hundreds, wearing costumes costing as much as $5000 each. Trained nurses, permanently hired, provided an essential service to the inner circle of fashionable families who wintered in Palm Beach, summered in Newport or Bar Harbor, and visited London and Paris. Such nurses were often accepted as traveling companions and helped to manage dozens of servants.

PRESIDENT McKINLEY AND HIS NURSES

In September 1901, President William McKinley was shot by an anarchist while visiting the Pan-American Exposition in Buffalo, New York. The nurses on duty in the emergency hospital on the exposition grounds when President McKinley was carried in performed an active part in the historic event that was about to unfold. Though scarcely more than a first-aid station, the hospital had an

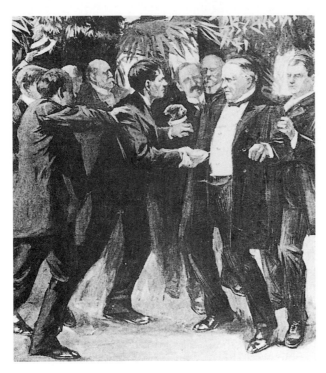

The shooting of President McKinley.

operating room, and the president was at once laid on the table. He was in severe shock but conscious and entirely composed. As the nurses undressed him, a bullet fell from his underclothing. The first shot had ricocheted off the breastbone, causing only an angry graze along the ribs, but the serious nature of an abdominal wound was immediately apparent to the physicians who gathered around the operating table. The president's lips were forming the words of the Lord's Prayer when ether was administered.

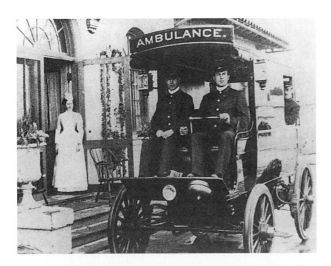

Entrance to the Pan-American Exposition Hospital, where President McKinley was taken.

Adella Walters, superintendent of the hospital and a member of the first graduating class of the Buffalo General Hospital Nurse Training School in 1890, was at her post, and Miss Morris and Miss Barnes were the nurses on duty when the distinguished patient was brought in. The other nurses, Miss Simmons, Miss Dorchester, Miss Baron, and Miss Shannon, arrived soon afterward and assisted during surgery. The nurses "worked well, every one of them," said Walters afterward. "I got all the things needed for the operation, for none of the nurses were as familiar with the places where the needed articles are kept as I, since the nurses change every month." Simmons and Barnes were the nurses who came in direct contact with the patient during the operation. They handled the instruments and dressings and prepared the president for the operation, Simmons standing at the head of the table, fanning him.

In the spotless little operating room off the main hall on the first floor of the hospital, Morris and Barnes told reporters from throughout the nation of their services to President McKinley. "They brought him right here from the ambulance," said Morris, placing her hand on the operating table, "and did not even lift him to remove the stretcher during the operation. I stood here and Miss Simmons stood over there"—indicating the opposite side of the table—"and Dr. Sasdin gave the anesthetic there," she said, pointing to the white-enameled stool at the head of the operating table. "He was the most admirable patient I ever saw," said Barnes. "When we were taking care of him that first night, sick as he was, there was not the slightest service performed for him that he did not recognize in some way. If he could not speak, he would just give a little 'umph-umph,' just to let us know that he noticed what we were doing for him."[11] Barnes admitted that she was shocked to see who the patient was: "I had no idea it was the President who was to be operated upon, when Miss Walters told me to get a hypodermic of morphia and strychnia. I looked at the face of the man on the table and said to myself: 'That looks like the President,' but it was some little time before I was quite sure about it."[12]

On opening the abdomen, the surgeons found that the assassin's second shot had passed straight through the stomach, puncturing the front and rear walls. The operation consisted mainly of suturing those wounds and cleansing the peritoneal cavity. The bullet was not found. No use was made of a Roentgen-ray machine, even though one of them was on exhibition at the fair, and an attempt to probe was abandoned because of the patient's dangerously weak condition. The assisting physicians and nurses used a looking glass to reflect the rays of the setting sun on the surgeons' work and succeeded toward the end in rigging an electric light. The incision was finally closed, without drainage, and covered with an antiseptic dressing.

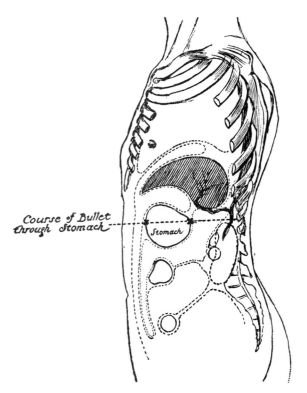

Course of Bullet through Stomach

Stomach

The course of the bullet through President McKinley's stomach.

Official bulletins issued to the press about the president's case were as follows:[13]

Friday, September 6

7:00 P.M.—The operation successfully performed. The President stood the operation well. Condition in general gratifying; justifies hope of recovery.

10:50 P.M.—Is rallying satisfactorily and resting comfortably.

Saturday, September 7

1:00 A.M.—Free from pain and resting well.

3:00 A.M.—Continues to rest well.

5:00 A.M.—Has passed a good night.

9:00 A.M.—No serious symptoms have developed.

3:30 P.M.—Continues to rest quietly; no change for the worse.

9:30 P.M.—Condition much the same. Responds well to medicine.

Sunday, September 8

3:20 A.M.—Has passed a fairly good night.

9:00 A.M.—Has passed a good night and condition is quite encouraging. Mind is clear and he is resting well; wound dressed at 8:30 and found in a very satisfactory condition. There is no indication of peritonitis.

12:00 P.M.—The improvement in the President's condition has continued since last bulletin.

4:00 P.M.—Since the last bulletin has slept quietly, four hours together since 9 o'clock.

Condition satisfactory to all physicians present.

9:00 P.M.—Is resting comfortably and there is no special change since last bulletin.

Monday, September 9

6:00 A.M.—The President passed a somewhat restless night, sleeping fairly well. General condition unchanged.

9:20 A.M.—Condition becoming more and more satisfactory. Untoward incidents are less likely to occur.

3:00 P.M.—The President's condition steadily improves and he is comfortable, without pain or unfavorable symptoms. Bowel and kidney functions normally performed.

9:30 P.M.—Condition continues favorable.

Tuesday, September 10

7:00 A.M.—The President has passed the most comfortable night since the attempt on his life.

9:00 A.M.—Condition this morning is eminently satisfactory to physicians. If no complications arise, a rapid convalescence may be expected.

3:20 P.M.—There is no change since this morning's favorable bulletin.

10:30 P.M.—The condition of the President is unchanged in all important particulars. When the operation was done on Friday last it was noted that the bullet had carried with it a short distance beneath the skin a fragment of the President's coat. This foreign material was, of course, removed, but a slight irritation of the tissues was produced, the evidence of which appeared only to-night. It has been necessary on account of this slight disturbance to remove a few stitches and partially open the skin wound. This incident cannot give rise to other complications. In consequence of this separation of the edges of the surface wound the healing of the same will be somewhat delayed. The President is now well enough to begin to take nourishment by the mouth in the form of pure beef juice.

Wednesday, September 11

6:00 A.M.—Passed a very comfortable night.

9:00 A.M.—Rested comfortably during the night. Decided benefit has followed the dressing of the wound made last night. Stomach tolerates beef juice well, and it is taken with great satisfaction. Condition this morning is excellent.

3:30 P.M.—Continues to gain and the wound is becoming more healthy. The nourishment taken into the stomach is being gradually increased.

10:00 P.M.—Condition continues favorable. Blood count corroborates clinical evidence of absence of any blood poisoning. Is able to take more nourishment and relish it.

The president's improvement was remarkable, but it did not indicate recovery. Gangrene was creeping along the bullet's track through the stomach, the pancreas, and one kidney. After an 8-day battle to keep the president alive, he died on September 14, 1901. The official bulletins of these events follow:[14]

Thursday, September 12
6:20 A.M.—Has had a comfortable night.
9:30 A.M.—The President has spent a quiet and restful night, and has taken much nourishment. He feels better this morning than at any time. He has taken a little solid food this morning and relished it.
3:00 P.M.—Condition very much the same as this morning. His only complaint is of fatigue. He continues to take a sufficient amount of food.
8:30 P.M.—The President's condition this evening is not quite so good. His food has not agreed with him and has been stopped. Excretion has not yet been properly established. The kidneys are acting well. His pulse is not satisfactory, but has improved in the last two hours. The wound is doing well. He is resting quietly.
12:00 A.M.—All unfavorable symptoms have improved since last bulletin.

Friday, September 13
1:50 A.M.—The President's condition is very serious and gives rise to the gravest apprehension. His bowels have moved well, but his heart does not respond properly to stimulation. He is conscious. The skin is warm and the pulse small, regular and easily compressible.
9:00 A.M.—Condition has somewhat improved during the past few hours. There is a better response to stimulation. He is conscious and free from pain.
2:30 P.M.—Has more than held his own since morning, and his condition justifies the expectation of further improvement. Is better than yesterday at this time.
4:00 P.M.—Only slightly improved since last bulletin.
5:35 P.M.—The President's condition is grave at this hour. He is suffering from extreme prostration. Oxygen is being given. He responds to stimulants but poorly.
6:30 P.M.—His condition is most serious in spite of vigorous stimulation. The depression continues and is profound. Unless it can be relieved the end is only a question of time.
9:30 P.M.—The President is dying.

Saturday, September 14
2:15 A.M.—The President is dead.

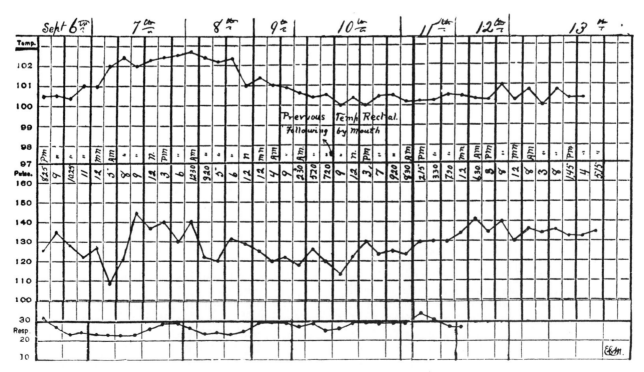

Nurse's chart of temperature, pulse, and respiration for President McKinley's case.

NURSE'S RECORD

Nurse's record, McKinley case.

REFERENCES

1. Massachusetts General Hospital, *Circular and Announcement by the Trustees of the Massachusetts General Hospital of a Two Years' Course of Training in General Nursing* (Boston: The Hospital, 1889).
2. Boston City Hospital Training School for Nurses, *Circular of Information for Candidates and Probationers on the Necessary Outfit on Entering Service, Course of Training with a List of Questions to Be Answered by the Candidate, and a Form of Agreement to Remain Two Years as a Pupil of the School* (Boston: The Hospital, 1889).
3. Emily L. Loveridge, "Reminiscences of Forty Years in Hospital Work," *Bulletin of the American Hospital Association*, vol. 4 (April 1930):48–52.
4. Lutheran Hospital, Cleveland, "The Good Old Days," *Bright Corridors*, vol. 8 (January 1963):1–4.
5. Mary Agnes Snively, "A Nurse's Day in a Hospital," *Trained Nurse*, vol. 13 (July 1894):8–12.

6. L. W. Quintard, "Limitations of Pupil Nurses in Caring for Male Patients," *Proceedings of the American Society of Superintendents of Training Schools for Nurses*, vol. 3 (1896):70.

7. "When Doctor's on the Floor," *Trained Nurse and Hospital Review*, vol. 16 (September 1896):90.

8. U.S. Department of Commerce and Labor, *Report on the Condition of Woman and Child Wage-Earners in the United States* (Washington, DC: Government Printing Office, 1911), vol. 9, pp. 24–25.

9. *New York Tribune*, February 18, 1890.

10. "Answering Dr. Catlin," *Trained Nurse*, vol. 16 (February 1896):121.

11. *Buffalo Express*, September 8, 1901.

12. Ibid.

13. P. M. Rixey, "Medical and Surgical Report of the Case of the Late President of the United States," *Report of the Surgeon General of the Navy for 1900–1901* (Washington, DC: Government Printing Office, 1901), pp. 297–311.

14. Ibid., pp. 312–318.

NURSES AND THE WAR WITH SPAIN

7

The Spanish-American War led to the emergence of the first large all-graduate nursing service and provided the first opportunity for incorporating the graduates of nearly 200 nurse training schools throughout the country into a single nursing corps. As a result of this war, trained nurses were accepted for the first time in military hospitals and thereby became forerunners of women in the armed forces.

The Spanish-American War, which began in April 1898 and ended in August of the same year, was one of the last minor wars fought before the devastating, cataclysmic struggles of the 20th century. The most important land fighting, which occurred in Cuba, lasted only a month. Enthusiastically reported by the press, this war produced enough heroes and slogans to supply a dozen larger ones. At the outbreak of hostilities, the regular army, only 28,000 men, was completely unprepared for war. There had been no brigade-sized formation of troops in the country for 30 years, and only a few officers had ever seen a unit as large as a regiment concentrated in one place. Because this force was inadequate for conducting a war against Spain, Congress authorized the president to increase the army to a standing force of more than 200,000 men.

THE DAUGHTERS OF THE AMERICAN REVOLUTION SECURES NURSES

Unable to supply hospital corpsmen for such vast numbers of soldiers, the War Department began to look elsewhere for assistance. When the National Society of the Daughters of the American Revolution (DAR) offered to serve as an examining board for the military nurses, Surgeon General of the Army George M. Sternberg immediately accepted. Directing the committee appointed by the DAR for this purpose was the young Dr. Anita Newcomb McGee.

Because hundreds of applications for service with the army were pouring in from trained and untrained nurses, they could not receive proper attention from the War Department, which was already overwhelmed with supervising the preparation of war material. Dr. McGee perceived that by examining and screening this mass of applications from women nurses, the DAR committee would be performing a valuable service for the government. Washington reporters raved that she was the ideal woman for the job because she was "young and charming, possessing unusual magnetism, vivacity, and a gift of language."[1]

The nurses of 1898 proved to be worthy successors to those of the Civil War. As the army grew, the sick rate rose in direct proportion, and the demand for nurses sharply increased. By working literally day and night, the committee succeeded in examining nearly 5000 applications. In one of her reports, Dr. McGee testified: "The work of separating the fit from the unfit was not so simple an accomplishment as it would appear, and the correspondence entailed was enormous. The visitors who made inquiries in person were also numerous. The officers were at their posts daily from 8 A.M. to 11 P.M."[2]

There were letters from eager, romantic young girls and from aged matrons who had served as nurses in the Civil War. Some appealed to the president, some to the secretary of war. Some had enough knowledge to direct their applications to the surgeon general, but their fitness for work ended there. A smaller number listed regular hospital training and service. Every one of these thousands of applications was examined, numbered, and filed in alphabetical order. Those applicants who had mentioned hospital training received the following letter in reply:

> Dear Madam: Your application of recent date has been received. All applications from women for hospital positions, whether addressed to the Surgeon General or to the director of the D.A.R. hospital corps, are placed on file in this office.
>
> The reserve list is composed, however, only of those who have had hospital training and who

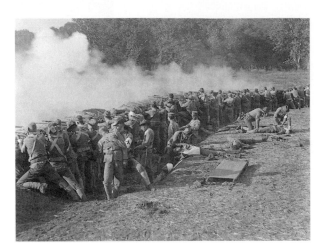

The Spanish-American War resulted in the first large all-graduate nursing service.

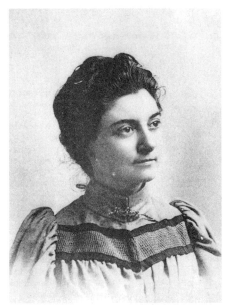

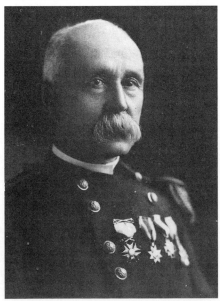

Dr. Anita Newcomb McGee and Surgeon General Sternberg.

answer satisfactorily to the enclosed questions. Nurses who receive appointment in the army must be between thirty and fifty years of age. They will be paid railroad fare to the place of duty and $30 a month with board. If practicable, lodging will be given, but other expenses must be met by the nurse.

Women may later be appointed to shore duty in the navy, but no provisions have yet been made therefor.

Endorsements as to good character and general ability should accompany the application, and it is requested that, if possible, such endorsements should include one from some Daughter of the American Revolution.[3]

A card was sent with the letter, requesting information such as age, state of health, and work experience. Significantly, the applicant was asked: "Have you had yellow fever?" and "Are you strong and healthy, and have you always been so?" Only graduates of training schools for nurses or of medical colleges were considered eligible. A physician's certificate that the applicant was in good health and strong enough for army duty was required. When the surgeon general received a requisition for more nurses, he referred it to the DAR office, which in turn sent the nurse her contract, transportation, and orders. The first call for nurses was received from the surgeon general of the army on May 7, 1898, and within a few days four women nurses were on their way to the general hospital at Key West, Florida.

In addition to the contract nurses selected as above, Mrs. Namah Curtis, wife of Dr. Austin M. Curtis, surgeon-in-chief of Freedman's Hospital in Washington, DC, was sent on July 13 by the surgeon general to New Orleans and other southern cities to secure the services of immune black women as nurses for yellow-fever patients. Mrs. Curtis registered 32 such nurses.

SICKNESS IN THE CAMPS

Of the more than 200,000 volunteers who enlisted in April and May of 1898, no more than 35,000 left the United States or were even assigned to expeditions during the war. The remaining soldiers sat out the war in military camps in the southern United States, where they spent many hours in target practice, drill, and large-scale combat maneuvers. In May, about 6.75% of the men were sick. In June, the sick rate climbed to almost 16%. By July this figure had risen to 20% of the army's total strength of 203,350. The climax came in August, when the sick rate increased to 30%. Malaria, typhoid, dysentery, and diarrhea accounted for 60% of the sickness in July, August, and September of 1898. Eighty percent of all deaths were attributed to typhoid.

Meanwhile, Surgeon General Sternberg downplayed the potential usefulness of female nurses on a large scale for the army. On May 3, 1898, he made the following comments to the secretary of war in regard to a joint resolution that had been introduced to authorize the greater use of trained women nurses in army general hospitals:

> In my opinion this would be very unwise legislation. Trained female nurses are out of place as regular attendants of sick and wounded soldiers in the wards of a general hospital. They may be very useful for certain cases and especially in the preparation and serving of special diets to such an extent as may be necessary and desirable, but the passage of this bill would greatly embarrass me in the administration of our general hospitals.[4]

Observers expressed their dismay at the pervasive filth in the military camps. Regiments often dug latrines and garbage pits within yards of their kitchens, hospitals, and living quarters. In rainy weather the shallow pits flooded and overflowed, spilling sewage throughout the camps. Regimental and company officers failed to enforce regulations controlling the use and maintenance of latrines, and the soldiers threw garbage on the ground near their tents and defecated in the surrounding woods. After viewing the camp of the Third United States Volunteer Cavalry at Camp Thomas, outside of Chattanooga, Tennessee, an inspecting officer reported:

> I have never seen so large an area of fecal-stained soil as that which we looked upon and walked over. This area was a checker board, marked with woody spots of irregular contour and open spaces, some of which had known cultivation. The woody lands were smeared with alvine discharges. As I have said, most of the soldiers had been removed before our arrival, but even then one could not walk under the trees without soiling one's shoes with human excrement. Behind every considerable tree it lay in heaped-up cones. The falling leaves and twigs did not suffice to hide it. The gentle winds had not wholly dispersed it; a hot September sun was drying it out. An occasional rain was sinking the pollution below the surface and down into the soil.[5]

FAILURE OF THE HOSPITAL CORPS

To provide the male nurses preferred by army surgeons at that time, the Medical Department tried to enlarge its small Hospital Corps. Strenuous efforts to attract civilian recruits and to persuade medically qualified volunteers to transfer from line regiments met with frustration. Even though the Hospital Corps

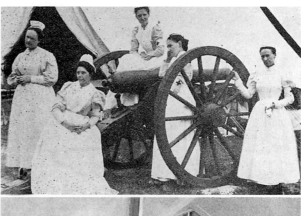

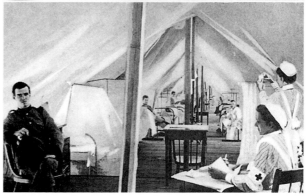

Nurses pose on a field gun and in a hospital tent.

had increased its ranks from a peacetime strength of 723 to almost 6000 men by August 31, 1898, it still had barely half the number required for the army of more than 200,000, and most of its recruits lacked training and experience. In their search for nurses for the camp hospitals, commanders temporarily detailed squads of infantry to ward duty. These detail men, often the dregs of the units, were grossly unqualified to care for patients, and their neglect of elementary sanitary precautions helped spread diseases, such as typhoid, through the camps.

The low status attached to the soldiers of the Hospital Corps accounted for much of their low morale and incompetence. The male army nurse, with his inadequate pay and enlisted rank, had little to expect but ingratitude from his fellow soldiers. The glory and distinction that might be gained on the battlefield was beyond the reach of the male nurse, although his duties were far more arduous and taxing than those of his comrades bearing arms. In constant contact with infectious diseases, he exposed himself to more danger than if he were on the battlefield.

A virulent outbreak of typhoid fever resulted in the more extensive use of women in the army hospitals. Driven to innovation by despair, Surgeon General Sternberg for the first time in the army's history employed large numbers of women nurses in military hospitals. Beginning in late July, typhoid cases increased the sick rate in every camp. The number of sick at Camp Thomas grew from about 2200 on

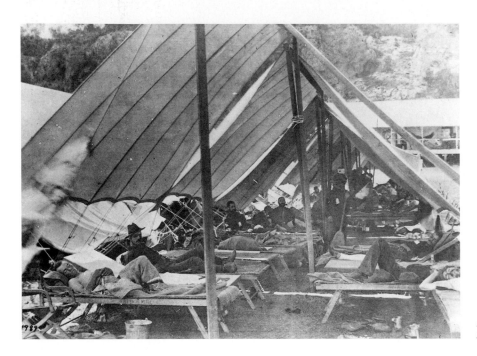

By July 1898, 20% of the army was suffering from disease.

July 25 to 3600 on August 8 and to 4400 on August 15. Typhoid patients sometimes lay in their own filth for as long as 24 hours because the hospitals lacked clean linen with which to change their beds. A medical officer at a Camp Thomas hospital wrote in panic:[6]

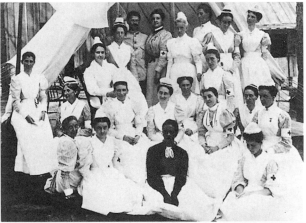

July 10, 1898

Leiter General Hospital
Chickamauga, Georgia
Dr. McGee D.A.R.

Dear Doctor:

Miss Dunmise, the nurse I recommended, arrived this A.M. much to our delight and I am much obliged for sending her so promptly.

We are in terrible distress for nurses and can't understand the delay in sending them—there ought to be 50 good nurses in Washington willing and glad to come here. We have now in the hospital 150 cases of typhoid fever and six trained nurses to take care of these and there are 100 more cases waiting to come.

We need 30 trained nurses and cannot do with less.

I understand from the Surgeon General that the matter has been turned over to you and I trust you will at once relieve our distress. There are three good nurses at Providence Hospl. that I think you can get. I am glad to see the Daughters are taking so active a part. I am Vice Prest. S.A.R. of the District of Columbia, and hence have a fellow feeling with you in the good work you are doing.

I hope you will pardon me for speaking so plainly about this matter but only those in the field can know the exigencies of the occasion.

Yours truly,
J. W. Bayne
Major & Brigade Surg. U.S.V.

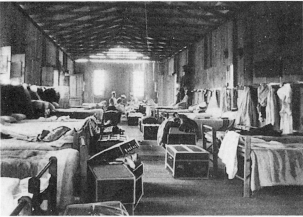

Nurses upon arrival at Camp Thomas; their living quarters.

BATTLING TYPHOID FEVER

"It was certainly a most harrowing sight to see the long narrow cots filled with what had been strong, splendid men, hollow-eyed, emaciated, muttering in the delirium of fever," reported Anna Maxwell, on leave as superintendent of nurses at New York's Presbyterian Hospital, after viewing conditions at Sternberg Hospital at Camp Thomas. She noted that "some of the men's bones protruded through their skin, and bed sores several inches deep were not uncommonly found on hips, back, elbows, and often on the head and ears."[7] All the energies and resources of the trained nurse were required to make the lives of these men less wretched and to restore them to health.

Ninety-one training schools from all parts of the United States were represented at the hospital. According to Harriet Lounsberry, who was on leave from her position as superintendent of nursing at Brooklyn Homeopathic Hospital, "it was curious and interesting to see representatives of so many training schools together." The nurses wore their own distinctive school uniforms during their work because the military had made no effort to outfit them in a standard dress. Lounsberry noticed that school badges, which reflected pride in one's alma mater, were prominently displayed. "Nothing would bring a nurse more quickly to a sense of her duty than to ask if in her training school she had

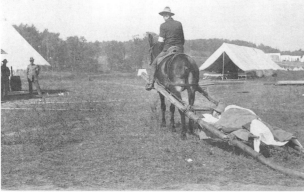

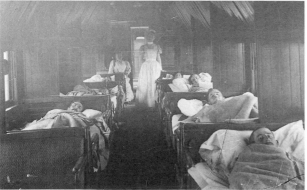

Transporting typhoid patients to hospital; hospital tent scene.

never been instructed as regards this or that," she recalled.[8]

Jean S. Edmunds of Rochester, New York, arrived at the Sternberg Hospital on August 17 along with 36 other nurses. She found that the nurses at Camp Thomas had been working day and night. As rapidly as tents were pitched and cots placed within them, more ambulances with fever-stricken men arrived. "Hastily donning our uniforms," related Edmunds, "but with skirts shortened and sleeves rolled up, we were each escorted to the tents where work had been assigned us by Miss Maxwell, who, while on the way thither, advised us of the need of strict discipline, as the eyes of America would be watching us."[9]

EXPERIENCES ON DUTY

The venerable Anna Maxwell constantly reminded the nurses that their work at Camp Thomas would forever speak for or against the women of America. During her first 4 weeks there, Edmunds cared each day for 42 men with typhoid fever. The men presented a dreadful sight when first brought to her. "Their poor tongues were swollen and cracked," she noted, "their lips raw with the fever sores; often the back was one raw bed sore, for the fever was of the most virulent type, and they had received little or no care in the Camp and Division Hospitals."[10]

Each of these men required several ice baths daily, besides nourishment every 2 hours and all other care. Some of the more delirious ones had to be watched almost constantly. Despite all this work, Edmunds had only one corpsman to assist her, and even he was replaced every few hours. Moreover, teaching each new aide the fundamentals of caring for the sick taxed the nurses' capabilities extraordinarily. Nurses worked at a frantic pace. For the first 4 weeks their working day lasted from 7:00 a.m. until 9:00 p.m., with a mere 20-minute break for lunch and the same for supper.

Helen B. Schuler and Florence M. Kelly, contract nurses from New York City, concluded that only by the grace of God did anyone survive the primitive, unsanitary conditions at Chickamauga Park, Georgia, during the summer and fall of 1898. Sternberg Hospital consisted of 13 rough board huts, bare, cold, and unfinished. The windows, mere holes in the walls without glass, provided the only means of ventilation and sunlight. Of course, these openings in the walls offered no protection against hordes of flies and mosquitoes that constantly streamed in. During a Georgia rainstorm, the nurses had to either close these openings with wooden doors and endure the foul, humid air of an overcrowded, unventilated ward or leave them open and contend with damp flooded huts. The interior of these huts was absolutely primitive, and the uncertain light afforded by lanterns made medical treatment hazardous.

Heavy, tropical air blanketed the nurses and their patients with "a suffocating pressure of steaming, smelly, deadening matter that passed for air." Attracted by all the sick men, flies and mosquitoes multiplied by the millions and spread infection between the sickbeds and the mess kitchen. The following passage illustrates a typical night:

> Two hundred suffering patients, mostly all delirious, were brought to the Hospital. Every one of them previously had been given a dose of Calomel and Jalop. There was not a bed "Utensil" to be had and we, the nurses, suffered the consequences. The soiled clothing and bedding had to be taken care of and we had no way or equipment to handle it, so as to reduce to a minimum the danger of infection for us. We had no disinfectant whatsoever to use.
>
> There was not even one wash basin in these wards for the nurses to wash their hands.
>
> At one time there was a shortage of water for several days [and] we were requested "not to wash at all."
>
> The three toilets which were supposed to be adequate for the needs of the two hundred nurses, were over 500 feet away from their sleeping quarters. Every one of the nurses had contracted Dysentery and under these fearfully unsanitary conditions, consider how inevitable it was, that the majority of the nurses left Sternberg Hospital Service with an intestinal condition which soon became chronic and which we shall suffer from the effects of, until the end of our life.[11]

Some of the nurses virtually worked themselves to death, as attested by a letter of August 18, 1898, from a Camp Thomas surgeon to Dr. McGee:[12]

> I am sorry to trouble you again. Your nurses arrived and are hard at work. Owing to the large percentage of sickness among the nurses I felt obliged to keep all six that arrived here. Unless some are able to return to duty I shall be obliged to telegraph on Sunday morning for six or perhaps 10 more.
>
> Could not some of mine who can not stand this climate be transferred to Fortress Monroe or Long Island? These nurses are very zealous—they over-work themselves from the highest and best motives and many of them take it awfully to heart when they are stopped and to be invalided away is very bitter to them. Now I have to send a number to the Mountains every week to recuperate. Now if I could hold out to these unselfish women the prospect of similar work in a more bracing climate I am sure they would not be so distressed at having to go away. It is really a very serious matter with them.
>
> Faithfully yours,
> E. C. Carter
> Major & Surgeon USV

Barbara U. Austin, a young nurse who had just finished her training and was assigned to Sternberg Hospital as one of the 166 women nurses on duty there during the summer of 1898, recounted her experiences as follows:

> We were ordered to prepare the tents for the receptions of patients. I recall distinctly the blistering July day we were hemming woolen blankets for the beds. I can see the tent section on the hill side. Ten tents to a section and ten sections each having from four to six beds in a tent. It was a long trek from morning til night. Our beds were filled with typhoid cases, and all desperately sick. Carrying ice and nourishment up and down the hillside. Rain failed to dampen our ardor if it did our uniforms and frequently left us soaked all day. How grateful the boys were for these services. It made no difference to us that we were forty to fifty in a shack when off duty, just room enough to stand between the cots. One lantern banging in the middle of the building for light.[13]

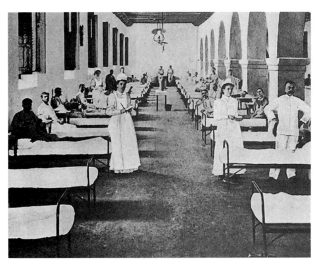

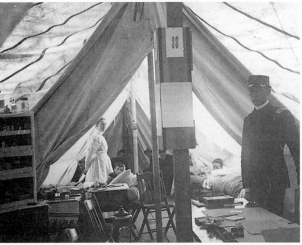

Army hospital ward and tent in Puerto Rico, 1898.

TABLE 7-1	NURSES LEAVING STERNBERG HOSPITAL FROM AUGUST 19 THROUGH SEPTEMBER 13, 1898			
NUMBER	FROM	DATE OF ARRIVAL	DATE OF DEPARTURE	REASON FOR DEPARTURE
1	Boston, MA	Aug. 7	Sept. 10	Overworked
2	New York City	Aug. 7	Sept. 8	Diarrhea
3	New York City	Aug. 7	Sept. 8	Diarrhea
4	Newark, NJ	Aug. 7	Aug. 19	Hysteria
5	Boston, MA	Aug. 17	Sept. 13	Typhoid fever
6	Rochester, NY	Aug. 17	Sept. 7	Exhaustion
7	Brooklyn, NY	Aug. 17	Sept. 7	Exhaustion
8	Brooklyn, NY	Aug. 17	Aug. 30	Exhaustion
9	Boston, MA	Aug. 17	Sept. 7	Exhaustion
10	Brooklyn, NY	Aug. 17	Sept. 13	
11	Pittsburgh, PA	Aug. 17	Sept. 7	High fever
12	Boston, MA	Aug. 17	Aug. 26	Broken down by night work
13	New York City	Aug. 17	Aug. 23	Diarrhea
14	New York City	Aug. 17	Aug. 30	Dismissed, not sick
15	New York City	Aug. 17	Sept. 6	Diarrhea
16	Rochester, NY	Aug. 17	Sept. 11	Diarrhea and suspected typhoid
17	Cincinnati, OH	Aug. 25	Sept. 2	Typhoid fever
18	Wilkes-Barre, PA	Aug. 25	Sept. 13	Typhoid fever
19	Boston, MA	Aug. 26	Sept. 13	Typhoid fever
20	St. Louis, MO	Aug. 27	Sept. 6	High fever
21	Wilkes-Barre, PA	Aug. 19	Sept. 13	Rheumatism
22	Chicago, IL	Aug. 23	Sept. 13	Diarrhea and high fever
23	Chicago, IL	Aug. 25	Sept. 13	Diarrhea and high fever

SICKNESS AMONG THE NURSES

One nurse who did not last long was Jane F. Riley of Boston. "When early in August, 1898, I read in the Boston papers that Miss Maxwell had sent out a call for nurses for Chickamauga Park . . . I immediately offered my services," remembered Riley. Shortly thereafter, "about September 8th Miss Moore had to give up duty on account of sickness, and I on the 10th, several others had already taken sick, some having been sent to the Mountains, others sent North."[14] Several doctors visited and examined them. The last physician was Dr. Jesse Lazear from Cuba, an expert on tropical diseases. He decided that the sick nurses had typhoid. Because they could not be cared for at Sternberg Hospital, he recommended that they be sent north immediately. They left on September 13, in the charge of a Brooklyn nurse who had asked to be released, and were taken by ambulance to an awaiting hospital train.

Later, Riley still remembered the jolting ride over rough roads. Their destination was Boston City Hospital. Sick as they were when they left Sternberg Hospital, the nurses did not forget to ask for their discharge. The medical officer, however, informed them that he could not discharge nurses taken sick on duty but would grant them a furlough for an indefinite period and await the results of their illness. After they had been patients in the Boston City Hospital for some time, they were propped up in bed and asked to sign some papers, which, they presumed, were annulments of their contracts. Riley was in the Boston City Hospital for 10 weeks, and for 6 months thereafter her weakened heart sapped her strength.

Harriet C. Lounsberry, who succeeded Maxwell as chief nurse at Sternberg Hospital, kept a list of all the nurses who had departed from the hospital (Table 7-1) and recorded the reason why each had left.[15]

TYPHOID INVESTIGATION COMMISSION

A team of medical officers, consisting of Major Walter Reed, Major Victor C. Vaughan, and Major Edward O. Shakespeare, was appointed by the secretary of war on August 18, 1898, to investigate the cause of the prevalence of typhoid fever in the various military camps within the United States. Before it could begin compiling statistical data, the typhoid investigation commission had to determine the minimum period of incubation in typhoid fever.

The arrival of 50 trained women nurses from Chicago at Camp Thomas soon enabled the commission to obtain the desired information. The commissioners assumed that all the new arrivals were free from typhoid infection when they began their hospital work. They watched each nurse carefully, and when the first nurse came down with typhoid fever 10 days after her arrival, they concluded that the minimum period of incubation in typhoid fever was

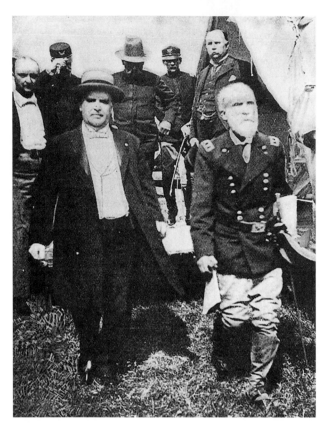

President McKinley and General Joseph Wheeler visit patients.

nated water supplies, infected food, and germ-carrying flies. The typical clinical picture revealed a disease of gradual onset, with vague anorexia and lassitude, low-grade headache, gastrointestinal upset, and pyrexia. Common specific symptoms, in order of frequency, were abdominal discomfort, joint and back pains, diarrhea without blood, slight cough, and vomiting. Good nursing proved absolutely essential, for the patients needed much rest, care of the skin and mouth, physiotherapy, and, most importantly, adequate fluid intake with a high-protein, low-roughage diet. Observers quickly realized that the desperately ill soldiers, many of them homesick, were acutely aware of how superior trained women nurses were to untrained male nurses. Under such circumstances, soldiers greeted the trained woman nurse as an angel of mercy in camp, on board ship, and in the hospital.

ADVENTURES ON A HOSPITAL SHIP

Realizing that military operations in Cuba would necessitate the evacuation of the sick and wounded by sea, the surgeon general urged the fitting out of a hospital ship. The steamer *John Englis* was purchased on May 18, 1898, rechristened the *U.S.S. Relief*, and supplied with the more important medicines and dressings, along with enough equipment to outfit a 750-bed hospital for 6 months.

something less than 10 days. This finding was later confirmed repeatedly. Vaughan wrote, "Of course with our present knowledge we would have vaccinated these girls and the probabilities are that all would have escaped the disease."[16]

The commission concluded that, had a conscious effort been made to demonstrate the epidemiology of typhoid fever, it could hardly have been better staged than at Camp Thomas.

> At first there were practically no trained nurses or hospital orderlies, either males or females. Before us every morning regiments were drawn up and so many men detailed from the ranks to serve in the hospitals as orderlies for the day. We followed these men to the hospitals and saw them handling bed pans in the awkward, ignorant way, often soiling their hands as well as the bedding, floors and the ground. At noon they went to lunch mostly without washing their hands, to say nothing of disinfecting them, handling their food, and passing it to their comrades. A like demonstration was repeated at supper. The next day a repetition of this cycle was re-enacted.[17]

The 20,926 cases of typhoid in the army during the Spanish-American War were precipitated by contami-

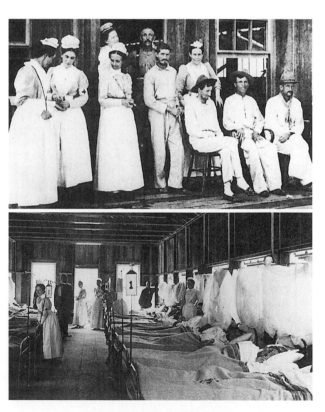

Army nurse with typhoid patient.

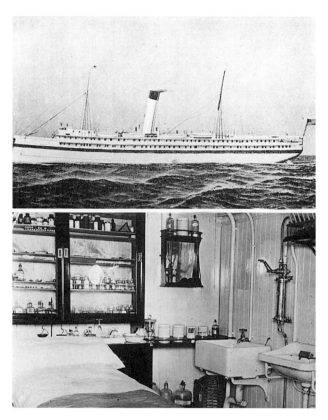

The U.S.S. Relief, *exterior and dispensary.*

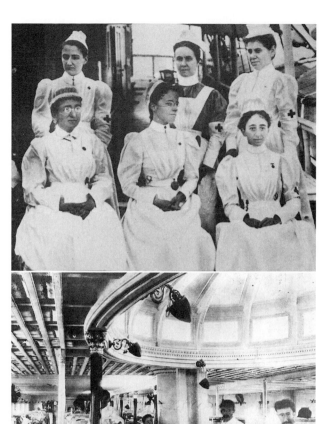

Hospital ship nurses; Ward 3 view of U.S.S. Relief.

Esther V. Hasson of New London, Connecticut, who later became the first superintendent of the Navy Nurse Corps, recalled that she experienced one of the greatest thrills of her life when she received a letter from Dr. McGee asking her to accept an assignment for surgical work aboard the *Relief.* A recent graduate of training school, she longed for something more exciting than private-duty nursing. "Therefore, with youth and enthusiasm sufficient to counteract the rather depressing prospect of $30 per month [and] one ration in kind, I started out on the Great Adventure," she wrote.[18]

It was July 3 before the *Relief* steamed out of Tampa harbor. The six women nurses aboard were immensely proud of their ship—beautiful in her fresh coat of white paint, with the green stripe of the Medical Corps encircling her hull, and flying the Stars and Stripes and the Red Cross flag. The space allotted to the hospital on two of the upper decks was divided into three large wards and one small ward of 30 beds, intended for officers but frequently used for overflow from the larger wards. The operating room directly to the right of the gangway was outfitted with the usual up-to-date equipment. Its crowning glory was the large X-ray machine lent by the Medical Museum in Washington.

"We made all possible speed to Cuba and upon arrival at Siboney, the hospital base of our army, were thrilled by the news of the naval battle [of Santiago

Bay], which had taken place while we were at sea," related Hasson.[19] On the morning of July 3, the Spanish squadron had steamed out of Santiago Bay, where it had been bottled up by the American fleet, and had turned sharply westward in a daring effort to escape. Because the commanders of all the American warships had specific orders concerning just such an escape attempt, they closed in on the enemy vessels and forced them to hold their course near the shore, where maneuver was impossible. With the *Brooklyn, Oregon,* and *Texas* in the lead, at the end of a 43-mile chase they had either destroyed or run aground the four enemy cruisers. The Spanish lost 323 killed and 151 wounded in this battle, while Americans suffered only 2 casualties. Although battle losses were small, rapidly deteriorating sanitary conditions were taking a toll. Yellow fever had broken out; malaria, typhoid, and dysentery were spreading. Hospital equipment and nourishment for the sick were in short supply, and incessant rain enveloped the nurses in seemingly endless vapor baths.

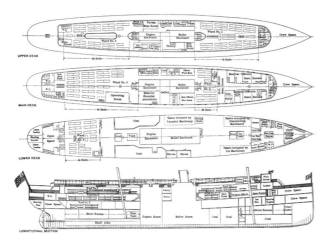

Layout of the hospital ship U.S.S. Relief.

The *Relief* nurses began admitting patients at once. For several days thereafter, boatloads of wounded, sick, and exhausted soldiers arrived on board. Many had not removed their uniforms for days, and, being too sick to care for themselves, they appeared in pitiful condition. After a bath, a clean bed, and sufficient nourishment, many regained enough strength to be shipped north on transports. Those in urgent need of medical or surgical attention remained on the hospital ship. During the 2 months from July 15 to September 15, 1898, the nurses aboard the *Relief* cared for 1234 sick, of whom 49 died, and for 251 wounded, of whom 16 died.

ON TO CUBA

Meanwhile, the destruction of the Spanish naval squadron had completely demoralized the beleaguered Santiago garrison, which, unable to secure reinforcements, had no choice but to capitulate. After 2 weeks of negotiations, General William R. Shafter accepted the unconditional surrender of the Spanish forces on July 17. It occurred at an opportune moment, inasmuch as the American expeditionary force was itself threatened with extermination by yellow fever, malaria, dysentery, and food poisoning. Ten days after the Spanish had surrendered, more than 4000 of Shafter's men were reported sick, and within a few more days Colonel Theodore Roosevelt stated that not even 10% of the men in his regiment were fit for active duty.

Physicians still had much to learn about the detection of yellow fever, malaria, and typhoid—the scourges that afflicted the army in 1898. Secretary of War Russell Alger told General Shafter, on July 13 and 14, to begin shifting camps and quarantining yellow fever suspects. When new yellow fever cases quit developing among the regiment, Alger said, the troops could be shipped back to the United States. Alger did not anticipate an early return of the army,

which he thought should remain at Santiago "until the fever has had its run."[20]

In response to urgent pleas from Shafter, the War Department dispatched 65 physicians, 729 women nurses, and a large quantity of medical stores to Santiago. Among this contingent of nurses was Lillian Kratz from Saint Louis, who described her arrival in Cuba as follows:

> So under order, we embarked from New York Harbor, across the Atlantic, and steamed into Santiago Harbor, our battleship proud and defiant as we passed the fleet of battleships, dotted here and there in close proximity in the harbor. As we neared our destination, I think our brave hearts fluttered a bit at the great uncertainty that awaited all of us. When we anchored and got foot ashore, the sun was just sinking to rest, and on board of one of the battleships, we could hear the familiar strains of the Star Spangled Banner, and My Country 'Tis of Thee. To the right of us was the desolate battlefield, and as the sun gradually sank behind the horizon, casting the reflection of its rays in purple and gold on San Juan hill where our dead and dying still lay, and as the sun's glow became fainter and fainter, it seemed to cast a benediction over all, it seemed to say, "God be with you and with thy spirit—peace be to thy soul." And so we landed with this sombre setting on one side, while on the left we could see the huge palm trees.[21]

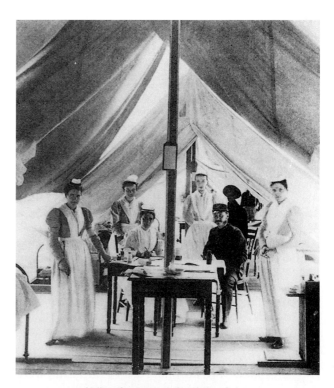

Yellow fever ward, Santiago, Cuba.

FIGHTING YELLOW FEVER

Anna Turner, a nurse from New York City, was asked by some of her friends in the United States to describe the symptoms and treatment of the yellow fever victims for whom she was caring. She told them that the patients first complained of a severe aching of the whole body, much the same as in other acute diseases, but that the nausea and vomiting became much more pronounced. The patient's temperature, which did not run as high as in typhoid, rarely exceeded 104 F°. As temperature rose, the pulse usually slowed—another symptom that one looked for when making a diagnosis. Because of their intense suffering, the men afflicted with yellow fever always appeared restless and rolled from one side to the other. In many cases, boards had to be put on the sides of their beds to prevent them from falling out.

The extreme nausea and vomiting continued until the crisis passed, a period of 6 or 8 days. Hemorrhage was nearly always present, the most common form being the bleeding of the gums. Next came that of the stomach, which caused the "black vomit" so often referred to. Turner had seen two cases of hemorrhage from the kidneys and a few in which the veins of the surface of the body ruptured and formed great knots under the skin. All the patients showed kidney dysfunction and produced urine loaded with albumin. Patients invariably suffered from constipation and usually had jaundice. The fever also caused a distinctive odor found in no other disease. Because the Cubans never seemed to contract the disease, nearly all of Turner's patients were either Spaniards or Americans.

The general care was much the same as for other acute diseases. Because of the supposed contagion, all patients received a daily soap-and-water bath and a complete change of linen. Cold sponges were applied to reduce the high temperature and restlessness. The patients' mouths had to be cleansed thoroughly and frequently owing to the constant bleeding of the gums. Because they could not take or retain medicine, patients received two enemas of plain faucet water daily. No nourishment of any kind was given until all nausea and vomiting had ceased, a period of about 1 week. But due to the condition of the kidneys and the large amount of albumin present in the urine, water was forced day and night, regardless of the nausea and vomiting.

When the patients could safely ingest food, the nurses began by giving them milk, 2 drams every 6 hours. In the absence of digestive disturbances, the quantity slowly increased until the patients received 4 oz every 3 hours. Then a dose of castor oil was administered. When they had recovered from its effects, they were ready for solid food. Three different buildings functioned as wards: one for suspected cases of yellow fever, one for acute cases, and one for convalescents. The extremely ill and dying patients had to be shifted constantly to keep them isolated.

With the orderlies so expert in moving patients easily and quickly, the nurses going off duty had to report the new location of the various patients. Every morning the night nurse had to total all the fluids taken in and excreted by the patients during the last 24 hours. Turner then recorded these figures on charts.

Later, when a camp was established a few miles from the city of Havana for the study of yellow fever, Turner became involved in the first experiments to prove or disprove that yellow fever was a contagious disease. The nurses were asked to set aside the sheets and pillow cases taken from the beds of their worst cases and put these on beds in screened tents. Uninfected men who had volunteered for the purpose then slept in these tents. When no cases developed during a period of several weeks, it was proved that yellow fever was not contagious.

It was then decided to test the theory of Dr. Carlos Finley of Havana, who maintained that a certain species of mosquito carried the disease. The physicians came to the hospitals daily, armed with test tubes containing swarms of the suspected carriers. These were allowed to bite infected patients and then were carefully released to bite uninfected volunteers, who shortly thereafter contracted the disease. These tests proved yellow fever to be a mosquito-borne disease transmitted by only one kind of mosquito. They also established the incubation period during which a mosquito that had bitten a yellow fever patient could transmit the infection to another man: Mosquitoes that bit fevered patients after the third or fourth day of the patients' illness were no longer capable of carrying the infection. Upon this discovery, newly diagnosed patients with yellow fever were soon kept in screened cages inside well-screened wards until the period of infection passed.

During these experiments, nurses displayed a heroism and devotion to duty equal to that of any soldier or sailor in battle. Among these courageous nurses, the example set by 25-year-old Clara Louise Maass of East Orange, New Jersey, deserves special mention. Moved by the suffering of her yellow fever patients and aware that scientific knowledge about the disease was pitifully inadequate, she volunteered to be bitten by a carrier mosquito to increase this knowledge. She was bitten on the hand, and when the subsequent attack of yellow fever was not considered sufficiently immunizing, she was bitten several more times. A martyr to science, she perished from these infections but helped prove that yellow fever was carried by mosquitoes.

DISEASE DRIVES THE ARMY HOME

Meanwhile, by August 1, the soldiers of the American expeditionary force were suffering more from disease than from Spanish bullets. Few precautions had been taken to safeguard the health of the men be-

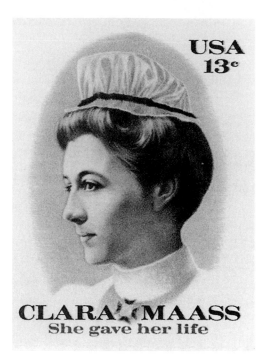

Clara Louise Maass.

cause the Medical Corps knew little about tropical diseases and because no effective measures had yet been developed to combat malaria and yellow fever. Theodore Roosevelt described the situation as

> horrible in every respect. I have over 100 men down with fever in my own camp out of my regiment of 400, 200 have previously died or having been sent to the rear hospitals. The mismanagement of the hospital's service in the rear has been such that my men will not leave the regiment if they can possibly help it; yet here we have nothing for them but hardtack, bacon, and . . . coffee without sugar.[22]

On August 3, 1898, a group of volunteer officers of the V Corps assembled and drafted a round-robin letter describing the wretched plight of the army. After this letter had been circulated and signed by all the divisional and brigade commanders, it was sent to General William R. Shafter, who forwarded it to Washington. Even before this document had reached Shafter, however, it had been leaked to the press, thanks largely to Theodore Roosevelt, now a brigade commander, who had been instrumental in composing it. The substance of this message was, "This army must be moved at once or it will perish."[23] Secretary of War Alger, who on the previous day had wired Shafter that there would be a considerable delay in moving troops from Cuba, quickly changed his mind on receipt of this news and ordered the immediate evacuation of the expeditionary force to Montauk Point, Long Island. The first shipload of troops left Santiago on August 7, fleeing from the scene of their triumph as if pursued by the enemy.

On Surgeon General Sternberg's recommendation, Secretary Alger had selected 5000 acres of rolling ground at Montauk Point, on the eastern tip of Long Island, as the expedition's rest and recuperation camp. Christened Camp Wikoff, it was remote enough for effective quarantine, and troops arriving from Santiago could disembark there without passing through any of the port cities. When completed, the installation comprised a detention camp, where newly arrived regiments were to be quarantined until proved free of yellow fever, and a larger general camp, where the troops were to rest and recover their strength. Each camp was to have a large hospital.

When the regiments from Santiago began disembarking on August 14, four fifths of the soldiers were ill and more than 10,000 required hospitalization. Most of the others were so enfeebled that they resembled walking scarecrows. Eighty-seven men had died aboard the transport ships, and about 200 more died after reaching the camp. Because the exhausted soldiers found no facilities ready for them, they were forced to sleep on the ground in tents without bedding. Sometimes they subsisted for days on short rations. In the half-completed, understaffed hospitals, sick men went untended for 24 hours at a time. Surgeon General Sternberg quickly authorized his subordinates at Wikoff to hire extra doctors and nurses without first having to send their requisitions to Washington for his approval.

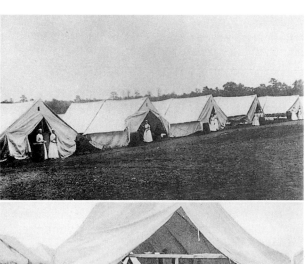

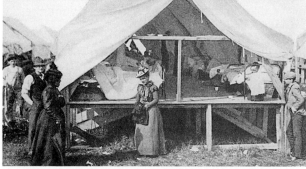

Nurses stand outside of hospital tents at Camp Wikoff.

NIGHTMARE ON A LONG ISLAND BEACH

As a result of this poor preparation and lack of trained personnel, chaos reigned at Camp Wikoff. Nurse Kate M. Walsh reported that her white clothing was not suitable because there were no laundry facilities. According to her, the nurses should have worn canvas frocks. In 2 days she was "filthy-looking and distressed." The patients' beds, placed only a foot apart, had springs of wire mesh that protruded from all sides and tore the nurses' clothes to ribbons. Walsh further stated that nurses "kept getting sick and some had to be sent away, some dying." One "convenience hut" was without a door for some time. Nurses fainted in this place and had to be carried away.[24]

Walsh confided that each night she felt she could not stand another day: "The heat was intense and I perspired freely from long hours of overwork, heat and flies, together with my anguish that our dear sick men were not half cared for."[25] In an attempt to relieve their overcrowded wards, surgeons at Montauk released hundreds of men prematurely; sick, sometimes dying, stragglers from Camp Wikoff collapsed in passenger cars and railroad stations across Long Island.

After this wretched beginning, conditions at Montauk slowly improved. The Medical Department enlarged its hospital facilities and brought in scores of contract surgeons along with about 300 women nurses. Numerous newspaper articles described the miserable conditions at the camp and mentioned the positive effect of women nurses on patient care. For example, a correspondent for *Harper's Weekly* wrote, "There is no exaggeration in the current stories of the starvation and utter neglect of these, our returning heroes." He further reported:

> I saw the Eighth (regulars) arrive at their camp. They came from the detention camp in army wagons. When the wagons stopped, many of the men fell headlong in attempting to get down, and lay just where they fell. One, a bugler, stood a little while, swaying and dazed, and then fell in a heap by the roadside. . . . It remains only to say a word of appreciation of the self-sacrificing Red Cross nurses and Sisters of Charity, who are working night and day in the hospitals, and to hope and pray that the like of the shameful spectacle of those poor famished lads gathered together after all their glory of achievement may never be witnessed in this country again.[26]

Each ward in the camp hospitals consisted of seven-section tents, with board floors, placed end to end. Soon there were 40 wards, each supposed to have four nurses and two orderlies on duty during the day and two nurses and two orderlies at night. Between the wards ran a boardwalk with kitchen and dining sheds at one end, where a large number of nurses, orderlies, and clergymen came for their meals.

At midnight a lunch was served for the night nurses, who took turns in going to the dining shed. Carrying lanterns, they would "follow along the boardwalk and watch the other lanterns flickering in the darkness, some coming, some going, and then in the none too well lighted shed we would eat our midnight meal." Miss Mary A. Quinn reported that her experience seemed a kind of dream, imaged by "the stream of faces coming in suddenly from the black night, the hurried meal, and the return to the darkness."[27]

By September 15, 281 nurses were on duty at Camp Wikoff. At this time, each of 43 hospital tents, designed to hold 30 cots, often contained 50 patients. Surgeons soon transferred more than 1000 of the camp's sick to hospitals in New York, Boston, Philadelphia, Providence, and other Northeastern cities. The shelter and care afforded to patients who remained at Montauk improved significantly. They were discharged as soon as possible, and by the end of October 1898, the former hospital sites at Montauk Point had reverted to empty sand dunes. Despite reassuring statements from authorities that everything possible had been done, thousands of citizens who had visited or read about Camp Wikoff formed the unshakable conviction that the soldiers who had risked all for their country had been betrayed by the government.

A GOVERNMENT INVESTIGATION

On August 12, 1898, the Spaniards signed an armistice that brought the Spanish-American War to an end. During the calendar year May 1898 through April 1899, the army suffered 968 battle casualties and 5438 deaths from disease. In stark contrast to the Civil War, in which 18% had fallen in battle, 15% had died of wounds, and 67% had died of disease, the Spanish-American War saw 10% slain in combat, 2% dead of wounds, and 88% killed by disease. These statistics provoked heavy criticism of the Medical Department.

On September 8, 1898, President McKinley, at the request of the secretary of war, appointed a commission to investigate the conduct of the War Department during hostilities with Spain. This commission, headed by Grenville Dodge, held 109 meetings and heard a vast amount of testimony concerning the work of female nurses.

The Dodge Commission published the following conclusions and recommendations in regard to army nursing: During the months of May, June, and July, the nursing force "was neither ample nor efficient, reasons for which may be found in the lack of proper volunteer hospital corps, due to the failure of Congress to authorize its establishment, and to the non-recognition in the beginning of the value of women nurses and the extent to which their services could be secured." What the Medical Department needed in the future was a corps of selected trained women nurses "ready to serve when necessity shall arise, but, under ordinary circumstances, owing no duty to the War Department, except to report residence at determined intervals."[28]

The number of women army nurses had reached a maximum of 1158 on September 15, 1898. After this date, many nursing contracts were annulled because the suppression of the typhoid epidemic and the mustering out of volunteer regiments rendered so large a nursing force unnecessary. Between the first appointments on May 10 and the close of 1898, the number of contracted women nurses totaled 1563. They had worked on 3 ships and at 42 places, 9 of the locations being camps that had contained several hospitals each.

UNWANTED WOMEN ARMY NURSES

The position of women nurses in the army was precarious, however, as indicated by a letter from Major L. M. Maus, surgeon and commander of the U.S. Hospital at Fort Hamilton, New York, to Surgeon General Sternberg, dated June 3, 1899:

> Should we expect to restore the Hospital Corps to that grade of efficiency that existed previous to the Spanish-American War, the employment of female nurses must be discontinued. As a result of the present state of affairs, the hospital private takes no interest in his duties as a nurse, nor can he be expected to, so long as he is brought in contact with the female nurse. There is a decided tendency on the part of the latter to ignore entirely the hospital corpsman's ability to care for his sick comrade, and to put him aside except for the menial duties of the ward.
>
> Divested of any responsibility in the way of taking temperature, attending the serious cases, administering medicine, dressing wounds, etc., the private soon becomes a willing party to the arrangement, and hence his utter worthlessness as a nurse in the course of a very short time. It is practically impossible to divide the ward work equally between nurses so radically different in class. I also find it difficult to preserve good military discipline with this mixed personnel.[29]

Especially severe was Major Maus's indictment against women nurses for "coddling" their patients:

> The "coddling process," which is characteristic of the female nurse in caring for male patients, has become more accentuated in her treatment of the sick soldier, through some maudlin sentiment; as a consequence, I find that many men apply for treatment, who under normal conditions would never think of going to the hospital.[30]

As a result of such hostile attitudes on the part of the military authorities, only 202 women nurses remained in army service by July 1, 1899.

MOVEMENT TO ESTABLISH AN ARMY NURSE CORPS

As early as December 1898, a committee of influential women, many of whom were prominent nurses, advocated passage of legislation to establish a permanent Army Nurse Corps. Mrs. Winthop Cowdin was the first chairman of this "Committee to Secure by Act of Congress the Employment of Women Nurses in the Hospital Service of the United States Army." Mrs. Whitelaw Reid, wife of the editor of the *New York Tribune*, contributed $500 in support of this movement, while others donated smaller sums. With the aid of these funds, the committee was able to recruit a sizable working force in Washington, DC, secure able counsel, and open offices in New York and Washington.

Adelaide Nutting, principal of Johns Hopkins Training School for Nurses, was charged with informing the nursing groups of the importance of the proposed reform. A bill providing for the establishment of a permanent Army Nurse Corps was introduced into the House of Representatives on January 24 by Congressman Michael Griffin of Wisconsin. On January 25 it was presented to the Senate by Senator Julius C. Burrowes of Michigan and referred by each body to its Committee on Military Affairs.

A delegation of the bill's supporters appeared before the House Military Affairs Committee on February 3, 1899. The bill's virtues were outlined in detail by Margaret Chanler, a wealthy young aristocrat of the Astor family, who had been selected as speaker because of her "heroic service last summer" during the war with Spain. She was accompanied by Mrs. Bayard Cutting and Mrs. Winthrop Cowdin, "both exquisitely gowned," according to the report.[31]

On the same day, at the Washington home of Mrs. John McLean, the wives of some senators and representatives held a meeting at which the nursing committee explained the full purpose of the bill. The lively discussion that ensued indicated that the nurses had many warm supporters among those present. The bill, reported on favorably by the Military Affairs Committee that same day, came before the House the following Monday, February 6. Although it passed by 40 votes, it lacked the full two-thirds majority necessary for it to be removed from the calendar. When the measure came before the Senate Committee on Military Affairs, it fell only one vote short of gaining approval.

In the belief that military medicine would derive much greater benefit from the services of graduate nurses than from those of the nonprofessional Hospital Corps, nursing leaders continued to agitate for a permanent Nurse Corps. Despite adverse opinions

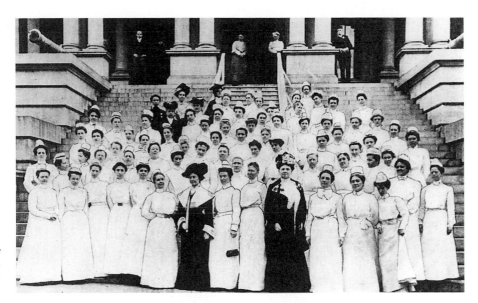

Dr. Anita McGee (in dark coat, front row, left) and a group of Spanish-American War nurses on the steps of the War Department in Washington, DC.

from several of his ranking officers, the once-reluctant surgeon general finally accepted the idea of women nurses as a permanent component of the Medical Department.

Because plans for a reorganization of the army already existed, Sternberg assigned Dr. Anita McGee the task of drafting a proposal for creating the Army Nurse Corps. This proposal, presented to Congress as part of a bill for a general army reorganization, was written in the War Department and received the approval of both the surgeon general and the secretary of war. Before passing this bill, the Senate added an amendment that the superintendent of the Nurse Corps had to be a hospital school graduate. Because Dr. McGee was not, she was forced to resign from the army when the Army Nurse Corps was established on February 2, 1901. Dita H. Kinney, head nurse of the U.S. Army Hospital at Fort Bayard, New Mexico, succeeded her as the superintendent of the Army Nurse Corps.

THE NAVY NURSE CORPS IS BORN

Surgeon General Presley M. Rixey of the navy also became convinced that women nurses were by natural endowment and special aptitude superior to male nurses for much of the duty required in the care of sick and injured men. He felt sure that their use would not conflict with the conditions arising from service in naval installations. Of course, the women nurses would have no place at sea except on hospital ships. But in the naval hospitals, where nine tenths of

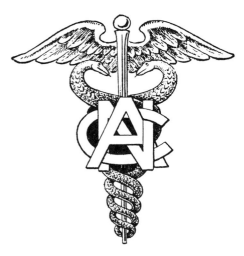

Insignia of the new Army Nurse Corps.

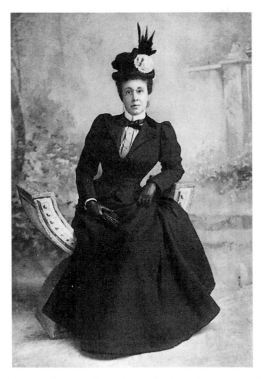

Dita H. Kinney, first superintendent of the Army Nurse Corps, 1901.

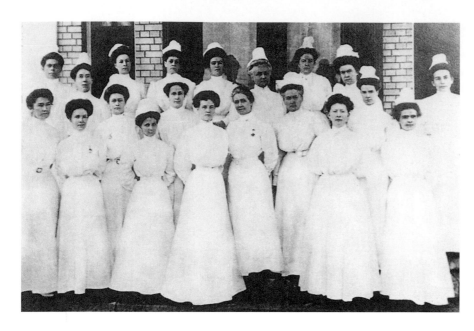

"The Sacred Twenty," the initial 20 members of the Navy Nurse Corps in 1908. Esther Hasson, the superintendent, stands in the front row, center.

the serious cases were treated, their exceptional capabilities for work in hospital wards and operating rooms made their services most desirable.

Congress was slow to act on the matter, and in his report for 1907, Surgeon General Rixey stated that he could not understand why it was so difficult to obtain congressional approval for such a worthy measure. He recalled that the desirability of using trained women nurses in the medical branch of the naval service had been urged on Congress for 5 years. The lack of female nurses was the most serious omission in the Medical Bureau.

His efforts finally bore fruit in 1908, when the Nurse Corps was established as an integral unit of the navy. The first group of nurses assigned to the Naval Medical School Hospital in Washington, DC, consisted of a superintendent, a chief nurse, and 18 staff nurses. Because the navy did not provide quarters for these nurses, they had to rent a house and cook their own meals.

Esther Hasson was appointed the first superintendent of the corps and served for 3 years. During her tenure the nurses proved their worth, and an additional 24 nurses were appointed. Early in 1909, nurses were sent to the naval hospitals in Annapolis and Brooklyn. Soon they were receiving orders for duty at Mare Island, California, and other naval hospitals. In 1910 the navy sent its first nurses to the Philippines and soon afterward to Guam, Honolulu, Yokohama, Samoa, the Virgin Islands, Haiti, and Guantánamo Bay, Cuba.

As the only women in the navy, the nurses formed a unique group. By congressional order they were designated as neither officers nor enlisted men, but they had military, as distinguished from civilian, status. Despite their nebulous rank, the nurses of the navy earned the unqualified praise of the surgeon general, who regarded their work as excellent and noted their positive effect in improving the level of nursing service in naval hospitals.

The official establishment of the Army Nurse Corps and the Navy Nurse Corps represented an important step in the professionalization of nursing. For the first time, two large nursing services were staffed entirely by graduate nurses. Student nurses, who represented the bulk of the work force in civil hospitals, had no place in this structure. Thus the military nursing services provided an opportunity for a unique demonstration in patient care.

REFERENCES

1. Unidentified newspaper clipping, May 17, 1898, McGee Papers, National Archives, Washington, DC, RG 112 (hereinafter cited as "McGee Papers").
2. Daughters of the American Revolution, *Second Report of the National Society of the Daughters of the American Revolution, October 11, 1897–October 11, 1898* (Washington, DC: Government Printing Office, 1900), Senate Document No. 425.
3. Application blank to applicants interested in nursing in the Army, McGee Papers.
4. Sternberg to Alger, May 3, 1898, McGee Papers.
5. V. C. Vaughan, *A Doctor's Memories* (Indianapolis: Bobbs-Merrill, 1926), pp. 385–386.
6. Bayne to McGee, July 10, 1898, McGee Papers.
7. A. C. Maxwell, "The Field Hospital at Chickamauga Park," *Trained Nurse and Hospital Review*, vol. 23 (July 1899):3.
8. H. C. Lounsberry, "Some Reminiscences of Sternberg Hospital," *American Journal of Nursing*, vol. 3 (November 1902):83.
9. J. S. Edmunds, *Leaves from a Nurse's Life's History* (Rochester: Press of the Democrat & Chronicle, 1905), p. 23.
10. Ibid.
11. Helen B. Schuler and Florence M. Kelly, "Reminiscences," McGee Papers.
12. Carter to McGee, August 19, 1898, McGee Papers.
13. Barbara U. Austin, "Conditions at Sternberg Hospital, Chickamauga, Georgia," undated, McGee Papers.

14. Jane R. Riley, "Sternberg Hospital," undated, McGee Papers.
15. U.S. War Department, Typhoid Commission, *Report (of Board) on Origin and Spread of Typhoid Fever in the U.S. Military Camps During the Spanish War of 1898. By Walter Reed, Victor C. Vaughan, and Edward O. Shakespeare* (Washington, DC: Government Printing Office, 1904), vol. 1, p. 283.
16. Vaughan, op. cit., pp. 386–387.
17. Ibid., p. 385.
18. E. V. Hasson, "The First Trip of the Army Hospital Ship *Relief*," undated, McGee Papers.
19. Ibid.
20. War Investigating Commission, *Report of the Commission Appointed by the President to Investigate the Conduct of the War with Spain* (Washington, DC: Government Printing Office, 1899), vol. 3, pp. 26–29.
21. L. Kratz, "Reminiscences of Santiago," undated, McGee Papers.
22. Henry Cabot Lodge, ed., *Selections from the Correspondence of Theodore Roosevelt and Henry Cabot Lodge, 1884–1918* (New York: Scribner's Sons, 1925), vol. 1, pp. 325–329, 331–334.
23. Russell A. Alger, *The Spanish-American War* (New York: Harper & Brothers, 1901), pp. 265–273.
24. K. M. Walsh, "Camp Wikoff, Montauk Point," undated, McGee Papers.
25. Ibid.
26. W. A. Rogers, "Camp Wikoff," *Harper's Weekly*, vol. 42 (September 10, 1898):890.
27. M. A. Quinn, "Montauk Point," undated, McGee Papers.
28. War Investigating Commission, op. cit., pp. 395–396.
29. Maus to Sternberg, June 3, 1899, copy in McGee Papers.
30. Ibid.
31. A. N. McGee, "The Army Nurse Corps in 1899," *Trained Nurse and Hospital Review*, vol. 24 (February 1900):119.

THE RISE OF PUBLIC HEALTH NURSING

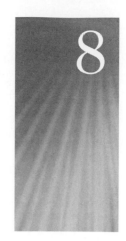

As the United States approached the 20th century, one of its most exciting developments was the rise of its cities. Their phenomenal growth eclipsed even the giant strides being made in industrialization. It was, of course, the rise of industry that made city growth possible, along with transportation improvements that enabled business to become national. Every city had its elegant mansions, the homes of fastidiously dressed socialites. In New York, they lined Fifth Avenue. In Chicago, they occupied two districts, the North Side and the South Side. The splendor carried over to monumental public buildings, formidable-looking banks, spacious churches, and luxurious hotels. Yet in every city the poor greatly outnumbered the well-to-do. Their hovels stood within a few blocks of the great mansions.

THE INFLUX OF IMMIGRANTS

During the 9 decades from 1820 to 1910, nearly 30 million immigrants entered the United States; of these, 91% came from Europe. Until 1883, about 95% of the movement from Europe originated in the United Kingdom, Germany, Scandinavia, France, Belgium, Holland, and Switzerland. Even as late as 1882, these countries furnished 87% of the total immigration from Europe. By 1907, however, 81% of the immigrants came from Austria-Hungary, Italy, Russia, Greece, Turkey, Spain, Portugal, Serbia, Romania, Bulgaria, and Montenegro. Thus, in less than one generation, the principal sources of immigration had shifted drastically, and with this shift came a host of new social, economic, and health problems.

In 1893, the foreign-born population in the city of Baltimore was 16% of the total; in the slum district, 40%. In Chicago, foreign-born persons in the entire city constituted 41% of the population but 58% of the slum district. In New York, the foreign-born population made up 42% of the total population and 63% of the inhabitants of slum districts. In Philadelphia, the foreign-born constituted 26% of the total and 60% of the slum dwellers. Thus the proportion of foreign-born was much higher in the slums of each city than in the total population pool.

Of all the great cities, New York was perhaps the most intimately concerned with the problems of immigrants. By the late 1880s, foreigners from southern and eastern Europe had become a large element in the city's population. Italians had moved into the old Irish neighborhoods and in 1890 were found massed in the wards west of the Bowery. Russian and Polish Jews were packed to the east of the Bowery and were scattered up the east side of the city to Harlem. Hungarians, a considerable proportion of whom were Jews, were gathered in a large colony east of Avenue B, around Houston Street, and Bohemians centered on the Upper East Side, near the river, from about Fiftieth to Sixtieth streets.

The following is an impression of New York's Italian colony in 1884:

> In Jersey Street exist two courtyards. Six three-story houses are in each. These houses are old and long ago worn out. They are packed with tenants, rotten with age and decay, and so constructed as to have made them very undesirable for dwelling purposes [even] in their earliest infancy. The Italians who chiefly inhabit them are the scum of New York chiffoniers, and as such saturated with the filth inseparable from their business. The courtyard swarms with, in daytime, females in the picturesque attires of Genoa and Piedmont, moving between the dirty children. The abundant rags, paper, sacks, barrels, washtubs, dogs, and cats are all festooned overhead by clotheslines weighted with such garments as are only known in Italy. Sorting is chiefly done indoors, but at times a ragpicker may be seen at his work in any convenient spot to be had. In each yard live 24 families (nominally only, because lodgers here as elsewhere are

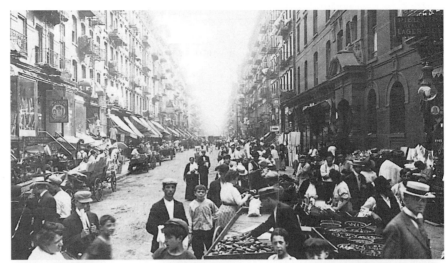

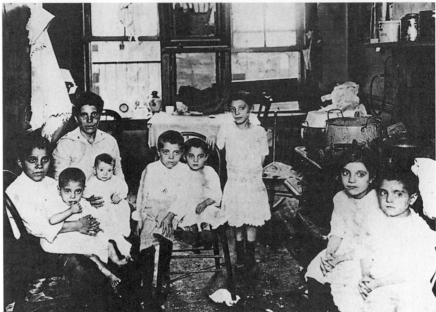

Immigrants from southern and eastern Europe required a new health care approach.

always welcome), paying rents of from $6 to $9 monthly for two rooms, the inner one being subdivided by a partition consisting perhaps of a simple curtain, and measuring when so arranged about 5 by 6 feet each.[1]

TENEMENT HOUSES

As space commanded more of a premium, tenement houses were constructed. In 1879, a new architectural design had accelerated their erection and greatly contributed to the congestion. A New Yorker had devised a dumbbell-shaped floor plan that could pack an amazing number of occupants into a narrow six-story building. The "dumbbell" tenement soon became the standardized type. It was supposedly an improvement because an air shaft gave each room some slight exposure to the sun. Actually, by concentrating a minimum of 24 families in a six-story walk-up building on a narrow lot of 25 by 90 feet without any play yard, the dumbbell multiple dwelling, which sometimes housed as many as 36 families, made congestion, clutter, and dirt more acute.

The usefulness of the air shaft as a means of ventilation was subverted by its typical use as a garbage dump. It was said in the course of a tenement house investigation that, due to the rotting garbage, the air shaft could be called a "foul air shaft" or a "culture on a gigantic scale," and that it was simply a "stagnant well of foul air emptying into each of the rooms opening upon it." Many people testified that "the air from these shafts was so foul and the odor so vile that they had to close their windows opening into them,

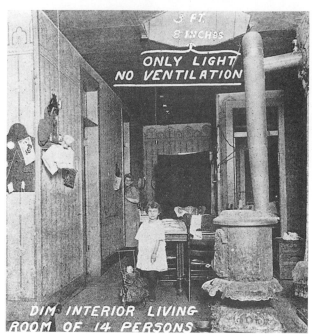

Typical tenement house environment.

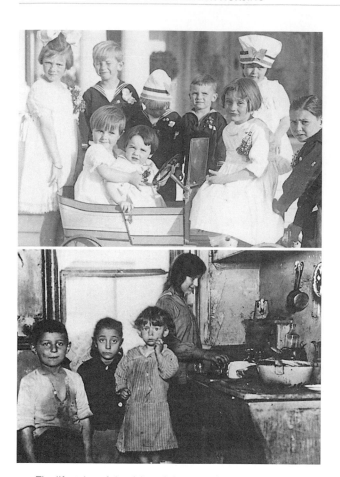

The lifestyles of the rich and the poor contrasted sharply.

and in some cases the windows were permanently nailed up for this reason."[2]

By the mid-1890s, about two thirds of the 3,500,000 people living in New York were packed into 90,000 tenement houses in districts without parks or recreation areas. In one New York block of tenements, 577 people were crowded into 96 rooms. In the 10th ward on Manhattan Island, the average population density was 747 people per acre. Boston developed its own characteristic form of "three-decker" wooden tenement. Slum colonies were found not only along the Eastern seaboard but also in interior cities such as Cincinnati and Chicago. To make matters worse, immigrant families often converted their apartments into sweatshops, where garments or cigars were manufactured amid the most unsanitary conditions.

Such slums endangered health. In 1880, New York City, with a population of 1.2 million, had a death rate of more than 25 per 1000 and an average of 16 people to a dwelling. London, a far larger city, with a population of 3.8 million, recorded a death rate of 21 per 1000 and averaged fewer than 8 persons to a dwelling. One especially crowded tract in New York had such a high death rate from tuberculosis that it was known as the "lung block." With vermin abundant and sanitary facilities inadequate and

often out of order, diseases were inevitable. Any that were communicable had an excellent opportunity to spread, often with a strong likelihood of fatality. Slum dwellers were ravaged by epidemics of typhus, scarlet fever, smallpox, and typhoid fever, and many of them died or developed tuberculosis or other communicable diseases.

ESTABLISHMENT OF VISITING NURSING

More than 20 years earlier in Great Britain, the wife of William Rathbone, a wealthy citizen of Liverpool, died in 1859 after a long and painful illness. She had been attended during her illness by a very competent trained nurse, whose care had brought her great relief. Rathbone, a philanthropist, had long been interested in helping the Liverpool poor. He had concluded that if skilled nursing could do so much for his wife, who had already had everything that wealth could procure, how much more might it do for the poor, whose illnesses were aggravated by the misery of their surroundings. Rathbone was a man of action as well as of vision, and his kindly thoughts quickly crystallized into a concrete plan for helping the needy sick of Liverpool: nurses should be sent to their homes. To test the idea, Mary Robinson, the nurse who had attended his wife, was employed for a 3-month term to visit the ailing poor of Liverpool.

Curiously enough, opposition to Rathbone's undertaking was based on the very lack of comfort and the unsanitary conditions that were so often found in the homes of the poor. One contemporary physician had this to say about Rathbone's experiment:

> It is evident that the essential conditions of rational and successful sick nursing such as good air, light, warmth, bedding, good food, etc., are altogether wanting in the homes of the poor. Of what use are the gratuitous supply and regular giving of medicines, if every necessity is wanting for ordinary healthy living? It is not that the nurse shrinks from the privations and injurious influences existing in the cottages and hovels, but it is the impossibility of being useful under such circumstances that renders home nursing unattainable for the poor. One can comfort them in their cottages, and give them food and medicine, but to nurse and heal them there with any prospect of success cannot be done.[3]

The general belief was that home nursing for the poor was not practical. Municipal and charity hospitals were available for such care. If the poor were seriously ill, let them go to those hospitals.

Rathbone quickly countered such objections. He noted that many patients with serious illnesses were either unsuitable for or not admissible to a general hospital. In addition, many sick persons objected to being taken to the hospital. Rathbone argued that "there are not enough and there never can be hospitals large enough and numerous enough to take in all cases of grave illness among the poor"; moreover, "the work done by district nursing is, in proportion to its results, far less costly than that done by the hospital." Rathbone's reasoning prevailed and funds were collected so that additional nurses could be employed. Thus, visiting nursing was firmly established in Liverpool.[4]

In the United States, visiting nursing began its development in 1877, when the Women's Branch of the New York City Mission sent its first trained nurses into the homes of the indigent. A little later, the New York Ethical Society placed nurses in several city dispensaries and afterward, in 1883, sent a nurse to Chicago to begin similar work there. Three years later the Boston Instructive District Nursing Association was organized to promote health education. In 1890, 13 years after the first nurse had been sent out by the New York City Mission, there were 21 organizations in the United States engaged in the work of visiting nursing, most employing no more than one nurse each.

LILLIAN WALD

Full recognition of the widespread benefits that this new role might yield were first recognized by Lillian Wald. Born in 1867, she spent her growing years in Rochester and was educated in Miss Crittenden's

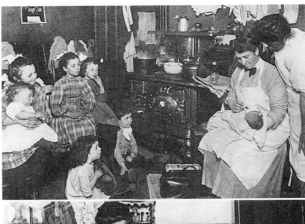
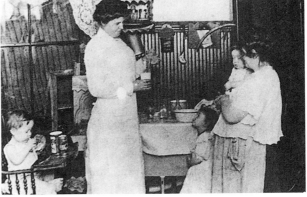

Visiting nurses brought care into the homes of the poor.

English and French Boarding and Day School for Young Ladies and Little Girls. Influenced by relatives who were physicians, Wald went to New York City to become a nurse.

After 3 years of training at the New York Hospital School of Nursing, from which she graduated in 1891, Wald spent a year nursing at the New York Juvenile Asylum. Unhappy with her scant medical knowledge, she entered the Woman's Medical College in New York. While attending medical school, she and a fellow nurse, Mary Brewster, were asked to go to New York's Lower East Side to lecture to immigrant mothers on the care of the sick. What they found there profoundly shocked them.

One morning in March 1893, Wald was showing a group of mothers how to make a bed when a child came in asking for help. He led her to a foul tenement, where nine pitifully undernourished people—most of them sleeping on the floor—were living in two rooms. On a bed lay a helpless woman who, although seriously ill, had not received care for 2 days. No one had ever told 26-year-old Lillian Wald that such suffering existed. As a nurse with a social conscience, Wald went to work; she bathed the woman, washed the linen, sent for a physician, and cleaned the filthy room. Hours later, visibly shaken by what she had seen, Wald left. She then resolved to forsake medical school and join with Mary Brewster in embarking on a career of offering nursing care to such needy people. The two women soon learned that

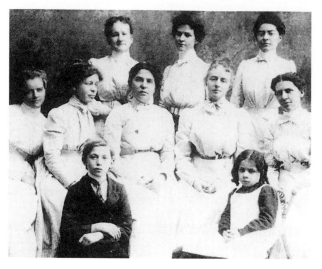

The Henry Street nurses (Lillian Wald, 2nd row center).

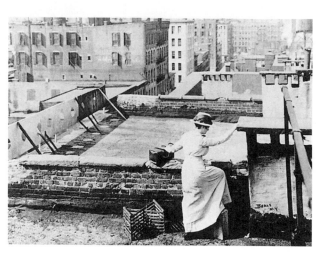

A visiting nurse traverses a tenement roof on the way to another case.

there were thousands of similar cases in that same little neighborhood alone.

To implement their resolve, Lillian Wald and Mary Brewster set up a Nurses' Settlement House in one of the slum sections of the Lower East Side to serve as a focal point for a visiting nursing service for the poor. They readily gave up a more comfortable living environment and moved into a little top-floor tenement on Jefferson Street. The motives underlying the settlement were no more fully defined than to seek out the sick and nurse them.

Wald and Brewster quickly established the concept of the nurse ready to give her services in the home to all who needed them, making no distinction between those who could pay and those who could not, allied with no religious group, seeking to educate as well as to heal. They simply permitted it to be known that their services were available to neighbors in need. At first, calls came almost entirely from families with someone fallen ill. In each case the nurses established communication with the physician, if one was already in attendance, and if not, they called one in. Sometimes hospital treatment appeared necessary, and the nurses arranged for admission. Often, the very poor needed bedding and other comforts, and the nurses met those needs with stores placed at their disposal by well-to-do friends.

Only during the first few days were patients sought out. After that, calls for the nurses came by the hundreds. They became known and trusted by their neighbors as friends who did not draw back from contact, no matter how demanding the situation, and who were glad to place their education and skill at the service of all in need. Gradually, too, the nurses' work came to be valued by the physicians of the neighborhood and by those in charge of the various hospitals. Whereas at first practically all the calls came from families, a steadily increasing number of patients were referred by physicians. Lillian Wald and her associates brought basic nursing care into the streets. Neatly dressed in modest suits with black ties and spotless white blouses, they made daily calls wherever needed, often traveling over tenement house roofs as the shortest distance from patient to patient.

Illness was not new to Jewish, Italian, Greek, Polish, and Russian immigrants, but in the New World, they found traditional methods for treating the sick insufficient. Many immigrants gradually abandoned folk remedies, or at least combined them with pills, ointments, diets, and bed rest made mandatory by the "nurse lady." Old superstitions did not die out altogether, however. A Jewish mother ensured the health of her growing children with fresh air, good diet, and regular milk—all the measures strongly recommended by the visiting nurse—but, just in case, she would also make sure that nobody inadvertently stepped over her child, an action that supposedly would stunt his growth.

From the beginning, one of the basic principles underlying Lillian Wald's work held nursing care of the sick in their homes as the primary aim, with health instruction secondary. Another guiding principle saw the visiting nursing service as analogous to the established system of private-duty nursing. Thus the visiting nurse was to respond to calls from the people themselves as well as from physicians and to act with as little delay as possible.

THE HENRY STREET SETTLEMENT HOUSE

Within 2 years, the volume of work had increased to a point where larger facilities and more nurses were urgently needed. In 1895, with the aid of banker and philanthropist Jacob H. Schiff and others, Lillian Wald and Mary Brewster moved the Nurses' Settlement to larger accommodations at 265 Henry Street, where it then became known as the Henry Street Settlement

House. Soon nine graduate nurses were living in the house, including Lavinia Dock, a vigorous figure who was to become a dynamic nursing leader.

The statistics of the Henry Street nurses' work for 1905 sheds light on the specific duties and responsibilities involved:[5]

Patients cared for in homes	5032
Nursing visits	43,503
Friendly visits	4372
First-aid treatments	13,791

Cases reported by:

Families	2398
Physicians	1881
Charitable agencies	753
Total	5032

Disposition of cases:

Cured	2624
Hospital	740
Dispensary	598
Investigations	342
Died	312
Special nurse	165
Department of Health	69
Carried over into 1906	182
Total	5032

Diagnosis of cases:

Unclassified medical	1735
Unclassified surgical	602
Pneumonia and bronchitis	956
Tuberculosis	296
Gynecological	212
Burns	197
Rheumatism	158
Obstetrical—normal and abnormal	155
Meningitis	123
Typhoid	122
Contagious	119
Ulcers	118
Cardiac	97
Eye diseases	90
Alcoholism	6
No illness	46
Total	5032

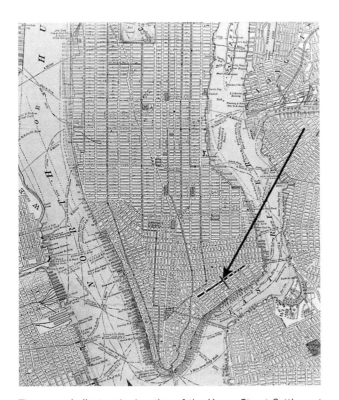

The arrow indicates the location of the Henry Street Settlement House.

By 1909, the Henry Street staff numbered 37 nurses, 5 of whom held administrative posts, with all the others providing direct nursing care. Of this group, the supervisors and 10 staff nurses lived in the Henry Street headquarters. A new nurse, except in case of emergency, began her work there and was assigned to one of the nearby districts under careful supervision. Even if the novice Henry Street nurse had the status of a former nurse training school superintendent who, weary of administrative duties, desired to spend some time in direct bedside care, she still had to undergo the same careful initiation process, so that misunderstandings of immigrant families and their curious customs might be avoided.

Although there was no established period of probation, nurses were not considered permanent until at least 3 months' satisfactory service had been completed. Some nurses showed early aptitude for the work. To others, the Henry Street point of view, and understanding the people living under conditions and with traditions foreign to their own experience, dawned slowly. Only nurses who proved capable of delivering empathic nursing care were retained, because the Settlement's leaders saw their purpose as not merely to maintain a staff of nurses but also to seize the rare opportunity to demonstrate the value of truly understanding the condition and problems of the immigrant. In her daily work among the immigrants, each nurse kept two sets of records: one, a bedside chart with notes for the physician to review during his visits; the other, a record for the Henry Street superintendent containing the main points of the nurse's work.

The nature of the work varied somewhat, according to the nurse's district. Acute cases predominated in the crowded Lower East Side, where the Settlement had made its initial foothold among immigrant families from southern Europe, who were both distrustful of hospitals and less familiar with the other resources of the city. Pneumonia had the highest incidence rate, followed by typhoid fever and meningitis. The nurse cared for many patients with severe pneumonia, with only one or two visits made by a physician, who was kept informed of the patient's progress through the nurse's records. This was especially true for patients unable to pay for physician's visits.

At first-aid homes established in several densely populated sections of the city, a daily nurse treated minor surgical cases, ear and eye problems, and other ailments. Most patients, many of whom were schoolchildren, were sent to the nurses by dispensary physicians. Small but well-equipped surgical dressing rooms were maintained at the main Henry Street office and at several of the branches to accommodate patients who came to have surgical dressings changed. Unlike the typical visiting nursing association, Henry Street had a small obstetric service, with a separate staff, that attempted to uplift the level of practice of scores of immigrant midwives. A daily supply of certified milk was sent to the Settlement every morning, where it was bottled under aseptic conditions and sold at market price to patients who could afford to pay or was distributed free to the indigent.

By 1909, the Henry Street Settlement House had grown from two nurses living on the top floor of a tenement, nursing the sick, to a highly organized social enterprise with many departments. The residents included a staff of nurses and other men and women engaged in various social and civic efforts. Florence Kelley, general secretary of the National Consumers' League, testified as one of the Henry Street staff:

> I have lived 20 years at the bottom of the pit, first eight years at Hull House, Chicago, and now at The Nurses' Settlement in New York City. All these 20 years I have been increasingly depressed—putting it mildly—at the waste of the precious gifts that the young immigrants bring with them, the possibilities we crush out by the living conditions into which we allow the children to come, the lack of educational facilities, and the pressure under which they work. Sometime ago a little boy came to the First Aid room at the Settlement from the tenement house where he lived and said he was making paper bags. He said he could not make any more until his head stopped hurting. The nurse held him at a safe distance, sheared and cleansed his head, and told him to send all his sisters and brothers to her. He was put on the list of candidates for the truant officer. He said he did not think his mother could spare him to stop work and go to school.
>
> A nurse followed him to his lair and found four brothers and a little girl five years old working with incredible rapidity turning out the little paper bags used for rolls and fruit and chestnuts, such bags as come from the grocer into the kitchens of all of us. The place in which this work was being done was a rear cellar bedroom. Not one of the children was tall enough to reach the window sill. They had lived there 18 months, and a charitable society paid their rent. Nobody had visited them but a series of doctors. The children had had the diseases of childhood. Different physicians had seen them through these, but no one had reported them to the truant officer. When the matter was taken up with the factory inspector, he said he never knew of any one occupying that room but had supposed their living place was a coal cellar.
>
> These children were being robbed of all their school years. The oldest boy had once known how to read a little, and when he got into school the knowledge came back to him. Here was a perfectly dead waste, due to the civic negligence of the physicians who had pulled the children through their diseases and left everything as it was before. The family was never before brought to the attention of the truant officer and the truant officers are not allowed, under a series of judicial decisions, to go into a dwelling against the wish of the parent. The two persons who have access everywhere are the nurse and the doctor.[6]

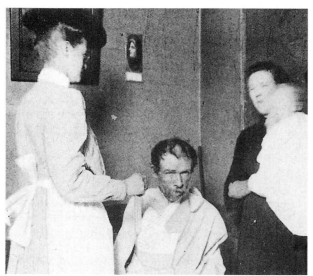

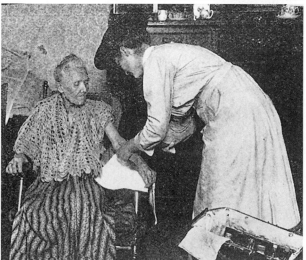

Injured and elderly receiving visiting nurse care.

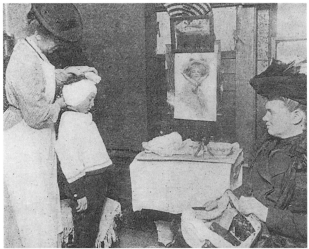

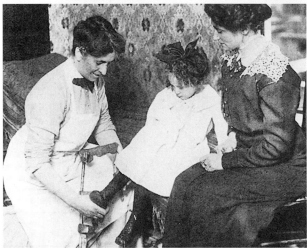

Boy and girl receiving Visiting Nurse Association services.

BEGINNINGS OF SCHOOL NURSING

The successful establishment of school nursing in America also owed much to the efforts of Lillian Wald. In 1902, an average of 15 to 20 children daily were sent home from each New York school for health reasons. When 300 children were excluded from one school in a single day, however, the problem assumed massive proportions. Wald suggested that placing nurses in the schools might help solve the problem because nurses could effectively supplement the work of local physicians who occasionally examined the school children. This medical examination only excluded the child from school; the physician did nothing to prevent recurring cases of exclusion and did not follow up the children during the period of exclusion. Wald offered the services of Henry Street nurse Lina L. Rogers for 1 month as a demonstration of what could be done.

The experiment proved an unqualified success. During the month of September 1902, 10,567 children had been sent home from the New York

schools, whereas in September 1903, with a school nurse in attendance, only 1101 were excluded. It was not difficult to account for this marked drop in the number of exclusions from schools. Many of the exclusions had been for minor illnesses such as pediculosis, ringworm, scabies, and other problems that were easily curable and did not legitimately require the pupil to stay out of school.

Before the inception of school nursing, teachers and physicians often had no choice but to send home children who seemed physically unfit to associate with others. Indeed, in some cities, such exclusions became a convenient method for easing the pressures of badly overcrowded classrooms. For example, the Henry Street Settlement nurse uncovered a boy aged 12 who had never been to school because he had a tiny sore on his head. When investigated, this situation was found to be typical.

The New York Board of Health, realizing the value of the nurse in the school, soon appointed dozens of school nurses to assist in carrying out the work. Dr. John J. Cronin of New York City wrote, "When I state that in the city of New York, during the period of three months, out of 24,358 children who were actually excluded from school for longer or shorter periods, only 400 had serious diseases, imperiling their own lives, the others being more of the character of 'nuisances,' it will be seen what an advantage this system may prove from an educational point of view."[7]

School nursing, however, sometimes caused riots. In New York City on June 27, 1906, excited mothers

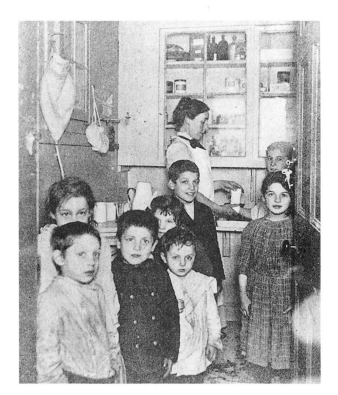

School nurse at work, New York City, 1905.

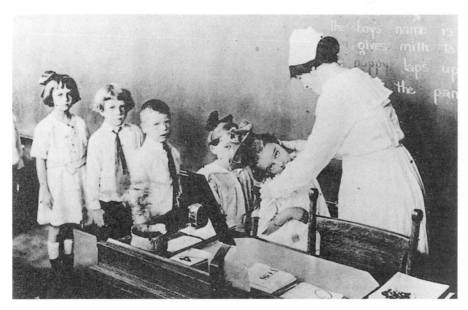

A school nurse giving health exami-nations in a New York City school.

stormed schools to demand their children. The cause of the riot was 83 adenoid operations that had been performed in the schools by three specialists, assisted by health inspectors and nurses. A rumor spread around the neighborhood that the children's "throats were being cut," and an excited mob demolished several windows and doors before the children could be dismissed.

A newspaper story of October 5, 1906, told of a similar riot in front of a public school near the Williamsburg Bridge in Brooklyn. According to the newspaper, this riot resulted from the initiation of active measures in the school for the eradication of trachoma. About 1500 Italian women fought the police desperately and actually attempted to batter down the doors of the school building. Again, the trouble followed from a misapprehension.

Insight into some of the problems encountered by school nurses can be derived from letters received from parents:[8]

Miss Eichler:

We received the note from the Doctor and will say that we give him medical attention when he needs it. We know that George had headaches but when he comes home from school he complains of a boy in the 3rd grade by the name of Andrew Aimeck who knocks him down and jomps on him. I wish you would give this your attention. I know boys are all alike but this boy is mutch larger.

Very Respectfully Yours,

S————.

To Whom This May Concern:

I received your letter stating that Edna Ross (my Sister) is in need of glasses. It is utterly impossible for me to purchase her any as my husband is out of work and her father does not contribute one penny towards her support and I am obliged to share the little I have with her and have two infants of my own. Her mother is dead and the Father placed the child on my hands.

Yours Respectfully,

H————.

To the Nurse:

Jennie was not born with here eyes crossed they were perfectly strait until after she was three years old and then they crossed. I could never tell what caused it unless it was from a fall down stairs which she got six months before.

Yours truly,

S————.

Miss Hill:

I received a note wich Martha brought home to instruct me to take her to a doctor now I want you to know that I or my can Judge wen Martha needs medical treatment if Martha is sick I keep her home. I send Martha to school to be instruction my wife has ask you to give Martha some lessons to bring home and my wife would instruct her you complain about Martha she keeps her mouth open well she does just as any other child would wen intrested or surprised it is more or less a habit with her and no catarrh she has a slight cold I will atmit but nothing more. So I hope you will give her some lesson to bring home and we will instruct her the best we can.

W————.

One mother, on being notified that her young son needed a bath, wrote: "teacher, Johnny aint no rose. Learn him; don't smell him." Another mother, on receiving a notice that her boy suffered from *astigmatism*, wrote that she had whipped him soundly and hoped that he would not do it again.[9]

METROPOLITAN LIFE EMPLOYS NURSES

In June 1909, at the suggestion of Lillian Wald, the Metropolitan Life Insurance Company organized the Visiting Nurse Department and entered into an agreement with the Henry Street Settlement in New York City, whereby the latter was to furnish the services of its visiting nurses to the company's industrial policyholders in a limited section of Manhattan. The service proved to be very satisfactory during the 3-month trial and was extended to other parts of the city. Two months later, it was introduced in Baltimore and in Washington, DC. By the end of 1909, policyholders in Boston, Chicago, Cincinnati, Cleveland, Dover, Harrisburg, Philadelphia, St. Louis, Trenton, and Worcester also obtained this service. By the end of 1909, there were 14 Metropolitan nursing centers; by 1912, there were 589. Wherever possible, the company contracted with the local Visiting Nurse Association to furnish the nursing service at a certain rate per patient. When that was impossible, the company hired its own nurses, under the direction of its field supervisors.

STANDING ORDERS

The proper scope of nursing practice in the community evoked considerable debate among physicians and nurses. Visiting nurses experienced more autonomy than their hospital nurse colleagues, yet the exact bounds of their responsibilities were not clearly defined. Some physicians believed the public health nurse should perform numerous procedures thought to be traditionally medical, whereas others viewed the situation quite differently. A physician in a Massachusetts town complained bitterly that "the nurse took the temperature, pulse, and respiration,

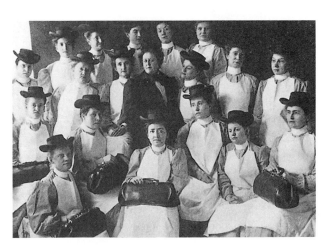

Visiting nurses with their famous black bags.

opened the windows and put the pneumonia patient on a milk diet, and left nothing for the doctor to do," while a young surgeon in a nearby city told nursing students that "they should be prepared for any emergency . . . , even to giving an intravenous or to religating slipped abdominal sutures."[10]

Because of these divergent approaches, in 1912 the Chicago Visiting Nurse Association prepared a list of standing orders for staff nurses. In this way, they hoped that thorough and speedy care could be given to every patient. No medication, however, not even castor oil, was included in this list. Bath orders were included, because many patients strenuously objected to taking a bath in cold weather and would more likely accept a bath when told that the physician had ordered it. The standing orders read as follows:

An Undiagnosed Case Running Temperature—Cleansing bath; liquid diet; low S.S. enema, P.R.N. when no abdominal pain or tenderness is present; sponge for R.T. 102.5°.

Sore Throat—Gargle and mouth-wash of baking-soda; liquid diet; children to be isolated if possible until physician sees case.

Colds—Cleansing bath; low S.S. enema, P.R.N.; liquid diet; for adults, plenty of hot water taken frequently.

Pneumonia—Cleansing bath; low S.S. enema, P.R.N.; sponge for R.T. 102.5°; liquid diet; cold-air treatment, if possible.

Typhoid Fever—Cleansing bath; low S.S. enema, P.R.N.; sponge for R.T. 102.5°; milk diet. Emphasize need for plenty of fresh air and cold drinking water (boiled if possible) and disinfection of stools.

Obstetrical Cases—For mother: cleansing bath; local cleansing with Lysol solution; abdominal binder; change pads; breast binder, P.R.N.; low S.S. enema, P.R.N. For the baby: alcohol dressing to cord; oiled and bathed.

Infants and Young Children (sick but not diagnosed)—Normal salt flushing, P.R.N.; diet, boiled water for twenty-four hours.

Infectious Diseases—Isolation; boric solution for eyes and nostrils, P.R.N.; Vaseline or cold cream for lips and nose, P.R.N.; oil rub, P.R.N. for all desquamating cases; liquid diet; sponge for R.T. 102.5°

Pleurisy—Apply tight binder to chest.

Infantile Diarrhea—Normal salt flushing, P.R.N.; no food; boiled water for twenty-four hours.

Infantile Convulsions—Same orders as diarrhea.

Burn Cases—Remove clothing; apply normal salt or boric solution dressings; if severe burn, get into hospital as quickly as possible.

Chronic Ulcers—Clean with Lysol or boric solution; apply wet boric dressings and firm bandage.

Minor Dressings—For cuts, scratches, bruises and infected fingers, apply hot boric packs and refer to dispensary.

> Discharging Ears—Cleanse the outer ear with moist boric solution swabs; do not irrigate; refer to dispensary.[11]

Any or all of these orders could be canceled or changed at any time by a physician who preferred to leave specific written orders. As suggested aids to both nurse and physician, standing orders were used in the absence of other instructions.

EARLY EFFORTS TO IMPROVE MATERNAL AND CHILD CARE

As a corollary to the visiting nursing movement, organized efforts to improve infant hygiene began. Early work concentrated on the improvement of milk and water supplies, such as the establishment by private agencies of milk stations for the distribution of clean, safe milk or modified milk at a nominal cost for infant feeding, along with the passage of city ordinances controlling milk production, care, and distribution. The first milk station in the United States was established in New York City in 1893, and by 1910 similar stations existed in 30 other cities. From milk dispensaries, these stations often evolved into preventive health centers as the emphasis swung toward educational activity and physical examinations for preventive care.

In the early 1900s, much innovative work was carried out in attacking maternal and infant mortality. For example, the Boston Lying-in Hospital's visiting nurses divided the city into four districts and cared for mothers in their homes. Five graduate nurses and two student nurses divided the workload into prenatal and postnatal cases. On her first visit, the nurse assessed the social conditions of the patient's family. If the patient had sufficient money to pay for medical care, she would be referred to a neighborhood physician.

For those poorer mothers, the visiting nurses of the Lying-in Hospital implemented the following plan of home care. First, an appraisal of the mother's general condition was made, with the physician notified if medical care was needed. The mother learned nutrition basics, with emphasis on milk-producing foods, because breast-feeding was encouraged. The second visit reviewed the articles of clothing needed for the baby and the special supplies required by the physician for the delivery. The number of preparatory visits varied with the necessity for instruction, but three were typical. Postpartum visits involved care of mother and baby. When the patients were discharged, the nurse encouraged the mother to attend well child-care classes offered by the Milk and Baby Hygiene Association.

Despite such efforts, however, the national rate of infant mortality remained distressingly high. An estimated 300,000 children under 1 year of age died each year in the United States, with perhaps half of those deaths preventable. A percentage breakdown of the cause of 154,373 infant deaths in the registration area of the United States in 1910 follows:[12]

Diseases of the digestive system	2.1
Diseases of early infancy (including premature birth, 13.1; congenital debility, 7.8; and injuries at birth, 2.4)	25.5

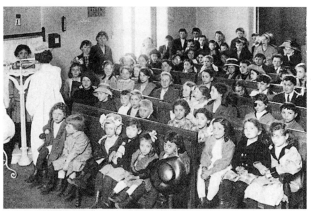

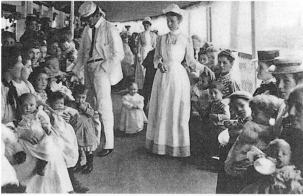

Examining infants and children at the clinic and aboard ship in Boston harbor, where poor mothers and infants were exposed to fresh air for the day.

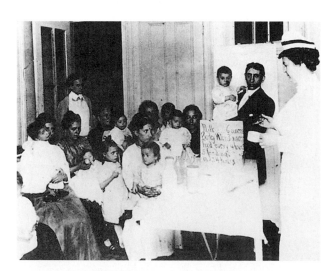

Instruction in nutrition basics.

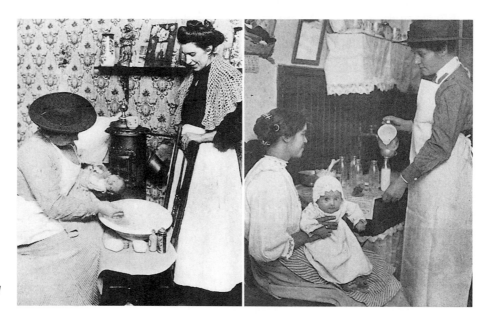

Demonstrations in bathing and feeding.

Diseases of the respiratory system
(including bronchopneumonia,
6.9; pneumonia, 5.5; and
acute bronchitis, 2.7)   15.8
General diseases (including all
forms of tuberculosis, 1.6;
syphilis, 1.1; and whooping cough,
measles, scarlet fever, diphtheria,
and croup, 4.0)   9.2
Diseases of the nervous system
(including convulsions, 2.6; and
meningitis, 1.5)   5.5
Congenital malformations   4.9
All other causes   7.0
Total   100.0

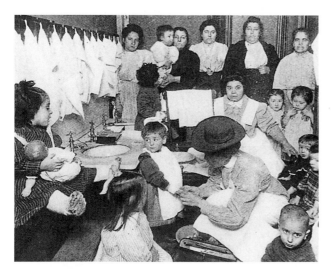

Child care instruction.

The death rate per 1000 infants younger than age 1 year in the larger cities of the registration area that same year revealed the following:

Oakland, CA	94.8
Seattle	100.4
Portland, OR	105.3
Los Angeles	110.7
San Francisco	113.6
Toledo, OH	125.0
Cambridge, MA	126.1
St. Paul	130.8
Birmingham, AL	133.0
Louisville, KY	134.0
Denver	134.7
Grand Rapids, MI	134.8
New Haven, CT	134.9
Nashville, TN	135.1
St. Louis	135.8
Chicago	139.5
Omaha	140.0
Columbus, OH	140.4
Spokane, WA	142.4
Indianapolis	144.8
Newark, NJ	145.8
New York	146.2
Paterson, NJ	146.7
Dayton, OH	146.8
Cleveland	147.2
Cincinnati	149.8
Jersey City, NJ	153.2
New Orleans	154.9
Atlanta	155.3
Bridgeport, CT	155.5
Philadelphia	162.2
Albany, NY	162.9
Boston	168.0

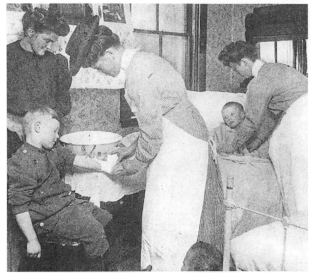

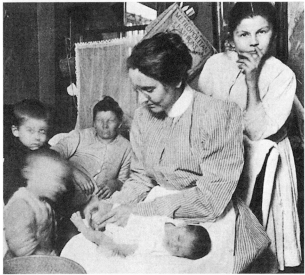

Visiting nurses effectively reduced infant and child mortality rates.

Worcester, MA	168.0
Kansas City, MO	170.4
Milwaukee	172.0
Providence, RI	173.7
Syracuse, NY	176.4
Pittsburgh	179.6
Buffalo	180.9
Washington, DC	194.6
Detroit	204.8
Baltimore	209.6
Richmond, VA	229.3
Fall River, MA	259.5
Lowell, MA	261.0

THE ATTACK ON TUBERCULOSIS

Through the 19th century, the mortality rates showed tuberculosis as perennially the leading killer among the myriad infectious diseases. Although bedridden

tuberculosis patients had been cared for by general visiting nurses from the beginning of the visiting-nurse movement, not until 1899 was the first attempt made to provide special home nursing service for tuberculosis patients. The first efforts in this movement were launched by a female medical student who had been assigned to follow up tuberculosis patients from Johns Hopkins Hospital. She investigated and reported on the patients' living conditions and taught families the care and precautions necessary for treatment and prevention of the disease. Believing that the problem of tuberculosis was a home problem and should be combated there, Dr. William Osler of Johns Hopkins initiated the Laennec Society of Baltimore "to systematize and stimulate work in tuberculosis and diffuse in the profession and the public a knowledge of the disease."[13]

The first work of the Laennec Society was to investigate the social conditions of a group of 190 tuberculosis cases. The first study of its kind, this study uncovered many tragic conditions. Patients in the last stages of tuberculosis were found living in one- or two-room apartments with six other people and poor or non-existent ventilation. Often they slept in the same bed with one, two, or sometimes three others, and they always ate with the family, sharing the same utensils and often giving the children sips of coffee from their cups or bites of food from their forks. Obviously, the disease spread swiftly in such fashion, and the need for assistance to these patients and their families was urgent.

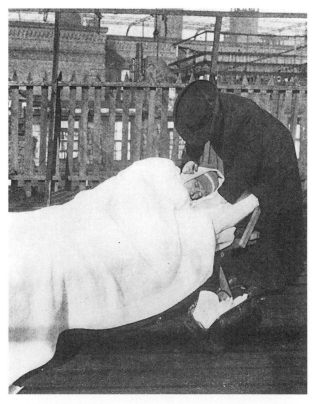

Tuberculosis patient taking fresh-air treatment on a roof.

The publication of this study led to the appointment in 1903 of a nurse who spent all her time following up tuberculosis patients in their homes. This nurse was instructed "to find 'lost patients' and get them back to the dispensary; to teach the doctrine of fresh air, good food, and rest; and not only report the home conditions, but to do all in her power with the help of relief agencies to improve them." She was also expected "to give bedside care to the sick and to establish the precautions necessary to avoid infection of others." In 1904, through contributions received from interested citizens, additional nurses were employed for tuberculosis work and assigned for supervision to the Visiting Nurse Association of Baltimore.[14]

General recognition of public responsibility in the control of tuberculosis had yet to emerge. Leading health workers, as early as 1897, had put forth the principle that a city health department should take responsibility for the control of tuberculosis as a communicable disease, and the New York Health Department had made significant strides in that direction. In 1895, the Massachusetts legislature made an appropriation for the first state sanatorium for the treatment of tuberculosis in the United States. By 1905, there were 19 public sanatoriums or hospitals for tuberculosis, including 3 federal, 4 state, 4 county, and 8 municipal institutions. All these institutions hired at least a few graduate nurses, and several began nurse training schools to assist in staffing rather than hire a large number of untrained attendants.

RED CROSS NURSING

Another growing movement was Red Cross nursing. The idea that led to the birth of the Red Cross had originated in June 1859, 3 years after Florence Nightingale had returned from the Crimea. An investment banker from Geneva, Switzerland, J. Henri Dunant, went to Italy with the intention of securing a meeting with Napoleon III of France, then on campaign, but instead found himself at Solferino, in the midst of the bloodiest battle of the war between France and Austria. Horrified to learn that some 6000 wounded men were being attended by only two physicians, he organized a makeshift nursing service and successfully persuaded the local people to bring water, bandages, and food to the men. Three years later, in his famous *Recollections of Solferino*, Dunant proposed the establishment of a permanent international relief society that could take immediate action in time of war. This idea was incorporated into the Geneva Convention guidelines, signed by 12 governments on August 22, 1864. On that day the International Red Cross was born.

Not until 1881, however, was the American Red Cross first organized, through the efforts of Clara Barton, a former New England school teacher who had

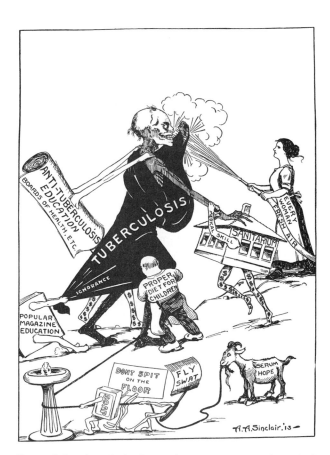

How to fight tuberculosis, the number one menace to the nation's health at the turn of the century.

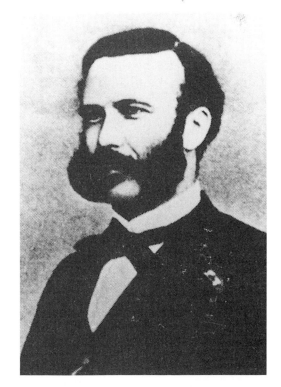

J. Henri Dunant, founder of the International Red Cross.

found a psychological outlet by attacking vast social burdens. In 1854, she had been appointed to a clerkship in the Patent Office in Washington, DC, perhaps the first time a government position was held by a woman. During the Civil War, Barton independently directed a large-scale war relief operation, arranging for huge quantities of supplies to be furnished to the army and the hospitals. She occasionally did personal nursing, and during this time she had ample opportunity to determine the need for an organization like the Red Cross.

In 1870, Barton served with the German Red Cross during the Franco-Prussian war; after her return to the United States, she organized the American Red Cross. She was instrumental in persuading Congress, in 1882, to ratify the Treaty of Geneva, so that in times of peace the Red Cross Society could continue to engage in humanitarian work. The charter committed the Red Cross "to continue and carry on a system of national and international relief in time of peace and to apply the same in mitigating the sufferings caused by pestilence, famine, fire, floods, and other national calamities, and to devise and carry measure for preventing the same."[15]

Barton joined in relief work with the Red Cross during a number of disasters, including the yellow fever epidemic in Florida in 1888 and the Johnstown flood of 1889. During the half-century following 1882, Red Cross nurses gave assistance in more than 1000 disasters in the United States, at a cost of $53 million. These disasters included 271 cyclones, tornadoes, hurricanes, and other storms; 152 floods;

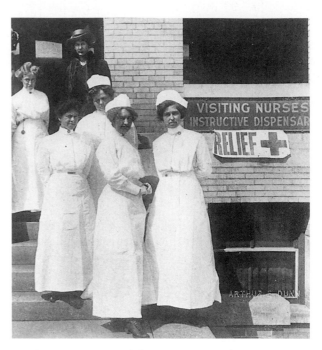

Red Cross nurses at a relief station after the Omaha tornado of 1913.

and 139 fires. The Red Cross also lent aid in the aftermath of mine cave-ins, explosions, epidemics, forest fires, steamboat wrecks, train wrecks, and numerous other types of catastrophes.

THE TOWN AND COUNTRY NURSING SERVICE

Rural public health nursing progressed slowly. With few exceptions, there was practically no nursing service available for the great masses of people living on farms or in isolated country districts. At the second annual meeting of the Association for the Prevention of Infant Mortality, held in 1911, Lillian Wald gave an address on rural problems. She reviewed the terrible health care conditions found in rural districts—the high prevalence of tuberculosis, hookworm, and fevers; the gross inadequacies in maternity care; and the extraordinarily high infant and maternal mortality rates. She compared the different attitudes in the United States with the work going on in Great Britain, Canada, and Australia, where nationwide nursing services for rural populations were provided. Wald asked, "Why should not our National Red Cross Society, with all its splendid organization and resources, support, direct and operate such a national service during the intervals of time in which there is no need for its emergency duty?"[16]

In 1912, the Red Cross endeavored to establish a rural nursing service, which provided nurses to care for the sick, gave instruction in sanitation and hygiene in the homes of the rural people, and attempted to improve living conditions in little villages

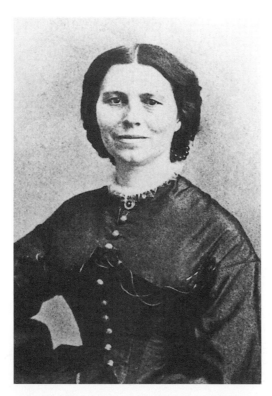

Clara Barton, founder of the American Red Cross.

and on lonely farms. The organization of the Red Cross Rural Nursing Services was made possible when Lillian Wald secured a generous gift of $100,000 from New York financier Jacob H. Schiff, together with $1000 annually from Mrs. Whitelaw Reid, wife of the editor of the *New York Tribune.*

This money paid for administrative and supervisory expenses, but the salaries of the nurses came from the communities they served. A superintendent of nurses was appointed, and a headquarters opened in Washington, DC. The next year, the name was changed from Rural Nursing Service to the Town and Country Nursing Service, to include the small towns with no visiting service. Although this effort in extending nursing service met a great need, it grew slowly. With a typical disdain for national supervision over what might be considered local affairs, many communities hesitated to call in the aid of the National Red Cross. Others could not raise the money for the nurses' salaries. Consequently, until 1915, only 40 or 50 Red Cross public health nurses worked throughout the nation.

Due to the vast unmet rural health care needs, in the town and country districts certain restrictions limited the visiting nurses' work. Almost invariably, the nurses reported the prevailing diseases to be tuberculosis, pneumonia, and typhoid. Other common ailments included grippe; rheumatism; gonorrhea; hookworm; pellagra; cholera infantum; malaria; and epidemics of measles, scarlet fever, tonsillitis, smallpox, and typhus, together with all the contagious diseases of children. Among miners and in foreign settlements, grippe, pneumonia, and other pulmonary diseases were conspicuous. To prevent epidemics, nurses engaged in setting up quarantine and enforcing the laws for smallpox vaccination. In only a few communities were contagious cases sent to hospitals. Under the jurisdiction of the local health authority, they were usually quarantined at home, in vacant houses, or sometimes even in tents.

An interesting phase of the rural nurse's work involved the remarkable degree of resourcefulness she developed out of pure necessity. Very few nurses had adequate stocks of medical supplies; many of those that a nurse had taken for granted during her training were nonexistent now, and it was up to her to contrive substitutes. Examples of such improvisations included using hot bricks, salt, or sandbags in place of hot water bottles; making bed rests out of chairs; soaping windows to give opaque light for surgical operations; fashioning a protective cradle out of three barrel hoops wound with strips of muslin; using wooden blocks for raising low beds; and constructing a stretcher out of boards padded with quilts. Sometimes the rural nurse had to make long trips for drinking water or perhaps melt snow to secure water to bathe patients. Boiled water was carried in fruit cans to maternity and surgical patients.

Early rural nurses recommended many practices that yielded improved living conditions, such as the screening of houses, the fumigation and whitewash-

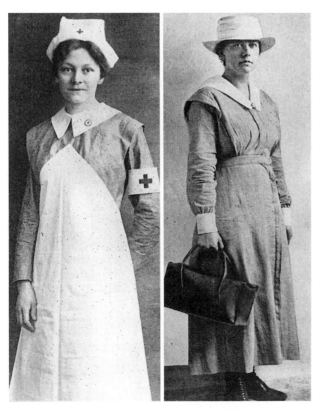

Uniforms of the Red Cross Town and Country Nursing Service.

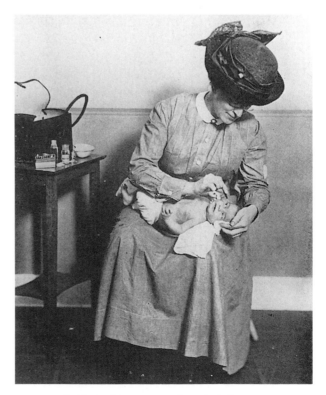

Public health nurse treating a baby's eyes.

ing of rooms after tuberculosis patients had occupied them, the reporting of bad conditions in outhouses and the careless disposal of garbage, and the improvement of sanitation ordinances. Nurses also instituted vigorous action against flies by promoting practices such as keeping garbage pails covered, emptying them more frequently, and discouraging the practice of throwing potato peelings out into the yard. In many homes, heavy, dirty, unwashable bed quilts were either replaced by new ones or kept covered with clean sheets. As a result, areas served by rural nurses showed decreases in infant mortality and the general death rate and overall improvements in cleanliness, nutrition, and sanitation.

THE BIRTH OF INDUSTRIAL NURSING

Industrial establishments also made use of early visiting nurses. In 1895 in Vermont, Fletcher D. Proctor, son of a governor and himself one-time governor of that state, introduced "district nursing" into several villages whose residents were mostly employees of his Vermont Marble Company. As president of this company, Proctor demonstrated unusual interest in the welfare of his employees. After observing the work of visiting nurses in several cities, he selected 24-year-old Ada Mayo Stewart, an 1894 graduate of the Waltham (Massachusetts) Training School, to do visiting nursing among the families of his workers at Proctor. A few months later, Ada's sister Harriet was hired to care for the company's employees and their families in the village of West Rutland and Rutland Center.

This early form of industrial nursing placed little emphasis on the care of injuries. It was essentially a

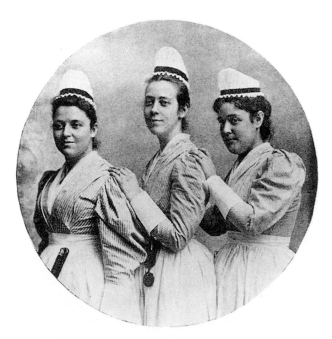

Ada Mayo Stewart (left) was the first industrial nurse.

home visiting service with patient referrals coming from physicians. The figures for 1896 through 1898 showed that obstetric patients topped Stewart's workload, with medical patients coming a close second, followed by a few surgical patients. Service was free to employees of the Vermont Marble Company and their families and to other townspeople who were unable to pay for medical care.

FORMATION OF THE NATIONAL ORGANIZATION OF PUBLIC HEALTH NURSING

Although the decade from 1900 to 1910 witnessed a rapid expansion and extension of visiting nursing, there had been no effort to organize and standardize this type of care or to establish recognized requirements for being employed as a visiting nurse. But on June 7, 1912, a handful of visiting nurses, who unofficially represented 2500 poorly prepared and unsupervised colleagues in 900 agencies, formed the National Organization for Public Health Nursing (NOPHN). This organization comprised nurses and laypeople engaged in the actual work of public health nursing and in the organization, management, and support of such work. Leading organizers included Lillian D. Wald, Ella Phillips Crandall, Mary Beard, Mary Lent, Edna Foley, Lystra Gretter, and Elizabeth G. Fox. Favoring the term *public health nurse* as more inclusive than *visiting nurse*, the founders declared that "the experience data available emphasized the urgency and practical necessity for the extension of public health nursing service to a much larger proportion of wage-earners and people of moderate means than now have the benefit of the same."[17] Lillian Wald was chosen as the first president of the NOPHN.

In 1909, an unpretentious little magazine entitled the *Visiting Nurse Quarterly*, the first American publication to deal exclusively with the subject of public health nursing, was initiated by the Cleveland Visiting Nurse Association. Three years later, the Cleveland Association offered this quarterly to the NOPHN on the very day the organization was founded. Under the new title the *Public Health Nurse Quarterly*, it quickly proved to be a valuable means of communication among the membership.

NOPHN founders soon noted that mortality statistics for the first 14 years of the 20th century showed an overall decline in the death rate, a development attributed to improved water supply, better methods of sewage disposal, cleaner streets, better housing laws, and more stringent regulation of food and dairy products as well as to recent discoveries in medical science, the work of visiting nurses, and an improved awareness among the public regarding the importance of health. The decline in the following most prevalent diseases, per 100,000 people, is shown in the figures below:[18]

	1900	1905	1910	1914
Typhoid fever	35.9	27.8	23.5	15.4
Diphtheria and croup	43.3	23.6	21.4	17.9
Tuberculosis of all forms	201.9	192.3	160.3	146.8
Pneumonia	180.5	148.8	147.7	127.0
Diarrhea and enteritis in children younger than age 2	108.8	97.0	100.8	66.0

However, certain other diseases were on the increase:

	1900	1905	1910	1914
Cancer	63.0	71.4	76.2	79.4
Organic heart disease	123.1	143.8	150.4	150.8
Cerebral hemorrhage	67.5	71.6	73.7	77.7
Nephritis	89.0	103.4	99.0	102.4

Also in 1912, an act of Congress created the U.S. Children's Bureau, a long-standing dream of Lillian Wald, as part of the Department of Commerce and Labor. Several years earlier, she had helped found the National Child Labor Committee to fight the ruthless exploitation of child labor. To ensure the promotion of all aspects of child health and welfare, Wald had repeatedly suggested to the government the need for such an agency and had been summoned to Washington by President Roosevelt in 1905 to explain her plan in detail. Four years later,

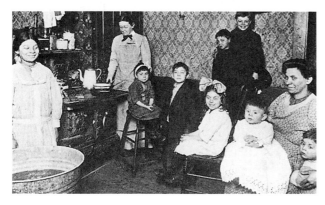

Establishment of the Children's Bureau in 1912 brought greater attention to child health.

the legislation passed, and President Taft chose Dr. Julia C. Lathrop, a resident of the Hull House settlement in Chicago, to head the new bureau. Nursing was related to most of the Children's Bureau functions, which included investigating and reporting on all matters pertaining to child welfare.

By 1912, the rapidly expanding public health nursing movement could look back nearly 20 years to the Nurses' Settlement on Henry Street, knowing that from humble beginnings a humanitarian ideal had grown into a substantial force, which was effectively attacking much human suffering and need. The noticeable decline in tuberculosis, diarrheal diseases of children, and typhoid fever—campaigns in which public health nurses had taken so active a part—inspired the confidence that better results were within reach.

REFERENCES

1. New York Association for Improving the Condition of the Poor, *Annual Report for 1884* (New York: The Association, 1884), p. 43.
2. New York Tenement House Commission, *Report of the Tenement House Commission for 1900* (New York: The Commission, 1900), p. 17.
3. W. Rathbone, *History and Progress of District Nursing* (New York: Macmillan Co., 1890), p. 7.
4. Ibid.
5. Henry Street Settlement, *Annual Report of the Henry Street Settlement for 1905* (New York: The Settlement, 1906), pp. 3–14.
6. Florence Kelley, *Medical Problems of Immigration* (Easton, PA: American Academy of Medicine Press, 1913), pp. 6–7.
7. Allen G. Rice, *Medical Inspection of Schools* (Providence: Snow & Farnham Co., 1912), pp. 48–49.
8. Unpublished letters, Records of the U.S. Children's Bureau, National Archives, Washington, DC, RG 102.
9. Ibid.
10. Edna L. Foley, "Standing Orders," *American Journal of Nursing*, vol. 13 (March 1913):451.
11. Ibid., pp. 451–453.
12. U.S. Department of Commerce and Labor, Bureau of the Census, *Mortality Statistics, 1910: General Death Rates; Specific and Standardized Death Rates; Infant and Child Mortality; Causes of Death* (Washington, DC: Government Printing Office, 1913), pp. 1–142.
13. Ellen N. La Motte, *The Tuberculosis Nurse: Her Function and Her Qualifications* (New York: G. P. Putnam's Sons, 1915), pp. 33–35.
14. Ibid., pp. 36–38.
15. J. E. Pilcher, "The Red Cross," *Military Surgeon*, vol. 20 (April 1907):230–237.
16. Mabel T. Boardman, "Rural Nursing Service of the Red Cross," *American Journal of Nursing*, vol. 13 (September 1913): 937–939.
17. Mary Sewall Gardner, "The National Organization for Public Health Nursing," *Visiting Nurse Quarterly*, vol. 4 (July 1912): 13–18.
18. U.S. Department of Commerce, Bureau of the Census, *Mortality Statistics, 1914* (Washington, DC: Government Printing Office, 1916), pp. 9–23.

9

IN QUEST OF REFORM, 1909–1917

The progressive era was a time of political, economic, and social reform in the cities, the states, and the nation. It gained its first impetus at the local level in the 1890s, reached the national scene with the succession of Theodore Roosevelt as president in 1901, and lasted until 1917, when the United States entered the First World War. As a reform impulse, progressivism was primarily an urban, middle-class response to the abuses and evils that had sprung up in the wake of uncontrolled industrialization and metropolitan expansion after the Civil War.

THE CRUSADE FOR REGISTRATION

Within nursing, reform was also needed. A large proportion of those who were practicing as "nurses" had never received any training, yet there were no legal restrictions against their presenting themselves to the public as fully trained graduates. Legislation to control the practice of nursing and the importance of having well-organized state associations to help secure it was recognized by the growing number of trained nurses. The idea of nurse registration to separate trained from untrained nurses was not a new one. It had been instituted in South Africa in 1891, and other countries had adopted it in the following order: Natal (1899), New Zealand (1901), and Great Britain (1902). For the United States, however, such legislation would have to be handled on the state rather than the federal level.

In 1898, Sophia Palmer made the first public statement on the subject of nurse licensure in a paper read before the New York State Federation of Women's Clubs. As a result, the federation passed a resolution favoring the establishment of a board of examiners chosen by the state society of nurses and recommending the inclusion of nursing in the list of professions supervised by the Board of Regents of the State University of New York.

An event that emphasized the need for immediate action by nurses to secure nurse registration occurred in 1900, when the Philadelphia County Medical Society and the College of Physicians of Philadelphia boldly announced that they were launching a school of nursing that would fully prepare students in only 10 weeks. Simultaneously, several correspondence schools began operations on a wide scale, advertising extensively with such promises as: "You can become a trained nurse by study at home. Send ten cents for handsome catalogue to the National Correspondence School of Health and Hygiene, 41 Telephone Building, Detroit, Michigan."[1] The advertisement was illustrated with a nurse's cap, apron, badge, bottle, and spoon. The 10-cent fee quickly bought eager applicants the "handsome catalogue," which stated that for about $13 and a few "extras," anyone, regardless of age or physical condition, could become a trained nurse by a mere few months' "study at home." Every graduate would receive an impressive-looking diploma—one that would often fool the public and discredit legitimate schools of nursing.

In September 1901, the first meeting of the newly founded International Council of Nurses (ICN) was held in Buffalo. Nurses in attendance were strongly encouraged to launch an effort to elevate and maintain the highest possible nursing standards. At one of the sessions, with many hundreds of nurses present, the following resolution in favor of state registration of nurses was proposed from the chair by Mrs. Bedford Fenwick of Great Britain, president of the council:

> Whereas the nursing of the sick is a matter closely affecting all classes of the community in every land; Whereas to be efficient workers, nurses should be carefully educated in the important duties which are now allotted to them; Whereas at the present time there is no generally accepted term or standard of training nor system of education nor examination for nurses in any

state nurses' association to present a bill before its legislature. The North Carolina nurse registration bill passed the State House of Representatives on January 20, 1903, with very little alteration. In the Senate a few weeks later, however, it met with strong opposition from the lobby of the state medical society, and finally a bill with much weaker provisions was substituted, which was passed in March of the same year. As signed by the governor, completion of a nurse training course was not required for registration. Any applicant, regardless of training or experience, who passed a state-administered examination was entitled to a certificate and a license to practice. The responsibility for developing the examinations and issuing licenses was assigned to a new board of nurse examiners, composed of two physicians and three nurses.

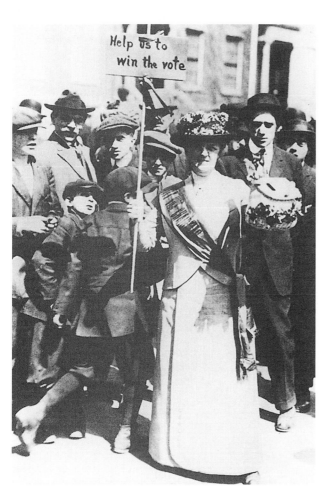

Public demands for social reform characterized the Progressive Era.

country; Whereas there is no method, except in South Africa, of enabling the public to discriminate easily between trained nurses and ignorant persons who assume that title; and Whereas this is a fruitful source of injury to the sick and of discredit to the nursing profession, it is the opinion of this international congress of nurses, in general meeting assembled, that it is the duty of the nursing profession of every country to work for suitable legislative enactment regulating the education of nurses and protecting the interests of the public, by securing State examinations and public registration, with the proper penalties for enforcing the same.[2]

Following the ICN congress, the introduction of nurse registration bills in the various state legislatures was generally preceded by the formation of state nurses' associations composed either of individuals or of individuals and organizations, such as alumnae associations. In North Carolina and New York, strong, widely representative graduate nurses' associations already in existence spearheaded the drive to gain passage of the legislation. North Carolina's was the first

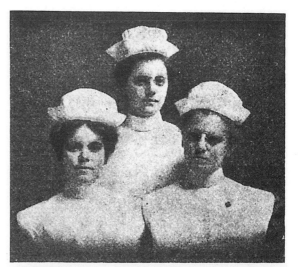

THREE SISTER NURSES

The Misses Avery, 735 West Central Avenue, St. Paul, Minn., graduates of this School

(The eldest Miss Avery, graduated in 1906, writes: "On my last case I received $25 a week.")

WE have trained thousands of women, in their own homes, to earn $12 to $30 a week.

The Chautauqua School's method of preparation has been proven—its success admits of no question.

Send today for 56-pp. Blue Book explaining our new method. Also interesting stories of experience by 100 graduates and physicians, just issued.

The Chautauqua School of Nursing

309 Main Street, Jamestown, New York

Hospitals, sanitariums and physicians in any part of the world supplied with well-taught nurses, experienced or juniors.

Advertisement for the Chautauqua School of Nursing.

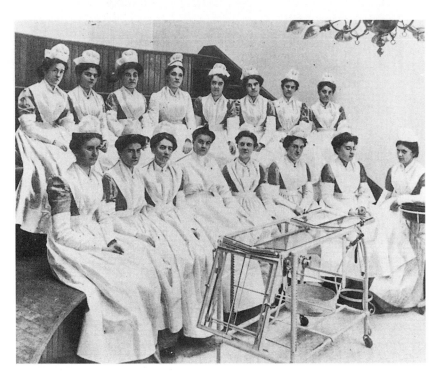

North Carolina enacted the first nurse registration law in 1903.

Among the initial state registration laws, New York State's legislation was considered the most progressive. To be eligible for registration in New York, nurses had to be graduates of training schools approved by the regents of the state university. Nurses who had been trained outside the state and who were engaged in institutional, private, or visiting nursing in New York were required to register in accordance with the law to continue their in-state work. Thus, schools from many of the other states in which these nurses had been trained soon applied to the board of regents for registration. In some instances, they altered their methods of teaching and expanded their curricula to conform to New York State requirements.

These requirements, as defined by the State Board of Nurse Examiners, established the minimum amount of practice and theory instruction in subjects considered essential to developing professional knowledge. A course in obstetrics, not offered by many nurse training schools, was early made a curricular requirement by the state board—bringing about new obstetric nursing courses throughout the East. One large hospital that had met all New York requirements except experience in the nursing of sick children opened a children's ward to enable its students to receive state approval. As the result of a hard-fought battle with New York medical societies, the nurse examining board in New York was composed entirely of nurses.

But even this law was not fully satisfactory. The need for tightening up the registration laws was glaringly apparent. In New York in 1909, for example, there were registered nurses who had completed 3-year courses, others who had finished 2-year courses,

and some who had received no formal nurse training at all, registering under a grandfather clause in the nurse registration act. Until the carryover of nurses from preregistration days slowly ran through the active labor force, the effectiveness of the registration laws was dulled.

POSTGRADUATE PROBLEMS

A second area of nursing in need of reform involved the nebulous concept of postgraduate training. The term *postgraduate* was applied indiscriminately to many clinical courses that were offered to diploma-holding nurses as substitutes for advanced nursing education. The level of achievement attained through many of these so-called postgraduate clinical courses could just as well have been gained through general staff nursing experience in a hospital offering good clinical experience together with an effective in-service staff education program. Most of these so-called postgraduate courses were characterized by service. The nurse went on duty at 7:00 a.m. and stayed until 7:00 p.m., scrubbing the ward in addition to caring for the patients. She was often used, for the benefit of the hospital, to fill in gaps or to help out during vacations.

There was a tremendous lack of uniformity in the postgraduate courses conducted by various hospitals. One 1905 postgraduate course gave no allowance, whereas another offered $20 per month. Still another provided no class work, gave no lectures, administered no examinations, yet awarded certificates. A 1902 postgraduate course offered by the Woman's

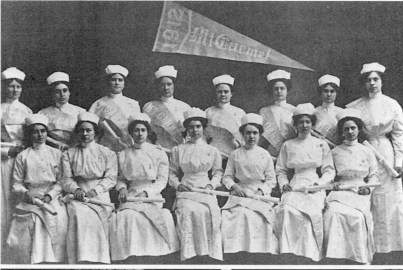

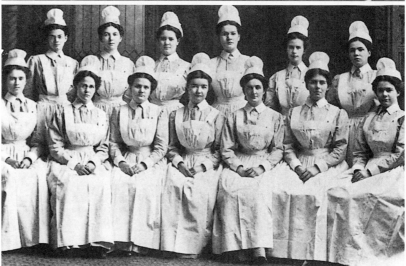

Few diploma graduates took the poor-quality postgraduate courses.

Hospital and Infant Home in Detroit included lectures by the specialists of the medical staff and classroom work with demonstrations given by the supervising nurse once a week. In addition, postgraduate students were allowed to attend the Farrand Training School lectures with the undergraduates.

An article entitled "My Impressions as a Postgraduate," published in the *American Journal of Nursing* in 1904, disclosed that

> there were classes and clinics both medical and surgical that we were privileged to attend.
> I went to a good many and liked going, but very often was too tired even when I had the time. . . .
> Could it not be possible to shorten the hours of graduates, giving them more time for study and making it compulsory to attend certain classes and clinics? To partly cover the expenses I would suggest that an entrance fee be charged.[3]

The results of a 1905 survey of postgraduate courses in 114 general hospitals and 20 special hospitals revealed that, among general hospitals of 100 beds or more, 26 gave a supplementary postgraduate course, only 3 of which made

> any provision for a regular course of lectures and class work. The others permit the graduates to attend the lectures and classes of the pupil nurses, but as many of the schools admit graduate nurses only during the vacation season, there are no lectures and classes to attend. . . . In one, a fee is charged of one dollar per day, while in others we find allowances given of varying amounts to as much as twenty dollars a month.[4]

Nurse training school superintendents who were finding it difficult to secure competent assistants and head nurses thought that postgraduate courses in which the nurse could secure expertise in the art of hospital housekeeping were essential. An ideal course would include information about the various hospital departments, including the kitchen and laundry and storerooms and linen rooms, as well as details such as cutting and making hospital garments, ordering supplies, and learning the business management of hospitals. Such training would allow hospitals to fill their nursing administration positions with qualified graduate nurses.

In 1899, as a result of this obvious need, a course in hospital economy was established at Teachers College, Columbia University, through the efforts of the American Society of Superintendents of Training Schools for Nurses, for the purpose of preparing graduate nurses to become teachers in training schools and superintendents of nursing in hospitals. Its eventual aim was to attain uniformity in training school methods so that nurses graduating from a school connected with any general hospital would be similarly trained.

The society appointed a board of examiners, whose duty was to select all candidates for the Teachers College course. The board required the aspiring superintendent to enter Teachers College for a full term of 8 months. It also stipulated that either before or after this term, she was to spend 3 to 4 months in private-duty nursing. After this year of extra education and experience, and if she passed the required final examinations, the nurse received a certificate, signed by the dean of Teachers College, Columbia University, attesting to her qualifications as a superintendent for either a training school for nurses or a hospital.

The general supervision of this course was in the hands of Anna L. Alline, instructor of hospital economics, who supplemented the work of the special lecturers and conducted excursions and fieldwork in various hospitals and health agencies. The course covered subjects such as the preparation of culture media, the isolation and culture of bacteria, and the preparation of antitoxins. Visits were made to laboratories preparing modified, sterilized, and pasteurized milk. A survey of various types of hospitals, including general, private, and special hospitals, mental institutions, and others, identified the unique nursing service demands of each. Special lectures were given on the following topics: hospital construction, the history of hospitals, hospital administration, and a practical exposition of training school administration.

In 1910, a $150,000 endowment by Helen Hartley Jenkins, a trustee of Teachers College, allowed the postgraduate course to be expanded in length and quality. This gift marked the first substantial financial provision for any part of the education of nurses. A new department of nursing and health was created at Teachers College, embracing three main divisions of work and preparing nurses for teaching and supervision in nurse training schools, for administration in hospitals and training schools, and for work in the social and preventive branches of nursing. Adelaide

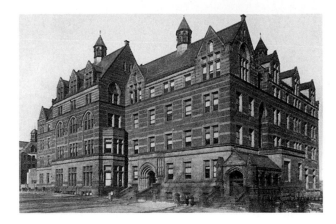

Teachers College, Columbia University.

Nutting, former superintendent of nurses and principal of the Training School for Nurses at Johns Hopkins Hospital from 1894 to 1907, who had come to Teachers College 3 years earlier as professor of hospital economics, was now appointed to head the new department of nursing and health. Under her leadership, the nursing program at Teachers College soon became the world leader in preparing nurse educators.

REFORM OF MEDICAL EDUCATION

Criticism of the low standards prevailing in the field of medical education had also been heard, but no one fully realized how shoddy conditions were until Abraham Flexner, with the support of a grant from the Carnegie Foundation, began a nationwide investigation. After a preliminary period of careful study and preparation, Flexner proceeded on a swift tour of medical schools in the United States and Canada. He had no fixed pattern and used no questionnaire in his investigation, yet he personally visited every one of the 155 schools and talked, in each instance, with medical school faculty members and their students.

Flexner soon came to realize that five points were conclusive in judging the quality and value of a medical school, all of which were just as pertinent for nursing education:

> First, the entrance requirements. What are they? Are they enforced?
>
> Second, the size and training of the faculty.
>
> Third, the sum available from endowment and fees for the support of the institution, and what becomes of it.
>
> Fourth, the quality and adequacy of the laboratories provided for the instruction of the first two years and the qualifications and training of the teachers of the so-called preclinical branches.
>
> Fifth, the relation between medical schools and hospitals, particularly including freedom of

access to beds and freedom in the appointment by the school of the hospital physicians and surgeons who automatically should become clinical teachers.[5]

The conditions depicted by Flexner in his 1910 report were shocking, and he pulled no punches in applying words such as "disgraceful" and "shameful." For example, Chicago, with its 14 medical schools, was described as "the plague spot of the country." He found that entrance requirements were enforced in only 10 of the 155 medical schools in the United States and Canada. Libraries were inadequate or nonexistent in 140 of the schools, and laboratory courses for the first and second years were deplorably equipped and poorly conducted in 139 of the schools.

Part 2 of the report lashed out at specific abuses found in each school:

> California Medical College (Los Angeles)—This school had led a roving and precarious existence . . . a disgrace to the state whose laws permit its existence.
> Georgetown University School of Medicine— There is no library accessible to students, no museum, and no pharmacological laboratory.
> Georgia College of Eclectic Medicine and Surgery (Atlanta)—Its anatomy room, containing a single cadaver, is indescribably foul. . . . Nothing more disgraceful calling itself a medical school can be found anywhere.
> Kansas Medical College (Topeka)—The dissecting room is indescribably filthy; it contained, in addition to necessary tables, a single, badly hacked cadaver and was simultaneously used as a chicken yard.
> Maryland Medical College (Baltimore)—The school building is wretchedly dirty . . . one neglected and filthy room is set aside for bacteriology, pathology, and histology: a few dirty test-tubes stand around in pans and old cigar-boxes.
> St. Louis College of Physicians and Surgeons— The school is one of the worst in the country.
> Pulte Medical College (Cincinnati)—Anything more woe-begone than the laboratories of this institution would be difficult to imagine. The dissecting room is a dark apartment in the basement.

Flexner's report contained such candid and drastic criticism of the defects of medical education in North America that the weaker schools were unable to continue. Of the recognized schools that survived, some merged for mutual strengthening, and most secured university connections. All became nonprofit institutions. In his preface to the Flexner report, Henry S. Pritchett, president of the Carnegie Foundation, anticipated such changes when he stated

that "progress for the future would seem to require a very much smaller number of medical schools, better equipped and better conducted than our schools now as a rule are; and the needs of the public would equally require that we have fewer physicians graduated each year, but that these should be better educated and better trained."[6]

The decade from 1910 to 1920 saw the establishment of medical education as a university discipline with definite educational standards, but only the better-financed and better-led schools were able to develop adequate laboratories and hospital affiliations to achieve the requisite quality of medical education. The number of inferior schools quickly dwindled.

A FLEXNER REPORT FOR NURSING?

Leading nurse educators were enthusiastic for a similar comprehensive survey of schools of nursing to be made. In 1911, the American Society of Superintendents of Training Schools for Nurses presented a proposal for such a study to the Carnegie Foundation in hopes of securing assistance. Adelaide Nutting reported the results of this effort in a report at the annual convention of the superintendents in 1912. She related to the group that President Pritchett "seemed much interested in the matter, but stated that the Foundation was at the time unable to take the question up [as] all of its energies were centered in work in other directions."

The following year Nutting told the assembled nurse educators, "Realizing the enormous benefit to medical education resulting from such an investigation of medical schools by the Carnegie Foundation, the Committee is confident that similar benefits must result from such an investigation of our much more complicated educational problems."[7] Meanwhile, Pritchett directed a considerable amount of Carnegie Foundation funds into "Flexner-like" studies of dental, legal, and teacher education and passively ignored the pleas of nurses.

TRAINING SCHOOL LIFE IN THE PROGRESSIVE ERA

According to the second edition of the *American Medical Directory*, by 1909 the number of general hospitals in the United States had increased to 4359—of these, 1006 operated nurse training schools. In addition, 90 mental institutions ran schools. A typical hospital school of nursing in a smaller city of the era required 2 years of high school for admission along with evidence of "careful home training" and a "definite knowledge of housekeeping duties." Students were admitted between the ages of 18 and 35 years.

When a candidate made application for training, she was sent the usual application and physician's certificate form. If her responses to these and the required references were satisfactory, arrangements were made for a personal interview. Except for maintenance, textbooks, and uniforms, the probationers received no financial compensation during the first year. The second year they received a monthly allowance of $7.50, and the third year it was raised to $15. The school had found that the absence of any allowance during the entire first year did much to discourage those who might have entered nursing for financial reasons.

Two classes of probationers were admitted yearly, one entering September 1 and the other February 1. The superintendent always met a new class of probationers personally and gave them an informal word of welcome and encouragement. This was followed by a weekly class in ethics, which covered many important and necessary dos and don'ts.

In the first 2 weeks after admission, probationers were not allowed to be on the wards for more than 1 or 2 hours a day. This orientation period was only long enough to permit them to become somewhat familiar with hospital customs. During this time, they were not assigned to care for patients but were shown how to keep a ward in order, how to care for flowers and patients' belongings, and other minor details. Their hours and duties on the ward were gradually increased during the next 2 months, until, at the end of their third month, they were in the wards 6 to 7 hours daily. During this time they attended classes in nursing and were taken by the assistant superintendent into the wards, where they were taught to put the latest lesson into practice.

During their third month, the head nurse, who was a third-year nursing student, supervised the work of these new students, as directed by the assistant superintendent. At the end of their third month, an examination was held on all subjects taught up to that time. If this was passed satisfactorily, and if her clinical performance and personality were also considered

satisfactory, the probationer was accepted as a student nurse.

The school gave a 3-year course of training, which included 3 months of probation, although the entire first 6 months were considered to be a preparatory course. The curriculum of this typical school was as follows:[8]

Preparatory Class

Anatomy and Physiology	15 hours
Solutions	7 hours
Practical Nursing	24 hours
Theoretical Nursing	24 hours
Preparatory Materia Medica	6 hours
Nursing Ethics and Hygiene	10 hours
Principles of Cookery and Dietetics	20 hours
Bacteriology and Urinalysis	12 hours

Junior Class

Anatomy and Physiology, continued	20 hours
Principles of Cookery and Dietetics	20 hours
Surgical Nursing and Bandaging	16 hours
Obstetrical Nursing	6 hours

Intermediate Class

Medical Diseases and Contagion	7 lectures
Surgery	10 lectures
Obstetrics	12 lectures
Gynecology	4 lectures
Pediatrics	5 lectures
Eye, Ear, Nose, and Throat	5 lectures
Materia Medica, Regular	12 lectures

Senior Class

Massage, Hydrotherapy	20 hours
Advanced Nursing, with lectures on nursing, topics of day and current events	12 hours

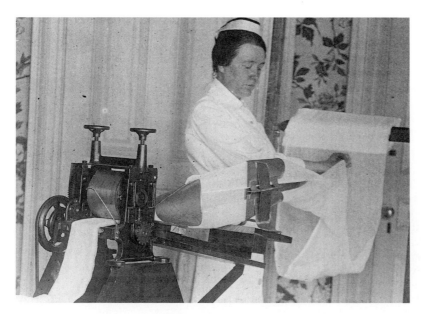

Surgical supervisor operating a machine used to make gauze bandages.

The course of instruction was taught according to the following arrangement:

Superintendent
Nursing Ethics
Hygiene
History of Nursing, with lectures on special nursing topics and current events

Assistant Superintendent
Theoretical Nursing
Practice Nursing
Solutions
Preliminary Materia Medica
Practical Obstetrical Nursing
Practical Ward Surgery

Surgical Supervisor
Surgical Technic
Bandaging

Special Hydrotherapy Nurse
Massage and Hydrotherapy

Instructor from the Manual Training School
Dietetics—chemistry of food
Cookery—preparing of invalid diet

Physician's Lectures
Anatomy and Physiology
Materia Medica—regular and homeopathic
Medical Diseases
Contagious Diseases
Surgery
Gynecology
Obstetrics
Bacteriology
Urinalysis
Eye, Ear, Nose, and Throat

The staff of the training school consisted of the superintendent of nursing for the hospital and training school, the surgical supervisor, and the night superintendent—all registered nurses—and one graduate dietitian. The school's enrollment averaged about 22 student nurses. There were no full-time teachers. The larger part of the teaching and actual nursing supervision was in the hands of the assistant superintendent. An authoritarian atmosphere was ensured by assigning one of the graduate nurses to be in charge of the students at all times. In the operating room, the instruction in surgical technique was given by the surgical supervisor, and while on night duty the nurses were entirely responsible to the night superintendent, receiving all necessary instructions from her.

The hospital used a 9-hour day, but the nurses were on actual duty 56 hours per week, each nurse being allowed 3 hours for meals and rest daily, a half day off on Sunday, and an additional half day off during the week. A student nurse assigned to a special patient was always given 8 consecutive hours of rest daily and 1 day off every 7 days on the case. Required night duty amounted to 6 weeks of continuous duty for juniors, with 3 days off when the service was terminated, and 8 continuous weeks for seniors, with a 4-day rest on completion.

In common with all other training schools, this institution had a strict set of rules, which were read to the probationers during their first week of training. As far as possible, the hospital superintendent tried to make the school self-governing. One of the first things she told a class of probationers was that every nurse in the school was on her honor—if it was found that a nurse could not or would not voluntarily act in an honorable manner, she would be expelled. There was also a special set of rules for the guidance of advanced students, who functioned in the role of head nurses:

The head nurse is to be on duty promptly at 7:00 A.M. and immediately to assign morning work to senior and junior nurses.

To take report from night nurse and see that charting room and lavatory are in order, and fresh towels ready for doctor's use, nurse's table in order, etc.

At 7:15 take charge of diet kitchen and at all times to *personally supervise and assist* in serving trays, making sure that all food is hot, nicely cooked and served, and that each patient is getting correct diet as prescribed by doctor; to carefully instruct juniors in proper tray service and to see that all helpless patients are fed; to make a room-to-room trip after trays are served to see that patients have eaten and enjoyed meals.

To give all medication occurring before and to 9:00 A.M. inclusive.

To take all T.P.R.'s up through that hour.

To make up all drug lists, requisition lists, etc.

To write up all charts to 9:00 A.M. inclusive.

To be entirely responsible for cleanliness of drug closet.

To prepare surgical trays and take charge of surgical dressings.

To make rounds with doctors and superintendent, reporting carefully about patients.

To see that all doctors' orders are carried out at the earliest possible moment, and to carefully supervise and direct nurses doing same, and to assume care of certain patients whenever necessary.

The head nurse is absolutely responsible for the comfort and welfare of all patients entrusted to her care.

She is to practice and to insist upon the greatest care and economy in the use of all hospital supplies.

She is to report any failure to carry out doctors' orders, with any reasons for same, at the earliest possible moment; also any sudden change in patients' condition or any high temperature to house surgeon and superintendent.

To inspect all beds and backs of all bed patients at least once daily.

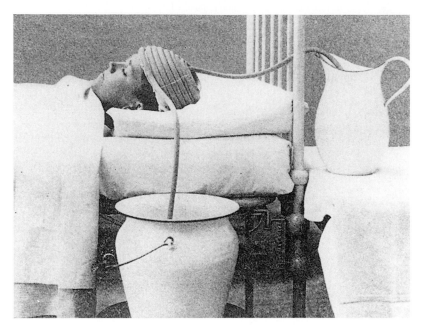

Procedure to reduce the temperature of a fever patient.

To *immediately* report any accident happening to any patient under her charge to house surgeon and superintendent.

To write up night orders and diet slips.

To give personal supervision to all work done by nurses and orderlies or ward maids; to see that work is arranged so that day nurses can get off duty promptly at 7:00 P.M., and never go off duty, unless told to do so by supervisor.

To report to dietitian immediately any unsatisfactory diet, shortage, etc., and, in the event of repeated trouble, to report to supervisor; to make out all diet lists, ordering only the probable amount of extras needed, and practice judgment and economy in ordering of food and supplies.

To get a signed order from superintendent for any rush or special work from laundry.

To see that linen is carefully used and to have all torn or ragged articles placed in a bag for repair or to be replaced; to see that all private room patients are bathed every day and ward patients twice a week; bed patients given alcohol rub every night.

In absence of the senior nurse, her duties are to be assumed or arranged for her by the head nurse.

One of the most important duties of the head nurse is to keep the assistant superintendent informed at all times about any matter of interest or importance on her floor; any reports or complaints from patients or doctors must *always* be immediately referred to assistant superintendent; also any shortages of working materials, medicines, linen, supplies, etc.

The head nurse is to insist upon order and quiet at all times, and must eliminate all unnecessary noises, such as loud talking, rattling of dishes, utensils, etc. The head nurse should stand out as a leader, from the standpoint of efficiency, ethics, and good breeding, by her own personal example and precept.

The duties of the senior nurse were somewhat less responsible than those of the head nurse, but still very demanding:

The senior nurse is to assume duties and responsibilities of head nurse when she is absent or off duty.

To take charge of the most ill patients as assigned by head nurse. (Probably three, in emergencies, four.)

To take all T.P.R.'s except those previous to 9:00 A.M.

To assist when necessary in making rounds with doctors and in preparing dressings, trays, and doing surgical dressings.

To give all unusual or special treatments.

To prepare patients for operation, and take them to operating room when necessary.

To be responsible for caring for work of juniors when they are off duty.

To see that all charting after 9:00 A.M. is kept up at all hours of the day.

To keep dressing trays set up and look after all surgical instruments and supplies, and see that all such supplies are left ready for the night nurse.

The juniors were charged with the following duties, which reflected the decreasing degree of authority:

The juniors will be responsible for any of the senior work during absence of senior, or any other work arranged by head nurse.

To care for patients as assigned by head nurse; to do work thoroughly and quickly, and have patients comfortable and well cared for at all times; also to have private rooms and wards in strictest order.

When two juniors are on a floor, one shall be responsible for the diet kitchen and linen closet, and the other for the bathrooms and utensils.

To give any medication or treatment directed by head nurse and, if directed to do so, to keep up patient's charge after 9:00 A.M.

To keep head nurse carefully informed as to patient's condition at all times. If any bed patient shows the least tendency to bed sores, same to be immediately reported to head nurse.

The lowly duties of the probationers demanded a strong back and very little thinking:

> Probationers are to dust rooms, arrange flowers, put empty beds and rooms in order, and care for bathrooms, diet kitchen, linen closets, and chart rooms; also to have such other duties concerning the personal care and treatment of patients as arranged for by superintendent with head nurse for the application of the principles of nursing as taught.[9]

The school taught the students to be prompt and careful in carrying out physicians' orders. The head nurse or senior on the ward made the rounds with the various members of the medical staff, waiting on them as necessary. Before leaving the floor, the physician wrote his own orders in the order book or requested the house physician to do so. The nurse who carried out the order initialed it in red ink and also noted the hour. By means of this simple plan, it could be immediately ascertained, should any question arise, which nurse had carried out the order.

Complaints from physicians were generally made personally to the superintendent or her assistant. When a patient's complaint reached the head nurse, it was immediately reported for investigation; when a complaint concerned a specific nurse, she was requested to reply in writing. If the mistake made was serious, the nurse was removed from duty by the superintendent until the matter had been fully investigated. In the third year of training, the students were given black bands for their caps, designating them as head nurses, and the greatest punishment that could possibly befall a third-year nurse was to have her black band taken away. The most common method of discipline for any serious misdemeanor was to extend the nurse's period of service from 2 to 4 weeks.

WASTE OF THE NURSE'S ENERGY

A great deal of unnecessary energy was expended by nurses on ward duty. In 1913, one enterprising physician attacked what he called a lack of cooperation on the part of training school authorities in implementing conservation of energy on hospital wards, especially in matters concerning the comfort of patients. He placed pedometers on nurses in several hospitals and discovered that in a single day one of the nurses walked 7½ miles, whereas the average nurse walked 5½ miles.

In one hospital, this investigator discovered that a ward was so long that the farthest bed was 120 feet from the ward kitchen. Worse still, hospital custom required that trays be carried individually to and from each bed three times a day. He added up the unnecessary walking required of the ward nurse and found that it amounted to about 2 miles a day. The food trays and their contents were found to weigh 15 pounds. Thus the nurse had to haul considerable weight for 2 extra miles. When he suggested that wheel trucks be used to carry all the trays at one time, the objection was that the food would reach the patients cold. Similarly, the bed screens weighed 31 pounds, and because it took three screens to surround a bed when a patient used the bedpan, the nurse had to carry 93 pounds to and from his or her bed and then, of course, carry the bedpan back and forth, walking a total distance of 480 feet.

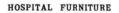

HOSPITAL FURNITURE

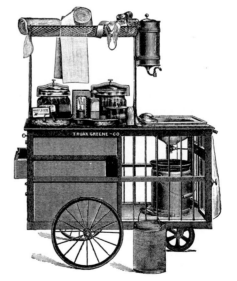

Fig. 1744. NECKER HOSPITAL WHEEL CARRIAGE.

Price, with wash bowl and slop bucket.....................................$100 00

These carriages are made from a model brought direct from Paris. It is the pattern in use in each of the wards in Necker hospital. After examining the patterns in use in most of the better equipped hospitals of the world, we selected this as being one of the most desirable. They are well made from hardwood, have rubber-tired wheels on steel axles. The bowl is of porcelain, while the upright rack for dressings is of wrought iron. The whole apparatus combines many desirable features in the one appliance.

Hospital wheel carriage used during the 1890s.

HOSPITAL SCREENS.

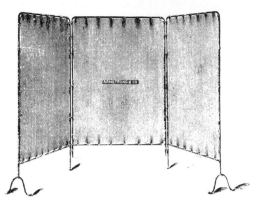

Screen No. 1.   For the operating room or for use in wards.   Threefold, of wrought iron, white
enamel finished.   Height, 60 inches; total length, 96 inches............ .... $10 00
Canvas cover, with eyelets and cords... 4 50   *Hospital bed screens.*

A WALK AROUND THE WARDS

Let us walk the wards of a big city hospital with one of the nurses of this period by leafing through the pages of her diary.

> February 10—Monday—My funny Irish woman, Mrs. Maloney, is much dissatisfied with the nurses and doctors. She says they ought to be middle-aged people. We had a horrid afternoon, a rushing, tumbling kind. I had to fly to get around, yet the patients were unusually kind. Bridget encouraged me in her rough way. Poor Alice had a sinking spell and was so sick.
>
> February 11—Tuesday—A probationer was put into our ward and under my special care. I am having good times teaching her, for she is so nice and quick to learn. We have a patient poisoned with carbolic acid, who is doing nicely. Alice is better.
>
> February 12—Wednesday—Chaos, rushing, and weariness! Another case of attempted suicide.
>
> February 13—Thursday—A little negro girl, one of my patients, died this morning. She had only been in a day and was very sick, poor child. She had told me while I was trying to clean her nails, against her express desire, that I was not a good nurse, being too determined. A new stretcher case was brought in. It is the worst morning we have had. Poor Miss Dunstan gave up and cried.
>
> February 14—Friday—Miss Thayer is back, and we are so glad. Things will go better now. Our nice little probationer has patients of her own and is doing beautifully. Poor Nellie is very much worse. I have had such a fancy for the child ever since she came in, and she has wanted me to do everything for her. She is delirious now, and knows no one; I do hope she will get well. I bathed five and one-half people this morning. One woman I fixed had a double nail on one toe and she told me she used to have six toes on her left foot, but one had been amputated.
>
> February 15—Saturday—We didn't half get through our work. We had four new cases, one on a stretcher and two in wheelchairs. Seven of the patients have to sleep on the floor. We have over sixty.
>
> February 16—Sunday—Was on in the morning and the work went beautifully.
>
> February 17—Monday—Alice gave me fifty cents to spend for her, and asked me to get two envelopes, two sheets of paper, two stamps, a can of honey, and some gingersnaps. Nellie knew me for the first time in ever so long, but she is no better.
>
> February 18—Tuesday—Miss Thayer called the nurses together and told us we must finish our work on time. Then she divided it differently and gave me two private rooms and four patients in the ward. That gives me ten patients in all; six are typhoids, and all are very sick. Nellie is my patient now, but is too sick to know it. I have a homesick little Bohemian, and a repulsive paralyzed woman. Two of my patients have bedsores that have to be dressed every day.
>
> February 19—Wednesday—We watched all day a threatened case of abortion, but it didn't come off before we came away.
>
> February 20—Thursday—Miss Dunstan, our senior nurse, is sick, so I have the senior work—medicines, temperatures, and the private rooms. Our ward is so full that eight sick patients have to sleep on the floor. We had to send away two of our best help, the night woman and the kitchen woman, because they fight so. Our case of abortion still hangs on.

February 21—Friday—I have Annie to care for now, and she is funnier than ever. She is a little delirious yet, and when she does anything horrid and I talk to her about it, she opens her big black eyes and says, "Forgive me, nurse." Miss Drake telephoned to Miss Thayer, who was taking her half day, that she must come back, and she did. Finally, Miss Fife appeared on the scene with uplifted hands and a look of horror, saying, "Really, Miss Thayer, Ward E will drive me distracted." When they had gone, we laughed, for we didn't feel a bit guilty; we had worked so hard and every necessary thing was done, though things did look horrid.

Washington's Birthday—Saturday—I was on in the morning and spent most of my time over Frances, giving her stimulants and hypodermic injections. We have sixty-five patients now. An extra row of beds has been put down the middle of the ward.

February 23—Sunday—I was on in the morning again and had a terrific time getting through. I had to keep up poultices and fomentations, besides fixing fourteen patients. Poor Frances died last night.

February 24—Monday—They have moved two very sick patients from the ward into my rooms and my hands are full. They have to have turpentine stupes kept up day and night. Nellie got out of bed today under the delusion that she had to move to Broadway. I had to tie her in bed after that. I tied one foot to the foot of the bed. Some time after, I found her looking sadly at the foot, and she said to me, "Nurse, won't you please release this prisoner? He has been tried and has proved himself clear; he was only one of a gang." It is very odd that though she is all the time delirious, she knows me, and though she won't answer one of my questions sensibly, she will take anything I give her, and makes a great fuss with any one else. Our abortion woman departed in pretty good health today.

February 25—Tuesday—A horrid, vile day. I was so tired my legs wouldn't walk, and my arms wouldn't work, and I had so much to do. In the afternoon Miss Thayer asked me to print some labels, and then when I started, she sent me on errands everywhere, and each time I went through the ward half a dozen patients would shout at me for something.

February 26—Wednesday—Poor little 43, a Swedish girl, with golden hair and blue eyes, is getting worse so fast. I have to give her milk every fifteen minutes and a stupe every hour; 41 is very sick too.

February 27—Thursday—41 died last night. I feel so sorry that I ever pulled her hair. It used to get so tangled I could hardly help it. The little Swedish girl is dying. Her doctor does not believe in stimulants, so we have just had to watch her grow worse and worse without doing anything for her. It does seem wicked. The two patients in my middle room always amuse me so much—Nellie, and Bohemian Mary. I made some lemonade for them today, and they were perfectly delighted. I used to think Mary was very stupid, but she talks a little now in her broken English and says I am "awfoo good," which makes me as happy as anything I have ever heard. She has a dreadful bed-sore.

February 28—Friday—Nellie grows more amusing every day. She begs me every morning to make her some "clarimot," which is as near as she can get to lemonade. She asked Miss Gault today to bring her a few squirts of water. Mary is ever so much better, but her back is dreadful. She says it is "no good." Sophie went away today; she has been one of my favorite patients, so pretty and timid and willing. She scrubbed my tables and chairs for me before she went. Annie was funny, too, today. When she did something she ought not and I said, "Oh, Annie!" she replied, "Poor little Annie's going to die." While I was changing the sheets, she tried to console me by throwing kisses.

I did not half finish my work today, but the patients have been so nice to me. One woman in the ward never fails to smile when I go by, because when she first came I would not let them cut her hair, which was fearfully tangled, but after a half hour's tug got it smooth.[10]

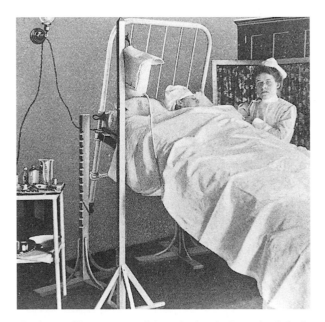

Device used by nurses to elevate the head of a patient's bed.

THE RISE OF WOMEN'S RIGHTS

Student nurses were classed as employees by the Bureau of the Census. According to the bureau, in 1909, 20.6% of the nation's 6,615,046 wage earners were female. Of the total work force, about 2.1% were children younger than 16 years of age. The number of women engaged in gainful occupations had increased steadily since 1870. In that year, only 13% of the gainfully employed workers were female, but by 1910 the number had increased to more than 20%. More than half the workers in 12 of the nation's 88 leading industries were women, and nursing was almost entirely in the hands of women. Large numbers of women were also employed in various aspects of the textile industry, in canning and preserving, in confectionery, and in the manufacture of tobacco products.

The fact that divorce had increased from 27 to 86 per 100,000 population from 1867 to 1906 reflected the liberalization of divorce laws. There had been fewer than 10,000 divorces in 1867, when divorce had meant social ostracism. By 1907, more than 72,000 divorces were granted in the United States—more than in all the rest of the Christian world. In part, this trend reflected the loosening of economic and religious bonds and the sharp increase in careers open to women who chafed against the restraints of unhappy marriages. The growing insistence on a single moral standard led legislatures to relax the procedural requirements of having to establish adultery, as well as desertion and cruelty, as grounds for divorce. The waiting period for divorces was usually a year, although ordinances in Reno, Nevada, cut this in half during the early 1900s.

Conservative churches, among them the Roman Catholic and Lutheran, tried to check the official divorce rate, but they could not halt the sensational increase in desertion, "the poor man's divorce." Desertion—at least four times more common than divorce—seemed to thrive in the unstable social environments of unemployed or migratory factory hands and broken immigrant homes. Many regarded increased divorce as evidence that unhappiness in marriage was greater than ever before. Others asserted that there had always been a great many unhappy marriages and that the high divorce rate meant only that more people were taking the legal way out of an unfortunate situation.

MATRIMONY AND THE NURSE

Whenever a nurse and her patient married, newspapers were inclined to treat the incident as a romance, and the reading public, forgetting that the atypical was always more newsworthy, often came to regard matrimony as the ultimate goal of all trained nurses. According to the eminent physician William Osler of Johns Hopkins University:[11]

> Marriage is the natural end of the trained nurse. So truly as a young man married is a young man marred, is a woman unmarried, in a certain sense, a woman undone. Ideals, a career, ambition, touched though they be with the zeal of St. Theresa, all vanish before "the blind bow-boy's butt shaft." Are you to be blamed and scoffed at for so doing? Contrariwise, you are to be praised, with but this caution—which I insert at the special request of Miss Nutting—that you abstain from philandering during your period of training, and, as much as in you lies, spare your fellow workers, the physicians and surgeons of the staff. . . . There is a gradually accumulating surplus of women who will not or who cannot fulfill the highest duties for which Nature has designed them. I do not know at what age one dare call a woman a spinster. I will put it, perhaps rashly, at twenty-five. Now, at that critical period a woman who has not to work for her living, who is without urgent domestic ties, is very apt to become a dangerous element unless her energies and emotions are diverted in a proper channel. . . . Such a woman needs a vocation, a calling which will satisfy her heart, and she should be able to find it in nursing without entering a regular school or working in ecclesiastical harness.

The reverse was true, according to a 1916 investigation published in the *Journal of Heredity*, which found that fewer than half of the graduates of the best nurse training schools had married. The lowest number of married graduates, 21%, was reported at the training school of Washington University in St. Louis, whereas the highest, 52%, was recorded at St. Luke's Hospital Nurse Training School in New York.

The *Journal of Heredity* investigator observed that no amount of optimism could bring one to conclude that the marriage rate of trained nurses—or at least of the graduates of the best training schools—was even reasonably high. Ironically, it was generally thought that the education of a nurse prepared her admirably for homemaking and motherhood. Although the investigator postulated that nurses should have been in great demand as wives, the extraordinary infrequency of marriages suggested that men did not use good judgment in selecting mates. It was possible that there was something in a nurse's education to which men objected; it was also possible that many nurses preferred to remain single. It was thought that their remaining single could not be largely due to a lack of opportunities to meet men, because such opportunities appeared to be plentiful.

Any attempt to analyze the causes of this low marriage rate was considered futile until more solid data were available; however, one simple cause was suspected—age. Ten or 15 years before this report, the age of admission to good training schools had often been from 21 to 25 years. The average age of nurses at graduation was not younger than 25 years. Nurses who graduated in classes before 1902 were already, therefore, well toward the end of the most marriageable period of a woman's life. More recently, training schools had been reducing the age standards, age 20 years perhaps being an average minimum, while many schools had begun to admit students at the age of 19 years. The average age of graduates at the time of the *Journal of Heredity* investigation was about 23 years. It was thought that this lowering of age alone would soon tend to increase the marriage rate of the more recent graduates.

THE PROGRESSIVE EFFECT ON NURSING

There were implications for nursing in the 1908 Supreme Court case of *Muller v. Oregon*, which involved a state law limiting women factory workers to a 10-hour day. The case was notable for the presentation made by Louis D. Brandeis of a heavily documented brief that forcefully argued from factual evidence rather than from legal deduction that long hours of work were detrimental to the health of women and to the general welfare. The "Brandeis Brief" became a landmark in the practical application of "sociological jurisprudence." The Court upheld the Oregon law and, by accepting the Brandeis Brief, gave judicial cognizance to a type of concrete presentation that other progressive lawyers learned to use to good effect.

Much of the data for the Brandeis Brief had been gathered by Josephine Goldmark, Brandeis's sister-in-law. Josephine, along with another sister, Pauline, did important work with Florence Kelley in the National Consumers' League, staying on to eventually become chair of the League's committee on the legal defense of labor laws. Goldmark's book, *Fatigue and Efficiency*, based on this experience and written in collaboration with Brandeis, was destined to become a source book of great value in framing protective legislation for women. The decision in *Muller v. Oregon* opened the way to a surge of protective legislation. Between 1908 and 1917, 39 states either passed new laws or strengthened old ones regulating the hours of women's work.

In 1910, a special federal investigation of occupations that were "morally dangerous" for women concluded that nursing was a job entailing moral risk. Five types of work were deemed morally dangerous by different social and rescue workers: domestic service, the work of hotel or restaurant waitresses, the low-grade factory trades, trained nursing, and the less-desirable stenographic positions. The report expressed some surprise at having found trained nursing to be a calling in which women were especially likely to "go wrong," but it had been so identified in several places,

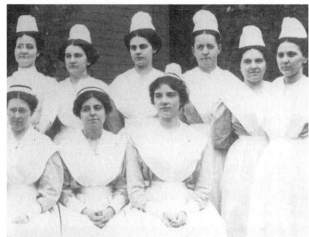
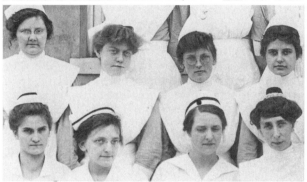

Nursing students were an exploited labor source.

all large cities. The investigators had therefore concluded that there seemed to be good reason to look at nursing as a somewhat dangerous pursuit.

The nurse was subjected to periods of long and exhausting mental strain along with much hard physical work. Her position made it convenient for her to secure drugs and liquor, and the nature of her work created a special demand for stimulants or restoratives. It was easy for her "to become a hard drinker or a drug fiend, and when a woman adopts either habit the chances of her going wrong in other ways are much increased." In addition, the nurse, like the domestic servant, was "in a position which makes it easy for men to essay advances toward her if they have any desire in that direction." She did not have the protection of working in public that was afforded by the factory or the department store, and when she was nursing a man, "opportunities for complications are evident."[12] In light of this kind of reputation, it is no wonder that the pendulum of morality swung to a nearly monastic extreme in many training schools.

CALIFORNIA LEADS THE WAY

Although progressive states attempted to minimize the most outrageous and indefensible forms of exploitation of the working population, they largely bypassed the hospitals. One notable exception to this indifference took place in California. In 1911, a bill was passed in the California legislature that was known as the "Eight-Hour Law for Women." This bill, which in the course of time became law, limited the working hours of women employed in any mercantile, mechanical, or manufacturing establishment or office to 8 hours a day for 6 days per week.

Early in 1912, the first indications of a movement to extend to student nurses the protection of the 8-hour law were revealed in certain communications between California progressives and several state nursing organizations. Such an amendment was introduced in the legislature in 1913 on behalf of the California Bureau of Labor. Investigation revealed that in many California hospitals, the hours of student nurses were excessive because it was general practice to use students as special private-duty nurses. It was said that the income of certain proprietary hospitals accrued almost entirely from this practice. For the benefit of the student nurse herself as well as for the good of the patient, it seemed essential that these young women have the same protection as that given to almost all other working women in California.

The bill was fought bitterly by commercial hospitals in the state. Even the Nurses' Association of Southern California sent a petition against its passage. In addition, hospitals submitted petitions signed by hundreds of undergraduate nurses opposing the measure. A small group of graduate nurses in San Francisco and Alameda counties provided the only visible support that proponents of the bill could garner from the nursing profession.

One reason for this was the argument, voiced by many hospital physicians, that the nursing profession would be debased by its inclusion in a law that could be enforced by the State Bureau of Labor. Many nurses agreed and were honestly incensed by the Bureau's action. The bill had the support of a few progressive physicians, but for the most part the medical profession vigorously opposed the measure.

The bill was introduced in the California Senate by Henry H. Lyon of Los Angeles and in the House by Assemblyman Walter McDonald of San Francisco. Debate in the Senate was heated, and the bill was impeded in its progress by a phalanx of opposition members. Senator Lyon, who championed the bill, reviewed the situation in the hospitals of the state, pointing out the long hours of labor required by student nurses, the money earned by them for their institution, and the pittance, barely enough to cover the cost of uniforms and books, paid to them. He urged speedy passage of the bill but was blocked at the outset by an amendment proposing that hospitals be exempted from the operation of the law. From that time, the fight centered on the amendment.

The spirited Lyon was followed by one of the northern California senators, who read several letters from prominent people asserting the critical need among student nurses for the protection of the 8-hour law. Senator Anthony Caminetti also made a vigorous objection to the amendment, pleading that the 8-hour legislation be backed by every man who had the cause of humanity at heart:

> We took a great step forward two years ago when we passed the Eight-Hour Law, and I don't know a man who fought against it at that time who would change it now. We cannot go backward. We must go forward. Our parties have pledged themselves to the uplifting of humanity; it was the slogan of our last campaign, and there can be no better example of putting into practice than by passing this bill by an almost unanimous vote.[13]

That evening, Senator Caminetti spoke again in support of the 8-hour bill, introducing statistics showing the detrimental effects of overwork. Despite vehement objections and an avalanche of opposing telegrams, the bill passed. The Senate chambers and galleries had been crowded all day with women interested in the passage of the bill. Many of the wives of assemblymen, some of whom had been student nurses, stayed on until passage of the bill was assured.

To provide for possible referendum, the bill was required to wait 90 days before final passage into law. There was a great deal of agitation on the part of hospital owners for such a referendum. Many errors of fact were circulated in an attempt to provoke such action, the most preposterous of which claimed that all graduate nurses would be included under the law and that families in need of private-duty nurses would have to circulate three nurses over 24 hours—an impossible financial burden for most people. What is more, the state hospital association sent delegates to the governor asking him to withhold his signature, thereby scuttling the bill. When the governor looked over the room filled with physicians and hospital representatives, he asked, "Where are the people in favor of this law?" Bessie Beatty of the *San Francisco Bulletin* told him that the people in favor of the law were the young women in hospitals caring for the sick who were unable to get away to present their claims. The governor signed the bill.

On October 14, 1913, in an attempt to halt enforcement of the new law, the trustees of the Associated Hospital Workers of Southern California filed a petition in the U.S. District Court for a restraining order. Two months later, however, the U.S. Court of Appeals upheld the California 8-hour law for student nurses as being constitutional and in no way impairing the right of contract guaranteed by the Fourteenth Amendment. Oakland's Merritt Hospital then took the law to the Supreme Court for decision.

In the case of *California v. Merritt Hospital*, the argument for the defense was presented by the attorney for the hospital, who attacked the constitutionality of the 8-hour law, while two briefs were presented by the representative of the labor organization defending the law. A decision was rendered on February 23, 1915, which held that "the same restriction as to the hours of employment of student nurses in hospitals is not an unconstitutional violation of the freedom of contract, as these persons, upon whom rests the burden of immediate attendance upon and nursing of the patients in hospitals, are also pupils engaged in a course of study, and the propriety of legislative protection of women undergoing such a discipline is not open to question."[14]

California hospital administrators viewed the new law unfavorably. It forced a larger payroll and bigger housing and operating expenditures because additional graduate nurses were required to supplement the work of the students. After passage of the law, these expenses were offset in the private institutions by an increase in rates and in the endowed institutions by a decrease in charitable work. According to the critics, an increased management burden fell on the hospital administrators, whereas greater expenses fell on the taxpayers for the maintenance of public institutions and on the patients themselves for the maintenance of private hospitals. The law also caused a decrease in the dividends of commercial hospitals.

The decrease in outside income generated by sending students into homes for private-duty work seriously affected the finances of some hospitals. In a paper on this subject read before the American Nurses Association in April 1914, Lila Pickhardt, superintendent of nurses of the Pasadena Hospital, reflected: "Just how great this revenue was may be estimated when we have reason to believe that in some institutions 40 percent of the student nurses were on special cases. Frequently, probationers were assigned to special duty, and some have estimated that two-thirds of the time while enrolled as a student nurse was given to special duty."[15]

The following extract from the letter of a California superintendent of nurses to a friend expresses the reactionary view of the establishment at that time:

> The eight-hour law is still a heavy burden, really the most cruel thing they have ever done in the nursing profession; I don't know when it is going to end. Patients are complaining, head nurses work day and night doing the student nurses' work, while the latter are constantly grumbling and in a state of discontent at not getting all the experience they should have; that is, the conscientious ones, while the others are running around, attending picture shows, theatres, etc., tiring themselves out before they begin their work. . . . I worked out a system of instruction— it worked beautifully, but the eight-hour law has smashed it all up, crippled us, for every time a head nurse wants to teach a student anything, she is off duty, and I have to form classes at night to give instruction that should be learned in the wards. The patients also complain of the

> constant change of nurses—the doctors, also, as orders are frequently overlooked or not properly attended to. We cannot keep a nurse on half-an-hour longer today and make it up tomorrow, even if it is in the middle of an operation or obstetric case she must drop everything and go. . . . The eight hours has compelled us to increase the number of nurses threefold, which also means more head nurses, maids, cooks, waiters, etc., etc.[16]

Anne A. Williamson, superintendent of nurses at the California Hospital, Los Angeles, complained that a young woman gave up 3 of the best years of her life to learning her profession, and it was unjust to deprive her of the work to which she was entitled. According to Williamson, nursing was a profession that belonged exclusively to women; it called for the highest in character and education; and it could not succeed without perseverance, determination, and self-sacrifice. But how could hospital schools instill those principles into the minds of their pupils when the first lesson they had to teach was the self-centered 8-hour law?

THE ELEMENTS OF SACRIFICE

Neither fresh ideas nor nurses who had them were welcome in the places where elderly, respectable superintendents of nursing held the levers of authority. The idea of labor control in hospital training schools was repugnant to most graduate nurses. They saw a grave danger in the entrance of labor laws into nursing and hospital affairs, because once the wedge was entered, no one could guess how deep it would go. The demand might be for 8 hours 1 year, but who could guarantee that it would not be 6 hours next year, and something else the year after?

Physicians generally agreed. Dr. Antonio D. Young, in a paper "The Nurse's Duty to Herself," claimed: "The element of sacrifice is always present in true service. The service that costs no pangs, no sacrifice, is without virtue, and usually without value." Conversely, a reform nurse, Lavinia Dock, argued: "I think nurses should stand together solidly and resist the dictation of the medical profession in this as in all other things. Many M.D.'s have a purely commercial spirit toward nurses (have private hospitals of their own, etc.) and would readily overwork them." She added, "If necessary, do not hesitate to make alliances with the labor vote, for organized labor has quite as much of an 'ideal' as the M.D.'s have, if not more."[17]

In the October 1913 issue of *Ladies' Home Journal*, the editor published a scathing criticism of the manner in which hospitals fed their student nurses. The editor noted that hospital superintendents all across the nation were voicing concern over the decreasing numbers of nurse-training applications and the

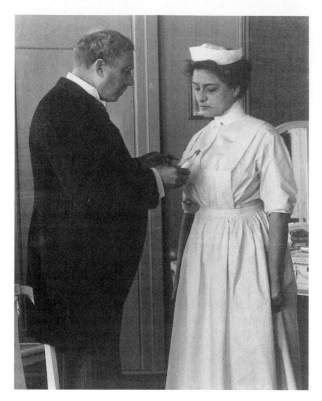

Physicians generally subscribed to the belief that, for nurses, suffering was a virtue and opposed efforts at nursing reform.

slipping personal standards of those who did apply. Yet how could administrators expect "women of better education and finer feelings" to come to a place where they would be "asked to sit down to rations of a kind and quality only a remove better than what we might place before a beggar?" The way the nurses at the average hospital were fed "was nothing short of an outrage upon womanhood," and this outrageous condition could be found in 7 of every 10 hospitals. Indeed, it was a common remark among resident physicians in hospitals that "they would not stand the stuff that is put before the nurses to eat." There was not "one scintilla of doubt that if those nurses were men the present order of things would soon change by compulsion," concluded the *Journal* editor.[18] Little complaint came from the student nurses, however, as such would be grounds for expulsion.

Recognizing that only healthy young women would be able to do the strenuous work required of them, schools of nursing routinely gave health examinations to entering students. At the time of entrance, careful health records were taken, and only the physically fit were admitted. Theoretically, the health training that was given the student should have placed her in a better situation to avoid infection. However, administrators of schools of nursing knew that the health of the average student did not improve during the years spent in the hospital; on the contrary, it tended to deteriorate.

In training hospitals that admitted tuberculosis patients, it was well known that most students who entered with negative tuberculins would have developed positive tuberculins on finishing their training. In the average general hospital carrying a tuberculosis service, approximately 80% of the student group graduated with positive tuberculins. Two investigators found that the frequency of tuberculosis infections contracted by student nurses in three general hospitals in Minnesota was five times greater than the frequency among girls who were attending regular colleges in the same communities.

Progressive nurses had begun agitating for educational reforms. Adelaide Nutting expressed this move forcibly in addressing the Superintendents' Society in 1911:

> From ecclesiastical control . . . nursing has by degrees passed over into the control of the hospital and the medical profession, quite as distinct a hierarchy as any ecclesiastical organization that ever existed. Under the control nursing has prospered in certain ways and has done valuable service, but that service has been strictly subordinated to hospital and medical needs.[19]

OBSTACLES TO NURSING REFORM

The obstacles to nursing reform were largely a product of the vested interests of hospital boards of trustees and medical societies who wanted to maintain the existing nursing conditions. At the 1912 meeting of the American Hospital Association, Dr. Henry M. Hurd, secretary of the board of trustees of Johns Hopkins Hospital, stated:

> The hospitals of the United States and Canada find themselves without adequate funds for the increased cost of operation because of the growing need of expensive apparatus for the diagnosis and treatment of disease; for the greater cost of all food supplies due to the high cost of living; for the increased cost of service in every department; for the increased scope of hospital service; for the need of doing more for the education of nurses and the training and education of physicians and hospital administrators; for more departments, better operating service, and better equipped hospital wards; and lastly, for ample resources to carry on social service and preventive work.[20]

Although more than 10,000 trained nurses were being graduated each year, health care for most of the population was inadequate. When a worker or one of his family got sick, the medical and nursing services available were few and comparatively simple. Illnesses

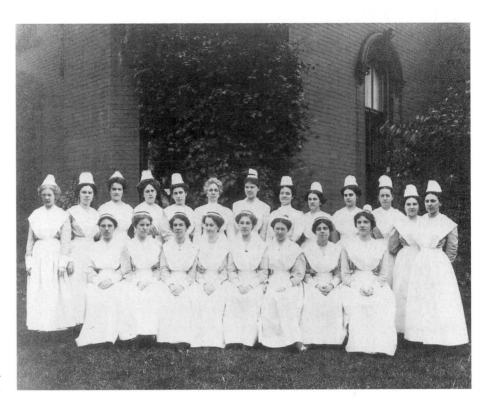

Black bands on students' caps defined those who were head nurses.

viewed as minor were still treated with home remedies and patent medicines. For severe illnesses, the family physician was called in. Among families with moderate and lower incomes, even this was not done without serious consideration of the cost involved and a determination as to whether the family resources could be stretched to cover the bill or whether the physician could be asked to wait for his fee.

Often, calling the physician was delayed until it was too late, especially in cases of childhood diseases. The wife still handled the nursing duties with what help she could obtain from relatives and neighbors. When she was ill, the family and friends did as much as they could, or a practical nurse was called in. In childbirth, untrained midwives often took the place of both physician and nurse. Although the dangers of this action were recognized and frequently publicized, this practice continued, particularly among families of recent immigrants and unskilled native-born laborers.

Hospitalization was still the exception among all groups. Aside from their high cost of treatment, many hospitals retained the stigma of the pesthouse. As to cost factors, George P. Ludlam, superintendent of New York Hospital, observed:

> It is, I think, an acknowledged fact that the per-diem cost of patients per capita is constantly increasing. Also, I think it will be admitted that this increase is not wholly due to advances in the market cost of supplies. It is due in large measure to the advance and development of

medical and surgical science which has revolutionized old methods and introduced such as are unquestionably more costly. To this fact may be added the other patent one that constant familiarity with these methods engenders a spirit of extravagance which permeates the whole establishment and which it is exceedingly difficult to check or control. I do not mean deliberate intentional waste. I suspect that does not exist. But the generous, liberal, and even extravagant use of supplies of all kinds leads to precisely the same results in the matter of the cost of maintenance, and this habit is, undoubtedly, prevalent in a controlling degree.[21]

The editor of the *Modern Hospital* deplored the presence of "disreputable hospitals" in a ringing 1914 editorial:

> There are many hospitals in this country that are a disgrace to everybody connected with them. Some are immoral in one way, some in another, and some of them are immoral in their very essence and in every way. Some are notorious abortion "parlors," some of them have a reputation for the immorality of the training school, some are distinguished by a reputation for shady transactions in their financial dealings.[22]

UPLIFT OF HOSPITAL CONDITIONS

Gradually, a few enlightened administrators began to see the necessity of adapting hospital service to community needs. The administrator of Johns Hopkins Hospital in Baltimore in 1916 declared:

> We need to study and to understand the broader relationships of the hospital to the community. That we have begun to appreciate this broader usefulness is evidenced by the inauguration of social service work, indicating that we are no longer content to ignore the relationship of the individual to his family, to previous environment, to the community, and to post-hospital environment and opportunities. . . . In the great public health movement the hospital, with its trained clinicians and investigators and its many points of contact with the community, occupies an important, indeed a strategic, position.[23]

There was an awareness of the need for properly trained hospital administrators. A speaker at the 1916 Conference of the American Hospital Association said:

> Whatever may have sufficed in the past, the institution for the sick, small or large, of the future, will need apparently for its administration an educator, a scientist, a sociologist, and a good businessman or woman, or one whose business it is to be a composite of all.[24]

One of the first considerations in maintaining high efficiency of personnel was to allocate duties properly. The complaint voiced in the following 1916 editorial was commonplace:

> Serious difficulties in hospital administration are often due to the lack of a proper differentiation of the regular duties of the several departments. Nurses, for example, sometimes cannot resist the impulse to regulate the kitchen or laundry. Matrons occasionally are found who have overwhelming desire to assume the responsibility and direction of the nursing work, to the neglect of their own duties. Physicians sometimes long to undertake the distribution of pupil nurses in ward duty, and seek to instruct them and some times to discipline them . . . . The watchword of every large institution should be departmental independence, coordinated through the office of the head of the hospital.[25]

The hospital's physical environment was generally bleak and uninviting for patients as well as nurses. In 1916, an architect said in an address at Johns Hopkins Hospital:

> While the medical profession and the hospital people consider it highly necessary that the sick should be surrounded by pleasant odors as against the older offensive smells of ether and iodoform, and while it is considered necessary that there be quiet in the hospital, yet no consideration is given to the patient's sense of

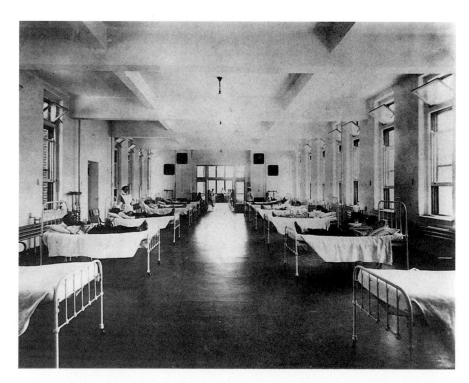

The hospital's interior environment was stark and uninviting: glaring white walls and bare furniture.

sight. Glaring white walls, severely simple furniture, and absence of draperies and curtains and the little incidentals of home comfort certainly impress the mind of the sick. Why would not pleasing sights and harmonious colors and agreeable forms serve to shorten the stay of the sick and influence their recovery?[26]

During this period, hospitals in America were administered haphazardly. There was no real organization and the management had no standard to follow. Some hospitals gained a good reputation because of the presence of a superior surgeon who required better organization, but such hospitals were considered unusual, and no effort was made to copy them.

When the American College of Surgeons was founded in 1913, its organizers understood the necessity for hospital improvement. In its earliest program of activities, this organization published its intention to study hospitals and to encourage improvements. By 1918, considerable analytical work had been done, and the college was ready to embark on a program of hospital standardization. During 1918 and 1919, field representatives visited 671 hospitals of 100 beds or more in the United States and Canada; of these, 89 in the first year and 198 in the second year were approved as meeting the minimum standard, and further progress was soon effected on many fronts. The 10 fundamental requirements of the "Minimum Standard for Hospitals" were:

A modern physical plant, properly equipped for the comfort and scientific care of the patient.
Clearly stated constitution, by-laws, rules and regulations setting forth organization, duties, responsibilities, and relations.
A carefully selected governing board having complete and supreme authority for the management of the institution.

A competent, well-trained executive officer or superintendent with authority and responsibility to carry out the policies of the institution as authorized by the governing board.
An adequate number of efficient personnel, properly organized and under competent supervision.
An organized medical staff of ethical, competent physicians for the carrying out of the professional policies of the hospital, subject to the approval of the governing board.
Adequate diagnostic and therapeutic facilities with efficient technical service under competent medical supervision.
Accurate and complete medical records, promptly written and filed in an accessible manner so as to be available for study, reference, follow-up, and research.
Group conferences of the administrative staff and of the medical staff to review regularly and thoroughly their respective activities in order to keep the service and the scientific work on the highest plane of efficiency.
A humanitarian spirit in which the best care of the patient is always the primary consideration.[27]

NATIONAL HEALTH STATUS IN 1920

What was the state of the nation's health by the end of the second decade of the 20th century? Whereas in 1901–1902 the average life expectancy of a white male child at birth was 48.23 years, it rose to 50.23 years in 1909–1910 and to 54.05 years in 1919–1920. The improvement in longevity held true until one reached the age of 40 (Table 9-1), after which the chances of increased longevity actually fell somewhat

	MASSACHUSETTS (%)	ORIGINAL REGISTRATION STATES (%)		
AGE (Y)	1890 (Males)	1901–1902 (White males)	1909–1910 (White males)	1919–1920 (White males)
0	42.50	48.23	50.23	54.05
7	51.15	53.76	53.85	55.34
12	47.64	49.72	49.56	51.02
22	39.97	41.44	41.13	42.69
32	33.39	34.15	33.33	34.93
42	26.70	27.03	25.99	27.32
52	20.09	20.08	19.02	19.91
62	41.15	13.76	12.85	13.38
72	8.88	8.56	7.95	8.17
82	5.08	4.81	4.56	4.53
92	2.37	2.69	2.70	2.10

TABLE 9-1 Comparison of Changes in Life Expectancy, 1890–1920

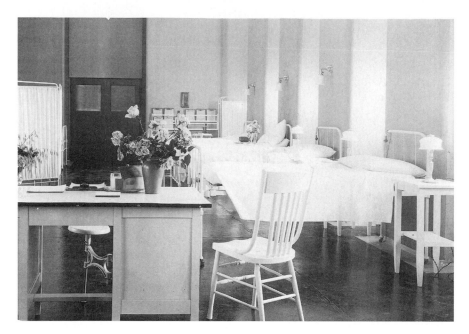

Hospital wards began to reflect the function of facilitating the best care of the patient.

below the expectations of 20 years before.[28] The same was true, to a lesser extent, for women. At the age of 40, the premature development of degenerative diseases of middle age set in, killing Americans much more rapidly than Britons, Swedes, Norwegians, Danes, Dutchmen, and Australians.

When in 1917, amid preparations for war, the Progressive Era in American history came to a close, perceptive nurses could see that the reform movement for nursing had largely been muted. The unique external constraints imposed on student and graduate nurses had prevented any large-scale alteration of either the educational or the work environment. Nevertheless, nurses of that era had achieved some important early insights into the developing conflict between nursing's professional idealism and the reactionary tendencies of the hospital and medical establishment.

REFERENCES

1. *New York Tribune*, April 16, 1900.
2. Lavinia L. Dock, "Secretary's Report of the Meeting of the International Council of Nurses, Buffalo, New York, September 16, 1901," *American Journal of Nursing*, vol. 2 (October 1901): 51–54.
3. Mary Allenson, "My Impressions as a Post-graduate," *American Journal of Nursing*, vol. 5 (November 1904):100–103.
4. Clara D. Noyes, "Postgraduate Study for Nurses," *Proceedings of the Annual Meeting of American Society of Superintendents of Training Schools for Nurses*, vol. 11 (June 1905):121–129.
5. A. Flexner, *Medical Education in the United States and Canada* (New York: The Carnegie Foundation for the Advancement of Teaching, 1910), pp. 3–185, *passim.*
6. Ibid., pp. vii–xvii, 185–319, *passim.*
7. M. Adelaide Nutting, "The Report of the Committee on Education," *Proceedings of the Convention of the National League of Nursing Education*, vol. 19 (June 1913):76–77.
8. Elizabeth A. Greener, "Organization and Administration of the Nursing Department," *Modern Hospital*, vol. 2 (March 1914):163–164.
9. Ibid., pp. 166–167.
10. Katharine DeWitt, "Hospital Sketches," *American Journal of Nursing*, vol. 6 (April 1906):455–459.
11. William Osler, *Nurse and Patient* (Baltimore: John Murphy and Company, 1897), pp. 14–15.
12. U.S. Department of Commerce and Labor, *Report on the Condition of Woman and Child Wage-Earners in the United States* (Washington, DC: Government Printing Office, 1911), vol. 15, pp. 87–89.
13. *San Francisco Chronicle*, May 2, 1913.
14. *San Francisco Examiner*, February 24, 1915.
15. Lila Pickhardt, "Recent Legislation Governing Hours of Duty of Pupil Nurses in Hospitals," *Proceedings of the Twentieth Convention of the National League of Nursing Education*, vol. 20 (June 1914):106–111.
16. "The Eight-hour Day for Nurses," *Trained Nurse and Hospital Review*, vol. 53 (July 1914):37–38.
17. "Nurses and Labor Laws," *Trained Nurse and Hospital Review*, vol. 52 (January 1914):37–38.
18. "Are Nurses in Hospitals Underfed?" *Trained Nurse and Hospital Review*, vol. 51 (December 1913):364–365.
19. M. Adelaide Nutting, "Address," *Proceedings of the Annual Convention of the American Society of Superintendents of Training Schools for Nurses*, vol. 17 (June 1911):18–22.
20. Henry M. Hurd, "President's Address," *Transactions of the American Hospitals Association*, vol. 14 (September 1912): 88–89.
21. *New York Times*, March 3, 1913.
22. Henry M. Hurd, "Disreputable Hospitals," *Modern Hospital*, vol. 2 (May 1914):296.
23. Winford H. Smith, "The Educational Function of the Hospital," *Modern Hospital*, vol. 6 (January 1916):1–4.
24. Annie W. Goodrich, "How Shall the Superintendents of Small Hospitals Be Trained?" *Transactions of the American Hospital Association*, vol. 18 (September 1916):359.
25. Henry M. Hurd, "Another Source of Friction in Hospital Administration," *Modern Hospital*, vol. 6 (February 1916):112.
26. Charles F. Neergaard, "Some Glaring Faults in Hospital Construction," *Modern Hospital*, vol. 6 (June 1916):408–410.
27. American College of Surgeons, *Manual of Hospital Standardization: History, Development and Progress of Hospital Standardization; Detailed Explanation of the Minimum Requirements* (Chicago: The College, 1938), pp. 61–67.
28. U.S. Department of Commerce, Bureau of the Census, *United States Life Tables, 1901–02, 1909–10, 1919–20* (Washington, DC: Government Printing Office, 1923), pp. 16, 48, 62.

10

DAYS OF TRIUMPH
Nursing in World War I

On June 28, 1914, a shot fired in Sarajevo, Serbia, set off a sequence of events that brought almost all Europe, and subsequently most of the world, into a long and terrible war destined to cost millions of lives and do incalculable damage. The United States was to enter it a little less than 3 years later, after a long struggle to maintain neutrality, and the nation's nurses were to be an important part of this involvement. They had already read of the execution of nurse Edith Cavell before a German firing squad on October 12, 1915. Cavell, the superintendent of a nurse training school in Brussels, Belgium, had been charged with harboring British and French soldiers and assisting them in escaping from Belgium. Cavell, who had nursed both German and Allied soldiers, could herself have escaped, but she stayed at her post until she was apprehended and sentenced to death.

The United States had never been in a war like the one it entered in April 1917, but few nurses realized this. It was a global conflict that set one coalition of nations against another. Much more so than either the Civil War or the Spanish-American War, it was a war of materiel, calling for the expenditure of vast amounts for supplies and demanding the organization of all the nation's resources for military purposes. It was also total in its effect on society, compelling the government to mobilize men, women, money, materiel, and even public opinion.

NURSES JOIN THE FIGHT

An American army of 3½ million men assembled, with more than 2 million of this force sent to France. At the same time, the size of the Army Nurse Corps rapidly expanded and soon began to approach a strength of 20,000. The Navy Nurse Corps expanded too, but because fighting was primarily on land, it grew much more slowly. Applicants for appointment for both military nursing services had to be between 25 and 35 years of age, unmarried, and graduates of

training schools for nurses that offered solid theoretical and practical courses and were attached to general hospitals of at least 100 beds. As the war continued, however, graduates of schools connected with hospitals not meeting the 100-bed requirement were also accepted.

To determine an applicant's qualifications, the army and navy requested certification of the nurse's moral character and professional qualifications from the superintendent of her school. Married nurses were unacceptable for appointment, and those who married while on active duty were dishonorably discharged.

Among the women of the United States, interest in nursing quickly began to increase after war was declared. Society girls and others with romantic notions—but without training—who were eager to go overseas to serve as nursing aides at their own expense quickly enrolled in intensive Red Cross courses. On April 8, 1917, Clara Noyes, director of the new Red Cross Bureau of Nursing, wrote to Adelaide Nutting in desperation:

> Surely we need your prayers. There are moments when I wonder whether we can stem the tide and control the hysterical desire on the part of thousands, literally thousands, to get into nursing or their hands upon it.
> Tell Annie [Goodrich] of Albany that if I were not convinced before, I should be now that the most vital thing in the life of our profession is the protection of the use of the word nurse. Everyone seems to have gone mad. I talk until I am hoarse, dictating letters to doctors and women who want to be Red Cross nurses in a few minutes, not knowing the meaning of the word nurse and what a Red Cross nurse is.[1]

Nurse educators were horrified that army nursing might fall into the hands of aristocratic socialites, as it had done under the auspices of the Red Cross in most European countries. Such women, including those of royal families, lusted to be near the glory of battle, confident that they could fully carry out the "angel of mercy" role merely by dispensing large quantities of morphine to the wounded.

NURSING RESOURCES AND THE WAR

Consequently, Adelaide Nutting, Annie Goodrich, and Lillian Wald met on June 24, 1917, to determine ways of avoiding some of the mistakes in providing nursing service to the military that had been made by other countries already in the war. Headed by Nutting, the Committee on Nursing also included Jane Delano, chairman of the American Red Cross Nursing Service; Lillian Clayton, president of the National League of Nursing Education; Dora Thompson, superintendent of the Army Nurse Corps; Dr. Winford H. Smith, president of the American Hospital Association; and several others. The announced purpose of the group was to devise "the wisest methods of meeting the present problems connected with the care of the sick and injured in hospitals and homes; the educational problems of nursing; and the extraordinary emergencies as they arise."[2]

Ten weeks later, on August 2, 1917, the Committee on Nursing was attached to the General Medical Board of the U.S. Council of National Defense and was granted federal status and backing. The government provided space for an office, secretarial service, and a few other items, but most of the committee's work was financed from funds contributed by friends of nursing and nurses themselves.

The committee estimated that there were about 200,000 active "nurses," both trained and untrained, in the nation in 1917. There were 115,000 (98,000 registered and 17,000 unregistered) fully trained nurses and 85,000 untrained and partially trained nurses. The only field that had a reasonable supply of nurses was private-duty nursing, which comprised approximately 150,000, or 75%, of the total active

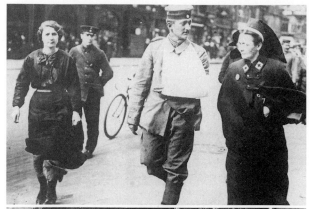

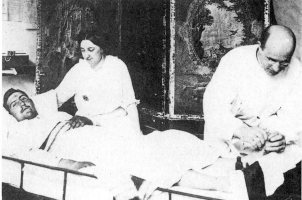

Wounded German soldiers with their nurses in Berlin.

number. In addition to this mixed pool of 200,000, there were about 45,000 student nurses in training. The challenge at hand was to maintain a steady supply of trained nurses for the care of acutely sick patients from both the military and civilian sectors. This was a tremendous undertaking, inasmuch as the original request for 10,000 nurses for the army soon rose to 20,000, then to 30,000, and finally to 35,000. Civilian needs also became acute, especially in industrial centers and in towns and cities adjacent to military installations.

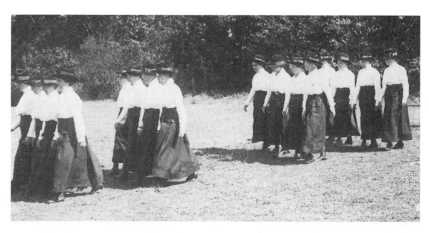

U.S. Army nurses in training before assignment overseas.

The United States, starting almost from scratch, swung into the war effort. A general conscription act was passed, after much opposition, on May 18, 1917, more than a month after the declaration of war. Housing and training this vast number of draftees required building 32 camps, each able to shelter more than 40,000 men. Despite great difficulties in supplying and equipping them, the camps soon resembled small cities, with running water, electric light, amusement centers, libraries, and hospitals. After 6 months of preliminary training, the troops went abroad for further instruction before being sent to the front. To motivate people at home to fully support the war effort, a massive propaganda drive was waged by the Committee on Public Information, established by Congress. Motion pictures, pamphlets, and posters proclaimed that Germans were depraved. Even German nurses were depicted as inhumane and cruel.

THE TRIP ACROSS

In May 1917, the first units embarked from this country, and from that time until the signing of the Armistice on November 11, 1918, nursing units came from every section of the United States to New York and Hoboken for embarkation at the port handling the American Expeditionary Forces.

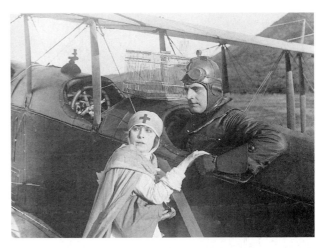

The young film industry was used to mobilize public opinion.

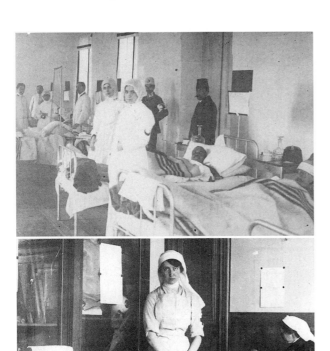

Turkish nurses (top) and British nurses attending wounded soldiers.

Embarkation was a difficult experience for these nurses. The great adventure, long anticipated, had begun. Early in June 1917, a mobilization center was established by the army for the nurses at Ellis Island. Three large buildings formerly used by the Immigration Department were turned over to the army. One nurse wrote:

> As our buildings were on the sea wall directly in front of the channel to the ocean, all the activities of a harbor given over to war went on in our front yard. Also there were a thousand interned Germans and imprisoned German agents under heavy guard on Ellis Island, and their presence produced rather a shadow of apprehension.[3]

In December 1917, the Old Colony Club in New York City was offered to the War Department and became a mobilization center for nursing units awaiting transportation overseas. Later, the Knott chain of hotels in New York City was taken over by the army for the nurses, and Hotel Albert became the administration center. From the beginning until the close of the war the Central Club for Nurses was a favorite social rendezvous of nurses from all the mobilizing units.

Crossing the hazardous Atlantic was often troublesome; the chief nurse of Base Hospital No. 8, which left New York on the *Saratoga*, wrote of her experience:

> Passing Staten Island, the S.S. *Saratoga* slowed up and finally dropped anchor off Tomkinsville. The day was desperately hot and after luncheon most of the nurses removed their heavy uniforms and were lolling about in their cabins in all degrees of dishabille. Suddenly there was a crash and a terrific shock—the S.S. *Panama* had rammed into the *Saratoga*, tearing a thirty-foot hole in her side. The ship immediately began to list and orders were given to abandon ship at once. There was no hysteria among the nurses.

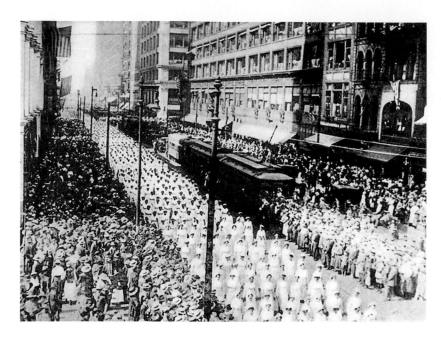

Nurses march in Chicago in support of the war effort.

Half-clad as they were, they took their places in the boats. All the smaller craft in the harbor rushed to our assistance and we were picked up and taken to various large boats scattered about the bay. A government boat finally collected and carried us back to quarters on board the *Finland*, which was then lying at her dock in Hoboken. We learned that seventeen minutes after the last person left the ship, the *Saratoga* submerged. With her went not only our own personal belongings, but our entire hospital equipment.[4]

Eight days after the sinking of the *Saratoga*, this unit, completely reequipped by the American Red Cross, embarked again on the *Finland*, and during the last 3 nights of the voyage across the Atlantic the nurses were not permitted to remove their clothing, and the life preservers were held constantly at hand. German submarines in search of allied ships bound for Saint-Nazaire plied the waters near Belle Isle, just off the coast of France, and the *Finland* was attacked. The chief nurse described the encounter:

Suddenly about nine o'clock on Monday morning, the signal came, six short blasts and the firing of a cannon. Each hurriedly took her place beside the boat to which she had been assigned, and during a tense hour and a quarter watched the battle. The roar of cannon and the shock of depth bombs brought to us a grim realization of naval warfare. Out of the five ships of the convoy, the *Finland* seemed to have been the best target. . . . We were off the coast of France when the attack occurred.

After the submarines had been routed, we proceeded on our way to St. Nazaire. When we arrived there at seven in the evening of August 20, the populace who had heard the news of the battle by wireless, was waiting to bid us welcome, and we docked amid round after round of cheers.[5]

OVER THERE

Six months after the United States had entered the war, nearly 1100 nurses were overseas, about half of them stationed in six British general hospitals. American troops were close on their heels. Vera Brittain, who served as a nurse behind the British lines, described her first sight of American troops:

I was leaving quarters to go back to my ward when I had to wait to let a large contingent of troops march past . . . though the sight of soldiers marching was now too familiar to arouse curiosity, an unusual quality of bold vigour in their swift stride caused me to stare at them with puzzled interest.

They looked larger than ordinary men; their tall, straight figures were in vivid contrast to the undersized armies of pale recruits to which we had become accustomed. . . . Had yet another regiment been conjured out of our depleted Dominions?

Then I heard an excited exclamation from a group of Sisters behind me.

"Look! Look! Here are the Americans!"

The coming of relief made me realize how long and how intolerable had been the tension, and with the knowledge that we were not, after all, defeated I found myself beginning to cry.[6]

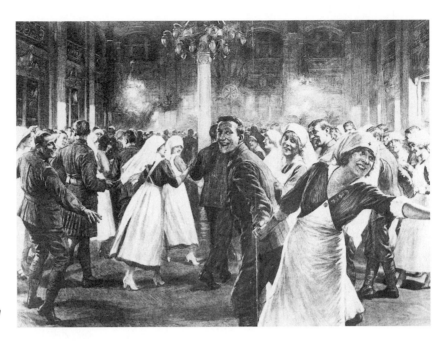

Red Cross nurses entertaining troops upon arrival in Paris.

Nurses enrolled in the American Red Cross constituted the unofficial reserve of the Army Nurse Corps for service in time of war or other emergencies. Consequently, when more nurses were needed, the Red Cross was called on to furnish them. In addition, entire medical and nursing forces were organized at many of the large medical centers in the United States. On May 7, 1917, the first base hospital unit, the Lakeside of Cleveland, with Grace E. Allison as chief nurse, sailed for Europe.

The organization of hospitalization in France was as follows: Wounded men were carried from the trenches to the first-aid dressing station immediately behind the firing line. After treatment they were moved by motor ambulance to the nearest evacuation hospital, which was 4 to 10 miles behind the first-line trenches and consisted of four separate hospitals. If immediate treatment was not imperative, the patient was taken by train to the nearest base. Those requiring quick aid or surgery were cared for at once at the evacuation hospital by surgical teams composed of two surgeons, an anesthetist, two nurses, and two orderlies sent from the various base hospitals nearest the station.

STEPPED-UP RECRUITING ACTIVITIES

The next challenge was to increase the actual supply of student nurses. The General Medical Board Committee sent out a torrent of posters, motion pictures, photographs, speeches, and pamphlets aimed at making Americans aware of nurses and creating a positive attitude toward the nursing profession. More than 70,000 copies of the 15-page pamphlet *Nursing—A National Service* appealed to the young women of the United States to prepare for nursing. It

stressed the need for student recruits, outlined the opportunities for service during and after the war, and listed the kinds of training available and the way to get in touch with good nursing schools. Additionally, 55,000 copies of the four-page brochure *State Sources of Advice and Information on Nursing* presented a list of names and addresses of nursing representatives in all the states, from whom information regarding nursing schools and other local nursing matters could be secured.

In addition to these direct measures, a widespread campaign of newspaper publicity was waged, and arrangements were made for magazine articles on nursing. Toward this end, the *Ladies' Home Journal*, with former President William H. Taft as editor, urged women to help "the boys over there" by enrolling in

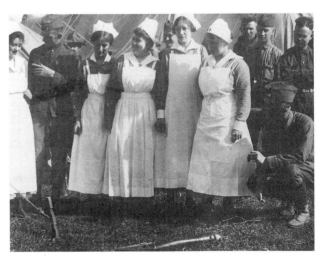

An unexploded German bomb dropped near a U.S. Army hospital in France.

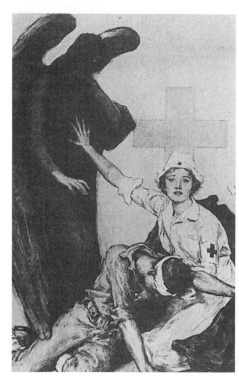
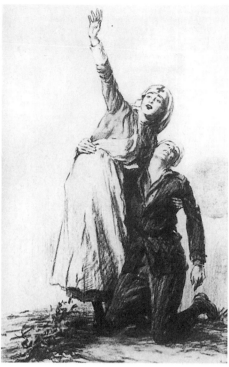

Nurse recruitment posters for the Red Cross.

schools of nursing. Entitled "A Distinct Call to Women," the editorial asked:

> Have you felt that you could best answer the war's appeal to you by entering the nursing service? Then this is the day of your opportunity, provided you are in earnest and wish to set your patriotic impulses free in the place where they will do the most good.
>
> That place is in a regular nurses' training school, such as is conducted in nearly every hospital in America. Many women, untrained in nursing, have been disappointed to learn that their services were not wanted on the field of battle, nor even in a base hospital.
>
> It is the professional nurse only who has been called and accepted, and more than a thousand of her are now in active service. More thousands will follow soon. They are the finest of their profession, and they go gladly; but do you realize that each one is leaving behind her important work in civil life, which must now be done by someone else?
>
> We have no right to expect—though we may hope for—a short war. We must put away makeshift methods and think of a year from now, two years, perhaps even three years. The woman who enters training today is the woman who a little later will be prepared to take the place at home of the nurse who has gone, or even to follow her to the Front.
>
> The Red Cross earnestly hopes that many young women, particularly those with the advantages of a good education, will let their desire to be of service take a most practical form and prepare to enter a profession which has been called upon to do so noble a work.[7]

Having done everything in its power to attract educated young women to enroll in schools of nursing, the General Medical Board Committee next appealed to the 700 leading nursing schools throughout the country to enlarge their schools immediately to the limit of their capacities, resources, and clinical facilities. To achieve this, they were requested to secure additional nursing dormitories and more supervisors and instructors and to shorten the lengthy working hours that had been an impediment to the entrance of more middle-class women into nursing. Where they were unable to find additional quarters, it was suggested that temporary arrangements be made to permit local students to live at home during at least part of their training.

As a result of these measures, the number of students entering schools of nursing during the year 1917–1918 increased by about 25%. This meant that instead of a yearly output of 12,000 to 15,000 graduate nurses, the nation would have 15,000 to 18,000 available in 1919 and 1920. By April 1918, approximately 7000 applicants over and above the normal 15,000 admitted annually were enrolled in nursing schools. The wartime publicity campaign for student nurses was the first to be organized on any large scale, and its effectiveness was due in large measure to its patriotic wartime appeal.

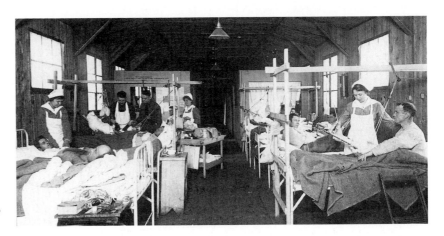

As more American troops were rushed into battle, more nursing students were needed.

NURSING'S IMAGE AMONG HIGH SCHOOL STUDENTS

Helpful relations were established with the Women's Committee of the Council on National Defense, which, through its state and local committees, publicized the importance of assisting hospitals in their recruiting efforts. Some outstanding work was done on the local level. For example, a women's group in Cleveland became eager to measure the average high school girl's interest in nursing as a possible vocation. With the help of the city's high school teachers, a regional survey was conducted.

The questionnaire was designed to yield a comparison between the amount of interest displayed toward a possible future college arts and science degree and a possible future course in a school of nursing. Chief among the objections to a nursing career that were raised by 1139 high school graduates were the long hours, hard work, severe discipline, lack of recreation and pleasure, and low quality of education. Among the objections and difficulties voiced were: "I can't stand it physically"; "It is a life of drudgery"; "The work is too strenuous"; "When you get old, nobody wants you"; "The nervous strain is too great"; "Too much scrubbing"; and "Too much standing on one's feet." Over 73% did not know of any positions that a graduate nurse could fill.

It was significant that although nearly half of the respondents had previously talked with a member of the nursing profession, fewer than one fifth considered nursing as a career possibility. Undoubtedly, school of nursing alumnae were not giving very glowing reports of their schools and of their work. A massive national effort was obviously needed to lessen hours of duty, decrease drudgery, and elevate nursing educational standards by expanding the theoretical portion of the curricula and by hiring full-time instructors and lecturers.

Many nursing schools did not have facilities for even a modest educational program, and their living and working conditions were nearly intolerable. Complaints soon began to reach the Committee on Nursing from some of the beginning students. To try to improve poor nursing school conditions, a letter was sent by the Women's Committee of the Council of National Defense to the 12,000 state and local committees of the Women's Committee, urging them to follow up the young women who had been placed in nursing schools in their vicinity, to take an interest in them, and to try to see that they secured their training under satisfactory conditions. They were especially asked to investigate students who had been admitted to low-quality nursing programs. Enclosed with this letter was a memorandum prepared by the Committee on Nursing entitled *What Is a Good Training School of Nurses?*

TAPPING THE COLLEGE WOMAN

The urgent need for a greater number of better-educated women in many areas of nursing led to an informal effort by the Committee on Nursing to see if some of the leading schools of nursing would be willing, in the national emergency, to reduce the term of 3 years for college graduates with satisfactory backgrounds in science. Most schools were willing to allow credit for 8 to 9 months of the usual 3-year course, and some would allow a full year. Other schools were more cautious, however, and some openly skeptical. Superintendents wanted to know what evidence existed to show that college graduates would make good nurses or that a longer period of academic education would be any special asset in the training of a nurse.

Using these reactions as a basis, the committee proceeded in a bold attempt to attract female college graduates into nursing through an experimental program at Vassar College. The objective was to use the plant and resources of Vassar College in an effort to interest numerous college women in nursing service by providing an intensive preparatory course of 3 months on the Vassar campus. A vigorous recruiting campaign was organized by the Vassar alumnae to secure enrollment.

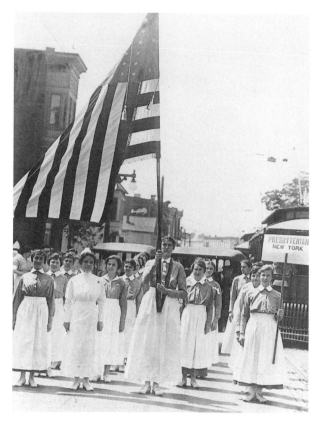

Student nurses in the experimental program at Vassar College parade for the public.

The summer school for nurses at Vassar opened auspiciously with 439 college graduates selected from a large number of applicants. They ranged in age from 19 to 40 years and represented 115 of the nation's colleges. More than half the women had been teachers, some with excellent positions. The next largest group comprised students entering directly from college, but a number of secretaries, so-

cial workers, newspaper women, librarians, and others were also in attendance.

There were two terms, with classes 6 days a week and a half-holiday on Saturday. The expenses amounted to $25 for tuition and $70 for room and board. All the usual preparatory subjects were covered, including courses in anatomy and physiology (60 hours), bacteriology (48 hours), chemistry (48 hours), hygiene and sanitation (30 hours), elementary materia medica (24 hours), nutrition and cooking (60 hours), elementary nursing and hospital economy (60 hours), and history of nursing (10 hours). In addition, all students who had not yet had psychology and social economy took a 30-hour course in each of these subjects.

At the end of the summer, students chose from a list of 33 cooperating hospitals a school of nursing in which the balance of their training would be completed in 2 years and 3 months. It was impressive that 418 of the 439 college graduates completed the Vassar course, and 399 of these entered the 33 affiliated schools, each of which had promised to admit a certain number of these students and to carry them through the remainder of the program. Fifty-seven went to Bellevue Hospital, New York; 21 to City Hospital, New York; 17 to Boston City Hospital; and 13 to the University of Michigan Hospital, Ann Arbor. Eventually, Vassar Training Camp graduates would help fill key leadership roles for the next 4 decades.

Soon, five other universities (Western Reserve in Cleveland, the University of Cincinnati, the University of Iowa, the University of Colorado, and the University of California) set up similar courses, to which high school students were also admitted. The prenursing or preparatory course that was given at Vassar College and at other universities during the summer of 1918 showed what might be done on a large scale in the way of cooperating with higher educational institutions for a part of nurses' training. The standard of teaching was much higher than that available in most nursing schools. It seemed to many nurse educators that even

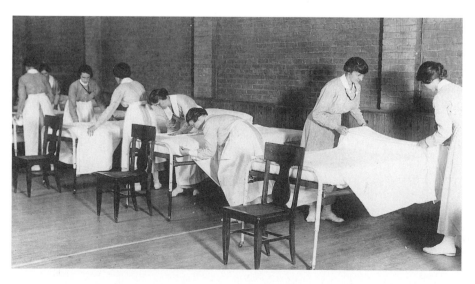

Instruction in bed-making, Vassar College.

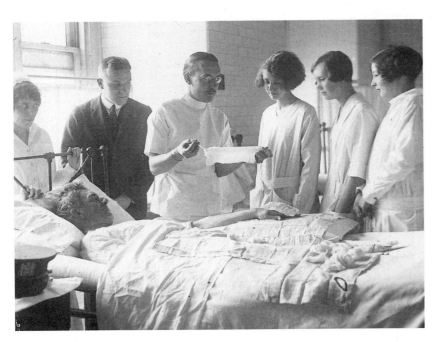

Teaching bandaging to college women recruited into nursing.

if the special incentives of the war period were eliminated, there would still be an advantage in having prenursing work conducted under the auspices of a recognized college or university.

INCREASED WAR DEMANDS

Meanwhile, since the declaration of war against Germany on April 6, 1917, the United States had been exerting a stupendous national effort in carrying out its responsibilities to the allied cause. Eventually, the total strength of the U.S. Army would reach 3,685,458 men. Of these, approximately 2 million would be equipped for combat, preliminarily trained, and sent to France to form the American Expeditionary Force. They would not participate in military action in Europe until the late spring of 1918—just in time to help stem the great German offensive. Then, they would serve in camps and in the field and fight great battles, from Château-Thierry in July to Saint-Mihiel in September and the Meuse-Argonne offensive from September 26 to the Armistice on November 11, 1918.

Because only graduate nurses were eligible for military service, by the winter of 1917–1918, the country's civilian nurse supply was seriously depleted. In European nations, the solution to the problem had been found in accepting as military nurses women who had undergone a short period of training as aides. For the United States, the question of Red Cross nurses' aides versus trained nurses for the military was full of emotion and controversy. Although members of the nursing profession eagerly sought financial and moral support from women of the leisure classes, they did not want to turn their profession over to those who hungered for tinsel glory.

Trained nurses were forced to fight large and highly vocal groups of society women anxious to serve as nurses but hesitant to enroll when a definite period of training was suggested. These lay women clung to the belief that the war had created a demand for a reduced standard of nursing service, which they themselves would be unwilling to accept in times of peace. They seemed to think that there was something especially patriotic in serving as a volunteer free lance rather than as a regularly enlisted member of the Army Nurse Corps. These socialites pointed to the huge numbers of amateurs who had served in hospitals abroad, and they clamored for an opportunity to show their patriotism and devotion in a similar way.

Although Dora Thompson, superintendent of the Army Nurse Corps, and Jane Delano of the Red Cross Nursing Service urged the use of nurses' aides to conserve the supply of graduate nurses in civilian hospitals, military personnel returning from overseas for War Department conferences encouraged Surgeon General William C. Gorgas to take a firm stand against use of the aide group. As the pace of war increased, Secretary of War Newton D. Baker asked the surgeon general to take a "long look ahead" to relieve the personnel situation. Somewhat alarmed, Surgeon General Gorgas temporarily abandoned his earlier opposition to aides and notified the Red Cross on February 9, 1918, that it could proceed with its nurses' aides plan. Such aides would be selected from applicants who had completed a 4-week course in elementary hygiene and home care of the sick, supplemented by a short practical training course of at least 1 month.

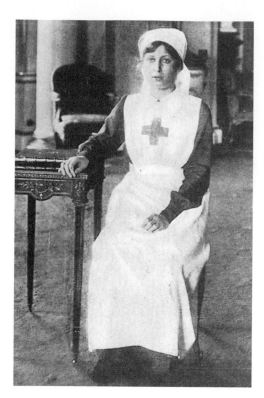

Princess Mary of England served as a "society-type" hospital nurse.

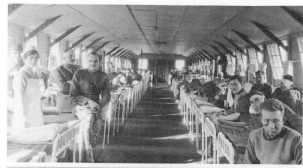

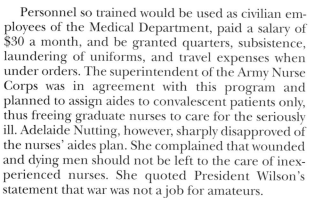

Annie Goodrich was critical of the quality of nurses at military hospitals.

Personnel so trained would be used as civilian employees of the Medical Department, paid a salary of $30 a month, and be granted quarters, subsistence, laundering of uniforms, and travel expenses when under orders. The superintendent of the Army Nurse Corps was in agreement with this program and planned to assign aides to convalescent patients only, thus freeing graduate nurses to care for the seriously ill. Adelaide Nutting, however, sharply disapproved of the nurses' aides plan. She complained that wounded and dying men should not be left to the care of inexperienced nurses. She quoted President Wilson's statement that war was not a job for amateurs.

After receiving reports critical of nursing conditions in American military camps, the Committee on Nursing asked that the surgeon general appoint Annie W. Goodrich to evaluate the quality of nursing service in military hospitals. Shortly thereafter, Goodrich, president of the American Nurses Association and an assistant professor in the Department of Nursing and Health at Teachers College, Columbia University, received an appointment as chief inspecting nurse of the army hospitals at home and abroad. She reported for duty at the War Department on February 18, 1918. Goodrich was considered especially well suited to this position because of her varied experience, including much experience in inspection of training schools. Assisting her was Elizabeth C. Burgess, the inspector of training schools of New York State.

On March 24, 1918, on completion of their tour of inspection, Goodrich and Burgess reported that the military base hospitals presented a sharply negative contrast to the best civilian hospitals. In civilian hospitals, the bedside care of the patient was given by a carefully selected group of student nurses under the constant supervision of highly qualified instructors and supervisors. In military hospitals, the trained nurses were unable to handle all the bedside care; much of their work was delegated to the continually changing hospital corpsmen, who, as enlisted men, did not approach the task with any desire to excel. Meanwhile, the patient struggled to help himself or to help others, to relieve the nurses and the corpsmen.

CONTROVERSY OVER AN "ARMY SCHOOL OF NURSING"

The unfavorable report on nursing conditions in the army was accompanied by a formal proposal on March 24, 1918, to establish an Army School of Nursing, which would provide for patients in army hospitals the kind of student care that was furnished in civilian hospitals. Goodrich recommended that the Committee on Nursing of the Council of National Defense act as an advisory group to the proposed school.

The Army School of Nursing was to be centralized in the surgeon general's office, under the supervision of a dean, with training units and teaching staffs in many camp hospitals. More than a mere effort to circumvent the Red Cross training program for aides, the plan represented Annie Goodrich's determination to implement an educational pattern new in nursing education. The school faculty would determine all aspects of instruction, administration, and professional training of students at the army camp hospitals. Each hospital would be an individual unit, with its own staff, supervision, and teaching equipment. Goodrich believed that the care given by army student nurses under expert instruction and supervision would far surpass that given by hastily trained aides. New units would be opened as needed, each offering a 3-year diploma course and meeting requirements for state registration.

Early in May 1918, the second joint annual meeting of the National League of Nursing Education, the American Nurses Association, and the National Organization for Public Health Nursing was held in Cleveland. The Germans had already struck their second blow on the Western Front at this time and were preparing for the third major offensive. Now, Cleveland became the battleground for the dispute over nurses' aides. Annie Goodrich, as president of the American Nurses Association, welcomed the group with a ringing proclamation: "We have come together in the most momentous period not in the history of this country, but in the history of the world, to consecrate ourselves anew to the service of humanity through our chosen profession."[8]

The two convention addresses of greatest importance were those presented by Colonel Winford H. Smith, which outlined plans for the Army School of Nursing, and by Dr. S.S. Goldwater, which advocated, under the title "A Nursing Crisis," the employment of nurses' aides. Colonel Smith's paper represented Goodrich's ideas. He told the audience:

> Under this plan, it is proposed to enroll young women between the ages of 21 and 35, who have received the equivalent of a high school

education, and to assign them to the schools in military hospitals. . . .

> We believe that the requirements of 21 to 35 age limits and the equivalent of a high school education will interfere less with civil hospitals than [would] a lower standard or acceptance of candidates for short courses. It will likewise guarantee to us a type mentally and morally best fitted to our service, and if we are to place these young women in our camps, they must work under and live under close supervision and control, and no better system can be devised than that which the civil hospital has found successful after years of experience. Recognize please that what we propose is, in our opinion, a better protection to the civil hospital training school than the short course system for nurses' aides.[9]

Conversely, Goldwater's argument was that the nation could not spare the necessary number of trained nurses from the civilian sector. He claimed that the proposed army school would divert large numbers of applicants from civilian nursing schools, that standards in civilian hospitals would very seriously suffer, and that an Army School of Nursing would leave the United States with a huge surplus of nurses at the close of the war. He asserted that women of the leisure classes were the only significant labor reserve of the country, that they were willing and eager to serve, and that they should be permitted to do so.

> I come finally to what appears to me to be the safest and best way out—in fact, the only way out; namely, the training of a large number of nonprofessional, voluntary war nursing aides, enlisted for the period of the war only and composed of a class which will not take up nursing professionally

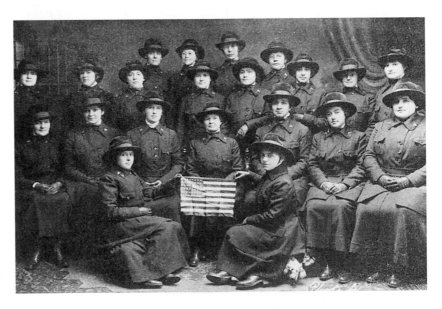

Some worried that army recruitment would strip nurses from the civilian sector.

under any circumstances, but which is willing to give gratuitous hospital service during the emergency. Such women can be obtained quickly, in large numbers. Among the 1,500 training schools of the country, there should be no difficulty in finding 300 which are capable of training and which can be trusted to train 12 nursing aides or nurses' assistants per month, or say, 150 per annum. With the moral support of the Army, the hospitals of the country can easily obtain and turn out 25,000 nurses' assistants before the end of the present year, or 40,000 by July, 1919.[10]

A lively discussion followed in which Frances Payne Bolton, a wealthy and influential citizen of Cleveland, supported Goodrich's plan for the army school. Adelaide Nutting then rose from her chair and strongly endorsed acceptance of the army school plan. When a vote was taken, the three nursing organizations backed the establishment of an Army School of Nursing.

Before the close of the convention in Cleveland, however, Annie Goodrich received an official telegram from the surgeon general's office stating that the plan for an Army School of Nursing had been rejected by the general staff of the War Department. The boards of the three national nursing organizations held an emergency meeting and appointed a committee to go to Washington and appeal to Secretary of War Baker to override the decision of the general staff. Recognizing the value of lay support, they named only one nurse to the committee, Annie Goodrich. The two other members were Florence Linden Brewster and Frances Payne Bolton.

The secretary of war granted a special hearing on the proposed Army School of Nursing on May 25, 1918. By courtesy of the surgeon general, Bolton, Brewster, and Goodrich were admitted to Baker's office, where they waited some hours for the weary secretary of war to return from a long session on Capitol Hill. Many years later, Bolton shed some light on the circumstances of the meeting:

At the time that the nursing situation in this country was exceedingly serious and some of us had joined with a number of the top nurses in the American Nurses' Association to establish an Army School of Nursing, we found nurses faced with formidable opposition. Secretary Newton Baker was very much inclined to the Army School, but it was apparent to all of us that someone, some organization, some group stood very much in the way. . . . There was no question in any of our minds that a few weeks or even a very few months of aide "training" could not take the place of skilled nursing care. Fortunately for our boys, the Secretary saw the wisdom of making possible transportation of our skilled women and the establishment of the Army School of Nursing.[11]

Indeed, at the May 25 meeting, Baker agreed to approve the Army School of Nursing and nullify the action of the army general staff. His consent came following assurances by Brewster that the Council of National Defense Women's Committee volunteers would exert every effort to recruit students for civilian nurse training schools, thus saving them from depletion at the hands of the army school.

SEEKING APPLICANTS FOR THE ARMY SCHOOL OF NURSING

The Committee on Nursing of the Council of National Defense set out in the summer of 1918 to recruit 25,000 women for the Army School of Nursing and other training schools, thus to provide an adequate supply of student nurses. The first literature concerning the army school, issued on June 7, 1918, announced that it offered to women desiring to care for sick and wounded soldiers a course leading to a diploma in nursing. Candidates had to be between 21 and 35 years of age, in good physical condition, and of good moral character. They were also required to be graduates of recognized high schools or present evidence of an educational equivalent.

Within 10 days after the first official announcement in the press, 981 letters of inquiry were received; 8 months later, more than 10,000 applications had

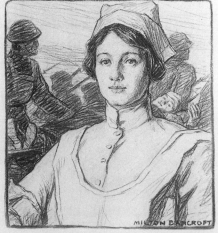

World War I student-nurse recruitment poster.

arrived in the surgeon general's office. When the first year's campaign ended, 14,000 applications had been received. Of these, 5380 applicants were admitted to the army school and 5185 were enrolled for entrance into civilian schools of nursing. The rest were put on a waiting list.

Annie Goodrich was appointed dean of the Army School of Nursing. She and her assistants carried on their activities from the army surgeon general's office. She saw in the army school plan an opportunity to establish an outstanding demonstration school in which the accepted principles of organization, administration, and teaching would be effectively applied. No tuition was required. The students were provided with board, lodging, laundry, and required textbooks.

The 3-year course was based on the new *Standard Curriculum for Schools of Nursing*, published by the National League of Nursing Education in 1917. The time allotted to the various subjects was divided between lectures and demonstrations by members of the medical staff, or among special lectures and classes, quizzes, and laboratory work under qualified nurses and other instructors. The hours of duty on the ward were arranged to accommodate required class work. Unlike the schedule in most civilian hospital schools, duty hours during the probationary period did not exceed 6 daily; after that, a period of 8 hours daily was the maximum. The military hospitals provided experience in surgical nursing, including orthopedic; eye, ear, nose, and throat; and medical nursing, including communicable, nervous, and mental diseases. Experience in children's diseases, gynecology, obstetrics, and public health nursing was provided through affiliations in the second or third year.

AT THE FRONT

On the front, contrary to expectations, the war offered no heroic glamour. The firepower generated by modern artillery was so devastating that armies could no longer stay on the surface of the battlefield. Consequently, trenches hundreds of miles long were dug. Then, to secure the trenches from surprise attack, each side spun hundreds of thousands of miles of barbed wire before its entrenchments. The art of offensive warfare shifted to wallowing, defensive action amid mudholes and barbed wire. Armies became cannon fodder as the glory of war disappeared in the mire of eastern France.

Military nurses soon saw the devastating effects of modern artillery fire. Fragmentation shells burst into a hail of small, deadly splinters that caused extensive, deep, and ragged wounds highly favorable to infection. The great lacerations caused by explosive projectiles required expert surgical specialists and good nursing. Shrapnel (consisting of jagged pieces of iron) often cut across different organs of the trunk or abdomen and produced multiple injuries at a single

impact: deep, penetrating wounds that were ready culture for infections and demanded the most careful nursing care. High-explosive blast concussion alone could destroy several parts of the body at once. "The wounds which you will be called upon to handle and dress are such that you have never imagined it possible for a human being to be so fearfully hurt and yet to be alive," exclaimed one nurse.

The soil of France and Belgium, manured and cultivated for centuries, was found to be heavily laden with pathogenic germs. Long periods of duty in the muddy, often filthy trenches made the soldier's skin, as well as his uniform, dirty and germ-laden, so that bits of the soil driven into a wound would almost inevitably produce infection. Consequently, nurses on the Western Front soon discovered that there was no such thing as a sterile gunshot wound.

These women also saw the effects of the new steel-jacketed bullets. Impact reduced soft body tissues to a devitalized pulp that quickly necrotized and was an ideal medium for the growth of pathogenic bacteria. Surgical asepsis under such conditions was impossible, and it became necessary to regress to fundamental listerism or antisepsis. It was soon found, however, that strong antiseptics applied to deep, infected wounds would not sterilize them. An added difficulty was that strong antiseptics were likely to kill both the infectious organism and the surrounding healthy tissue.

Medical researchers attempted to find a substance that would kill the germs without causing injury to tissue. An answer to this problem was found by surgeon Alexis Carrel and chemist Henry Dakin, who developed an effective method of disinfecting wounds by using a weak chlorine solution in continuous irrigation. Continuous irrigation was secured by Carrel's device of inserting into the wound a series of rubber supply tubes through which was fed the chlorine solution. In this way it became possible to disinfect a wound and thus permit more rapid healing. After use of continuous irrigations, the progress of the wound was checked biologically by the laboratory as

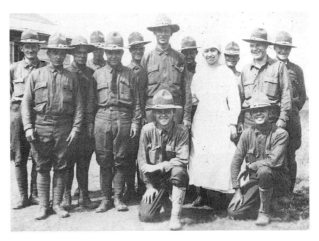

Nurse and American soldiers on the Italian Front.

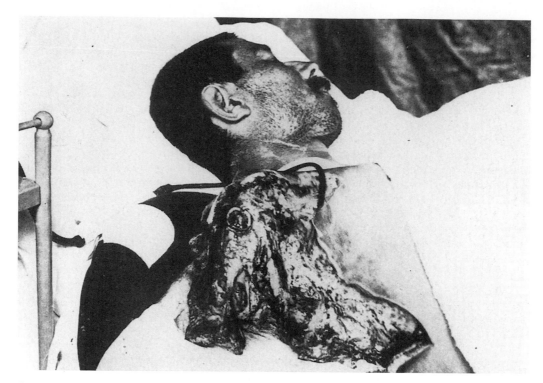

Continuous irrigation of deep wounds with a weak chlorine solution proved an effective disinfectant.

to the kind and number of bacteria. When the dangerous kinds had disappeared and the ordinary types were present in very small numbers, the surgeon practiced what was called secondary suture, and healing progressed with a new rapidity.

SUPERHUMAN DEMANDS

Given the new challenges of patient care, it was common for nurses to work 14 to 18 hours a day for weeks at a time, and some hospitals had only 70 or 80 nurses caring for up to 2100 patients. One hospital reached a patient load of 5000, with only 70 nurses to furnish patient care. There were many other hospitals with equally disproportionate figures. A nurse at Crézancy described her situation:

> About 2 o'clock Monday morning the journey's end was reached. No place to lie down. All lay down with suits, coats and raincoats on, with gas masks and helmets near at hand, and in spite of the soft drizzle of rain slept, forgetting the war, until 8 A.M. That day several nurses appropriated a tiny house by the side of the road; and others got a cot in barracks or little tents. Later, marquise tents were provided for all the nurses.
>
> The drive was on, the wounded poured in, the nurses forgot themselves in a combined effort to do their share to check the crimson tide which was so terrible at this place. The nurses with operating teams as well as those attached to the hospital worked, not caring how hard nor how long the hours. The object of all was to save.
>
> The dead about Crézancy were still unburied, and the flies and yellow jackets were too terrible for description. Many of the nurses were ill. Sanitary conditions here were most pitiful.
>
> The weather was extremely hot—especially were the tents extremely hot—the blazing sun beat down on the tents at day. The combined smell of ether, blood, stale air and heavy atmosphere from the steam sterilizers is one to be not easily forgotten after fifteen or eighteen hours of work.[12]

The work of the army nurse was exceedingly strenuous. Emma Quandt, a nurse from Chicago, wrote:

> A hypodermic of morphine was given the patient so that he would rest until morning, provided his condition or the nature of the wound did not need surgical attention in the operating theatre. I shall never forget my first convoy of wounded soldiers, twenty-seven stretcher cases, almost every one had to have an amputation of some member of the body. A number of my patients died from exposure in the trenches, because it had been about thirty-six hours before any aid could reach them. It was a pitiful sight to see these strong, healthy, young men, blind or crippled for life.[13]

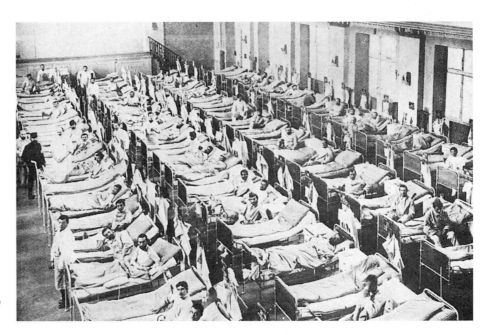

An overcrowded military hospital in France.

The 8587 nurses with the 184,000 wounded and sick American soldiers in the 153 base hospitals, 66 camps, and 12 convalescent hospitals in Europe in mid-1918 became familiar with many dramatic scenes. As the wounded were brought in, their packs, gas masks, and helmets were thrown on the salvage heap to be carted away at any slack hour. There was no time to remove the clothing from the men. The wounds were hurriedly fluoroscoped, and places where shell fragments or bullets were lodged were marked with a cross in indelible pencil as a guide to the surgeons. The stretchers were placed directly on the operating room table to save time, and the clothing cut away from around the wound. As the patient was given chloroform and ether, the wound was cleansed with gasoline, then iodine was applied. Each wound was laid open and the injured tissue cut away—an operation called a débridement.

EXPERIENCES IN WAR

One nurse described the scene at a large allied hospital in France:

> Eleven P.M. The whistle sounds three times. Six newcomers.
> "This leg is bleeding badly. Don't jolt him. Take him carefully to the operating room. Hurry."
> "Your wound is in the head, I see. Doctor, to which ward shall he go?"
> "Wash him and warm him. Then let them take him to Salle III. It is Nourier's turn tomorrow. He will operate."
> "And this one, ma soeur?"
> "A bullet in the abdomen; hardly any pulse and he has been vomiting."

"When was he wounded? Twenty-four hours ago? It is a scandal. We must operate at once. You say that none of them have had antitetanus serum? What criminal neglect. An inquiry must be set afoot. Such things cannot be allowed to pass. Where is he from?"

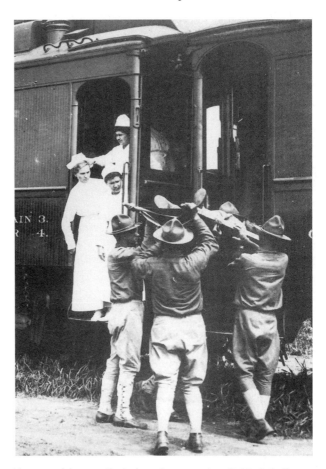

Nurse receiving a patient aboard an army hospital train in France.

"From Bosinghe."

"Our section. How can they expect us to save them if they keep them so long before sending them on? What with poisoned ammunition and exposure, the odds are all against them."

"This man, doctor, is wounded in the neck. His card says the bullet went through the neck and is probably lodged in the base of the skull or in the spine."

"When was your last dressing done, mon ami? I can hardly hear what you say—two hours ago? Two? (Holding up two fingers.) You have come all that way with your head over the end of the stretcher like that? I see, you could not breathe with it otherwise? Get him warm, nurse, and send him to the operating room. Then we will see."

"How terrifyingly blue his face is. Such a nice face, too. He has hardly any pulse."

"Here, my friend, let me put this cushion under your head and raise it a little. And the hot-water bottles will soon make you feel better. Thank you for that smile."

All bad cases tonight.

In the operating room the boy with a bullet in the abdomen lies on his stretcher on the floor, apparently dead. They do all they can to bring him round. He revives. They chloroform him, open the abdominal cavity. Floods of dark blood well out.

We are too late.

"If they could only send us these abdominal cases at once. A fine, handsome young chap like that, too."

"Yes, appalling. It's war. Now for that leg; it cannot wait.[14]

Shirley Millard was assigned to a field hospital in France. The carnage was on a scale beyond anything she had imagined. "Day after day we cut down stinking bandages and expose wounds that destroy the whole original plan of the body. One man had both buttocks blown off, one arm had been amputated at the elbow, and he had a host of smaller wounds from flying metal. Another lay propped on sphagnum moss to absorb the discharge from two large holes in each thigh."[15] Like other healthy young women, she felt somehow guilty in the presence of so much suffering and such majestic pain:

No matter what we did, how hard we worked, it did not seem to be fast enough or hard enough. More came. It took me several days to steel my emotions against the stabbing cries of pain. The crowded, twisted bodies, the screams and groans, made one think of the old engravings in Dante's *Inferno*. More came, and still more. . . .

My hands tremble as I pull at sodden boots and uniforms. The weather is cold and wet and most of their garments are caked with mud from head to foot, so that to get the things off without causing excruciating pain is almost impossible. "Leave me alone, will you," they scream wildly and resist my ministrations. Many of them have nothing on their wounds but a strip of coat sleeve or an old muffler or a muddy legging wrapped on quickly by a comrade in the field. Some have only newspaper tied on with a bootlace. I remove blood-and-mud-soaked bandages and find an arm hanging by a tendon. . . .

Gashes from bayonets. Eyes torn by shrapnel. Faces half shot away. Eyes seared by gas; one here with no eyes at all. I can see down into the back of his head. Here is a boy with a gray, set face. He is hanging on . . . too far gone to make a sound. His stomach is blown wide open and only held together by a few bands of sopping gauze which I must pull away. I do so, gently as I can. The odor is sickening; the gauze is a greenish yellow. Gangrene. He was wounded days ago and has been waiting on the grounds. He will die.[16]

The high-speed butchery of the operating theaters after a battle had its own horrors. The leg that one of the nurses was holding came off with a jerk, and she fell down still clasping the foot. She stuffed the leg into the dressing pail beside the other arms and legs. The emergency was so great that surgery was performed right on the wards, and amputated legs were stuck in buckets in the corridors outside. Still the casualties kept coming:

Here is an unconscious lad with his head completely bandaged. The gauze is stiff with blood and dirt. I cut carefully and remove it, glad he is unconscious; much easier to work when they cannot feel the pain. As the last band comes off, a sickening mass spills out of the wide gash at the side of his skull. Brains. I am stunned. I cannot think what to do. No time to ask questions. Everyone around me is occupied with similar problems. Boldly I wrap my hand in sterile gauze and thrust the slippery mass back as best I can, holding the wound closed while I awkwardly tie a clean bandage around the head. It does not occur to me until afterwards that he must have been dead.

A boy from Idaho, a big round boy, had his head all bound up and the tag around his neck, put on at a dressing station, said: "Eyes shot away and both feet gone." I talked to him and patted him on the shoulder, assuring him that everything would be all right now. He moaned through the bandages that his head was splitting with pain. I gave him morphine. Suddenly aware of the fact that he had other wounds, he asked: "Sa-ay, what's the matter with my legs?" Reaching down to feel his legs before I could stop him, he uttered a heartbreaking scream. I held his hands firmly until the drug I had given him took effect.[17]

In *Finding Themselves: The Letters of an American Army Chief Nurse in a British Hospital in France*, Julia Stimson's letters give a lucid, intriguing, honest look at the war, providing extraordinary personal insight and a haunting perspective on human tragedy. The collection is preceded by a brief note, written by Julia's father, which indicates that the letters were composed "as the daily record of the work of a Unit of Red Cross nurses who were sent to France in May, 1917, in response to the request of the British authorities."

Though her letters suggest a thoroughgoing patriotism, they rarely slip into propaganda; her willingness to view the war through a less biased and more humanistic lens is evident in letters such as the following, from July 1917:

On the fourth of July, we thought how like a home Fourth it was, but here the popping and the shots sound every day. And it is not fireworks that are being shot off. At neighboring camps there are experts in bayoneting, experts in gassing, experts in Hate Talk. There are actually special men who sometimes talk to as many as three thousand men to make them feel that their chief business is to kill. It is incomprehensible. Whenever will this toppling world right itself?[18]

In another letter, dated August 8, 1917, Stimson notes her reaction to a day of "gas training":

We had our masks tested first in a room filled with lachrymating gas; we were drilled in putting them on any number of times, for speed is a very important element, so each motion is counted and timed. We were lectured for an hour, the most interesting and barbarous lecture I ever heard in my life. It is at one and the same time the refinement of science and civilization, and of hideous barbarism.[19]

Stimson wrote that the bravery of the wounded is hardest to bear, making her "so ashamed for all the complaining we have done." She describes her first encounter with a triple amputee: "It seemed as though my throat would burst, and I had to think very quickly how absurd it would be for the new Matron to weep before all those heroic, stoical men."[20] The juxtaposition of Stimson's observations with private chatter—often gauged to provide

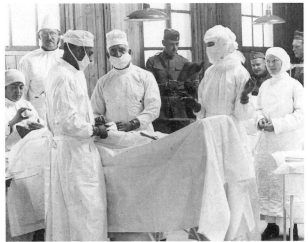

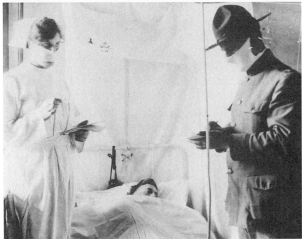

Infections from wounds and disease required heroic nurses.

reassurance to worried family members—reveals a tenacious, sensitive personality:

Our hospital again is almost full to capacity, and such badly hurt men—amputations, two or three of them, every day out of sixteen or seventeen operations every afternoon. Day after yesterday they had a man on the operating table before they decided which of his legs they had better take off! Such a price as is being paid for the new world— but it is not too big to make the new world and liberty and peace and brotherhood and democracy mean something. And how small a share we are having in that price and how we'd give more if we could. I wish E. wouldn't think that anything we are doing is worth admiration—it isn't—we are doing so little. We love being here and would not leave our jobs for anything that could be offered us. I am writing in bed; it is very late but I don't feel like sleeping yet. It is very comfortable here in my little bed with my good light hanging beside me. The light is such a comfort. I have bought an oil stove to try and heat this room. I think it will make things more comfortable.[21]

Stimson and her nurses not only sacrificed but also accomplished much, doing so with compassion and humility, courage and skill. Given enormous medical responsibilities, Stimson and her colleagues did "such surgical work as they never in their wildest days dreamed of." Nurses of front hospitals were assigned "no mere handling of instruments and sponges, but sewing and tying up and putting in drains while the doctor takes the next piece of shell out of another place."[22]

A NEW WEAPON—GAS

As if wounds from bullets and shrapnel were not enough, an even more terrifying and gruesome weapon of war emerged with cataclysmic results—poison gas. It was first used on April 22, 1915, in the vicinity of Langemark, near Ypres. On that fatal day, after bombarding the French forces with high explosives at early morning, the Germans halted their fire about 2 hours before sunset. Then they opened more than 500 cylinders containing 168 tons of pressurized chlorine gas and waited as the light wind bore it steadily toward the opposing forces. The effect was devastating—chlorine, a greenish yellow gas with a sharp, acrid smell, causes intense irritation of the lungs; if inhaled in a concentration of more than 1:10,000 for a minute or two, death ensues. The same concentration is incapacitating if inhaled for only a few seconds. The Germans had released the gas over a 4-mile front on an enemy totally unprepared for this kind of attack. All resistance was eliminated on the front to a depth of several miles. There were more than 15,000 casualties, including 5000 fatalities.

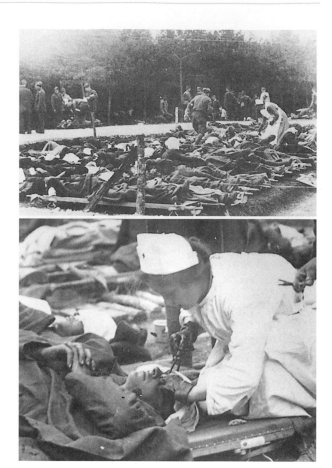

Gas casualties (above); nurse bathing eyes of gas patients (below).

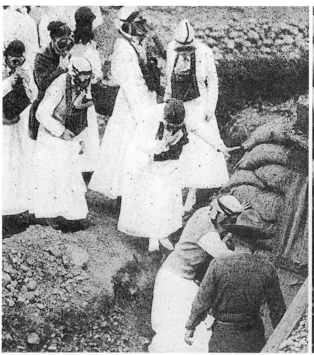

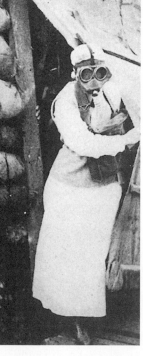

Nurses preparing for an attack of poisoned gas.

Even more feared was dichloroethyl sulfide, better known as mustard gas, from the odor of its impure, liquid form, first used by the Germans in July 1917. Like many of the toxic "gases," mustard is liquid at ordinary temperatures, boiling at 217°C. It evaporated slowly; when collected in the soil, it took weeks to evaporate completely. The liquid itself was harmful, quickly penetrating clothing and causing severe, deep burns on the skin, which were difficult to heal. The effects themselves took a few hours to appear but were often widespread. The eyes became inflamed and the lungs irritated. Large doses caused severe vomiting, nausea, fever, and side effects, among them shock, which resulted from the severe trauma to the body. Even diluted to 1:100,000, the gas still produced its effects after only 1 or 2 minutes' exposure. These began to appear about an hour after contact and would be fully developed after perhaps 5 hours.

The nurses at the base hospitals could easily understand why mustard gas was so effective: practically colorless, its garlic or mustard smell lasted only a few minutes. Provided that the means of delivery remain undiscovered, there was no reason why the gas would be detected until the effects had begun to appear some hours later. By this time, massive doses would have been received. Furthermore, the liquid and vapor would linger, making any position that had been attacked by mustard gas untenable for some time. During the last year of the war it accounted for 16% of the British casualties and 33% of the American ones.

Margaret Dunlop, chief nurse of the Pennsylvania Hospital Unit, recalled that their first hard experience in nursing came shortly after their arrival in France, when the field hospital received an exceedingly large convoy of mustard-gas victims.

> These patients were horribly gassed and were pictures of misery and intense suffering. They poured upon us in great numbers—600 in less than forty-eight hours—and their sufferings were pitiful to see, but their bravery, unselfishness, and fortitude were impressed upon us very fully. The nurses worked hard and faithfully during this short period, but the awfulness and immensity of suffering and cruel barbarity of war upon the individual were a soul-harrowing experience to them all. It was a tremendous strain on mind, heart, and body, being untrained to the handling of such large numbers and not yet inured to the immensity of the work. During that summer of 1917, we had our baptism of horror and work, but after a few months the whole Unit settled down to the inevitable, and as the handling of large numbers of severely wounded was efficiently expedited, the fear of not being equal to the task gradually disappeared.[23]

After a gas attack, the burned and sightless eyes made all the faces look like a ghastly row of masks, and the utter silence completed the illusion of one's being surrounded by puppets:

> November 8th, 1918
>
> More and more Americans in the death ward. Gas cases are terrible. They cannot breathe lying down or sitting up. They just struggle for breath, but nothing can be done . . . their lungs are gone . . . literally burnt out. Some with their eyes and faces entirely eaten away by the gas, and bodies covered with first degree burns. We try to relieve them by pouring oil on them. They cannot be bandaged or even touched. We cover them with a tent of propped-up sheets. Gas burns must be agonizing because usually the other cases invariably are beyond endurance and they cannot help crying out.
>
> One boy today, screaming to die. The entire top layer of skin burned from his face and body. I gave him an injection of morphine. He was wheeled out just before I came off duty.[24]

Shock, hemorrhage, infected wounds, and the care of gassed patients challenged the powers of observation and the technical skills of nurses. Barbara Thompson recalled:

> Gas was very disastrous in this war. I went on night duty during an artillery barrage, and I prepared morphine shots for twelve hours to ease the severe pain of the wounded. These patients suffered severe shock and pain and many died before first aid could be given. Working conditions were primitive. Not at all like the conditions in the operating rooms in the U.S. I was on night duty during the Château-Thierry drive. One night as I was giving a soldier an anesthetic when almost under he yelled, "I am the strongest man in America," and off the table he went with me hanging fast to his chin with the ether mask over his face.[25]

THE GREAT INFLUENZA EPIDEMIC OF 1918–1919

Meanwhile, another insidious force was at work. This phenomenon, a massive influenza epidemic that would cause many more deaths than did the fighting, burst on the nation and the world without warning. The continual movement of the troops created avenues of travel for the disease, and the mingling of people from home and abroad was probably the facilitating element in the development of the highly

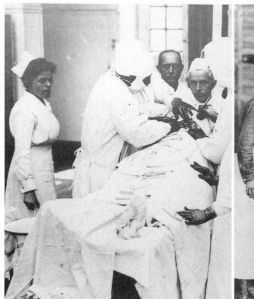
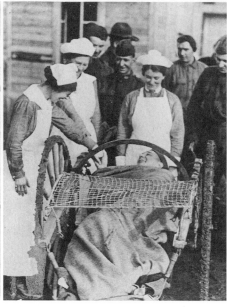

Shock, hemorrhage, and infected wounds challenged the skills of nurses.

virulent strain of influenza that emerged. Soldiers and civilians alike faced an unseen and unconquerable enemy, a microscopic virus—not photographed until 1933—in many ways more formidable an adversary than the armies themselves.

During this great epidemic, from September 1918 to August 1919, the United States experienced the highest excess death rate in its history. Ninety-two percent of all the excess deaths were directly attributable to influenza and its colleague in death, pneumonia. When it was over, incomplete data revealed that the death toll in the United States alone for the last 4 months of 1918 and the first 6 months of 1919 was 548,452—five times greater than total World War I American military deaths.

Nurses were expected to perform the more everyday chores of caring for influenza patients and to deal with situations of life and death. Often physicians were unavailable, and in the final analysis the nurses were the heroines of the fight of hundreds of thousands of human bodies against the epidemic. Shockingly, estimates of the number of influenza deaths worldwide ranged from a low of 15 million to a high of 30 million, with most estimates running around 22 million.

The influenza epidemic in the United States was in full force by the time news of the Armistice came. On November 11, 1918, there were 193,000 patients in hospitals in France and 70,000 patients in army hospitals at home. The larger hospital centers in France, such as Allerey, Bazoilles, Toul, Mesves, Mars, and Savenay, were originally 1000-bed units, but in times of heavy casualties had become huge installations with an emergency capacity of 10,000 to 40,000 beds. For example, the Mesves Hospital Center had, in November 1918, 25,000 beds, with 20,186 patients and 394 nurses.

A SUMMING UP

Though the ideal ratio was 1 nurse to every 10 patients, records show that at one time the army hospital in Savenay, France, had 59.5 patients to every nurse. In another hospital, 150 women were caring for 9000 wounded. During the great Meuse-Argonne drive, all the hospitals in France were shorthanded, while the demands of the great influenza epidemic in the United States were even more serious. Often the nurses worked until they themselves became patients, sometimes with fatal results. American nurses also helped staff the hospitals of the Allies, who continually asked for more of them.

Nearly 300 military nurses laid down their lives. None was killed in action, though three were wounded by enemy fire. Two lost their lives and one was seriously wounded in a premature explosion during target practice at sea on an American transport. One hundred

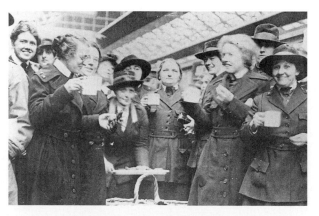

Armistice celebration by army nurses, November 1918.

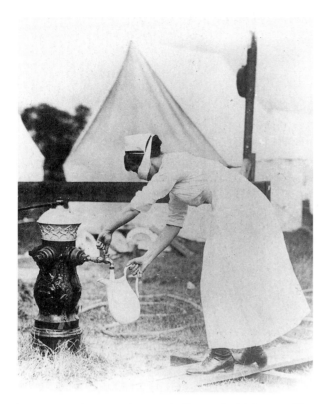

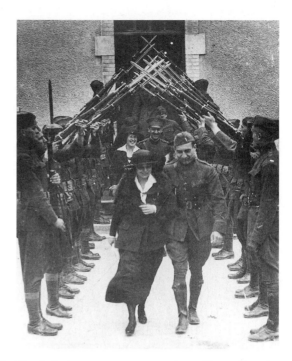

Wedding bells for an army nurse and an officer, somewhere in France.

A nurse, wearing a mask as protection against influenza, fills a pitcher from a water hydrant.

others narrowly escaped with their lives when their transport collided and sank in New York harbor. More than two thirds of the nurse casualties resulted from pneumonia and influenza, induced largely by overwork, exhaustion, and poor living conditions.

The war gave the Navy Nurse Corps its first major opportunity to impress on any remaining skeptics its importance to the navy. Assigned to hospitals in England, Ireland, and Scotland and on the French coast, navy nurses firmly established their value through devotion to duty, high-quality patient care, and effective instruction of hospital corpsmen. The demands of World War I on the Medical Department

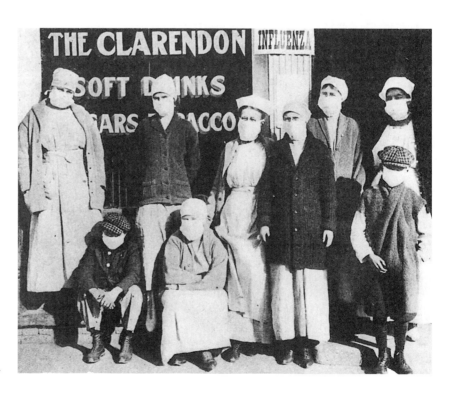

Attempts to protect against influenza.

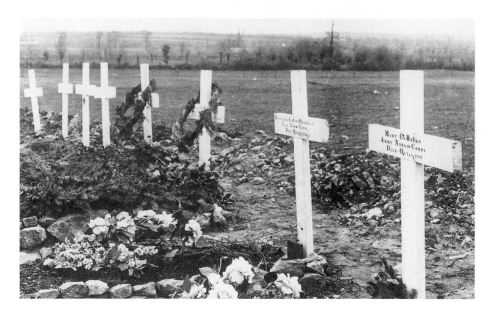

Graves of American military nurses near Mars-Sur Allier, Nievre, France.

of the navy were reflected in the strength of the Nurse Corps, which increased its ranks to a peak strength of nearly 1500.

After the Armistice, most of the nurses returned to their homes and to civilian nursing or marriage. But for many of those who had witnessed the carnage of battle, life would never be quite the same. The vivid images of the destruction caused by war and by the influenza epidemic lived on in their minds, and many of the nurses probably felt as did Dante in the *Inferno*—that the multiple horrors they had beheld defied description:

> *Who even in unrhymed words*
> *Could ever fully tell in many narrations*
> *Of the blood and the wounds I now saw?*
> *Every tongue certainly would fail*
> *Because our language and our memories*
> *Are insufficient to contain so much.*[26]

Although nurses would never forget the nightmare of treating mass casualties of the fighting and the accompanying diseases of World War I, they would remember with pride their own crucial and dramatic battles to save endangered lives and to lighten the toll of war and pestilence.

REFERENCES

1. Noyes to Nutting, April 8, 1917, Nursing Archives, Teachers College, Columbia University, New York.
2. U.S. Council of National Defense, *First Annual Report of the Council of National Defense, Fiscal Year 1917* (Washington, DC: Government Printing Office, 1917), pp. 1–5.
3. Letter of Bessie Baker to Jane A. Delano, June 6, 1917, Johns Hopkins University, American Red Cross Archives, Washington, DC.
4. Letter of Daisy D. Urch to Jane A. Delano, August 30, 1917, Northwestern University, American Red Cross Archives, Washington, DC.
5. Ibid.
6. Vera Brittain, *Testament of Youth: An Autobiographical Study of the Years 1900–1925* (New York: Macmillan Co., 1933), pp. 420–421.
7. William Howard Taft, "A Distinct Call to Women," *Ladies' Home Journal*, vol. 34 (September 1917):5.
8. Annie W. Goodrich, "Report of the Survey of the Nursing Resources of the Country," *American Journal of Nursing*, vol. 18 (August 1918):959–961.

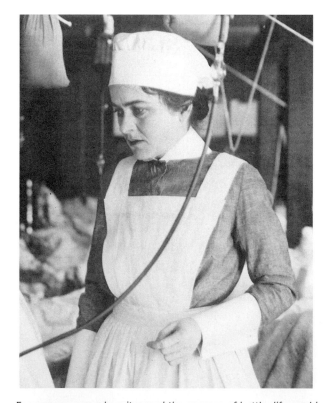

For many nurses who witnessed the carnage of battle, life would never be quite the same.

9. Winford H. Smith, "How Nurses Are Meeting the Present Needs," *American Journal of Nursing*, vol. 18 (August 1918): 979–986.

10. Ibid., pp. 983–986.

11. Interview with Frances Payne Bolton, Cleveland, Ohio, July 31, 1972.

12. "War Nurse's Diary," *Trained Nurse and Hospital Review*, vol. 60 (February 1918):90–91.

13. Emma Quandt, "Active Service on the Western Front," *American Journal of Nursing*, vol. 18 (March 1918):388–389.

14. Maud Mortimer, *A Green Tent in Flanders* (New York: Doubleday, 1918), pp. 173–174.

15. Shirley Millard, *I Saw Them Die: Diary and Recollections of Shirley Millard* (New York: Harcourt, Brace, & Co., 1936), p. 12.

16. Ibid., pp. 14–15.

17. Ibid., pp. 15–16.

18. Julia C. Stimson, *Finding Themselves: The Letters of an American Army Chief Nurse in a British Hospital in France* (New York: Macmillan Company, 1918), pp. 72–73.

19. Ibid., pp. 94–95.

20. Ibid., pp. 40–41.

21. Ibid., p. 154.

22. Ibid., pp. 134, 142.

23. Margaret A. Dunlop, "History of the Nursing Corps of Base Hospital No. 10, U.S.A.," in *History of the Pennsylvania Hospital Unit in the Great War* (New York: Paul B. Hoeber, 1921), p. 85.

24. Millard, op. cit., p. 108.

25. Interview with Barbara Thompson Sharpless, World War I nurse, Ventura, California, July 31, 1973.

26. Dante Alighieri, *The Divine Comedy*, trans. H. R. Huse (New York: Henry Holt & Co, 1954), p. 133.

11

BOOM AND BUST, 1920–1933

As the 1920s dawned, the nation's nursing staffs were still disorganized and depleted. Hospitals had not yet recovered from the double strain of war and influenza. Many graduate and student nurses had died in the epidemic, and the long-term effects of the disease forced many more to give up their work. The entire educational program in most schools of nursing had been suspended for weeks because of the absence of instructors and the critical situation in hospitals. World War I had enabled women to enter new areas of activity, and 1919 brought the passage of the Woman Suffrage Amendment in the United States. Once women became an integral part of the work force, they gained new status. As working wives, they helped support the family, or they could be self-supporting if unmarried. Spending much of their time outside the home, economically, they became part of a previously all-male world. Since the 1890s, middle-class single women had worked before marriage, but, after marrying, they faced either forced or voluntary unemployment. By 1920, the number of working women had nearly doubled since the turn of the century, so that women represented more than one fifth of the total working population.

A quest for private fulfillment, motivated by the new advertising industry and national prosperity, yielded an upheaval in social mores, often called "The Flapper's Revolution." It was an age of unheard-of freedom for women, hard won in World War I. Women had proved they could take the place of men on countless fronts when the latter went off to war and could work beside them in the uniforms of nurses, motor-corps chauffeurs, or canteen hostesses. One might almost say that the idea of equality with men had gone to a woman's head as she bobbed her hair to look like his; borrowed his shirt, tie, and felt hat to appear on the golf links; and flattened her curves with a bandeau that reduced her to subteen straightness.

The defense of the new clothes and hairstyles on the grounds of practicality had a solid basis; the loosened,

dropped waistline was more functional than the tightly bound middle that demanded time-consuming, strong, painful corseting. Women felt freed from the necessities of such formality and inhibition and preferred the nonrestraint of the loosened waist. Women increasingly objected to being "placed in restraints" when engaging in the same activities as men. The campus as well as the white-collar professions of secretary, typist, and salesgirl provided occasions for men to work with women, and women's clothes reflected this new status.

SHORTAGE OF STUDENTS

During the war, applications to nursing schools had greatly increased, and, in response to appeals from the Committee on Nursing, extra classes had been admitted to help meet wartime needs. Consequently, it was estimated that in the 1755 schools of nursing in the United States, several thousand of the 54,953 student nurse enrollees would not have been attracted to nursing without the war-induced stimulation. A fairly large proportion of these young women had been drawn from other occupations and had patriotically entered the schools "for the duration of the war." Most young women with such motivation who were physically fit remained through the influenza epidemic. Shortly afterward, however, they thought their war service was over, and large numbers dropped out of the schools.

The United States faced a shortage of approximately 55,000 trained nurses in 1920. The Public Health Service, which was temporarily handling all the hospitalization for war veterans, needed 10,000 more nurses than could be recruited. According to statistics compiled by the National Organization for Public Health Nursing, 70,000 American babies died in 1920 because their mothers did not have proper prenatal or postnatal care. Of those deaths, 5000 occurred in New York City. Physicians everywhere

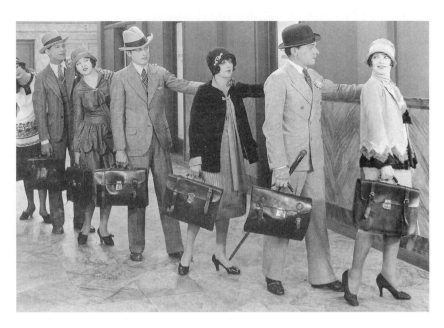

Women entered business occupations in the 1920s.

complained that they were greatly handicapped because they could not get competent nurses for serious cases. Hospitals were unable to provide adequate nursing service for their patients for this same reason.

Schools of nursing could not recruit enough students to fill their classes. In Connecticut, the schools were short 700 student nurses. In New York State, the roster was 2500 short. At the Lenox Hill Hospital, New York City, where the quota of nursing students was 125, the classes totaled only 56. Recruitment prospects had grown so hopeless in Indiana that some hospitals in the smaller towns were closing their doors.

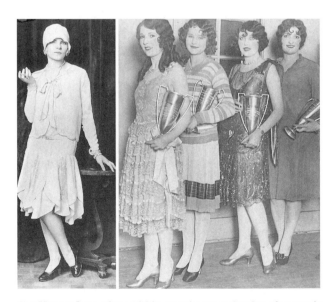

The "flapper" era of the 1920s saw the emancipation of women's dress.

THE EFFECT OF WORLD WAR I

In 1921, Isabel Stewart, assistant professor in the Department of Nursing and Health at Teachers College, Columbia University, summed up the effect of the war years on the nursing profession in a bulletin issued by the U.S. Bureau of Education, *Developments in Nursing Education since 1918.* She observed that through widespread publicity the number of young women entering nursing schools during 1917 and 1918 had been increased by 25%. Every effort had been made to attract the more serious and better-educated women for this service, and as a result the average educational level of entering students had increased noticeably. Despite the disruptions caused by the war, the epidemic, and the disorganization of teaching and supervisory staffs in hospitals, the educational status of nursing schools was in certain ways better at the end of the war than it had been at the beginning. Stewart concluded:

> Probably the greatest contribution to nursing of the war experience lies in the fact that the whole system of nursing education was shaken for a little while out of its well-worn ruts and brought out of its comparative seclusion into the light of public discussion and criticism. When so many lives hung on the supply of nurses, people were aroused to a new sense of their dependence on the products of nursing schools, and many of them learned for the first time of the hopelessly limited resources which nursing educators have had to work with in the training of these indispensable public servants. Whatever the future may bring it is unlikely that nursing schools will willingly sink back again into their

old isolation, or that they will accept unquestionably the financial status which the older system imposed on them.[1]

THE IMAGE PROBLEM

From the point of view of the hospital administrators of the 1920s, student nurses were a necessity and could be secured only by an apprenticeship system of education. Financially, the institutions were well repaid, because student nurses furnished nursing care at very low cost. As a result, numerous additional schools were established, as the figures surged from 1755 in 1920 to 1964 in 1923 and to 2286 in 1927. Student enrollments soared from 54,953 in 1920 to 77,768 in 1927. Too many nurses were soon being graduated, many without adequate training. From the student nurses' point of view, their own exploitation was rarely considered, because an overriding consecration to service was taken for granted among those who entered the profession.

After the glamour of service in the war, the overall prestige of nursing declined sharply. Nursing's lower prestige was partially related to the fact that 95% of the active nurses in the nation were women. In a culture that was predominantly "a man's world," any occupation made up primarily of women was considered to be feminine and therefore inferior. Added to this was the social phenomenon that most nurse leaders were unmarried; therefore, they lacked the social prestige that marriage brought in the society of the time.

An unforgettable picture of middle-class American sex-typing was presented in the sociologic study *Middletown*, by Robert S. Lynd and Helen M. Lynd. Here, as depicted in 1924, men and women belonged to two different subcultures: the man's world involved professional leadership, whereas the woman's involved the care and training of small children. Male authority always loomed in the background. This role differentiation was based on an assumption that men and women were different kinds of people. Men were portrayed as stronger, bolder, more logical, and more reasonable, but in need of coddling and reassurance from women. Women, although more delicate physically, were considered stronger morally and more refined, sympathetic, and sensitive. What held in *Middletown* was postulated as true of the nation as a whole.

The fast-growing motion picture industry, with its myriad depictions of nurses on the screen in such productions as *Goodnight Nurse* and *When a Woman Sins*, was of little help to hospitals in stimulating nurse recruitment. In 1921, Edwin P. Haworth, superintendent of Wilcrest Hospital and Willows Sanitarium, Kansas City, Missouri, noted that "nursing life" had always been looked on by the laity "as a Florence Nightingale or Clara Barton sort of life— something ideal, with a purpose."[2] It was the model profession for the humanitarian, one that might often be enhanced by altruistic or religious commitments. It was a nonworldly profession. For the non-Catholic world, nursing was the substitute for the Sisters of Charity, an opportunity to give one's life in service to society. As such, nursing had had its own distinct and lofty appeal.

"Why do movies have such unreal stuff when they attempt to present a drama of nursing or hospital life?" Haworth asked. He had just seen Mary Miles Minter in the 1920 film, *Nurse Marjorie*. Minter skillfully acted the part she had to play, but it was clear that she was not a nurse. "No nurse would do the things she did," Haworth complained. No hospital of standing would tolerate the actions of such a nurse. It was not typical of nursing or hospital life.[3]

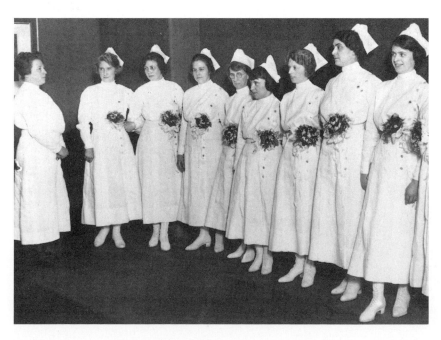

The overall prestige of nursing declined in the early 1920s.

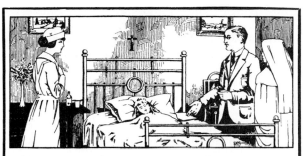

Nurses Training Schools

For the Training of Young Women In the Noble Profession of Nursing

We believe that many young women would be eager to enter Nurses' Training Schools as pupils, in the state of Wisconsin, if they appreciated the splendid opportunity for service to their fellow-man offered by the greatest profession open to women. There is a large number of such training schools for nurses connected with the many excellent hospitals of this state.

Hence, the subjoined Catholic hospitals of Wisconsin, as members of the Wisconsin Conference of the Catholic Hospital Association of the United States and Canada, present the following facts for the careful consideration and sympathetic appreciation of the young women of Wisconsin who are seriously thinking of what their future life work shall be.

(1) Nursing is a profession whose great purpose is to help the medical profession in the prevention, alleviation and cure of disease in human beings. According to state law each applicant must have finished two years in an accredited high school or the equivalent following the eighth year of the grade schools, and must be of good character and sound health. The nurses' curriculum is of three years' duration and embraces regular courses in the necessary sciences along with daily practice in the technique of service to the sick. It is, therefore, an intellectual profession based on the sciences and arts called for in the highly specialized care of patients.

(2) Nursing is a noble profession because it involves consecrated service based upon the high purpose of caring for fellow human beings in need of watchful and sympathetic regard for all the wants of body and mind and soul.

(3) This deeply human and truly altruistic profession has a serious ethical intent which looks to the securing for the patient of all his God-given rights that affect the life and welfare of life in every contingency of human existence when life and health are involved.

Such a profession can have a strong appeal only to such young women as have an earnest and sympathetic appreciation of the deeper meaning and needs of individual and social welfare, and a strong urge within their own character to render this generous and conscientious service to ailing human beings which is peculiarly distinctive of a woman. The call is an urgent one and our young womanhood will not fail.

The following hospitals offer a course in nursing that is complete in its scientific and technical training, while it embraces with special emphasis the ethical and religious principles and motives which give such depth and satisfaction to one who serves the health needs of her fellowman. The spirit of these schools is beautifully expressed in the words of Florence Nightingale.

"I do entirely believe that the religious motive is essential for the highest kind of nurse. There are such disappointments, such sickenings of the heart, that they can only be borne by the feeling that one is called to the work by God, that it is a part of His work, that one is a fellow worker of God."

Wisconsin Conference, Catholic Hospital Association

ASHLAND	**GREEN BAY**	**MILWAUKEE**
St. Joseph's Hospital	St. Mary's Hospital	St. Mary's Hospital
		Trinity Hospital
DODGEVILLE	**JANESVILLE**	
St. Joseph's Hospital	Palmer Mercy Hospital	**OSHKOSH**
		St. Mary's Hospital
EAU CLAIRE	**LA CROSSE**	
Sacred Heart Hospital	St. Francis' Hospital	**PORTAGE**
		St. Saviour's Hospital
FOND DU LAC	**MANITOWOC**	
St. Agnes' Hospital	Holy Family Hospital	**RACINE**
		St. Mary's Hospital

Address, Chairman Publicity Committee, Catholic Hospital Association, 208 Montgomery Bldg., Milwaukee, or Communicate Directly with the Hospital in which you are interested.

Hospitals in New York City and elsewhere had difficulty recruiting nurses after the war.

He worried that with the film presenting the nurse and her profession in this light, the nursing standards of earlier years would not be preserved for the eyes of the world. He perceived that movies were beginning to elicit school-of-nursing applicants who came with the "wrong ideals." In the meantime, young women with the proper ideals were not choosing nursing in the proportion they once did. Haworth concluded:

> Perhaps I am wrong in thinking the movies are treating the nursing profession worse than other kinds of life. Perhaps it is merely the unusual and farfetched method of handling all lines of life and thought. If so, so much the worse for the movies. If they are as abnormal and unrealistic as that, then they are a more demoralizing

influence for civilization than I had thought. But the life of the nurse, pupil and graduate, is subject to worthwhile dramatization if presented faithfully. There are details in her life that appeal to the imagination and show her to be a character worth spending an hour with in the movies. Why can't we see the real nurse on the screen, instead of the movie-actress, play-nurse! Both the personality and the dramatic motive would then be improved, much to the advantage of our ideals, and the future of the nursing profession.[4]

INADEQUATE FINANCIAL SUPPORT

According to Isabel Stewart, there was no hope for any substantial advancement in nursing education until nursing schools were removed from hospitals and placed on a separate standing. This did not mean that pupils should not be trained in hospitals but that the nursing school, "like the medical school, should have an independent financial status and the power to work out its own system of education, unhampered by the complicated and often crushing demands of the hospital."[5] She maintained that if some form of endowment could not be found for nursing schools, they should be supported by state or municipal funds. Stewart boldly put her finger on the core of the problem:

> The plain facts are that nursing schools are being starved and always have been starved for lack of funds to build up any kind of substantial

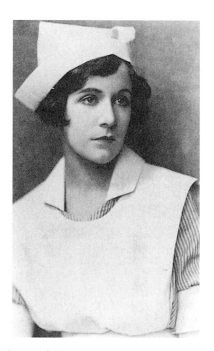

The proper image of the nurse became a matter of concern during the 1920s.

educational structure. As someone has recently said, the nursing school has been literally buried in the hospital, and few people have been aware of its existence. It has fed on the crumbs that fell from the hospital table—a very frugal table, as everyone knows. The educational interests of the school have had no chance whatever against the pressing economic interests of the hospital, and it is probable that even if the hospital recognized its educational obligations, which it has never done, it would find considerable difficulty in meeting them as they should be met.[6]

THE GOLDMARK REPORT

In 1918, Adelaide Nutting approached officials of the Rockefeller Foundation in an attempt to secure an endowment for her alma mater, the Johns Hopkins School of Nursing. During the interview, she stressed the need for improvements in the education of public health nurses. This meeting resulted in the appointment, in January 1919, of the Committee for the Study of Nursing Education, which was to investigate "the proper training of the public health nurse." Financial support was provided by the Rockefeller Foundation.[7] The committee of 19 chaired by C.E.A. Winslow, a professor of public health at Yale University, included six nurses: Adelaide Nutting, Annie Goodrich, Lillian Wald, S. Lillian Clayton, Mary Beard, and Helen Wood.

Also included were 10 physicians, among whom were two hospital superintendents. Two lay representatives, Julia C. Lathrop, of the United States Children's Bureau, and Mrs. John Lowman completed the committee membership. It soon became obvious to the committee that the fundamental problem in public health nursing education was the condition of hospital training schools. Therefore, the scope of committee inquiry was broadened to a study of nursing education in general.

The committee secretary was social worker and author Josephine Goldmark, best known for her 1912 study of the relationship between fatigue and industrial efficiency, who was placed in charge of the survey research. Under her direction, opinions from leading nurse educators were gathered and synthesized. In addition, surveys were made through scientific sampling of representative conditions in schools of nursing and in public health and private-duty nursing. An extensive survey of the more than 1800 hospital training schools in the United States was obviously beyond the resources of the committee. It was therefore decided to select a small group of schools for intensive study. Twenty-three such schools were finally chosen, representing large and small, public and private, general and special hospitals in various sections of the United States. These schools were undoubtedly well above the medium grade, and their average could be taken as fairly

representative of the highest standards of nursing education. Each school was studied in detail by two special investigators, one a practical expert in nursing education and the other an experienced educator from outside the nursing field. The investigation of these schools covered the records of 2406 students.

After the release of the general findings in 1922, the exhaustive 500-page study by Josephine Goldmark, on which the conclusions of the committee were based, was at last made public in 1923 to form the initial landmark in the evaluation of nursing education. Entitled *Nursing and Nursing Education in the United States*, this document emphasized the desirability of establishing university schools of nursing to train nurse leaders. It pointed out the fundamental faults in hospital training schools and identified the primary obstacle to higher standards as the lack of funds set apart specifically for nursing education.

The committee concluded that although training schools for nurses had made remarkable progress and although the best schools reached a high level of educational attainment, the average hospital training school was not organized on a solid enough basis to be compared favorably with the standards required in other professions. Formal instruction in schools of nursing was too casual and uncorrelated, and the educational needs and the health and strength of students were often sacrificed to hospital service demands.

"From our field study of the nurse in public health nursing, in private duty, and as instructor and supervisor in hospitals," said Goldmark, "it is clear that there is need of a basic undergraduate training for all nurses alike, which should lead to a nursing diploma." She concluded that postgraduate training in any one of these three nursing specialties should be given after the completion of basic undergraduate courses and should lead to an advanced diploma or degree.[8]

The reasons for the failure of some schools of nursing and the factors contributing to those failures were reported, including:

Tradition.
Continuance of the apprenticeship system.
Needs of sick predominate; the needs of education must yield thereto.
Lack of a paid group of graduate nurses to meet the hospital need, relieving the student body of non-nursing duties.
Irregular assignments.
Failure to extend the education promised in catalogue.
Failure of superintendent to show the board the impossible nature of task.
No training school committee.
School remains as a department of the hospital.
Many schools accept low educational entrance standards.
Failure to include all services, such as communicable and mental and nervous.
Understaffing of wards.

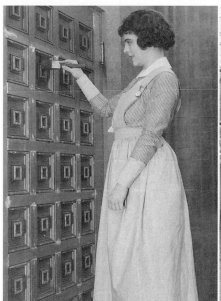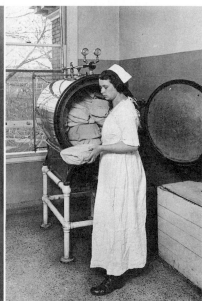

Service demands dominated students' lives.

Lack of adequate supervision.

Careless techniques.

Lack of sufficient and proper affiliations.

Need of appointment of full-time instructors.

Poor planning, in that instruction does not precede technique.

Theory and practice often taught by different women, differently trained, without conferences.

Lack of well-qualified teachers.

Neglect of suitable laboratory instruction and equipment.

Insufficient allowance of time for study.

Overcrowded character of courses.

Waste of student's time.

Lack of endowments.

Lack of graded training.

Use of students as head nurses.

Lack of conferences.

Lack of adequate records.

Lack of correlation between practice and theory.

Failure to use dispensary and clinics as teaching field.

Too much stress placed upon curative medicine to the detriment of preventive medicine.

Psychology, public health and social service not included in curriculum.

Excessive length of hours on duty.

Classwork in evening hours.

Lack of recreational facilities for students.

Failure to provide students with one day's rest in seven and to notify students of days off.

Assignments of night duty service disproportionately long and too close together.

Class hours interrupt sleep, when on night duty.

In commenting on several of these problems, the report stated that in most hospitals the major services—medical, surgical, obstetric, pediatric, and communicable—were too often staffed by students who lacked instruction in the diseases or conditions of patients committed to their care, other than for nursing procedures that were given by the clinical instructor. After her preliminary period of 4 months, the student nurse was usually assigned to one of the main hospital services, either medical or surgical. It was important that the medical and surgical lectures be given during this period. Yet in 75% of the small- and medium-sized hospitals, the students nursed medical and surgical patients after only 4 months of preliminary instruction; they received instruction in medical and surgical diseases during the second and third years. These students were assigned to night duty after only 6 months. They cared for critically ill patients both during the daytime and at night, without adequate teaching or supervision.

Too often the pressure of getting the work done removed any possibility of either good teaching or good supervision. It was determined that in most schools:

The sciences and the theory and the practice of nursing were frequently being taught by unprepared instructors in poorly equipped basement classrooms.

Hospitals controlled the total teaching hours or reduced the ground covered to the barest outline or might omit some subjects entirely.

Lectures were often given to students at night after a day of hard work.

The student's practical experience was usually limited to those services which were found in the hospital. The student learned to nurse those patients for whom the hospital cared.

The practical experience might be under the direction and guidance of graduate nurses who had neither preparation nor time to teach.[10]

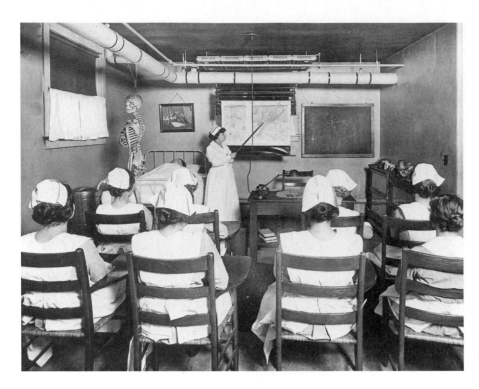

The Goldmark study pointed to the critical factor of the quality of the instructional staff in schools of public health nursing.

The survey made by the Goldmark committee concluded that the training of nurses was a serious educational business that must be directed by those who were primarily committed to quality nursing education. The Goldmark committee emphasized the fundamental need to recognize the hospital school as a separate educational department, dedicated to giving students not a course of training but a thorough liberal education in nursing.

THE FIRST UNIVERSITY SCHOOLS OF NURSING

In 1909 Richard Olding Beard successfully maneuvered to have the new nurse training school at the University of Minnesota organized as an integral part of that institution. Though it was subsumed under the college of medicine and offered only a 3-year diploma, the Minnesota program was still a great step forward. Previously, schools of nursing on college campuses had functioned as offshoots of the university hospitals and had been in no way part of the academic organization.

In 1916 Annie W. Goodrich reported that 16 colleges and universities maintained schools, departments, or courses in nursing education. A growing development in several universities combined an academic and professional course of 4 to 5 years, leading to a nursing diploma and a bachelor of science degree. The usual arrangement admitted the student upon completion of her high school course for 2 years of preliminary work in the university and then

gave her 2 years of nurse training in the hospital, followed by a year of clinical work and study, during which she would specialize in some particular branch of nursing.

By the early 1920s, Simmons College, Northwestern University, Columbia University, and the universities of Cincinnati, Minnesota, Michigan, California, Colorado, Indiana, and Washington had introduced courses of this type. Only a few students took the longer course leading to a degree, although it was open to any who could meet the requirements. By 1926, although there were 25 colleges and universities conducting nurse training schools that granted A.B. or B.S. degrees in nursing, total enrollment in these schools was only 368. The small number of students in these courses attested to the continued dependence of the affiliated university hospitals upon the student body for the nursing care of its patients and the necessity of stressing the 3-year course for almost all students. Not surprisingly, then, the findings of the Goldmark study concerning the influence of the university relationship in raising the standards of nursing education were disappointing.

The prenursing or preparatory course that had been given at Vassar College and at several universities during the summer of 1918 had demonstrated what might be done working with colleges and universities for at least a portion of the nurses' training. The standard of teaching at Vassar had been much higher than that which prevailed in the majority of nursing schools. It was thought, however, that the great weakness of such detached courses was the absence of any organic connection with the hospital in

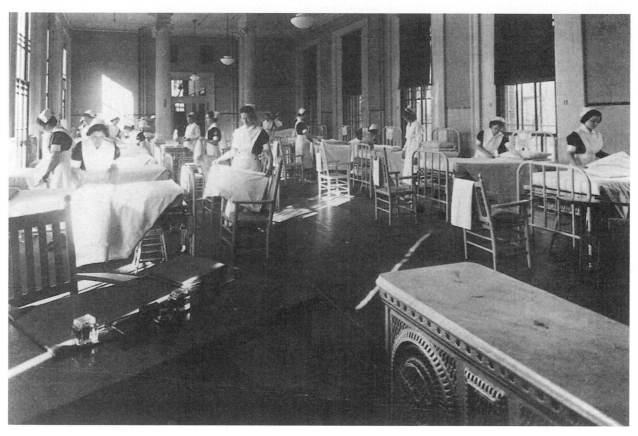

Students' practical experience was often limited to the work needs of the hospital.

which the student acquired her clinical experience and subsequent training.

YALE SCHOOL OF NURSING: FIRST AUTONOMOUS COLLEGIATE SCHOOL

Shortly after the Goldmark report came out, the Rockefeller Foundation, prodded by the Committee for the Study of Nursing Education, awarded a 5-year grant to Yale University to establish a truly collegiate school of nursing. Founded as an experimental and pioneering venture, this school was epoch making in that, for the first time in the history of nurse training, the financial means were provided whereby the content of nurse education might be developed according to curative and preventive needs. The grant was contingent upon the university's implementation of a course that would consolidate nursing theory and practice in the shortest feasible curriculum and eliminate traditional non-nursing assignments. Nursing theory was to be correlated with practical experience, and emphasis throughout the course was to be placed on the preventive aspects.

The Yale School of Nursing, which opened in February 1924, was the first in the world to be established as a separate university department with an independent budget and its own dean—Annie

W. Goodrich. Hospital affiliation was arranged with the New Haven Hospital, which discontinued operation of the venerable Connecticut Training School for Nurses. Undertaken on an experimental basis, the Yale program demonstrated its effectiveness so markedly that in 1929 the Rockefeller Foundation assured the permanency of the school by awarding it an endowment of one million dollars. The 28-month course led to the degree of Bachelor of Nursing, followed a definite educational plan, and included public health, community work, and hospital service. Applicants for the course had to have completed at least 2 years of work in a college of established standing, and their credits had to show at least 15 hours of academic work per week in relevant subjects of study, including courses in elementary chemistry, psychology, and the biologic sciences.

The professional training of the student in the actual care of the sick was strengthened by in-depth exposure to the underlying theory of disease as well as to the social, psychological, and physical aspects of patient welfare. Courses in the various hospital services were supplemented by observation and assistance in the dispensary clinics and follow-up work through the local visiting nurse association and other health and welfare groups. The program of clinical experience was designated as the "case assignment method," with the students assigned to the care of one or more patients rather than to a series of hypothetical nursing procedures. By employing this approach, it was believed possible for the student not only to master the required skills but also to attain an intelligent understanding of the patient and his or her mental and physical needs. Such an approach fostered attainment of a high degree of technical skill and an understanding of the underlying principles of the required procedures, together with an insight into the social and economic forces that inevitably bore heavily upon any patient.

Every student received a balanced curriculum, something rare in the traditional school of nursing. The carefully planned clinical experience, whether surgical, medical, pediatric, or obstetric, included all aspects of the particular subject. For example, the course in medical nursing included periods in the general medical, tuberculosis, syphilis, and skin clinics of the outpatient department, in the wards for communicable diseases, and in the general mental disease wards at the Butler Hospital in Providence, Rhode Island. Included in the comprehensive course in pediatrics was brief but intensive study in a nursery school directed by child psychologists, allowing the students to observe the development of the well child as compared with that of the ill child.

The Yale School of Nursing won quick success, 5 years later elevating its admission requirements to demand a bachelor's degree in arts, science, or philosophy and offering a 30-month course leading to a Master of Nursing degree. The 128 women nursing students, plus 300 other coeds, were surrounded by nearly 5000 male students.

OPPOSITION TO THE COLLEGIATE NURSING MOVEMENT

Widespread emulation of the Yale program was not forthcoming, although there were a few other positive developments. In 1923 a collegiate school of nursing that later offered the M.N. degree and B.S. in Nursing degree was endowed by Frances Payne Bolton at Western Reserve University. Seven years later, the hospital school of nursing at Vanderbilt University was upgraded to a full-fledged academic unit of the university with the aid of a $1 million endowment from the Rockefeller Foundation and additional assistance from the Carnegie Foundation and the Commonwealth Fund. In 1925 the University of Chicago founded a nursing school, absorbing about $500,000 in assets of the discontinued Illinois Training School for Nurses. Chicago added few resources to its nursing program, however, and 10 years later, the school had only four faculty.

Overall, the growth of truly collegiate programs lagged. Opposition came from many private physicians, who argued that nurses were overtrained, that the service they gave was too costly, and that women

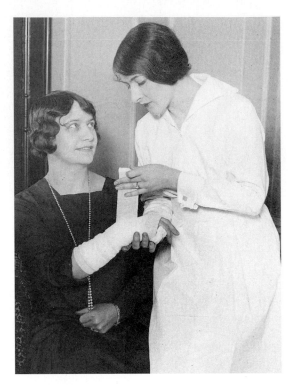

Many physicians continued to worry about the "over-trained nurse."

with brief training in bedside routines would be just as satisfactory. A number of hospital training schools continued to insist that nursing education meant acquisition of technical skills and manual dexterity only. They believed that intelligence and sound knowledge of theory were unnecessary and might handicap the prospective nurse. But the same people, opponents of this view argued, would demand the services of a highly competent nurse when some member of their own family became seriously ill. Unfortunately, most of those successful in getting their views into the public press belonged to the reactionary group. They viewed nursing as a form of simple manual work requiring a limited degree of dexterity and a smattering of elementary medical knowledge.

Veteran nurses pointed out that the old-fashioned training of the nurse had been simple and rigorous, stern and even. There had been no great variations in quality. Only women of high moral and physical stamina had survived the hardships of that earlier day. By contrast, students from schools in the 1920s represented every degree of quality. Some came from schools that chose their students with care, while others came from "schools" that were only interested in obtaining many strong hands and feet and accepted virtually every young woman who walked in the door.

An editorial in one of the prominent medical journals, entitled "Autocracy of the Sick Room Has Become Vested in the Despotic Realm of the Nurse," had this to say:

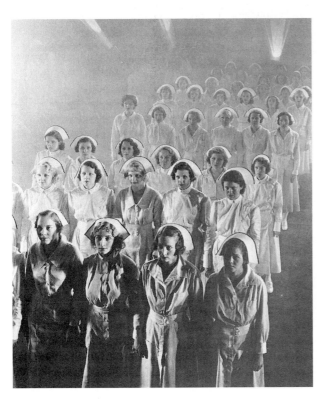

Nursing graduates represented a wide range of quality.

The nursing problem is becoming increasingly an example of the frequent paradox that where illness is concerned "the cure is worse than the disease."

As an example of efficiency "hoist by its own petard," the trained nurse situation is one of the most appalling. The medical profession views this Frankenstein of its own manufacture with positive unbelief.

Autocracy of the sick room has become vested in the despotic realm of the nurse who has become a positive czar and who is as luxurious an expense as any Romanoff ever dared to be. Sickness is an expense that no family budget can afford to carry under the best of circumstances, but under the present conditions insisted upon by a trained nurse before she will accept a case, the employment of such assistance in illness becomes enough to actually bankrupt a family.

The registered nurse situation today illustrates perfectly the process of refusing to render service in accordance with hire received. The shift system being forced upon the public makes the patient of less importance than the number of hours a day that a nurse stays under the patient's roof. Yet this discounting of wisdom, skill, and directive science upon the part of the physician is made a weapon of argument by the already overtrained and over-authoritative nurse in her fight for the greatest pay and the least service.[11]

Under the weight of such attacks, efforts to improve standards in nurse education lagged in many states. In regard to the educational requirements for nurses' registration of the early 1920s, the laws of no two states were in agreement. In most states registration was permissive rather than mandatory. Of those nurses who wished the R.N. title, little was required. South Dakota overlooked preliminary education entirely, registering all graduates of nurse training schools who had completed a 2-year general hospital course. Vermont required a grammar-school certificate and training of 2 years and 3 months in a general hospital. In Virginia the Board of Health examiners required no preliminary education, simply mandating 2 years of hospital training. In Ohio the registered nurse was required to have 1 year in high school along with graduation from a training school approved by the State Medical Board. California demanded a high school education or its equivalent and a 3-year nurse training course. New York mandated 1 year of high school and 2 years of training, with examination by the Board of Nursing Examiners. In Massachusetts nurses were registered after passing the examination of the State Board or upon presentation of registration certificates from other states. Most states placed absolutely no restrictions on the scope or quality of the training-school curriculum.

PERILS OF PRIVATE DUTY

By the mid-1920s the private-duty nurse was also in serious difficulty. Her counterpart of an earlier day had dealt with a common scope of diseases in patients. Only when people were acutely ill did they call the physician and nurse. Through supportive nursing care, they hoped to help save a life that was close to death. Typhoid-fever nursing of 6 to 8 weeks per case was one of the private-duty nurse's typical assignments. Influenza, pneumonia, and other contagious diseases were regular events. Surgical emergencies demanding operative procedures under primitive conditions in the home were commonplace.

Medical advances had changed this picture. Typhoid fever and most other contagious diseases had receded into the background, and a major area of private-duty nursing had disappeared. Screens, clean milk and water, and assistance from new laboratories and technologic innovations helped close still other areas. Good roads, telephones, and motor cars had moved many medical and surgical patients into general hospitals, where they were cared for by student nurses. For the remaining home cases, shorter units of nursing time were being used because less continuous nursing care was needed as a result of therapeutic advances. Consequently, the private-duty nurse lost ground in her field.

The slackening demand for private-duty nurses was noted in hundreds of nurse registries all over the

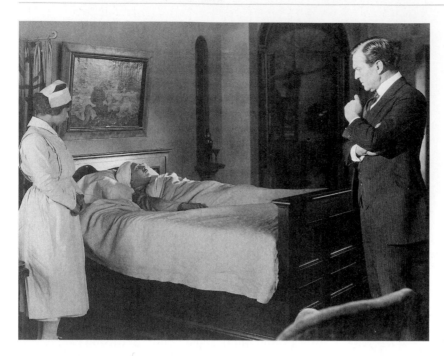

Patients who once employed private-duty nurses now went to hospitals for care.

nation. The early development of nurses' agencies dated from the time when, for the benefit of the graduates of a school of nursing, a list of the names of those wishing to do private-duty nursing was kept on file by the superintendent of the training school. The objective was to help supply work to the graduates of a particular school of nursing as well as to serve as a convenience to the hospital. The registry functioned only as a center for the distribution of nurses and the registrar was anyone who happened to be on duty in the training-school office when the call for the nurse was received. Records were simple and consisted of cards on which the nurse listed the cases she would not take or was "registered against." No other records were needed because the student history of the graduate nurse was on file in the school of nursing office.

Nurses were sent out on cases in rotation unless the patient or the physician expressed the wish for a particular nurse. In some instances the alumnae association was privileged to make certain recommendations to the superintendent of the training school relative to the management of the registry. So-called outside graduates were seldom seen on private-duty assignments in the hospital because each institution exercised its responsibility to its own graduates. Each registry was an isolated unit and standards were variable.

As schools grew older and the list of graduate nurses increased, the problems associated with the registry also increased, until it became necessary to take steps to centralize this important activity. Because many of the hospital registries had been sponsored by the alumnae associations, the next step was to see what could be done to amalgamate these alumnae activities, and the state nurses' association district organization was the logical unit to approach

to assume control of the registry. Soon the proliferation of competing commercial nursing enterprises necessitated the selection by the district registry of a name that would identify it as a functioning unit of the district nurses' association. "Official" was accepted as a term that would so identify the registry, and many registries at once became incorporated as the Nurses' Official Registry. Because of the interest of the American Nurses Association in the development of these registries, in 1929 the headquarters staff formulated a tentative minimum standard for official registries.

While the demand for private-duty nursing was decreasing, schools of nursing were expanding rapidly to staff newly enlarged hospitals. Where the private-duty nurse of earlier years had experienced limited competition, the private-duty nurse of the mid-1920s was overwhelmed by a fresh deluge of graduates every year. Nurses found themselves waiting longer and longer for cases, and their number of idle days soared alarmingly. It did not seem feasible for the private-duty nurse to raise her fees because the majority of the public had low or modest incomes, and the effect of such a change would cause many people to do without nursing, except in crises. Adequate income for the private-duty nurse could only come through more work—work that did not exist because her former patients were going to hospitals for care.

HOSPITAL SERVICE IMPROVES

The modern hospital of the 1920s contained a large amount of scientific equipment and a degree of specialized service not available in the office of the private practitioner or in the home with a private-duty nurse. Of 6830 hospitals surveyed, more than 44%

maintained clinical laboratories and more than 41% maintained x-ray departments. Used in common by a number of practitioners, equipment and services were available for the diagnosis and treatment of serious illnesses in ambulatory and bed patients, at a cost considerably below that which would be necessary were these provided independently by each practitioner. All told, there were 7370 American hospitals in 1924, with a total bed capacity of 813,926. These included institutions for special groups of disabled persons, such as children, convalescent patients, and maternity cases, and also for special diseases, such as mental disorders, tuberculosis, contagious diseases, disorders of eye, ear, nose, and throat, orthopedic defects, skin diseases, cancer, and venereal diseases.

The growing number of clinics was important in bringing patients out of homes and physicians' offices. The clinic was defined as an institution that organized the professional skill of physicians and nurses and provided special equipment for the diagnosis and prevention of disease or for the promotion of health among ambulatory patients. It corresponded to the ward service given to bed patients in hospitals, and, when attached to a hospital, the clinic was frequently called the outpatient department. In a few cases the term *dispensary* was still used because the early clinics had been opened primarily to provide free medicine for physicians' charity patients.

The number of clinics in the United States in June 1926, was 5726. Of these, 1790 were outpatient departments of hospitals, 2793 were unaffiliated clinics, 923 served special groups only, and 220 were general group clinics. At that time there were 197 clinics attached to hospitals for the treatment of nervous and mental disorders, and 70 of the unaffiliated clinics were for mental cases. Hospitals and sanatoriums for the treatment of tuberculosis had 107 clinics attached to them, and there were 585 unaffiliated clinics for tubercular patients. One thousand unaffiliated clinics for baby and child care were reported in addition to the 52 clinics connected with children's hospitals. The 350 clinics for the treatment of venereal diseases were all independent of hospitals.

The growth of health care resulted in a marked increase in the number of people affiliated with it. By 1920 in the United States alone, over one million people were employed on a full-time basis in some phase of the promotion of health (Table 11-1).[12]

THE GRADING COMMITTEE BEGINS WORK

Close on the heels of the Goldmark effort came that of the Committee on the Grading of Nursing Schools, which had its origin in two separate movements. One was an attempt by the American Medical Association to study the education and employment

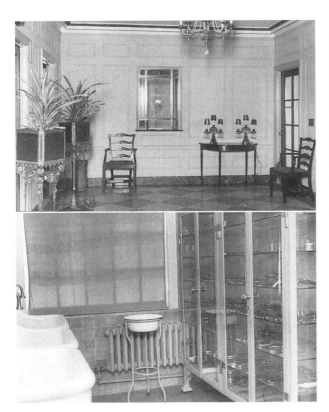
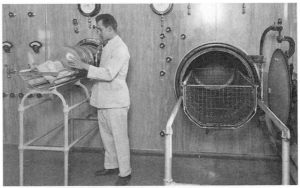
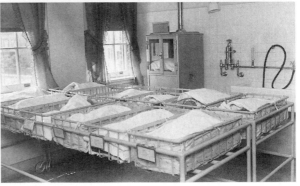

Lobby, operating room, sterilizing room, and nursery at New York City Hospital in 1926.

TABLE 11-1	Number of Health Workers Reported by the 1920 Census
Physicians and surgeons	147,000
Attendants of physicians and surgeons	24,000
Retail drug dealers	80,000
Dentists	64,000
Dental hygienists and dentists' assistants	8,700
Trained nurses and student nurses	149,000
Untrained nurses	152,000
Midwives	44,000
Hospital superintendents	2,800
Hospital attendants	330,000
Clinic attendants	5,000
Health department personnel	11,500
Total	1,018,000

of nurses to arrive at methods for improving the nursing service available to the members of the medical profession. The other, apparently begun earlier, was initiated by the professional nursing associations and contemplated a study of nursing education, especially as it related to the need for qualitative grading of schools. These two approaches to the nursing problem eventually led to an amalgamation of forces and the formation of the Committee on the Grading of Nursing Schools.

Frances Payne Bolton, who had generously endowed the new school of nursing at Cleveland's Western Reserve University in 1924 and who had been a friend of nurses and nursing since World War I, was asked to serve on the committee as a representative of hospital trustees and consumers. Her strong commitment to the objectives of the committee was expressed through a gift of $93,000. This sum, combined with the financial contributions of thousands of nurses, allowed the committee to embark on the first comprehensive survey of the nation's nursing schools.

The committee appointed May Ayres Burgess, Ph.D., as director of the study at a meeting in April 1926. Dr. Burgess was a well-trained statistician with many years of practical work, much of it learned from her brother, Colonel Leonard P. Ayres, chief of the statistics branch of the War Department General Staff. Nurses and other hospital workers had a great deal of confidence in her because she had worked in the field of education and with the Committee on Dispensary Development of the United Hospital Fund. Dr. Burgess had also demonstrated her interest in nursing through her studies of private-duty nursing in New York.

In fall 1926 the committee embarked on an ambitious program of three separate studies: (1) an inquiry into the supply of and demand for graduate nurses; (2) a "job analysis" of what nurses did and how they might be taught; and (3) the actual grading of schools of nursing. The supply-and-demand study resulted in the 1928 publication *Nurses, Patients, and Pocketbooks*. This investigation demonstrated that there was an oversupply of graduate nurses and that this oversupply was increasing much faster than the general population. Unemployment among graduate nurses was serious and chronic. Annual earnings, especially for private-duty nurses, were inadequate and educational standards were low. What is more, because nurses were concentrated in the cities, their geographic distribution was uneven. Although physicians and patients were, in general, pleased with their nurses, and although many nurses were happy with their work, there remained a critical proportion of nurses who were rendering unsatisfactory service and an even larger proportion of nurses who were chronically unhappy because of the inadequacy of their training or because of the conditions under which they were working.

POORLY PREPARED STUDENTS

In 1925 there were approximately 2100 schools of nursing in the United States. Of the 1500 schools that responded to an American Nurses Association

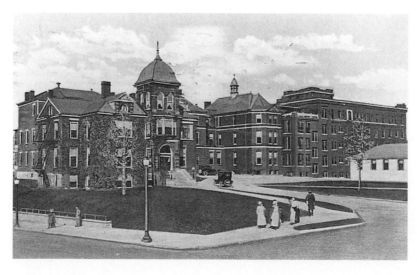

Hamot Hospital, in Erie, PA, was one of 7370 institutions in 1924.

TABLE 11-2	Minimum Educational Entrance Requirements of 1500 Schools of Nursing	
EDUCATIONAL LEVEL	NUMBER OF SCHOOLS	PERCENTAGE
8th grade	38	3
1 year high school	813	54
2 years high school	406	27
3 years high school	19	1
4 years high school	224	15
Total	1500	100

TABLE 11-3	Distribution of Students Among 1500 Schools of Nursing
STUDENTS	NUMBER OF SCHOOLS
0–9	104
10–19	336
20–29	334
30–39	210
40–49	128
50–59	86
60–69	86
70–79	60
80–89	39
90–99	26
100 +	91

survey, only 224 revealed a minimum entrance requirement of 4 years of high school. In half the nursing schools, one of every three students had been admitted to training without having finished high school. In some schools, none of the students had gone beyond the eighth grade (Table 11-2).[13]

Educational entrance requirements were not the only criteria for good schools. Many schools were so small that they could not provide adequate instruction. Of the 1500 schools responding, there were 104 in which the entire student body numbered 9 or fewer and 440 in which the entire student body was composed of 19 or fewer individuals (Table 11-3).[14]

POOR EDUCATIONAL ENVIRONMENT

Not only were many of the schools too small to make adequate instruction feasible, but all too frequently the hospitals themselves were too small to

be effective as teaching centers. One hundred eighty-five schools were connected with hospitals having a daily average of fewer than 25 patients; 562 schools had a daily average of fewer than 50 patients, making one third of the schools hopelessly below standard. Another 467 schools had a daily average of 50 to 99 patients, which was below the recommended minimum of 100 considered essential for satisfactory clinical instruction. Perhaps the greatest shock came when Dr. Burgess showed the great variation in the required hours of duty in the nursing schools that responded (Table 11-4).[15] The average was 55 hours. When these figures were compared with the 38-hour work week required of most factory workers or with the 42-hour week required of visiting nurses, one could see

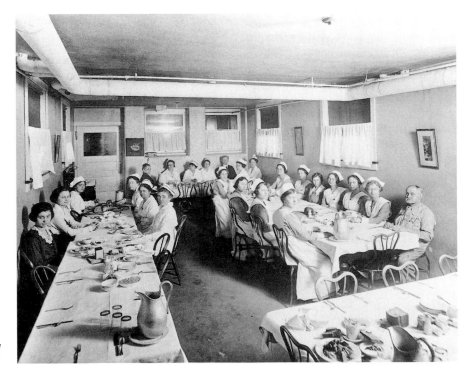

Most nursing programs of 1925 had fewer than 40 students.

TABLE 11-4	Required Hours of Duty per Week Among 1500 Schools of Nursing
HOURS OF WORK PER WEEK	**NUMBER OF SCHOOLS**
25–34	2
35–44	23
45–54	659
55–64	736
65–74	73
75–84	7

why young middle-class women were thinking twice about pursuing nursing careers.

Defining a teacher in the school of nursing as a person whose main job was instructing, Dr. Burgess compiled the figures in Table 11-5.[16]

There had been an increase of 102.5% in all hospital beds from 1910 to 1927, with an increase of 138.2% in student nurses for the same period. It was significant that the 4322 general hospital nursing staffs in the United States included fewer graduate nurses than the nursing staffs of British or most European hospitals. In this country student nurses carried the greater portion of the general hospital nursing load.

Because the training school had been successful, its growth was extraordinary, reaching a zenith during the late 1920s. The contrast between medical schools and nursing schools was amazing. In 1880 there had been 100 medical schools; in 1890, 133; in 1900, 160. Following publication of the 1910 Flexner report, which attracted nationwide attention to problems of medical education, there had been a widespread campaign by the medical profession to raise the quality of medical education and lower the number of schools. By 1927 only 79 schools of medicine remained. Nursing schools, on the other hand, showed a totally different picture. In 1880 there had been 15 schools of nursing; in 1890, 34; in 1900, 448; in 1910, 1121; in 1920, 1755; and in 1927, 2286.[17]

With the increase in nursing schools came an increase in nurse graduates. Medical schools in 1880 had produced a little over 3000 graduates; by 1900 there were over 5000. Then came the reorganization of medical education, and the number of graduates dropped rapidly, until by 1920 there were barely

TABLE 11-5	Teachers in 1500 Schools of Nursing
NUMBER OF TEACHERS	**NUMBER OF SCHOOLS**
0	549
1	639
2	208
3	57
4	21
5	8
6	18

3000; by 1926 this number had increased to about 4000. Medical educators were projecting that the numbers of graduates each year through the next 40 or 50 years would probably remain at about 4000. In nursing in 1880 there were 157 graduates for the entire country. In 1890 there were over 500; in 1900, over 3700; in 1910, over 7700; in 1920, about 15,000; in 1927, over 18,000; in 1931, just about 26,000. In 1931, with over 100,000 students enrolled, the numbers of nursing graduates were predicted to continue rising with startling rapidity and at a rate far beyond that of the increase in the general population.

APPRENTICESHIP VERSUS EDUCATION

Nurse education of the late 1920s was essentially functioning on an apprenticeship level. In the main, training schools were being conducted primarily to provide student nursing service for the care of patients in hospitals, instead of being operated with the objective of giving the students the best possible nursing education. There was unquestionable value in the apprenticeship method of teaching, and the committee thought that it should be retained in *any* system of nurse training, because much more depended on repetition and on practice in learning nursing procedures than on didactic instruction. There was, however, no question that hospitals had exploited student nurses in an attempt to avoid the expense required in employing graduate nurses.

Bearing out these findings, Dorothy Dunbar Bromley, in a 1930 article on the nursing crisis published in *Harper's Magazine*, vividly reminded the public:

> High school principals, when called upon for vocational advice, have been known to suggest nursing as a possible career for girls unfitted to do anything else. One principal recently wrote the head of a training school saying "Mary Blank's parents are too poor to support her; she is a hopeless failure in her studies, and she is not attractive enough to marry. But I think she would make a good nurse. Won't you take her in?"
>
> That nursing should have so fallen in the esteem of a portion of the community is largely the fault of those training schools which, in their anxiety to get the work of their hospitals done as cheaply as possible, have enrolled whatever young women were at the moment available.

She concluded that nursing was

> in short, the one line of work open to the uneducated girl which will not only raise her social status and pay her comparatively high wages but will provide her with a living while she is training and perhaps even a monthly allowance. If the standards of nursing are to be

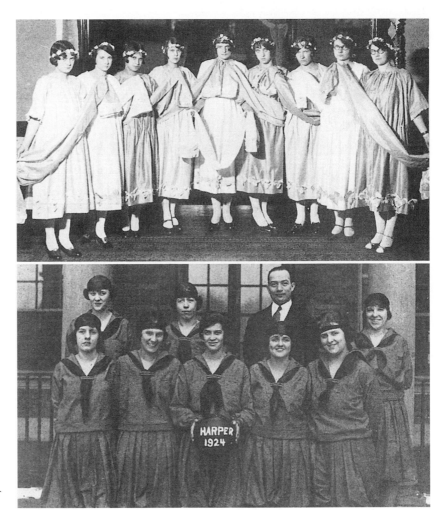

Student activities in 1924—May Flower Drill and basketball teams.

salvaged, a good many of the 2,200-odd training schools now in existence will have to be discontinued, and this will include most of those conducted by privately owned hospitals. When there are fewer schools and when the requirements for entrance have been raised, there will be fewer graduates and these of a much higher type.[18]

The grading committee's findings were published in a series of reports and in a final summary, published in 1934, called *Nursing Schools Today and Tomorrow,* which described weaknesses in nursing education and recommended specific improvements. This report reiterated the belief that providing adequate financial support was the most fundamental problem in placing nursing education on a higher level. In other forms of professional education, it was a firmly established principle that funds be supplied to provide teaching personnel and facilities for instruction. The nurse was the only worker whose professional training depended essentially on the service that she rendered in a hospital. This problem and the difficulty of finding faculty with scholastic qualifications for teaching created a serious deficiency in nursing education. Grading-committee statistics showed that 42% of teachers in schools of nursing were not even graduates of high school, and that only 16% had completed 1 or more years of college.[19]

Dr. Burgess and her associates insisted that it was imperative, if the educational program for a nursing student was to be administered in an effective manner, that an honest attempt be made to correlate classroom instruction and clinical experience. The reason the average hospital training school did not correlate practice with classroom work was that doing so necessitated rotation of a student from one hospital service to another, a program that would provide superior education but interfere with the hospital's freedom to place the student according to ward nursing needs.

INADEQUATE FINANCING OF NURSE TRAINING

There were few adequately financed hospitals. When the hospital was forced to budget for nursing education, the school of nursing received a minimal allotment. The administrator had a certain amount of

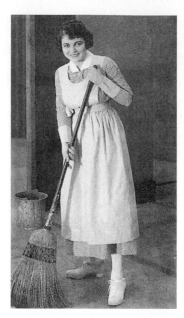

Labor needs of hospitals often subverted educational needs of the students.

money to spend in all departments of the hospital, and the board of directors usually agreed to expenditures that showed tangible assets, such as new buildings and equipment. First consideration was rarely given to the school of nursing by either the hospital administrator or the hospital board.

A central question was: how much did the pupil nurses earn—how much did their employment save the patient, the philanthropic donor, the taxpayer, and the proprietary hospital owner? Phoebe Gordon, an instructor at the school of nursing at the University of Minnesota, studied this matter for the University Hospital and for the Miller and Northern Pacific Hospitals of St. Paul. The results of Gordon's studies indicated that the then-current system of student staffing was least expensive. For a hypothetical school of 30 graduate nurses and 130 students the total hospital cost was $84,382. Substitution of graduates for students almost doubled the cost of the nursing service, to $167,977.

Against these charges the hospital executives and administrators argued that schools of nursing and nursing care of patients accounted for the high cost of hospitalization. According to Dr. Bert Caldwell, the executive director of the American Hospital Association, part of the cost of hospitalization was the result of expenses incurred by training a nurse over a 3-year period. While the 3-year training period cost the hospital $2,000, by Caldwell's figuring, the student returned only $1,000 in the form of service. Yet each student gave approximately 7000 hours of service to the hospital during her 3-year course; if these hours of service were worth only $1,000 to the hospital, as Caldwell mentioned, then student nurses were indeed inexpensive labor, for the hospital credited them at the rate of 14 cents an hour.

STUDENTS VERSUS GRADUATES IN HOSPITAL NURSING SERVICE

According to progressive nurse educators, graduate nurses were the logical people to provide nursing care in a hospital. A registered nurse could furnish more skillful nursing than could a student, was better prepared to adapt procedures to the individual patient, and had a better basis for judgment because her training and experience made her familiar with the various changing clinical pictures of diseases. A graduate nursing staff assured the patient of competent, safe nursing care. Hospitals might argue that students provided a service that was as good or nearly as good as a graduate service, but if semi-trained students were as well qualified for general duty nursing as graduates, there was little justification for maintaining a 3-year course in nursing education.

The conclusions announced in an address given by Dr. Malcolm MacEachern, associate director of the American College of Surgeons, on February 15, 1932, were of interest to many:[20]

Graduate Nurse Service

Advantages:
1. Older nurse—more mature—therefore take responsibility better.
2. The white uniform nurse gains the confidence of the patient more easily.
3. Can work more rapidly because she knows better how to carry out treatment orders.
4. Can do more work on her own initiative—less supervision required.
5. Better health—less lost time.

Disadvantages:
1. Does not like general duty—indifferent to this type of nursing.
2. Objects to discipline.
3. Insists on using her own methods.
4. More extravagant with supplies.
5. Chronic complaints—food, housekeeping, laundry.
6. Uses short-cut methods, thereby becoming careless.
7. Resents criticism.
8. Large salary.
9. Large turnover of help; doesn't stay in one place long.

Student Nurse Service

Advantages:
1. More enthusiastic.
2. More cheerful.
3. More amenable to discipline.
4. More conservative with supplies.
5. More sympathetic.
6. Less turnover.

7. Small salary.
8. Contracts business for hospital with friends and relatives.

Disadvantages:
1. Needs constant supervision.
2. Cost of theoretical education, instructor, etc.
3. Cost of recreational activities.
4. Less experience in handling patients.
5. Wastes time.
6. More mistakes.
7. Does not have as much emotional stability.
8. Less continuity of service.

Resistance to the use of general staff nurses in hospitals had become strongly entrenched. These attitudes were held both by the employer and the employee. The grading committee asked 500 superintendents of nurses: "If you had your choice, which would you rather have to take care of your patients—student nurses or graduate nurses?" Seventy-six percent replied emphatically that they would prefer student nurses, and only 24% voted for graduate nurses. That this preference was actually put into practice was evident in the disclosure that 73 of these same hospitals had no general staff nurses, 5% had one general staff nurse, 4% had two general staff nurses, 3% had three, and 15% had four or more.

GRADING-COMMITTEE CONCLUSIONS

The findings of the grading committee did little to alter what leaders of the nursing profession had long believed, although it did furnish data that could be used to strengthen arguments for reform. Such reform, it was decided, should have four basic goals:

To reduce and improve the supply. To make a decisive and immediate reduction in the numbers of students admitted to schools of nursing in the United States, and to raise entrance requirements high enough so that only properly qualified women would be admitted to the profession.

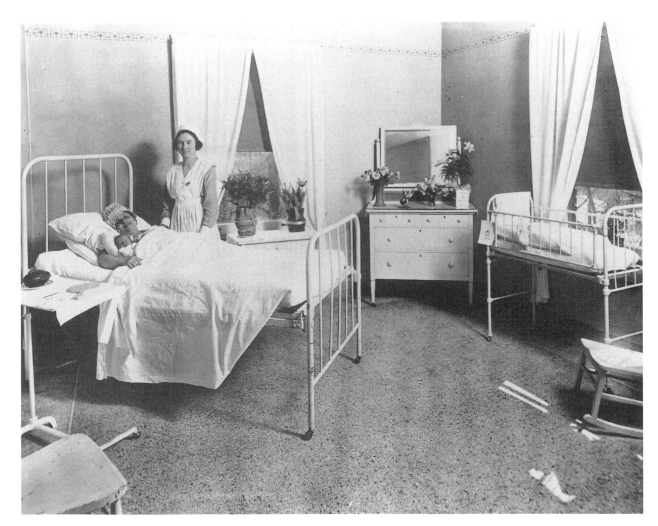

Hospitals with student nurses had little need for staff nurses.

To replace students with graduates. To put the major part of hospital bedside nursing in the hands of the graduate nurses and take it out of the hands of student nurses.

To help hospitals meet costs of graduate services. To assist hospitals in securing funds for the employment of graduate nurses and to improve the quality of graduate nursing so that hospitals would desire to have it.

To get public support for nursing education. To place schools of nursing under the direction of nurse educators instead of hospital administrators and to awaken the public to the fact that if society wants good nursing it must pay the cost of educating nurses. Nursing education is a public and not a private responsibility.[21]

The struggle for better nurse education and the debate over its proper role in American health care would focus once again on a question that had recurred elsewhere and would continue to bedevil the hospital for the next half century. In some ways, the central problem of hospital care was nothing less than the question of the true meaning of nursing. Was a good system one that allowed exploitation of students to subsidize the cost of patient care, or was it a system designed to maximize the preparation of quality nurses? Did "quality" imply the kind of quiet, submissive servant that the training schools produced in large numbers, or did it mean much more?

One outstanding attempt to elevate nursing-school standards had been the National League of Nursing Education's *Standard Curriculum for Schools of Nursing,* which had appeared in 1917 under the leadership of Adelaide Nutting and Isabel Stewart. Its purpose had been "to arrive at some general agreement as to a desirable and workable standard whose main features could be accepted by training schools of good standing throughout the country," and it had been hoped that "in this way, we may be able to gradually overcome the wide diversity of standards at present existing in schools of nursing and supply a basis for appraising the value of widely different systems of nurse training."

In 1927, following the general trend to deemphasize standardization, a revision entitled *A Curriculum for Schools of Nursing* was published, introducing "changes needed to keep in line with the newer developments in the field of nursing and the newer ideas in nursing education."[22] Among the alterations were the inclusion of psychology as a regular course, emphasis on mental health nursing and on public health nursing, and greater stress on a solid scientific background.

THE CASE OF NEW YORK STATE

In 1933 analysis of the curricula in the schools of nursing in New York State (Table 11-6) showed an amazing lack of agreement on what was essential.[23]

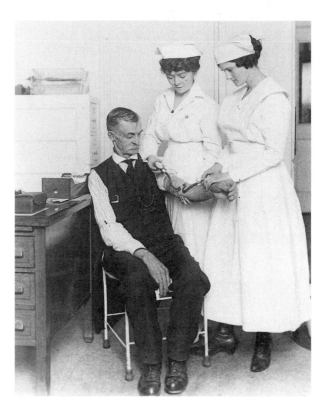

The 1927 National League of Nursing Education curriculum guide placed additional emphasis on public health nursing.

In the range of hours allotted to the various subjects taught, the extremes of variation in the theory component were astonishing.

Examination of school records indicated that students received experience according to what the individual hospital had to offer. Because schools of nursing were located in all sizes and types of hospitals, the clinical experience offered to students varied markedly (Table 11-7).[24]

THE HOSPITAL ASSOCIATION PRESENTS QUESTIONS

Lewis A. Sexton, M.D., president of the American Hospital Association, told the 1931 AHA convention that those who were most responsible for both nursing care and the support of the schools had begun to wonder what the nurse of the future would be like and just where her place would be in the scheme of things. Each year additions were made to nursing-school curricula, which were bulging with desirable general education courses but, year after year, were squeezing out the essentials on which the profession had been founded. Dr. Sexton said that he was for education and training that would fit nurses for their greatest sphere of usefulness, but that a feeling had grown among nurse leaders that unless hospitals freed their nursing students from the menial aspects of caring for the sick, their educational duty would not be fulfilled.

TABLE 11-6	Curricula, New York State Schools of Nursing, 1933
SUBJECTS	**HOURS**
Anatomy and physiology	48–270
Bacteriology	20–120
Bacteriology and pathology (combined)	32–94
Pathology	0–59
Personal hygiene	8–58
Nutrition and cookery	24–180
Drugs and solutions	15–64
Elementary nursing procedures (including bandaging and hospital housekeeping)	79–325
History and social aspects of nursing	8–34
Chemistry	0–315
Advanced nursing	0–174
Dietotherapy	0–81
Materia medica	16–88
Massage	0–40
Ethics	0–36
Psychology	0–120
General medicine (including skin)	10–130
General surgery and gynecology	15–164
Pediatrics (including infant feeding and orthopedics)	11–116
Communicable (including tuberculosis and veneral)	4–72
Operating room technique	5–62
Obstetric nursing	10–76
Public sanitation	8–42
Diseases of eye	2–18
Diseases of ear, nose, throat	2–22
Hydrotherapy	0–22
Nervous and mental	9–110
Occupational therapy	0–50
Occupational diseases	0–9
Professional problems	0–30
Public health	0–58
Private duty	0–9
Institutional work	0–8
Modern social conditions	0–60
Case study	0–15
Mental hygiene	0–12
Social service	0–43

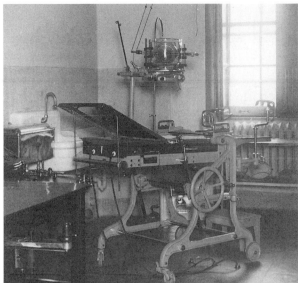

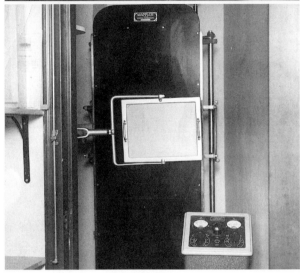

More nursing students were assigned experience in new hospital x-ray services.

He declared that he was old-fashioned enough to believe that one could overeducate people beyond their sphere of usefulness. Some institutions of higher learning seemed to think that unless a nurse had her Ph.D she was no longer worthy of her place in the profession. Dr. Sexton warned that if, for the next 25 years, all hospitals adhered to the flurry of new recommendations that were being made, there would be no one blessed with a sufficient amount of humility to do the actual nursing necessary for patients' recovery. More than one empire had collapsed under the weight of its own greatness, he noted.

Dr. Sexton pleaded for nurses to enter the profession for the love of the work and the good that they might do; for nurses who were willing to give of themselves to make the long, weary hours of illness less irksome; for nurses the sight of whom was an inspiration and a joy to all who needed their services. Theory in a nurse's training was desirable and essential, he maintained, but the man or woman whose needs called for a gentle, soothing touch cared little whether a nurse knew the solubility of salicylic acid or the atomic weight of sulfur.

TYPICAL STUDENT AND IDEAL GRADUATES

About this time, Clara D. Noyes, former president of the American Nurses Association and long-time director of nursing service of the Red Cross, was asked to depict the ideal nurse. She said that her ideal candidate would be a young woman about 24 to 26 years of age, of medium height, 130 to 135 pounds. She would be physically fit and would carry herself well.

TABLE 11-7 Range of Experience in Various Hospital Services

SERVICE	DAYS
Surgical	92–453
Operating room	35–145
Pathology laboratory	0–34
Medical	89–475
Tuberculosis	0–130
Communicable	0–114
Pediatric	56–379
Psychiatric	0–483
Physiotherapy	0–56
Occupational therapy	0–41
Obstetrics	62–197
Diet kitchen	24–82
Dispensary	0–103
Pharmacy	0–28
Public health	0–92
Administrative	0–150
Social service	0–58
X-ray	0–36

While a nurse with a lovely face was good to look at and might be a considerable comfort to a patient—provided she possessed the other necessary qualifications—this combination was not often found. Extremes were undesirable. Noyes went on to say that if she were to paint the portrait of a nurse, it would comprise "a rather low, broad forehead, brownish hair, with a natural wave or straight, parted in the middle in a more or less Madonna-like fashion." Her eyes would be "gray or blue, with eyebrows not too heavy, with a nose, mouth, and chin not necessarily classical, but at least possessing character, well-cared-for teeth, a skin smooth and free from blemish." Her face would "radiate cheerfulness and kindliness." She would also possess dignity and poise. Her voice would be well modulated and her enunciation clear.[25]

As to the ideal nurse's educational background, Noyes reflected that her preliminary education should be as broad as possible. Whether she was a high school or college graduate or the product of a private school did not matter as long as her education was sufficient to enable her to meet practical requirements. The broader and sounder the education the better, and a cultural background of reading, travel, and social experience was essential. The ideal nurse should possess courage, patience, and willingness to make sacrifices. Self-reliance, self-respect, self-control, steadfastness, and honesty were other indispensable qualities.

Examination of several yearbooks produced by graduating classes of three hospital nursing schools in 1929 and 1930 provides an amusing yet provocative glimpse of the nursing graduate's mentality—her values, aspirations, and sense of place in the world of health and disease. From the doggerel, inside jokes, cloying, inspirational messages, and the stale "humor" section emerges a standard understanding of what the graduate of 1930 hoped to achieve. The several annuals exhibit a few important differences. *The Stethoscope*, published by the senior class of Allegheny General Hospital in Pittsburgh, Pennsylvania, was apparently underwritten by the hospital itself. A hardbound book with a handsome embossed design of the new hospital on the cover, the yearbook served as a public relations organ of the hospital as well as an outlet for senior enthusiasm.

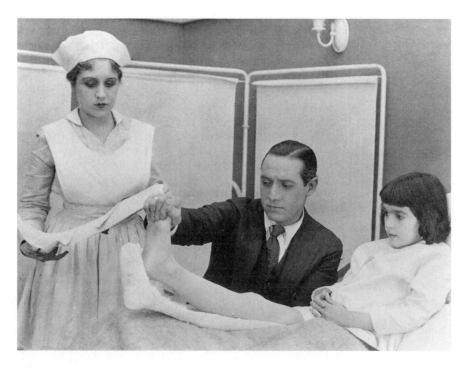

According to Clara Noyes, the ideal nurse should be physically fit, carry herself well, and possess dignity and poise.

The Nightingale, published by the graduates of St. Agnes Hospital School, Fond du Lac, Wisconsin, received some financial support from the medical staff; concomitantly, the medical staff received a glowing tribute and photographic representation at the beginning of the book. In addition, the students collected advertisements from area merchants to support the cost of the publication, which retained a more amateur and student-oriented viewpoint than that of *The Stethoscope*. *The Crescent*, published by the Warren General Hospital Training School, Warren, Pennsylvania, was liberally adorned with photos of various hospital buildings, rooms, and nursing residences. Warren General Hospital, with only nine graduating nurses, had a much smaller school than the other two, but this small size contributed to the annual's more sedate tone.

The fact that these nursing schools prepared and published yearbooks speaks to a certain development in the philosophy of nurses' training. From the perspective of both the school and the students, the yearbook served real or imaginary needs; considering the expense involved in any publication, these needs must have been considered important. The hospital and school had a vested interest in recruiting qualified students; thus the sense of fun and sorority and the expression of idealism conveyed by these annuals might have been a means of attracting students. In noting the names and whereabouts of the school's past graduates, *The Stethoscope* provided continuity and reinforced the hospital's claim on the affection and loyalty of its alumnae; they, in turn, proved valuable to Allegheny General Hospital by raising a considerable amount of money for the new hospital building fund.

The appearance of a yearbook added authenticity to the nursing school's academic identity; nursing students, although wearing uniforms and performing many hours of menial service, saw themselves as schoolgirls first and apprentices second. The workhouse atmosphere and sense of indenture common to nursing schools in the 1880s and 1890s had been eradicated by the 1930s. Yearbooks revealed that nursing students, despite increasing clinical responsibilities, remained firmly in the transitional student world. They lived away from home and worked hard, but retained enthusiasm and relished their last days of deferred maturity.

Yearbooks also expressed the belief that nursing school was more than a mere vocational or technical school where a young woman learned a skill. Reminiscences and reflections indicated that nursing school shaped the student's character and outlook. For example, this class song (sung to the tune of "If I Can't Have You") expressed the sentiment found in any school alma mater:

> *We have memories*
> *Of our classmates true.*
> *Think with joyful soul*

> *Of all the friends we knew.*
> *A.G.H. we'll strive,*
> *Honor give to you*
> *To do as you have taught*
> *To your ideals be true.*
> *We will close our book of dreams*
> *And seal it with this vow,*
> *We'll lock your image in our memory;*
> *We'll keep loving you,*
> *And to you we'll show*
> *Alma mater, we're all true blue.*[26]

Whatever benefits a hospital school might receive from the existence of a yearbook, the students undoubtedly derived the keenest pleasure and satisfaction from the annual publication. The inside jokes and personalized verses could only be appreciated by the graduates; they alone understood the mystifying remarks and prophecies written about each other, thereby establishing a veritable sorority closed to outsiders. The sense of sorority and shared identity apparently arose from the school experience rather than from the students' identification as nurses. Furthermore, they sought to idealize and fix in time memories of their nurses' training, emphasizing the positive and enjoyable aspects of the 3 years. Although all the books recalled back-breaking work, boring lectures, intolerable discipline, and saddening events, the students emphatically understated these aspects of their education in order to praise their school and, more important, themselves, for having completed their training.

These yearbooks allowed students to announce their self-confidence and independence. Jokes about medical staff, instructors, and supervisors were attempts to reduce the distance between students and superiors, but loyalty and gratitude transcended this innocent fun. The students' confidence was rooted in traditional hospital organization; that is, nurses worked under the usually benevolent dictatorship of physicians. As graduating seniors, the students might dare to treat the medical staff with familiarity. For example, *The Stethoscope*, 1929, printed an in-house verse entitled "The Interns," in which each of the young doctors was identified in complimentary quatrains: "Dr. Scull so they say/Goes a courting every day/Soon a wedding there will be,/Oh! what a lucky girl is she." Yet this same issue printed the "Graduate Nurse's Creed," in which she recited her credo: (1) belief in her hospital's superiority, (2) recognition of the medical staff's virtues—"a group of men of high ideals, chosen for their positions because of their character and professional ability" and "worthy of my help," and (3) belief in the "moral and professional standing" of the hospital's nursing graduates, who are as "sincere and hardworking" as older graduates. Thus were the medical virtues recognized as consisting of "high ideals" and "character" while the nurses were known for their moral standing, sincerity, and hard work. Three of the books listed physicians as advisors to the yearbook, each of which carried a "tribute" to the hospital's physicians—often in glowing terms of the doctor's selfless and untiring efforts.[27]

Students strove to achieve the competence demanded and exhibited by the graduate nurse. Nurses at all levels shared the same ideals and goals, thus cementing them into a single group divided by authority only temporarily. The yearbooks express the belief that an ideal nurse should have every conceivable virtue; however, while expressing esteem for their profession, the students were unsure of what exactly makes a good nurse. For example, in the short essay "Relationship between Head Nurse and Student Nurse" from *The Stethoscope*, 1929, the following virtues are mentioned: insight into human nature, initiative, foresight, executive ability, a personality that doctors and supervisors will admire and patients will love, competence, dignity, refinement, enthusiasm, a desire to learn, submissiveness, attentiveness, curiosity, willingness, and industriousness. "The Perfect Nurse," in *The Crescent*, lists energy, guile, innocence, wile, naivete, nerve, courage, sweetness, deceit, frailty, passion, love, wisdom, weakness, thoughtfulness, caring, humor, cussedness, spice, and goodness. Thus the students reveal no critical sense of what constitutes a good nurse; instead, they fall back on cliches and exaggerated ideals to substitute for a clear sense of the dimensions of their profession. They are to be all things to all people—pleasing everyone and expecting nothing in return, save an occasional word of thanks.

A good number of predictions and prophecies include expectations of marriage and motherhood. Nurses who specified a nursing field rarely mentioned general duty in a hospital; instead, they mentioned public health, pediatrics, obstetrics, or industrial nursing. A comparison of the nurses' stated ambitions with occupations listed by alumnae reveals great disparity. The most frequent occupation of graduates was private-duty nursing, which accounted for 58% to 65%.

These young nurses claimed to aspire to a noble, idealistic, altruistic profession offering service and adventure; yet their strongest loyalties were to their hospitals and local communities. For example, an essay in *The Nightingale* describes loyalty as the nurse's keynote in her psalm of life—to be loyal to her patients, her school, the physician, her co-workers, and her profession. Furthermore, from what can be gleaned about the real prospects of these students upon graduation, they probably remained in the general vicinity of their training school and worked in private duty or general duty at their hospital, at least until they married. Despite their ambitious and lofty notions about their profession, these nurses revealed little inclination to extend their professional experience or to promote themselves as autonomous professionals.

FAILURE TO ACCREDIT

Many nurses had been eager to have the training schools graded and viewed the publicizing of such information as a way in which hospitals might be stimulated to offer a higher level of education. They also saw listings of accredited schools as a means by which a prospective student could be guided in her choice of nursing school. No schedule of accreditation was attempted by the grading committee, however, largely because of "the advice of the representatives of higher education." The committee also felt that "the accuracy of a list compiled without personal visits to the schools might be questioned."[28] They explained that a firsthand visit to each school, valuable as it would have been, was not financially possible.

Concerned by the lack of accreditation action, in 1931 Isabel Stewart warned that nursing's biggest problems were still those of bringing some order out of the chaos of unregulated and widely differentiated schools, of reducing the overproduction of poorly prepared nurses, and of providing supplementary

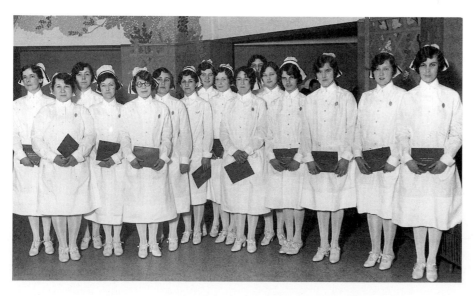

These graduates of the late 1920s hoped to become private-duty nurses.

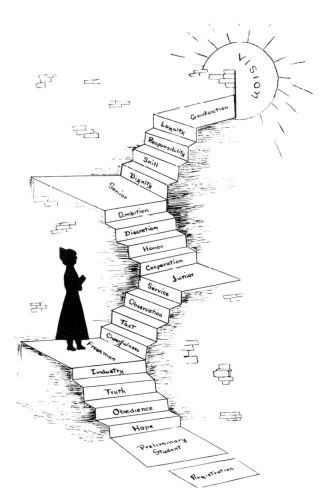

The steps to professional nursing as portrayed by the Allegheny General Hospital class of 1930.

Stewart later identified three 20-year stages through which nurse education had passed. The first, from 1873 to 1893, was a pioneering era, in which a few Nightingale schools had been founded in the United States. The second, from 1893 to 1913, was a period of phenomenal expansion, regulated to some degree by legal and professional controls. The third, from 1913 to 1933, was a time of stress and turmoil, of experimentation and painful self-examination.

The facts bore out her analysis. The population of the United States had doubled from 1873 to 1933, but the number of hospitals had increased more than 42 times. In 1873 the United States had 149 hospitals and allied institutions; at the close of 1933, 6334 hospitals offered over one million beds. The two factors primarily responsible for this amazing growth were the development of support services and the greater public confidence in hospital care. Comparative studies showed that the average per capita period of hospitalization had decreased from 24 days in 1900 to 12 days in 1933.

Meanwhile the confidence essential to prosperous American business had been swept away by the financial panic of October 1929; soon banks were unable to lend and businesses began to collapse. Small-business bankruptcies followed bank failures with dismal regularity. Hospitals and public health agencies began to lay off personnel. By the beginning of 1933 the unemployment rate had risen to 25% and business was at a near-standstill. During the same time the nation fell into crisis, nurses found the integral structure of their profession in chaos.

educational offerings to nurses who had been trained in substandard programs. She insisted that the public had to be made to face this situation and to see that nursing schools needed the same kind of public support that had been given to normal schools and agricultural colleges. Stewart lamented:

> In all these years, the public has done very little for nursing education. It has cost the public practically nothing to produce the hundreds of thousands of nurses who have spent their lives in its service. Nurses have paid for their own education, and through their services as students they have contributed in all these years millions of dollars toward the care of the sick in hospitals. They have also put a good deal of money into private pockets. Compare the public cost of training teachers or soldiers or stenographers or workers in agriculture and home economics to the cost which the public has borne for the training of nurses. Without some kind of radical treatment, it is doubtful if the nursing body can ever get back into a healthy condition.[29]

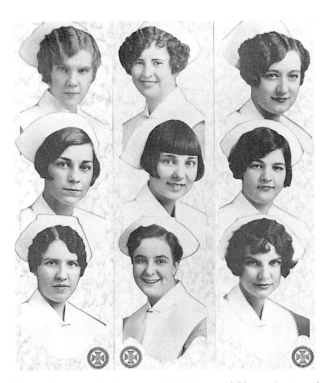

Uncertain economic times awaited these 1930 graduates of Allegheny General Hospital in Pittsburgh.

REFERENCES

1. Isabel M. Stewart, "Developments in Nursing Education Since 1918." *U.S. Bureau of Education Bulletin* 20:6, 1921.
2. Edwin P. Haworth, "Nursing in the Movies," *Modern Hospital*, vol. 16 (February 1921):156.
3. Ibid.
4. Ibid.
5. Stewart, op. cit., p. 17.
6. Ibid., pp. 17–18.
7. "Rockefeller Foundation and Nursing Education," *American Journal of Nursing*, vol. 20 (April 1920):525.
8. Josephine C. Goldmark, *Nursing and Nursing Education in the United States* (New York: Macmillan Co., 1923), pp. 1–36.
9. Ibid., pp. 187–472.
10. Ibid., pp. 310–312.
11. Quoted in "Why Not Be Fair?" *Bulletin of the American Hospital Association*, vol. 6 (September 1932):6–8.
12. U.S. Department of Commerce, Bureau of the Census, *Fourteenth Census of the United States, 1920* (Washington, D.C.: Government Printing Office, 1923), vol. 4, pp. 42–43.
13. "Some Problems in Grading Our Schools of Nursing," *Trained Nurse and Hospital Review*, vol. 77 (November 1926):507–509.
14. Ibid., p. 508.
15. Ibid., pp. 507–508.
16. Ibid., p. 509.
17. Shirley C. Titus, "The Present Position of Nursing in Hospitals in the United States," *Nosokomeion*, vol. 2 (April 1931): 288–310.
18. Dorothy Dunbar Bromley, "The Crisis in Nursing," *Harper's Magazine*, vol. 161 (July 1930):159–160.
19. May Ayres Burgess, "What the Cost Study Showed," *American Journal of Nursing*, vol. 32 (April 1932):427–432.
20. Malcolm T. MacEachern, "Which Shall We Choose—Graduate or Student Service?" *Modern Hospital*, vol. 38 (June 1932):97–98, 102–104.
21. May Ayres Burgess, "Nurses, Patients, and Pocketbooks," *Proceedings of the Thirty-fourth Annual Convention of the National League of Nursing Education*, vol. 34 (June 1928):237–256.
22. National League of Nursing Education, Committee on Curriculum, *A Curriculum Guide for Schools of Nursing* (New York: The League, 1927), p. 8.
23. Harlan Hoyt Horner, *Nursing Education and Practice in New York State, with Suggested Remedial Measures* (Albany: University of the State of New York Press, 1934), pp. 19–23.
24. Ibid., p. 20.
25. Clara D. Noyes, "How Some Nursing Leaders Visualize the Ideal Student Nurse," *Hospital Management*, vol. 23 (January 1927):53.
26. Allegheny General Hospital, School of Nursing, *The Stethoscope, 1930* (Pittsburgh: The Hospital, 1930), p. 10.
27. Allegheny General Hospital, School of Nursing, *The Stethoscope, 1929* (Pittsburgh: The Hospital, 1929), p. 15.
28. A. C. Bachmeyer, "Systems of Accreditment for Schools of Nursing," *American Journal of Nursing*, vol. 36 (April 1936):375–381.
29. Isabel M. Stewart, "Trends in Nursing Education," *American Journal of Nursing*, vol. 31 (May 1931):601–611.

PUBLIC HEALTH NURSING, 1912–1930

Despite the rapid growth of hospitals and other institutions for the care of the sick in the United States, the American public was slow in recognizing the parallel obligation to those who, for whatever reason, were unable to go to hospitals and therefore had to be cared for in their homes. By 1915, no more than 10% of the sick received care in institutions. Aside from the small proportion of the unhospitalized sick who could afford to employ private-duty graduate nurses at $25 a week, most people had to be cared for by either untrained practical nurses or well-prepared visiting nurses.

PUBLIC HEALTH NURSING SKYROCKETS

As late as 1891, there had been only 58 associations and 130 nurses throughout the country engaged in visiting or public health nursing. During the next decade, a national public health movement took form, creating a steadily increasing demand for nurses. Public health nursing surged ahead, so that in 1919 nearly 9000 trained nurses were devoting their entire time to this type of work (Table 12-1).[1]

The first visiting nurses had limited their work almost entirely to bedside care. They soon discovered that the giving of medicine had little effect if there was no food in the house; that to ensure cleanliness required more than just an order from the physician or nurse; and that health care and preventive measures required not only technical skill but also a high degree of communicative ability. The nurse soon found that she was making a certain number of visits that were entirely psychosocial in character and that to improve the health of a particular patient, her work might require a knowledge of economic, industrial, cultural, or social conditions—knowledge far removed from the therapeutic principles taught in the hospital. Thus the specialty of public health nursing emerged in strength.

Although it was essential that the public health nurse first be formally trained in hospital nursing, she also needed preparation in the public health aspects of her field. She could acquire this by special fieldwork in connection with her hospital training, by postgraduate studies in public health at a college, or by on-the-job training with one of the district nursing associations. Some excellent nurses had received their public health training through practical fieldwork under the instruction of a trained supervisor, but generally, such education was inferior to the combined theory and practice received in public health nursing courses offered by colleges and schools.

Special courses on the elements of public health nursing soon appeared. By 1916, there were at least eight different colleges, universities, or other institutions offering graduate courses for public health nurses—in Atlanta, Boston, Boulder, Chicago, Cleveland, New York, Philadelphia, and Santa Barbara—along with special courses offered by the state health departments of Kansas and Ohio. The Department of Nursing and Health directed by Professor Adelaide Nutting at Teachers College, Columbia University, was the strongest and most fully developed of these schools. It had a departmental faculty of five professors, with eight special lecturers attached to the staff. It offered 1- and 2-year programs of study on teaching in schools of nursing, administration of schools of nursing, hospital administration, public health nursing, school nursing and teaching, and supervision in public health nursing. In Boston, the District Nursing Association gave both 4- and 8-month courses; the public health, household economics, and educational aspects were offered at Simmons College and the sociologic aspects at a nearby school for social workers. In Chicago, a 16-week course was given by the School of Civics and Philanthropy and included classroom work, visits to social agencies, and fieldwork under the supervision of local public health nursing organizations.

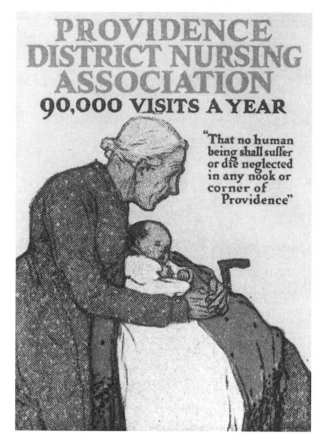

Public health nursing experienced spectacular growth between 1912 and 1930.

In addition to their usual work, public health nurses were being called to serve as sanitary inspectors, tenement-house inspectors, probation officers, hygiene teachers, hospital social service workers, agents of charity organizations, and welfare workers in large industrial plants. For example, Adelaide Nutting, at the opening of the 1916 fall term, received letters that reveal the type of work that was expected of the public health nurse of that period:

> I have just been talking with _____, superintendent of schools at _____. He wants a school nurse. . . . This is a new position, and he is inclined to give the right woman quite a free hand. He says they have 1,800 children in the

school and practically no foreigners [and] wishes this school nurse to assist the physical education instructor in medical inspection. During the year they conduct some chautauqua work, where the nurse would have an opportunity to deliver lectures to the farmers' wives. They also have a summer school, where they emphasize domestic science, domestic art, and general industrial activities, but this could be arranged later on. Mr. _____ wants to find a woman who is adaptable and who would be interested in remaining for some time. [He] emphasizes social training, and would like to find a woman of considerable enthusiasm as well as special training.

A letter received from a staff physician at a hospital in one of the large eastern cities stated:

> During the past year I have been developing a clinic for the investigation and treatment of diseases of metabolism in one of the large hospitals. . . . Our work thus far has been confined to the treatment of diabetes mellitus and nephritis. The board of managers of the hospital are [*sic*] very much interested in the work, which has been productive of the most gratifying results. Thus far I have been greatly handicapped because of the lack of knowledge on the part of the pupil nurses of the principles of dietetics and the elementary principles of metabolics, and even more handicapped by the fact that we have no teaching nurse who is able to instruct the pupil nurses. It is my plan to secure an educated trained nurse who will come into the hospital, supervise the care of the patients in this ward, and also act as a teacher in the nurses' training school. The position will be one of dignity and will carry with it a reasonable salary. The board of managers of the hospital has instructed me to negotiate for such a teacher. I am appealing to you for assistance in securing such a person. Will you kindly let me know if any of your graduate or present students are or will be available for such work?[2]

In 1916, Mary Sewall Gardner, director of the Providence, Rhode Island, District Nursing Association and author of the book Public Health Nursing, observed the attitude of the medical profession toward public health nursing. The more broadminded physicians had always recognized the work of public health nurses who helped them produce results that would have been impossible if they had been forced to work alone. The narrow-minded members of the medical profession, however, regarded public health nurses with suspicion and continually feared their interference. There was apt to be a certain amount of antagonism from physicians in any community contemplating the establishment

TABLE 12-1	Growth of Public Health Nursing in the United States	
YEAR	NUMBER OF ORGANIZATIONS	NUMBER OF NURSES
1891	58	130
1905	200	400
1914	1922	5152
1919	3094	8770

of a public health nursing service. This antagonism could be greatly diminished if the service was started with the cooperation of the medical profession and if the nurses made special efforts to assure everyone that the physician and not the nurse was in charge and that the nurse would not assume the duties and responsibilities of the physician.

Gardner interpreted the rules of professional ethics to mean that the public health nurse "should not diagnose, should not prescribe, should not recommend a particular doctor or a change of doctors, should not suggest a hospital to a patient without the concurrence of the doctor, and should never criticize, by word or unspoken action, any member of the medical profession." These severe rules were sometimes modified so that a nurse would not be compelled to serve under a physician who was professionally incompetent or dangerously careless. In such cases, the nurse was to report the problem to her supervisor, who, if she was experienced and resourceful, usually found a way to correct the situation.

THE METROPOLITAN LIFE NURSES

By 1920, a program instituted by the Metropolitan Life Insurance Company for its industrial policyholders had gained national attention. This service, started in 1909 in conjunction with the Henry Street Settlement in New York City, had been limited to company policyholders, most of whom were employed in industrial occupations. The service had increased rapidly and was extended to all industrial policyholders who were ill and required bedside treatment. In cities outside the New York City area, visits were made by company nurses, but as a rule Metropolitan Life employed the nurses of the local

visiting nurses' association. The total company cost of service during 1918 was more than $810,000, the average cost per visit was 53 cents, and the average number of visits per patient was 4.9. Based on the entire number of industrial policies, the cost per policy was 4.6 cents.

Metropolitan Life actuaries prepared a table showing the influence of the nursing service and other health and welfare activities on the mortality rate of their policyholders,[3] which revealed an average decline in the mortality rate of more than 7% in 7 years (Table 12-2). The decline was most marked and most significant during the early years, being more than 19% in the first year of life. When the rates for the principal causes of death of policyholders were compared with the general death rates for the community at large as obtained from government sources, the results were distinctly in favor of the policyholders. The company thus considered it fair to assume that a significant part of the decline in mortality and the accompanying improvement in general health was due to the program of visiting nurses established in 1909.

ACTIVITIES OF PUBLIC HEALTH NURSES IN THE 1920s

Meanwhile, nurses were becoming increasingly common in state health departments. Until 1907, no state recognized the public health nurse as a legitimate employee of an official health or education agency. As early as 1898, Los Angeles had employed a few municipal nurses, and in 1902 the New York City Health Department employed several nurses to assist in the control of communicable diseases, but these instances were experimental and were not authorized

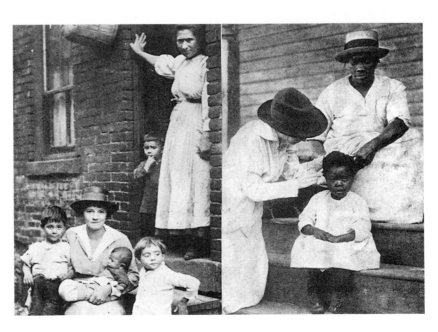

Health promotion and disease prevention services for children were important components of public health nursing.

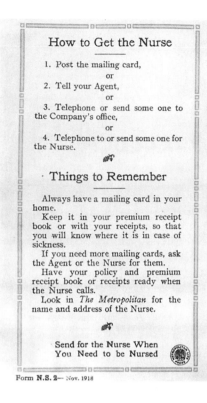

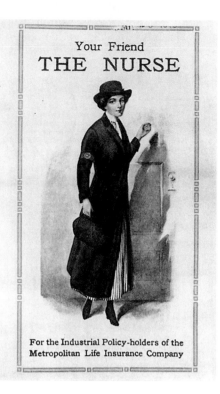

How to Get the Nurse

1. Post the mailing card,
   or
2. Tell your Agent,
   or
3. Telephone or send some one to the Company's office,
   or
4. Telephone to or send some one for the Nurse.

Things to Remember

Always have a mailing card in your home.

Keep it in your premium receipt book or with your receipts, so that you will know where it is in case of sickness.

If you need more mailing cards, ask the Agent or the Nurse for them.

Have your policy and premium receipt book or receipts ready when the Nurse calls.

Look in *The Metropolitan* for the name and address of the Nurse.

Send for the Nurse When You Need to be Nursed

Form N.S. 2— Nov. 1918

Your Friend
THE NURSE

For the Industrial Policy-holders of the
Metropolitan Life Insurance Company

Bulletin on the nursing service for Metropolitan Life Insurance policy-holders, 1918.

by legislative action. Recognition of public health nursing as a desirable and necessary function of government came gradually in the first quarter of the 20th century.

Alabama was the first state to approve the employment of public health nurses by governmental agencies. The County Health Law passed in 1907 specifically mentioned nurses as "employees necessary to accomplish the work of a county health department." The following year, New York State passed a law that permitted the employment of nurses to aid in the control of tuberculosis. Ohio was

The Visiting Nurse

F YOU are an Industrial policy-holder of the Metropolitan Life Insurance Company, living in a place where we have a Metropolitan Visiting Nurse, you may have her services, if you are sick enough to need a doctor.

No charge of any kind will be made to you, nor will any deductions be made from the face value of your policy when it matures.

The Metropolitan Nurse is paid by the Company for each visit made to an Industrial policy-holder.

The Nurse will carry out the instructions of the physician. She will stay from fifteen minutes to one hour, according to the treatment required.

The Nurse will nurse you after confinement if your policy has been in force nine months or more. Usually she will come eight times. If you are going to have a baby, she will visit you before confinement and instruct you about your diet, clothing, rest, etc., and will tell you how to get ready for your confinement.

METROPOLITAN NURSES DO NOT ATTEND AT TIME OF CONFINEMENT

Policy-holders may not call in at the expense of the Company any nurse but the regular Metropolitan Nurse.

Read the Following Carefully

1. The Nurse may care for you only when your policy and premium receipt book or receipts are shown to her on her first visit.

2. The Nursing Service may not be given to members of the family who are not Industrial policy-holders.

3. The Nurse may care for you only when you have a regular physician or will send for one.

4. The Nurse may not attend at operations, or give special treatments, such as "massage," "electricity" or hypodermic treatments unless you are confined to bed and are not able to visit a hospital, dispensary or physician's office to receive such treatment.

5. Where the Company employs but one Nurse it is not generally possible for her to visit you if any one in the home has a contagious disease.

6. A Visiting Nurse may not stay in your home. She will visit you as required, remaining long enough to do what the physician has directed and to instruct some member of your family, or a neighbor, how to take care of you between visits.

7. Send for the Nurse when you are sick enough to have a doctor. Should your sickness become chronic, the Nurse will make a few visits to teach some member of your family how to care for you.

Rules for requesting the services of a Metropolitan visiting nurse.

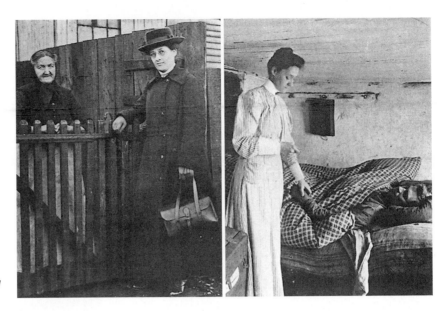

Public health nurses at work in the early 1920s.

the third state to recognize the public health nurse by specifying her in its school health inspection law, which was passed in 1909. Two years later, Massachusetts permitted certain cities to employ visiting nurses, and Pennsylvania authorized the employment of school nurses.

By the early 1920s, the scope of public health nursing was unclear. Experts who had carefully studied the public health nursing problem appeared to favor a generalized service combining health instruction and bedside care. The Committee on Nursing of the Rockefeller Foundation concluded:

> The question of whether the public health nurse should or should not render bedside care has been hotly debated during the past few years.

TABLE 12-2	Industrial Policyholder Experience of the Metropolitan Life Insurance Company, 1911–1917, in Deaths per 1000		
AGE PERIOD (Y)	**1911**	**1917**	**PERCENT DECLINE**
All ages	12.5	11.6	7.2
1–4	12.8	10.5	18.0
1	25.2	20.4	19.1
2	16.6	13.5	18.7
3	9.3	7.7	17.2
4	6.6	5.6	15.2
5–9	2.7	3.4	3.7
10–14	2.7	2.6	3.7
15–19	4.7	4.8	2.1*
20–24	7.3	6.6	9.6
25–34	9.5	8.4	11.6
35–44	13.7	12.4	9.5
45–54	19.8	19.6	1.0
55–64	36.0	35.8	.6
65–74	74.5	76.4	2.6*
74 and older	139.3	142.6	2.4*

*Percent increase in 7 years

The arguments for purely instructive service rest mainly on two grounds—the administrative difficulties involved in the conduct of private sick nursing by official health agencies and the danger that the urgent demands of sick nursing may lead to the neglect of preventive educational measures which are of more basic and fundamental significance. Both these objections are real and important ones. Yet the observations made in the course of our survey indicate that both may perhaps ultimately be overcome. Several municipal health departments have definitely undertaken to provide organized nursing service for bedside care combined with health teaching, while in other instances instructive nurses, under public auspices, combine a certain amount of emergency service with their fundamentally educational activities. So far as the neglect of instructive work is concerned it results from numerical inadequacy of personnel and can be avoided by a sufficiently large nursing staff.

On the other hand, the plan of instructive nursing divorced from bedside care suffers from defects which if less obvious than those mentioned above are in reality more serious, because they are inherent in the very plan itself and therefore not subject to control. In the first place, the introduction of the instructive but non-nursing field worker creates at once a duplication of effort, since there must be a nurse from some other agency employed in the same district to give bedside care. In the second place, the field worker who attempts health education without giving nursing care is by that very fact cut off from the contact which gives the instructive bedside nurse her most important psychological asset. The nurse who approaches a family where sickness exists and renders direct technical service in mitigating

> the burden of that sickness has an overwhelming advantage, then and thereafter, in teaching the lessons of hygiene. With a given number of nurses per unit of population, we believe that the combined service of teaching and nursing will yield the largest results.[4]

A census taken by the National Organization for Public Health Nursing in 1924 revealed a total of 3629 agencies, with a total of 11,171 full-time graduate nurses, in the United States. About one half of these agencies, employing more than one half of the nurses, were official branches of the federal, state, county, or municipal governments. Among the private agencies listed were 398 public health nursing associations or similar organizations, which had 2516 nurses; 473 local clinics and branches of the American Red Cross with 574 nurses; 128 tuberculosis associations with 125 nurses; and 424 other nonofficial agencies employing 1194 nurses. Of the 3045 counties in the United States, 866 had a local nursing service available in 1924 for the entire area and 379 for part of the area, leaving 1800 counties totally unprovided for.

During the 1920s, the primary duties of the public health nurse moved more toward advising and instructing—to advise and show others how to care for the sick, to secure adequate care for them, and to instruct people on how to avoid sickness by attention to personal hygiene. Bedside nursing of the sick poor was no longer the primary function of the public health nurse.

The actual work of dealing firsthand with communicable diseases, inspecting milk and other food, maintaining a pure water supply, conducting clinics, providing nursing service, reaching the people with health instruction, and grappling in other ways with the many problems of disease control rested with local health departments. It was important, therefore, that they be provided with adequate staffs and funds for their work. Yet of 818 municipal health departments in cities of 10,000 population or more listed by the U.S. Public Health Service in 1923, only 41% had full-time health officers. Similarly, a 1925 study by the Bureau of the Census of public expenditures in 247 cities having a population of 30,000 or more showed that only $.91 per capita was used for the conservation of health that year, whereas more than $14 per capita was spent for education and $7.53 for police, fire, and other protection to person and property.

SICKNESS SURVEYS

The most glaring weakness of the nation's total health care system had less to do with individual health professionals than with social and economic realities. A revealing study was made in 1915 by the New York

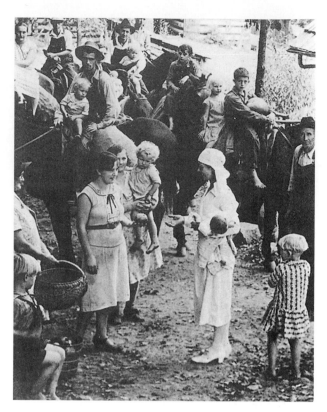

A child-health demonstration in rural Kentucky.

State Charities Aid Association (Table 12-3). All the recorded illnesses involved some degree of temporary or permanent disability.[5]

Another pertinent study, conducted in 1918 by the Public Health Committee of the New York Academy

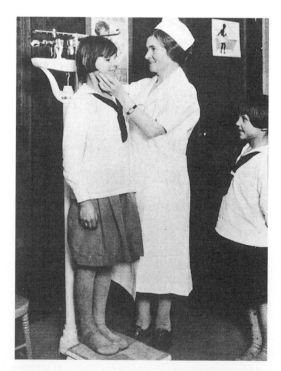

School nurses identified developmental problems.

TABLE 12-3	Modes of Health Care in 1600 Cases, Dutchess County, New York	
MODE OF CARE	**NUMBER**	**PERCENT**
Medical care provided by a physician at home	11,058	66
Medical care given outside the patient's home, either in a hospital or in other homes	159	10
No medical care rendered	383	24

TABLE 12-4	Treatment Used by Families in New York City, 1918
FORM OF TREATMENT	**PERCENT**
Private physicians at home	37.7
Lodge physicians at home	4.1
Charity physicians (sent to home from an institution)	0.8
Medical care in hospitals	11.6
Medical care in outpatient clinics	13.2
Midwives at home	10.8
Self-treatment or medication on advice of druggist	21.8

of Medicine, investigated the care secured by families in New York City (Table 12-4). It found that among the 8645 people surveyed, 3140 were reported as having suffered from 3536 illnesses during 1918.[6] This included partial and complete disabilities. It is significant that the proportion of sick people without direct medical care was about the same as in the Dutchess County survey.

In a third survey carried out from 1921 to 1924 in Hagerstown, Maryland, by the U.S. Public Health Service,[7] information was obtained for 17,217 illnesses (Table 12-5). The Hagerstown cases included a larger proportion of minor illnesses than did the other two studies. But, significantly, 100% of the cases of typhoid fever and cancer and 97% of the pneumonia patients were treated either in homes or in hospitals, whereas almost one third of the patients with measles reported "no medical care." Of the mass of sore throats, colds, and bronchial conditions constituting more than 7000 of the 17,217 total illnesses, fewer than 20% received outside medical care.

THE SCANDAL OF SELF-MEDICATION

Despite its danger, self-treatment through the use of patent medicines was still widespread. Americans consumed more drugs and used more patent medicines than any other country in the industrialized world. Self-medication had grown to tremendous proportions. Everywhere—in street cars, on trolley transfer tickets, on billboards, in magazines, in newspapers, in the mail—were advertised medicines to cure disease and devices to promote health. In addition to the classic patent medicines, such as Lydia Pinkham's Vegetable Compound, castoria, and cod liver oil, came promises of "Colds Cured in One Day" or remedies like "Appendixine" and an array of health foods, massage vibrators, violet rays, "Porosknit" underwear, sanitary tooth washes, soaps, and vitopathic, naturopathic, and assorted faith cures.

New panaceas appeared every day. One product, "Soothing Sirup," recommended for colicky infants, often permanently doped its small recipients or soothed them into a sleep from which they never

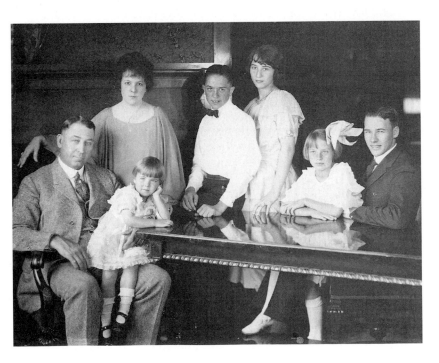

Most families in the 1920s received all health care in their homes.

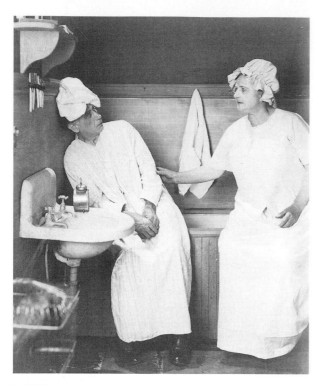

In 1916, Americans relied on self-medication to the exclusion of professional health care.

awoke. In New York, a visiting nurse encountered a group of frenzied women in the hallway of a tenement. Nearby a baby lay on a bed, gasping and "rolling its eyes up into the top of its head." The nurse asked the frightened mother what she had been giving the baby. "Nothing at all," said the woman, but a telltale "soothing" bottle indicated that the child was dying of morphine poisoning.

The prevalence of ill health and the widespread demand for "cures" also fostered the proliferation of quacks. These were unscrupulous charlatans who, with humbug promises and practices, extorted money from the simpleminded and the credulous. Samuel Hopkins Adams, in his exposé of this sordid business entitled *The Great American Fraud*, observed:

> No peril in the whole range of human pathology need have any terrors for the man who can believe the medical advertisements in the

newspapers. For every ill there is a "sure cure" provided in print. *Dr. This* is as confident of removing your cancer without the use of the knife as *Dr. That* is of eradicating your consumption by his marvelous new discovery, or *Dr. Otherwise* of rehabilitating your kidneys, which the regular profession has given up as a hopeless job.

The more deadly the disease, the more blatantly certain is the quack that he alone can save you, and in extreme cases, where he has failed to get there earlier, he may even raise you from your coffin and restore you to your astonished and admiring friends. Such things have happened—and pitiful gropers after relief from suffering believe that they may happen again, otherwise charlatanry would cease to spread its daily cure.[8]

Through their advertising, quacks spread a pall of fear over the country. "Have you a little pain in your back—look out for Bright's Disease! Have you a neglected cough?—look out for consumption!" This artificially created fear drove victims into physicians' offices as well as into the drugstore, and perfectly healthy patients paid needless fees. Elsewhere, quick-cure artists traded on a fundamental human want—the desire to be free from pain and from the fear of pain. Frequently, this desire was so urgent that price was no object, and often the sufferer passionately hoped to be cured in the privacy of his or her bedroom, without friends, family, or even a physician discovering the ailment.

TABLE 12-5 Health Care Providers, Hagerstown, Maryland, 1921–1924	
TREATMENT PROVIDER	**PERCENT**
Private physicians	46.00
Medical care in hospital	1.34
Chiropractors and osteopaths	0.41
Self-medication	2.25
No form of care reported	50.00

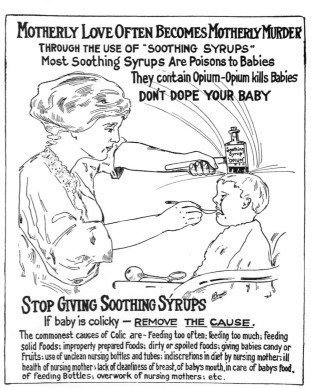

The dangers of soothing syrups for infants and children.

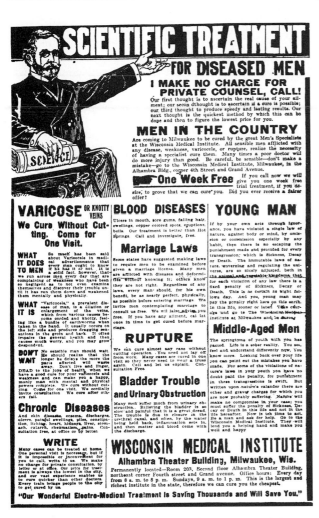

This "medical institute" promised cures for ruptures and rheumatism.

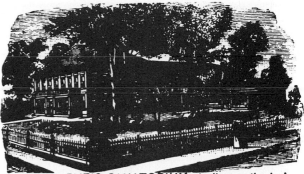

DR. B. F. BYE'S SANATORIUM, Indianapolis, Ind.

Cancer

Cured With Soothing Balmy Oils.

Cancer, Tumor, Fistula, Eczema and skin diseases. Cancer of the nose, eye, lip, ear, neck. breast, stomach, womb—in fact, all internal or external organs or tissues, cured without knife or burning plasters, but with soothing aromatic oils. Send for an illustrated book on the above diseases. Home treatment sent in most cases. Address as above.

Sellers of patent medicines exploited the fundamental human desire to be free from pain and illness.

IMMIGRANTS' HEALTH PRACTICES

Clare Terwilliger, a public health nurse assigned by the Henry Street Nursing Service to a block on East 39th Street, New York, furnished more than a year's impressions of the segment of life within her jurisdiction, under the title "How Thirty-ninth Street People Secure Care in Sickness." She also showed why they sometimes did not secure care. Terwilliger concluded:

> Uncertainty about the nature of the disease which a person seems to have appears to play a greater part than the severity of the illness in determining whether or not to call a doctor. If the disease is recognized, remedies are used which are suggested by some older member of the family or some neighbor who "always knows what to do." If a child with measles, for example, instead of growing better, begins to feel as if it were burning up and breathes very rapidly, that element of uncertainty provides a reason for

calling a doctor. If the family belongs to a group of friends or neighbors in which there is one person who has a family doctor, that person is consulted and her doctor is called. The use of a single doctor as the regular family doctor is, however, unusual. If the family does not belong to such a clique the nearest doctor is called.

> If the family is Irish and the patient grows better, the doctor's fine qualities are lauded up and down the street for months. If the patient does not grow better in a very short time, another doctor is called. As many as three different doctors have been called in a case of acute illness lasting only four days. If the patient dies, the members of the family and the interested neighbors are likely to state publicly as frequently as the opportunity arises that the doctor killed the patient.

> If, on the other hand, the family is Italian and illness is severe, the doctor is requested to bring a "professor" and the money is gathered somehow to pay him before he leaves the house.[9]

In a 1921 study by Michael M. Davis, entitled *Immigrant Health and the Community*, a Latvian immigrant was reported to have declared that he did not "trust hospitals or dispensaries, especially city hospitals, which many of the men from the factory had been to when different accidents happened. One or two of them had died and the family and neighbors looked upon all hospitals as a place where one goes to die."

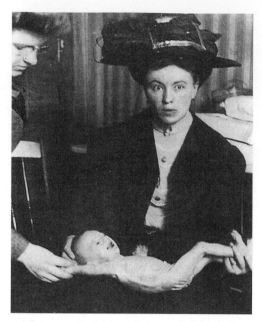

Immigrant families were often reluctant to seek health care from hospitals.

A statement from the same survey concluded:

> Most hospitals give even the sophisticated visitor
> a sense of being surrounded by very busy,
> presumably very efficient doctors, nurses, and
> employees, who are passing rapidly from one
> duty to another and have no time for him.
> The attitude towards hospitals revealed in one
> hundred and fifty interviews with (foreign-
> born) doctors, and about an equal number
> with individual immigrants, could be
> summarized in the following opinions:
> A strange place.
> A place in which I cannot understand what
> people say, or be understood.
> A place where doctors practice on you, especially
> young doctors.
> A place where people die.
> A place where I cannot get the food I like or am
> used to.
> A place where I either have to take charity or pay
> more than I can afford.[10]

A Lithuanian's testimony suggested how the neighborhood drugstore was patronized even without the urge from national advertising, because it was familiar and neighborly, whereas the hospital was distant and aloof:

> All hospitals are the same to Mr. M. "When
> men are hurt in the factory they are sent there,
> and if the young doctors do not practice on
> them they live, but otherwise they die."

Mr. M. had no other occasion to use doctors.
When he had a cold and sore throat he told the
druggist what the trouble was and he gave him
some medicine. "Of course the druggist knows
what is good for you."[11]

HEALTH DEMONSTRATIONS

Large-scale health demonstrations were extremely helpful in showing what could be done to improve community health during the 1920s. These intensive programs of health education in carefully defined areas were temporarily supplied with a modern public health service under the direction of trained and experienced personnel. The object of the demonstration was to show the benefits of such services, with the hope that they might become so widely appreciated that they would be permanently adopted by the demonstration community as well as a large number of similar communities. Financial support for health demonstrations came from philanthropic foundations, insurance companies, local contributions, and, in some cases, state funds.

The first public health demonstration in America was sponsored by the Metropolitan Life Insurance Company. In 1915, that company paid out $4 million in policies for deaths from tuberculosis alone. Such a serious situation warranted an effort to find means of early detection of the disease and of preventing its spread to other members of the community. The task of selecting a typical locality and planning and carrying out the demonstration was entrusted to the National Tuberculosis Association, which selected the town of Framingham, Massachusetts.

With the $100,000 contributed by the company, a 3-year study was launched. After it became apparent that it would be impossible to fight tuberculosis effectively without carrying on a general health program for the community, the project budget was doubled and the demonstration was extended to 7 years. Diagnostic standards were developed, and for the first time, accurate knowledge of the amount of tuberculosis existing in a given community was determined. As a result of this work, the tuberculosis death rate of Framingham fell from 97.5 per 100,000 in 1917 to 38.2 in 1923 and declined to two thirds of the rest of the state's tuberculosis rate.

From 1923 to 1929, the Commonwealth Fund conducted demonstrations in Fargo, North Dakota; Clark County, Georgia; Rutherford County, Tennessee; and Marion County, Oregon. From the experience thus gained, fund directors believed that state departments of health needed to give direct aid and guidance to rural health areas and that the efforts of all local health providers needed to be coordinated to secure satisfactory results. This included extensive use of local physicians as well as public health officers and public health nurses in programs of mass screening and health assessment.

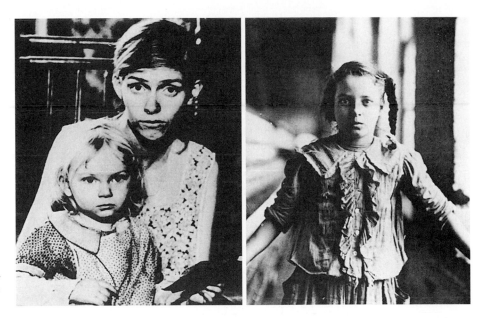

A tubercular mother with daughter and an overworked young factory girl.

THE KENTUCKY FRONTIER NURSING SERVICE

A practical demonstration in uplifting the health status of a remote rural area was also launched, in the form of the Frontier Nursing Service, organized by its director, Mary Breckinridge. In May 1925, Breckinridge had recognized the need for such work and had secured training at the St. Luke's Hospital School of Nursing in New York and at a nurse-midwifery program in London.

Several years earlier, Breckinridge had interviewed 53 of the area's midwives and had assembled her data in a manuscript report entitled "Midwifery in the Kentucky Mountains." All but one of the midwives were white, and they ranged in age from 30 to 90 years, with the average midwife being 60 years old. Only 12 of the 53 could read or write, and none had taken any formal training in midwifery.

As a group, these untrained midwives were grossly superstitious and knew nothing of prenatal or postnatal care. Only 7 of the 53 carried any equipment

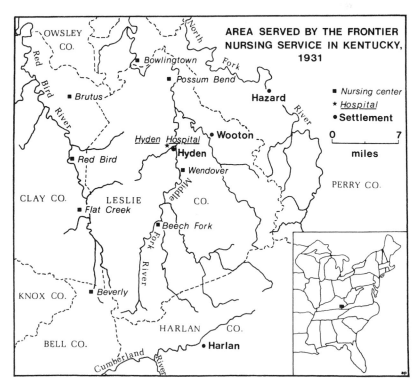

Map of the Frontier Nursing Service area, 1931.

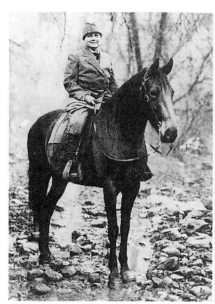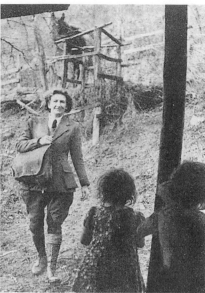

Mary Breckinridge on horse; a frontier nurse making a visit.

with them; the rest "counted on finding at the patient's home the hog grease which is their almost universal requisite." If complications in delivery occurred, the midwives would almost never call for a physician, considering such action to be a reflection of their competency. Instead they would attempt to stop hemorrhage by repeating a certain Bible verse or by making tea from black gum bark from the north side of a tree mixed with the bark of sweet apple tree from the south side of the tree. Soot was used extensively as a medication, some of the midwives preferring chimney soot, others, soot from pots and pans. Generally recommended preventive procedures included placing an ax under the delivery bed with the blade straight up.

Breckinridge's field of work was centered in Leslie County and parts of adjacent Clay and Owsley counties in southeastern Kentucky. Overwhelmingly rural in population, Leslie County's 10,000 inhabitants constituted a density of only 27.1 persons per square mile, the second lowest in the state. The only settlement of any size was Hyden, with 313 inhabitants. The area's poor economy supported only a fragile existence for the population. The absence of highways necessitated travel by horse or mule only. The area was divided into eight districts of about 78 square miles each. In a log cabin in the middle of each district lived two nurses who were responsible for the health of all the people who lived there. They provided midwifery and public health nursing to the approximately 200 families who lived in the general area.

The work plan was based on one used in the Highlands and islands of Scotland, whose systems had been observed by Breckinridge. A generalized service and a decentralized system of organization were the key elements of the plan. A fee of $1 per year for complete nursing and public health care was charged

and, as necessary, an additional $5 for maternity care—the same fee charged by "granny midwives."

A 12-bed general hospital, the Hyden Hospital and Health Center, was established and operated at near capacity with 375 patient admissions and 31 births in 1935. Assisted by a superintendent and two nurses, the medical director had his headquarters there, taking responsibility for the hospitalized patients and answering calls from the nurses in the various centers.

The bulk of the care offered by the Frontier Nursing Service was delivered by nurses working out of the centers at Wendover, Beech Fork, Possum Bend, Red Bird, Flat Creek, Brutus, Bowlington, and Beverly. All the nurses were required to have had preparation in midwifery in addition to their general nursing and public health training. Because there were no quality nurse midwifery programs in the United States until the early 1930s, the early nurses received their training in England or Scotland. Staff nurses were required to have a certificate from the Central Midwives' Board in either of those countries. These nurse midwives gave antepartal, intrapartal, and postpartal care to women in their districts. They visited their patients at least twice a month until the seventh month of pregnancy and then every week until the time of delivery. Normal deliveries were handled by the nurse midwives; for complicated cases, the physician was called. The nurse took care of the patients for 10 days after delivery.

In 1932, Dr. Louis I. Dublin of the Metropolitan Life Insurance Company studied the first 1000 cases of the Frontier Nursing Service and summarized the results. He found that the proportion of complications that occurred during pregnancy and delivery was lower among the patients cared for by the frontier nurses than among the general population.

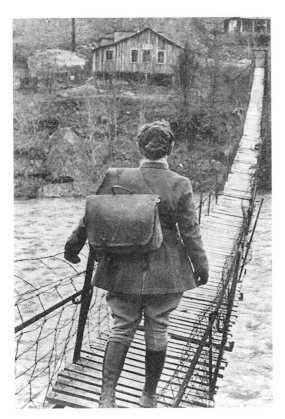

Frontier nurse approaching the cabin of a mountain family.

Regarding the mortality rate among the 1000 cases analyzed, Dublin wrote that "not one of the women died as the direct result of either pregnancy or labor. There were two deaths in the series; but in one the cause of death was a chronic kidney and heart disease, and in the other it was chronic heart disease. Neither of these two cases could probably be ascribed to the maternal state." There were one third fewer stillbirths and one third fewer deaths among babies in the first year of life than among the general white population of Kentucky. Dublin concluded:

> The study shows conclusively what has in fact been demonstrated before, that the type of service rendered by the Frontier Nurses safeguards the life of mother and babe. If such a service were available to the women of the country generally, there would be a saving of 10,000 mothers' lives a year in the United States; there would be 30,000 less stillbirths and 30,000 children alive at the end of the first month of life.[12]

The Frontier Nursing Service also offered care for infants and children. Babies younger than age 1 year were examined twice a month, preschool children from age 1 to 6 years were seen every month, and schoolchildren were examined once every 3 months. During these visits, mothers were taught about diet, cleanliness, health habits, general sanitation, and preventive care. Inoculations against typhoid and diphtheria and vaccinations for smallpox were also given.

The work of Mary Breckinridge and her frontier nurses constituted a vivid demonstration of the greatly expanded role that nurses could play in dispensing a primary form of health care. Although some nurses hoped that this type of service might be emulated elsewhere with the same successful results, the necessary mix of social, economic, and leadership elements failed to materialize, and the Frontier Nursing Service continued as a unique institution.

TRACHOMA ERADICATION

Another health demonstration was the trachoma eradication project carried out by nurses of the U.S. Public Health Service. The cause of trachoma, although it had been intensively sought after by capable bacteriologists, had not been discovered at that time. The disease seemed to be furthered by unusual exposure to wind, dust, and sun and by careless habits of personal cleanliness and the use of the same towel by several or many people—the "common towel." Trachoma first attacked the conjunctiva (the membrane lining the eyelids), causing granulations to form, which thickened the lid and irritated the eyeball. Later these granulations were replaced by scar tissue, which contracted, deforming the lids and bending them inward so that the eyelashes would rub against the front of the eye. The irritation thus caused was not only very painful but was commonly followed by partial or complete blindness.

To combat epidemic trachoma in the Appalachian Mountains, the Public Health Service established special hospitals at Hindman, Hyden, and Jackson, Kentucky, and at Coeburn, Virginia, in 1914 and 1915. Additional hospitals were set up later in the rural areas of West Virginia, Arkansas, and Missouri. Several dozen nurses were selected by the Public Health Service superintendent of nurses, Lucy Minnigerode, for appointment to the trachoma project. The trachoma eradication project was aimed at the very primitive mountain districts, where roads were impassable for automobiles. Thus one U.S. Public Health Service nurse making instructive visits and hunting for cases rode 3000 miles on muleback in a single year.

By 1925, U.S. Public Health Service nurses were working in trachoma hospitals at Rolla, Missouri; Russellville, Arkansas; Knoxville, Tennessee; and Richmond, Kentucky. At Rolla, a laboratory had been established so that bacteriologic studies could be performed in connection with the treatment. These temporary hospitals housed about 25 patients. In addition, there were a number of outpatients who also came for treatment. There were wards for all types of patients, together with treatment rooms, operating rooms, mess halls, kitchens, and bathrooms. The patients were seldom in bed, because they were able to take care of themselves. Generally two nurses were assigned to each hospital.

The treatments alone kept the nurse busy. All eyes were cleansed and irrigated before breakfast. At 9.00 a.m., the physician in charge gave his treatment and orders for the day, for example, atropine for one ailment and silver nitrate for another. The nurse again, before dinner, irrigated all eyes and carried out the orders. The physician made another call at 2:00 p.m. and the nurse made another round at bedtime, making a total of five treatments each day for each patient.

The work was rewarding for the nurse, because she knew she was preventing blindness and alleviating much suffering. A daily report of Blanche Pegg Allen, R.N., special fieldworker for the U.S. Public Health Service at Hazard, Kentucky, gives a typical example of this important assignment:

Wednesday: Left John Turner Home 8:30 A.M. To home Sam Turner. Mrs. Turner said her husband said their children could not go to hospital. Mr. Turner works in Hazard and I have seen him several times about his children going to hospital and he said he wanted them to go and have their eyes treated. He told Postmaster at Wolfcoal Sunday that I didn't need bother going to his place, that his children were not going to hospital. The children had been sent away from home and I did not see them. To home Allen Herald, saw Willie Turner, who has been to hospital. Asked him how he liked it there, said he didn't like it as they kept you in too close. He wanted to get out and run around. To home Elizabeth Turner, trachoma case. Said she couldn't go to hospital on account of her two children. Husband works two days a week and said he couldn't manage with wife gone. To home Mahala Raleigh, cicatricial trachoma with entropion. Examined four members of family, trachoma negative. To home Dora Turner, former Jackson patient. Lids in good condition. To home T. T. Herald to get some one to take me across Middle Fork River. Too high to ford. To home Elliott Turner, following six children suspicious trachoma cases, Bill, age 10; America, age 8; Dullseen, age 5; Johnnie, age 4; Sarah, age 11; Millie, age 16 months. I asked Mother to take part of children now and go to hospital. Said her husband would have to decide. Two older girls said they wanted to go but the boy didn't. To home Wm. Baker, son Alex, former Richmond patient. Lids in good condition. Examined seven members of family—paternal grandfather, age 80; has trachoma, almost blind and aunt cicatricial trachoma, others negative. To home Timothy Herald, have child five years old with bad-looking eyes. Youngster cried and would not let me see her eyes and mother just sat and didn't bother herself about having the child's

eyes examined and I naturally couldn't force her if the mother didn't. Examined three members of family, trachoma negative. To home Green Deaton, who is one of the outstanding members of the community. He said, "Oh, these people here are a sight and can't do anything with them." Walked three miles from Middle Fork River to Wm. Baker, Herald and Turner homes and return. Horseback five miles. Returned.[13]

PROMOTION OF MATERNAL AND CHILD HEALTH

Measures to improve maternal and child health as a phase of public health in general did not begin until organized prenatal nursing services and prenatal medical clinics were developed in the first decade of this century, following the more widespread recognition of the tremendous value of prenatal care. The greatest advance in maternal care in the early 20th century was the recognition of the importance of careful nursing and medical attention throughout the prenatal period. The development of prenatal clinics resulted in a decrease in mortality and morbidity from toxemias of pregnancy and cardiac, renal, metabolic, venereal, and associated complications. Consideration of adequate vitamin, mineral, and caloric content in the diets of pregnant women not only decreased the morbidity but also enhanced the health of all the mothers and children who received competent maternity care.

Effective federal investigation of the special problems of child health dates from the creation of the Children's Bureau in 1912. Investigations of the Children's Bureau fell into three main groups: (1) maternal and infant welfare (including the health and education of the preschool child); (2) the care of special groups of children handicapped by physical or mental problems or through delinquency, dependency, or neglect; and (3) problems relating to the child in industry. Field studies to determine the causes of the existing high rate of infant mortality were performed in industrial and rural communities, and these investigations, particularly in rural areas, gave special attention to the care provided mothers during pregnancy and at childbirth.

Under the direction of Julia C. Lathrop, the first chief of the bureau, and Grace Abbott, her successor, nearly 200 studies were performed during the following 15 years, and the results were presented in 195 special bulletins. Besides conducting research in the field, the bureau compiled, analyzed, and tabulated laws relating to child labor, juvenile courts, illegitimacy, sex offenses against children, mothers' pensions, and interstate placement and adoption of children and actively cooperated with child welfare and children's code commissions in the revision of state laws.

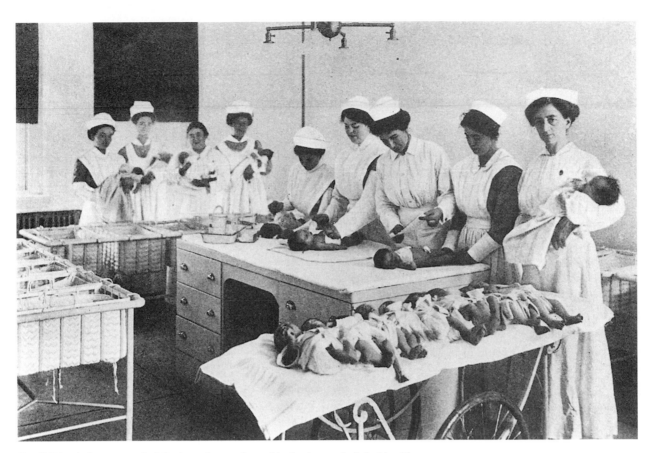

The Children's Bureau studied the importance of a well-trained nurse to infant health.

Early field studies and analyses of statistics indicated that preservation of the lives of mothers and babies depended on expansion of available prenatal care as well as on improvement in care at the time of delivery. Surveys showed that many births were attended by untrained, unskilled, and none-too-clean midwives. Many other mothers had no trained attendants at childbirth and did not understand the desirability of placing themselves in the hands of a physician or trained nurse for health supervision during pregnancy.

The failure to obtain competent prenatal care was reflected in the number of maternal deaths and also in the neonatal death rate, which peaked during the first month of life, largely due to prenatal conditions or events during delivery. The second most important cause of infant mortality was the gastrointestinal diseases, caused primarily by contaminated milk and water supplies, unhygienic surroundings, and improper feeding methods. Corrective measures included improving milk and water supplies and encouraging breast-feeding, a safer source of milk.

THE SHEPPARD-TOWNER ACT

Increasingly, a massive federal aid program was discussed as an approach to infant and maternal mortality problems. On April 21, 1921, Senator Morris

Sheppard of Texas introduced a bill (S. 1039) for the public protection of maternity and infancy and providing a method of cooperation between the U.S. government and various states. At a hearing before the Senate Committee on Education and Labor, Elizabeth G. Fox, the national director of the Red Cross Public Health Nursing Service and vice-president of

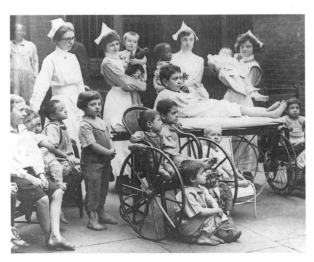

Child mortality statistics dropped significantly owing to the work of the Children's Bureau.

the National Organization for Public Health Nursing, spoke effectively for the bill:

> I am speaking from a knowledge of public health nursing gained from eight years' experience as a public health nurse and from three years' experience as executive officer in charge of 1,300 public health nurses. As much of the field work provided in the Sheppard-Towner bill will be performed by public health nurses, it is fair to suppose that it will be done according to the high standards and in the thorough manner now prevailing among public health nurses, some of whom are engaged in just the kind of work which is anticipated in this bill. There are now something like 10,000 public health nurses at work in the United States.
>
> It has been said by some of the opponents of this bill that maternal instinct and general intelligence are sufficient to guide a mother safely through pregnancy and in the care of her babies. Those who are familiar with the modern science of medicine and hygiene realize the fallacy of such an argument. . . . The point has also been made by our opponents that agencies would be allowed by this bill to enter private homes. I should like again to describe the practice prevailing among public health nurses. Their work lies entirely in the homes. Sometimes they are called to these homes by members of the family, sometimes by relatives and friends, sometimes by doctors or social workers, and sometimes by other agencies.
>
> When making a first call upon a family, they always explain who they are and why they have come. The family is at liberty to refuse them admittance if it chooses. It has been said that this bill will send large numbers of untrained individuals into private homes. Public health nurses cannot be called untrained individuals. They are not looked upon as nuisances by the people of this country. On the contrary, they are so sought after that they cannot begin to accomplish all the work which they are called upon to do.[14]

The bill's proponents pointed to the high infant and maternal death rates in America, especially in rural areas, compared with other countries. They showed that the latest medical advances were not being extensively used and argued that federal grants would greatly encourage improved care. Senator William S. Kenyon led the fight for the bill, stating: "There are about 250,000 infants who die every year in this country during their first year of life, and approximately 20,000 mothers. The comparison of the infant mortality and maternal mortality of the United States with that of other countries is not pleasing to an American citizen."[15]

Senator Sheppard also spoke strongly in favor of the bill. He noted that it had wide bipartisan support and had been endorsed in 1920 by both presidential candidates. He concluded, "If this Nation declines to take the necessary steps to end the appalling waste of the lives of mothers and children in America, a destruction exceeding every year our total casualties in the most stupendous and terrible war of history, it will invite severest censure."[16]

Opposition to the bill was led by Senator James A. Reed of Missouri. In discussing the leaders of the Children's Bureau who would be administering the program, Reed attacked the "absurdity of putting in charge of a question of maternity and child rearing a band of women who have never had any experience and who have chosen to remain in a condition of single blessedness," because it seemed to him "that they are the last people in the world to whom a position of that kind ought to be consigned." Senator William Borah also opposed the bill because, whatever its merits, he thought it "one of those measures which under the present economic conditions in this country can wait."[17]

After some minor amendments were adopted on the Senate floor, S. 1039 was finally passed by a vote of 63 to 7. On passage of this bill, opposing Senator Reed suggested an amendment of the title of the bill to read, "A bill to authorize a board of spinsters to control maternity and teach the mothers of the United States how to rear babies."[18] The Reed amendment was rejected. The bill was passed by the House of Representatives with only a few amendments. On November 21, the Senate concurred with the House version of the bill, and on November 23, 1921, President Harding signed it into law.

A separate division of the Children's Bureau was organized to administer the Sheppard-Towner Act. Three physicians, two nurses, an auditor, and a few clerks made up the staff of the Division of Maternity and Infancy at its headquarters in Washington. The Board of Maternity and Infancy met three or four times a year to act on the plans submitted by the states. There were no standards for state guidance, and the states were simply required to use federal and matched funds "in promoting the welfare and hygiene of maternity and infancy."[19] Usually physicians were in charge of the state programs, but in nine states the work was directed by nurses.

WORK OF THE SHEPPARD-TOWNER NURSES

Attempts were made to demonstrate the value of maternity and infancy care to local communities by sending a nurse to a community for a specified period to initiate a maternity and infancy program. It was more common for states to provide funds to communities to employ additional public health nurses as part of a general public health nursing

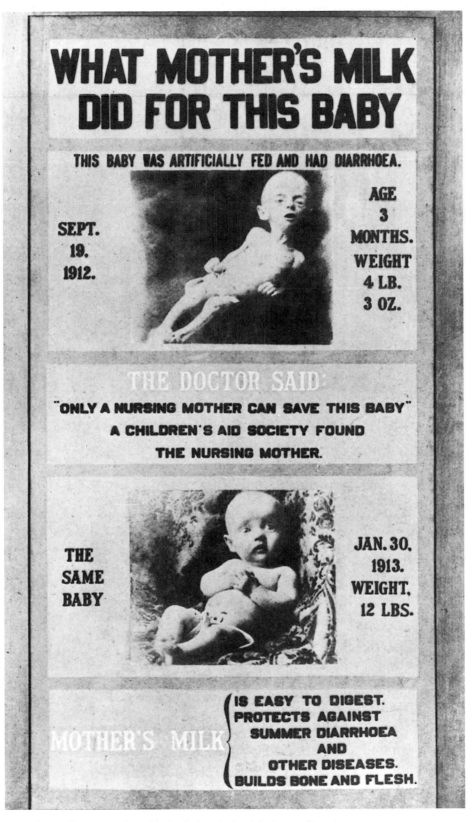

Educational efforts played a critical role in reducing infant mortality rates.

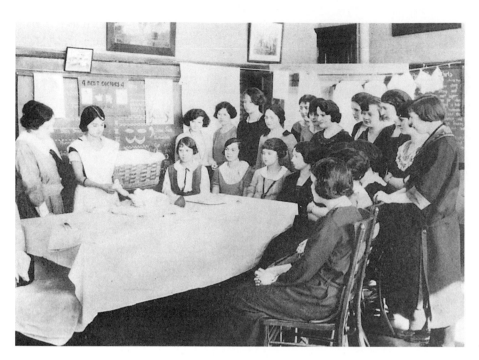

A demonstration in infant care.

program, which included maternity and infancy work. Under this plan, the share of the expense paid by maternity and infancy funds was prorated according to the time given to this phase of the program.

Home visits formed an important part of the work of child hygiene nurses. These informal visits provided mothers with excellent opportunities to ask questions and discuss their problems. The nurses used this time to assess the child for possible physical defects and to suggest that the family physician be consulted if problems were evident. The need for medical attention during pregnancy was constantly stressed. Surprisingly, many women had no concept of the value of a physician's care during this critical period and had to be taught that proper prenatal supervision lessened the possibility of complications during pregnancy and promoted the health of mother and child.

One of the problems experienced by the nursing supervisors was difficulty in recruiting trained and experienced nurses for county assignments in maternity and infancy. State directors attempted to deal with this roadblock in various ways. One method was to teach nurses who had been out of school for some years about the newer methods of maternity and child care, particularly in the areas of nutrition, infant feeding, and the routine to be followed in prenatal care. The directors also drew on the experiences of nurses who had organized successful clubs, classes, and consultation centers for mothers. Statewide meetings and institutes for maternity and infancy nurses were held in conjunction with state nursing association meetings. Regional and group conferences on local problems were arranged, and newsletters, lending libraries, and other devices were

used to maintain the professional standard of rural maternity nursing. Members of the state staffs also gave lectures on maternity and infancy care at training schools and public health nursing classes.

ALLEVIATING THE THREAT OF INCOMPETENT MIDWIVES

Another serious problem that existed in several sections of the country was the supervision and training of lay midwives. An astonishingly large percentage of

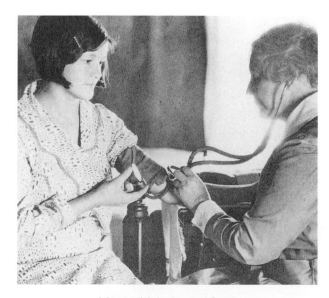

A home visit in the rural South.

births were attended by midwives. They were employed extensively throughout the United States, especially by mothers of foreign birth and by those living in isolated communities. It was estimated that in Iowa fewer than 1% of births were attended by midwives, whereas in Louisiana and Mississippi approximately 50% were attended by midwives. In the nation as a whole, midwives attended about 30% of all deliveries.

The extensive employment of midwives was due in part to objections by the prospective mother or her husband to having a male physician at delivery and also to the family's inability to pay the obstetrician's or general practitioner's fees. "Twenty-five dollars for confinement, if without complications, will be about the average country physician's minimum charge," wrote Samuel Hopkins Adams. "Reasonable though this is, it is still a heavy tax upon a struggling family. A local woman with some little reputation as a 'helper' will come in, more out of kindness than with an expectation of reward, and be quite satisfied with a 'present' of two or three or perhaps five dollars."[20]

A study made by Anne E. Rude of the Children's Bureau indicated that in 31 states in 1923 there were 26,627 midwives authorized to practice, and in those and other states more than 17,000 were practicing without authorization. It was useless to prohibit them from practicing. Any woman had the right to call in a neighbor to help her during confinement, and that

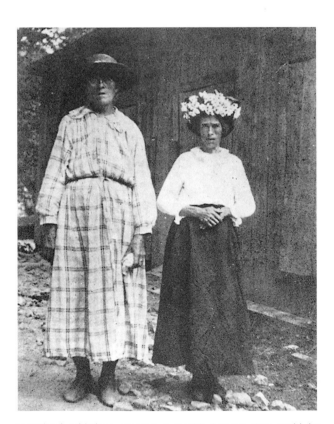

Untrained midwives created a health hazard that could be reduced through educational activities.

neighbor became a midwife. Many were illiterate and superstitious and thus were not receptive to training; yet it was imperative to teach them the importance of cleanliness, if nothing else. Thus classes for midwives were held regularly, with the support of Sheppard-Towner funds, in at least 19 states.

IMPACT OF THE SHEPPARD-TOWNER ACT

Before the introduction of the Sheppard-Towner bill, 12 states had established child hygiene divisions or bureaus. At the expiration of the act in 1929, 45 states and Hawaii had child health agencies. These states reported that for the period from 1924 to 1929, 144,777 health conferences for expectant mothers and children had been held by nurses and physicians, and 2978 permanent prenatal and child health centers had been established. During the last 6 years of the Act, public health nurses had made more than 3 million home visits to mothers and babies, and during the last 5 years of the Act, a total of 19,723 classes for high school girls, mothers, and midwives had been conducted. More than 22 million pieces of literature on infant and maternal care had been distributed, and approximately 700,000 expectant mothers and 4 million infants and preschool children were reported to have been reached in one way or another.

The effect of the Sheppard-Towner Act and other measures on the decline in the infant death rate was well documented. In 1928 it had fallen from the 1915 rate of 100 for each 1000 births to 69 per 1000 births. The greatest decrease was in the death rate from gastrointestinal disease—a direct result of informing the public about proper methods of infant care and feeding.

Strong efforts were made to renew the Sheppard-Towner Act after Congress allowed it to lapse in 1929, but these were unsuccessful in the face of the reigning political conservatism. The American Medical Association opposed its continuation in the sweeping terms of a resolution of its House of Delegates: "Resolved that the House of Delegates condemns as unsound in policy, wasteful and extravagant, unproductive of results and tending to promote communism, the federal subsidy system established by the Sheppard-Towner Maternity and Infancy Act and protests against a renewal of that system in any form."[21] Public health nurses supported a renewal and watched the course of debate with deep interest and anxiety, but their concern was of no avail.

MARGARET SANGER: NURSE ACTIVIST

The attack on maternal and infant mortality was given additional support by the birth control movement. In the United States the birth rate per 1000 women aged 15 to 44 years declined precipitously,

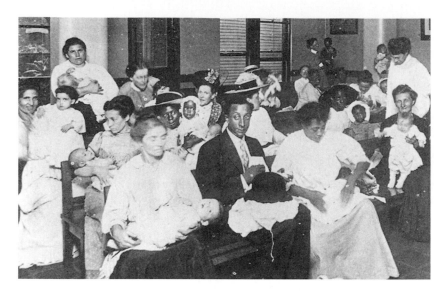

An infant and child clinic, New York City.

from 127 in 1910 to 89 in 1930, a decline of 38% in a single generation. Despite the unfavorable legal situation for birth control advocates, many Americans considered the declining birth rate a healthy development, asserting that a prime cause of poverty would be removed if birth control were practiced by the poor as well as by the well-to-do. Braving legal opposition, Margaret Higgins Sanger, a determined public health nurse in New York City, spearheaded this movement.

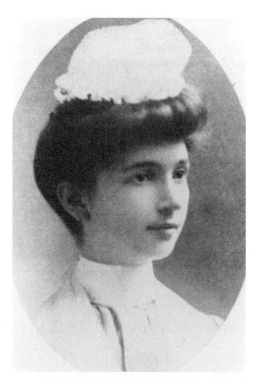

Margaret Sanger as a nursing student at the White Plains Hospital near New York City.

Born on September 14, 1883, in Corning, New York, Margaret Higgins attended the White Plains Hospital, a 25-bed facility where, according to her autobiography, the experience was rigid and sometimes inhumane. She recalls that in her second year she underwent surgery and just 2 weeks later was assigned to night duty. With her right shoulder still bandaged, she could use only her left hand in caring for the patients, all of whom were in serious condition. Higgins received part of her training through an affiliation with the Manhattan Eye and Ear Hospital, where she met William Sanger, an architect and aspiring artist, whom she later married. For the first few years of their married life, the Sangers lived in prosperous Westchester County, and her husband commuted to New York to work. During these years she gave birth to three children and devoted herself to homemaking.

Shortly thereafter Margaret Sanger began to develop an empathy for the millions of Americans who were living a hand-to-mouth existence. Particularly, she was drawn to the plight of industrial workers, such as those in Lawrence, Massachusetts, where, according to a 1912 United States Labor Commissioner's report, the median family income, with both parents working, was approximately $12 to $14 per week. When only the father worked, the median family income was barely $8. In "high-income" families, the children always worked.

Thus, it was not surprising that a labor strike during January and February of 1912 took 30,000 Lawrence workers away from their jobs in the cotton and woolen mills. Bound to affect the entire textile industry of the United States, the strike was seen as a clash between the radical forces of labor and the reactionary agents of big business. Because the primary reason for the failure of previous walkouts had been the near starvation of the strikers' children, it was decided that the children should be sent to the homes of labor sympathizers in New York until the issue was settled.

Because Sanger's interest in the plight of underpaid workers was well known among militant New York laborers and because she was a trained nurse, she was asked to direct the evacuation of the children from Lawrence. Their condition appalled her:

> We found the boys and girls gathered in a Lawrence public hall, and, before we started, I insisted on physical examinations for contagious diseases. One, though ill with diphtheria, had been working up to the time of the strike. Almost all had adenoids and enlarged tonsils. Each, without exception, was incredibly emaciated.
>
> Our hundred and nineteen charges were of every age, from babies of two or three to older ones of twelve to thirteen. Although the latter had been employed in the textile mills, their garments were simply worn to shreds. Not a child had on any woolen clothing whatsoever, and only four wore overcoats. Never in all my nursing in the slums had I seen children in so ragged and deplorable a condition.[22]

By the next week the situation in Lawrence had deteriorated to the point where violence broke out, and some of the parents had been beaten and arrested by the police. In Washington, Representative Victor Berger of Wisconsin was instrumental in securing a congressional investigation of the conditions responsible for the strike. The House Committee on Rules called Sanger to Washington to testify on the physical condition of the children:

> *Rep. Edward E. Pou:* Did you talk with those children about their manner of living in Lawrence and about the food they got?
>
> *Mrs. Sanger:* Yes, sir. I am a trained nurse, and I was especially interested in the condition of the children.
>
> *Mr. Pou:* Now, as a rule, is it true that the children of the working people in Lawrence—the class we are investigating—now only got meat once a week?
>
> *Mrs. Sanger:* Those were the assertions of not only the children but of the parents that I interviewed.
>
> *Rep. Martin B.:* You say you are a trained nurse?
>
> *Mrs. Sanger:* Yes, sir.
>
> *Mr. Foster:* And what was the physical appearance of these children that you took to New York? You know something about how they should look; were they properly nourished?
>
> *Mrs. Sanger:* Well, the condition of those children was the most horrible that I have ever seen.
>
> *Mr. Foster:* Tell the committee something about how they looked.
>
> *Mrs. Sanger:* In the first place, there were four little children who had chicken pox that we kept there; we would not allow them to go away; and then one of the children had just gotten over chicken pox, and the father begged us to let the child come; he had one

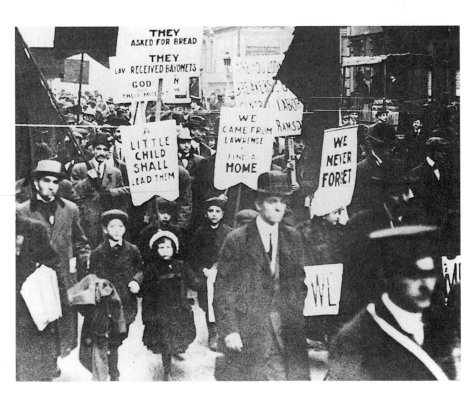

Sanger was appalled by the condition of the children of the striking mill workers of Lawrence, MA.

two-year-old and another 3 1/2 years old, I believe, and he begged us to let those children come because he was a widower and had no wife or anyone to take care of these children; he left them with the neighbors during the day. So I took these little children, and we isolated them on the way to New York, and when we got there they were placed under doctor's care. All of these children were walking about there apparently not noticing chicken pox or diphtheria; one child had diphtheria and had been walking around, and no attention paid to it at all, and had been working up to the time of the strike. Out of the 119 children, four of them had underwear on, and it was the most bitter weather, we had to run all the way from the hall to the station in order to keep warm; and only four had underwear.

Rep. Robert L. Henry: Kindly read the letter I now hand you to the committee.

Mrs. Sanger (reading):

New York, February 1, 1912

To whom it may concern:
    We, undersigned Italian doctors invited to make a preliminary physical examination of the Lawrence strikers' children, verified that all children were of poor physical build, defective, and underfed. The majority of them had enlarged glands, throat, nose, eyes, defective and affected. All were poorly clad even against the rigor of the season.

(*And signed by six physicians.*)

Rep. William W. Wilson: Where did those doctors live?

Mrs. Sanger: They were physicians of the Italian Federation of New York City, who volunteered their services to take charge of the children while in New York.

Rep. Irvin W. Lenroot: Have you had an opportunity to become familiar with the condition of the children of other workers in other places?

Mrs. Sanger: Yes, I have.

Mr. Lenroot: Can you give the committee any information as to how the condition of these children compared with that of other children in similar circumstances of life?

Mrs. Sanger: Yes. I have been brought up in a factory town where there are glassblowers and children of glassblowers, and I must say that I have never seen in any place children so ragged and so deplorable as these children were. I have never seen such children in my work in the Italian districts of New York City; in the slum districts, I must say, there are always a few of them who are fat and rugged, but these children were pale and thin.[23]

After nearly 2 months had elapsed and the workers had failed to return, the mills began to offer concessions. The strike committee, seconded by the cheers of an outdoor mass meeting, voted to accept. Within a few days almost everyone was back in the factories, with substantial wage increases all along the line.

After her involvement in labor strife, Sanger, in the spring of 1912, returned to her nursing career, working as a public health nurse. She was assigned to care for maternity cases on New York City's crowded Lower East Side, where she found that:

> Pregnancy was a chronic condition among the women of this class. Suggestions as to what to do for a girl who was "in trouble" or a married woman who was "caught" passed from mouth to mouth—herb teas, turpentine, steaming, rolling downstairs, inserting slippery elm, knitting needles, shoe hooks. When they had word of a new remedy they hurried to the drugstore, and if the clerk were inclined to be friendly he might say, "Oh, that won't help you, but here's something that may." The younger druggist usually refused to give advice because, if it were to be known, [he] would come under the law; midwives were even more fearful. The doomed women implored me to reveal the "secret" rich people had, offering to pay me extra to tell them; many really believed I was holding back information for money. They asked everybody and tried anything, but nothing did them any good. On Saturday nights I have seen groups of from 50 to 100 with their shawls over their heads waiting outside the office of a five-dollar abortionist.[24]

In mid-1912 Sanger took care of a 28-year-old mother of three who had attempted to abort herself. After 3 weeks under Sanger's care, the woman recovered and regained her health. When the physician made his last call, he admonished: "Any more such capers, young woman, and there'll be no need to send for me." "I know doctor," the convalescent replied, "but what can I do to prevent it?" The physician laughed good-naturedly. "You want to have your cake and eat it too, do you? Well, it can't be done. Tell Jake to sleep on the roof." She pleaded with Sanger: "Tell me the secret and I'll never breathe it to a soul, please!" Sanger could only remain silent. Three months later, the husband called and begged her to come at once. When she arrived, the wife was in a coma and death followed within minutes. Stunned and heartbroken, Sanger walked for hours through the New York streets. In years to come she would cite this experience as a turning point in her life. It was then that she decided to devote herself to learning about and disseminating information on contraception.[25]

First, she learned everything she could about methods of preventing pregnancy. There was very little such information available to the American public (although contraception was practiced widely in many European countries), largely because the Comstock Act of 1873 had classified contraceptive data with obscene matter and prohibited its passage through the mails. After 6 months of research at the Boston Public Library, the Library of Congress, and the New York Academy of Medicine, Sanger concluded that there was no practical medical information on contraception available in the United States. After a visit to France to study methods of birth control, she returned to the United States and published a journal, *The Woman Rebel*, which carried information on contraception and family planning along with a variety of other subjects pertaining to women's rights.

In 1916 Sanger opened the first birth control clinic in the United States, located at 46 Amboy Street in the Brownsville district of Brooklyn, a predominantly Jewish neighborhood. The clinic was operated by Margaret, her sister, Ethel Byrne (also a nurse), and Fania Mindell. Some 150 women sought assistance on the first day alone. For the next week everything went well, until a policewoman, disguised as a patient, arrested the sisters and Mindell and wrote down the names of the angry and frightened clients. To publicize the clinic's closure, Margaret Sanger refused to ride in the patrol wagon and walked the mile to the courthouse.

When she faced her charges in court several weeks later, Sanger found the courtroom filled with friends and supporters, and many reporters. It was difficult for the public to believe that the attractive woman seated with her two young sons was either oversexed or mentally ill, as her enemies would have it believed. Sanger did not deny the charge of having distributed birth control information; rather, she challenged the law that forbade such activity. The judge would have been lenient had she agreed to follow the law, but her response was: "I cannot respect the law as it stands today."[26] She was sentenced to 30 days in the workhouse.

Multilingual handbill advertising the first birth control clinic in America.

After serving her sentence, Margaret Sanger continued her crusade for many more decades. She allied herself with wealthy women, using their contacts and financial backing to further her cause. She gave lectures and organized meetings, such as the Birth Control Conference in New York City in 1921. That year she also helped establish the American Birth Control League, serving as its president until 1928, after which she founded the National Committee on Federal Legislation for Birth Control, a forerunner of the Planned Parenthood Federation. Her many books included *What Every Girl Should Know* (1916); *What Every Mother Should Know* (1917); *The Case for Birth Control* (1917); *Women, Morality, and Birth Control* (1922); *Happiness in Marriage* (1926); *Motherhood in Bondage* (1928); and *My Fight for Birth Control* (1931).

The opposition to Margaret Sanger's crusade for the free dissemination of birth control information continued for decades, the most vehement criticism coming from conservatives and various religious groups. Protestant churchmen disagreed on the moral issues involved in birth control. The Committee on Marriage and the Home of the Federal Council of Churches recommended in 1930 that the church should not seek to impose its point of view on the use of contraceptives by legislation or by any other form of force, and should not seek to prohibit physicians from imparting such information to those who in the judgment of the medical profession were entitled to receive birth control information. The general assembly of the Presbyterian Church, however, criticized this policy statement as morally dangerous. The Roman Catholic Church was uncompromising in its condemnation both of divorce and of birth control. The papal encyclical *Casti Conubii*, issued by Pope Pius XI in 1930, asserted that contraceptive devices were "an offense against the law of God and nature."[27] But despite strong opposition by many religious denominations, the effort to inform the public about ways of limiting families met a real social need and flourished. And, along with this crusade, the period from 1912 to 1930 saw a great surge in the number of public health nursing agencies in the United States, and this specialty quickly took its place as one of the most socially relevant occupations for graduate nurses.

REFERENCES

1. A. M. Brainard, *The Evolution of Public Health Nursing* (Philadelphia: W. B. Saunders Co., 1922), pp. 429–432.
2. Letters in Nutting Papers, Nursing Archives, Teachers College, Columbia University, New York.
3. Louis Dublin, *The Effect of Life Conservation on the Mortality of the Metropolitan Life Insurance Company* (New York: The Company, 1917), pp. 1–11.
4. Josephine C. Goldmark, *Nursing and Nursing Education in the United States* (New York: Macmillan Co., 1923), p. 9.
5. New York State Charities Aid Association, *Sickness in Dutchess County, New York: Its Extent, Care and Prevention* (New York: The Association, 1915), pp. 87–98.
6. New York Academy of Medicine, Public Health Committee, "Problems of Disease," *Modern Medicine*, vol. 2 (March 1920):1–23.
7. Edgar Sydenstricker, "Extent of Medical and Hospital Service in a Typical Small City," *Public Health Reports*, vol. 42 (January 14, 1928):121–131.
8. Samuel Hopkins Adams, *The Great American Fraud* (Chicago: American Medical Association, 1907), p. 70.
9. Clare Terwilliger, Unpublished report, Records of the U.S. Children's Bureau, National Archives, Washington, D.C., RG 102.
10. Michael M. Davis, *Immigrant Health and the Community* (New York: Harper & Brothers, 1921), pp. 308–309.
11. Ibid., pp. 309–310.
12. Louis I. Dublin, *The First One Thousand Midwifery Cases of the Frontier Nursing Service* (New York: Metropolitan Life Insurance Company, 1932), pp. 1–2.
13. Blanche Pegg Allen, Weekly report, Records of the U.S. Public Health Service, National Archives, Washington, D.C.
14. U.S. Congress, Senate, Committee on Education and Labor, *Protection of Maternity. Hearings Before the Committee, April 21, 1921* (Washington, D.C.: Government Printing Office, 1921), pp. 148–149.
15. *Congressional Record*, June 28, 1921.
16. Ibid.
17. Ibid., June 30, 1921.
18. Ibid., July 22, 1921.
19. U.S. Department of Labor, Children's Bureau, *Annual Report of Administration of the Maternity and Infancy Act* (Washington, D.C.: Government Printing Office, 1923), p. 23.
20. Samuel Hopkins Adams, "The Vanishing Country Doctor," *Ladies' Home Journal*, vol. 40 (October 1923):23.
21. American Medical Association, House of Delegates, *Proceedings of the Eighty-first Annual Session of the House of Delegates, June, 1930* (Chicago: The Association, 1930), pp. 35–41.
22. Margaret Sanger, *Margaret Sanger: An Autobiography* (New York: W. W. Norton Co., 1938), p. 81.
23. U.S. Congress, House, Committee on Rules, *The Strike at Lawrence, Massachusetts. Hearings before the Committee, March 2–7, 1912* (Washington, D.C.: Government Printing Office, 1912), pp. 226–229.
24. Margaret Sanger, op. cit., pp. 88–89.
25. Ibid., p. 92.
26. Ibid., pp. 93–96.
27. Ibid., p. 237.

DEPRESSION DOLDRUMS, 1930–1939

Whether the stock market crash of October 1929 precipitated the Great Depression or vice versa is still debated by economists. What is unarguable, however, is that in the 3 years following the crash, the whole American economy ran steadily downhill at a quickening and disastrous pace. Virtually every important industrial group suffered the same devastating erosion. Each responded in the only way it knew how: by cutting dividends, reducing inventories, laying off help, lowering wages and salaries, abandoning capital improvements, and going on reduced schedules.

Unemployment, increasing rapidly and continuously after the stock market crash of October 1929, created a major relief problem in the United States. In January 1930, almost 4 million people were unemployed. The number rose to about 7 million by December of that year, and this figure was doubled by early 1933. It was difficult to exaggerate the utter collapse of national economic life that had occurred before Franklin D. Roosevelt took the oath of office on March 4, 1933. Business had sunk to 60% below the normal level. Exports were close to the lowest point in 30 years. More than 1400 banks had failed during 1932, and in the 2 weeks preceding Roosevelt's inauguration, at least 21 states and the District of Columbia had either declared a banking moratorium or were allowing their banks to operate under special regulations. To a nation waiting with tense expectancy, Roosevelt urged confidence and courage. "The only thing we have to fear," he asserted, "is fear itself." He promised a special session of Congress to deal with the emergency and declared that "our greatest primary task is to put people to work."[1]

UNEMPLOYED NURSES

Nurses were affected by the massive unemployment: An estimated 8000 to 10,000 graduates were out of work. Announcements such as the following became commonplace in the *American Journal of Nursing*:[2,3]

> Nurses who are contemplating coming to Binghamton, New York, to work, are advised not to do so as there is not enough work for nurses already here.
>
> Secretary, Alumnae Association
> Binghamton Training School

> District 1 (Birmingham) of the Alabama State Nurses' Association does not wish to be inhospitable but advises nurses planning to come here to do private duty, that unemployment is a serious problem in that branch of nursing here, many local nurses not making enough to live.
>
> Catherine A. Moultis

> To nurses contemplating coming to Miami we wish to present the following facts: There are several hundred nurses out of employment in Miami at the present time. There is less work here now than there has been at any time during the past eleven years. Florida has passed a state law that all nurses practicing their profession in this state pay a tax of $15, this being county and state tax. This, added to the state registration fee, makes a total of $25 that has to be put out in order to nurse in the State of Florida.
>
> Arrie Allen Lambert, Registrar

In 1932, a campaign to promote the hiring of graduate nurses and discontinue training schools along with provision for an 8-hour day for nurses was launched by the American Nurses Association. This move met with considerable resistance. J. A.

271

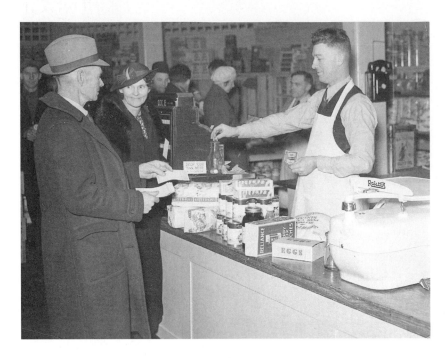

As the economic depression moved into 1933, business had sunk to 60% below normal.

Diekmann, superintendent of the Bethesda Hospital in Cincinnati, reported:

> There are today 68 Bethesda graduates in this city, victims of unemployment. To remedy this movement the national and state nurse organizations are forcing an issue that looks toward eliminating nurse schools from a large percentage of hospitals, and to employing only graduates for all hospital nursing work.
>
> But what would that mean in point of expense? We have made a careful study of what it would mean to Bethesda. The maintenance of our 112 students costs us $95,036 a year, or $848.53 a student. To do our nursing work through graduate nurses would cost us $132,107, or $37,071 more than student nursing. If we are compelled to give up our nurse school, where would we get that additional $37,071? Hospital rates cannot be raised. There is universal complaint of their being exorbitant now. Will the friends of the hospitals defray that additional large expense by more liberal contributions? The above movement would solve the nurse problem only to create an additional finance problem for the hospitals, most of whom now are in financial desperation.[4]

NURSES WORKING FOR ROOM AND BOARD

The suggestion that unemployed graduate nurses be hired by hospitals as graduate floor-duty nurses met with two general arguments. First, graduate floor duty as then organized was not considered respectable by many nurses; second, in the better hospitals, to which

graduates would naturally be attracted, there were virtually no positions available. Fifty-nine percent of the beds for sick patients were in hospitals that conducted training schools. The hospitals without schools were heavily staffed by so-called attendants. Of the hospitals with schools, 73% did not have a single graduate nurse on floor duty, and only 15% employed four or more.

The few graduates who were employed on floor duty in these hospitals were often looked down on by students. There was a general feeling among students that graduates on floor duty were unsuccessful private-duty nurses who were working in hospitals as a last resort. Floor duty was considered student work and in some schools not even student work, because the seniors who acted as head nurses thought their function was not bedside nursing but administration of the ward. Nurses who wanted to do bedside nursing after graduation found little encouragement. Few positions were open to them where they could render quality bedside care while retaining professional standing and dignity.

Amid dismal economic conditions, as 6000 to 8000 nurses found themselves unemployed, dignity became a luxury. Indeed, the question of the month for January 1933 in *Modern Hospital* was, "Should or should not graduate nurses be allowed to work for their board, room, and laundry?" Many penniless graduate nurses had applied to hospitals for work and were willing to accept room and board for their services. Should hospitals take them in? The nurses were not replacing other graduates but were probably replacing nursing students.

This query was sent to seven eminent hospital administrators representing various types of hospitals in different sections of the United States. The replies of

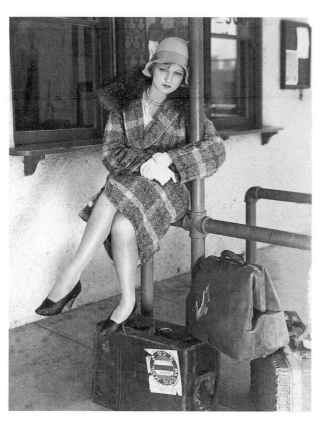

Many unemployed private-duty nurses headed to California for work.

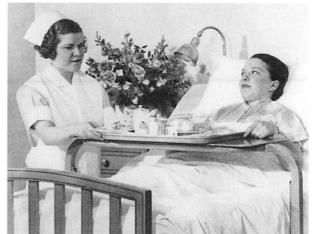

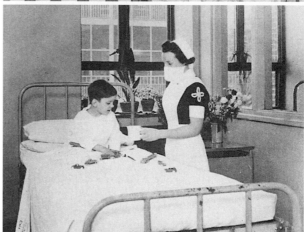

Hospital administrators debated whether graduate nurses were worth room and board.

these authorities were diverse. Dr. Donald C. Smelzer, director of the Graduate Hospital of the University of Pennsylvania, thought that this question should be settled primarily by the nurse and secondarily by the hospital. He thought that if the nurse voluntarily applied for work under such conditions, the hospital was justified in accepting her services. In return, the hospital should give her the type of work that would materially benefit her career. She should be placed on duty in a specific department (e.g., the operating room or the eye, ear, nose, and throat; medical; or bronchoscopic department) and thus have every opportunity to "brush up." Meanwhile, the hospital administration should not reduce either graduate or student nurse staffs to compensate for this additional service.

Dr. Maurice H. Rees, director of the Colorado General Hospital in Denver, answered that his hospital did not favor giving room, board, and laundry to unemployed nurses in return for limited amounts of service. His objections were, first, that nurses working only for room, board, and laundry as a rule gave inferior service and often were not even worth their food and lodging, and second, that he was sure no hospital budget could bear the expense of the additional board and laundry that these extra graduate nurses were sure to cause.

Grace Crafts, superintendent of Madison (Wisconsin) General Hospital, believed that the period of unemployment was a difficult time for the nursing

profession as a whole and for the private-duty nurse especially. Economic conditions called for close cooperation between the graduate nurse and the hospital. She felt strongly that hospitals should be helpful and sympathetic and should not take advantage of the unemployed nurse. To accept from her a full day's work in exchange for room, board, and laundry was in her opinion taking most unfair advantage of the graduate nurse's helpless situation.

Nonetheless, the Great Depression failed to reverse general long-term trends in women's employment. Indeed, by almost every measure, women's participation in work outside the home increased during the 1930s. Women's share of the labor force grew from 22% to 25%, while the percentage of all adult women who were in the work force rose from 24.3% to 25.4%. The proportion of married women who were employed grew from 12% to 15% during the decade, while married women increased their share of the female labor force from 29% to 35.5%. Such changes were consistent in direction, if not in rate, with trends that had been evident since the turn of the century.

Fashion considerably altered the female silhouette from the beginning to the end of the 1930s.

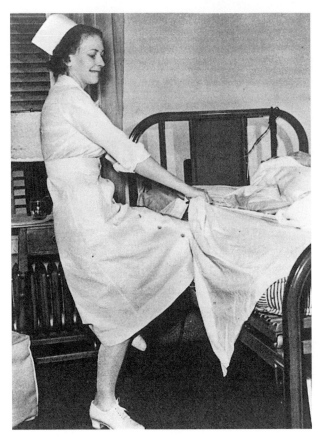

Graduate nurses moved into jobs on hospital staff.

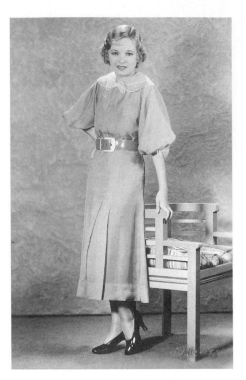

Hemlines dropped during the negative economic mood of the 1930s.

Early in the decade, hemlines were uneven, often with flounces or drapery that dipped below the basic skirt line or sometimes high in front and low in back. In reaction to the knee-high styles of the 1920s, hemlines went down almost to the ankles and then remained about 10 or 12 inches above the floor during the early 1930s. Gradually, the hems went up until they were 15 to 17 inches from the floor in 1939.

NURSES TAKE TO THE SKY

As the Depression deepened, a new field opened up for a limited number of nurses as airplane travel became common. In 1926 there had been about 50 so-called airlines in existence within the United States, but the onset of the Depression had forced widespread consolidation. United Airlines was put together by Boeing Aircraft through an amalgamation of smaller carriers. Other corporations molded competitors: American Airlines by Avco, TWA by Curtiss Wright, and Eastern by General Motors. Delta was the outgrowth of a Georgia crop-dusting company. By the early 1930s, the airline passenger market was not increasing to any noticeable degree because of the number of airplane crashes and the attendant publicity. The president of one airline admitted that he never flew in his company's plane whenever he

could possibly avoid it and further revealed that his wife refused to fly at all. What is more, the Department of Commerce reported that in 1930, the airlines on average were only filling 5 of 12 available seats per aircraft. The larger carriers realized that to survive they must improve their image and counter the widespread fear of flying.

The determination of air transport companies to make their mode of travel appear to be as safe and healthy as possible by having a trained health provider on hand for all emergencies created a new role for the nurse. There were few other lines of work open to the nurse that offered such thrilling experiences as the post of nurse-stewardess on one of the early passenger planes of the major air transport lines. Beginning in mid-1930, the major airlines would employ only graduate nurses of proven ability, and although the field was new and positions were relatively few, the work had a strong appeal. This was evidenced by the fact that in the first few months of 1931 there were more than 5000 applications from nurses for positions on the transcontinental passenger planes of United Airlines alone. The title "stewardess" was used even though it was considered inadequate. "Nurse" was a term too suggestive of the occurrence of illness en route, a contingency that arose much less frequently than was generally supposed.

The transcontinental planes of the early 1930s carried 14 passengers and a crew of three—pilot, copilot, and stewardess. With an average speed of 155 miles

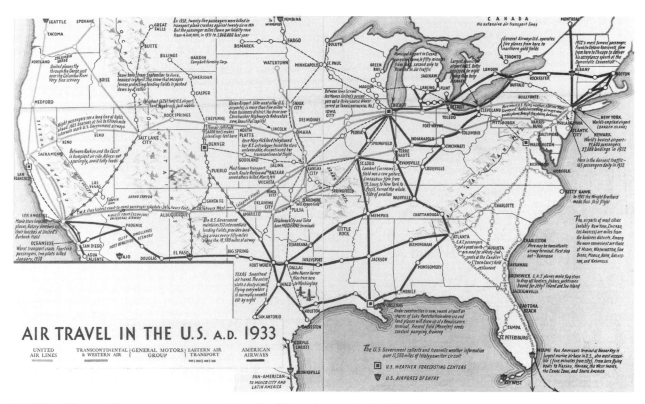

In 1933, airlines could transport a passenger from New York to Los Angeles in 28 hours.

per hour, the passenger planes never flew in bad weather, and it took 2 days of good flying conditions to go coast to coast. The cabin looked a little like a small Pullman chair car, but everything was made of the lightest material possible. The wicker chairs adjusted to comfortable couches for night runs, and each had its window with an arrangement for regulating the amount of air admitted, together with a coatrack and an individual electric light. The heating system ran off the engines.

The nurse-stewardess was responsible for the passengers' pillows and blankets, pillow slips, seat-back covers, towels, napkins, trays, vacuum bottles, and, most important, the first-aid kit. She also had supplies of stationery and airmail stamps, recent magazines, and in-flight literature issued by the company.

Early passenger planes did not have pressurized cabins, and when the planes climbed higher than 12,000 feet, many passengers experienced nausea. Airsickness could, in most cases, be prevented by systematic alkalinization before starting on a trip, and when it occurred, the use of an alkaline effervescent was often sufficient to overcome it. If there were signs of faintness, the patient might be entirely relieved by inhalation from a crushed ammonia ampule. The nurse-stewardess also carried amobarbital, which helped to induce sleep in nauseated passengers and was also useful in caring for extremely nervous travelers. Persons fearful of high altitudes were assured that fatalities among passengers from that cause were unknown.

To allay the passengers' fears of air travel, the nurse-stewardess thoroughly informed them about the precautions taken to prevent crashes. She regularly pointed out to the passengers the beacon lights and emergency landing fields that were situated 20 to 30 miles apart along the transcontinental route, explaining that a pilot was never more than a few minutes from a place where he could land the plane in case of emergency. The nurse-stewardess was instructed to always remain calm and composed, no matter how grave the crisis.

Many pilots looked on the young women as rank intruders. The hard-working newcomers won their respect before long, however, and came to be regarded as valuable members of the crew. The common belief was that stewardess service was merely a fad, but this was disproved as more and more nurses were employed.

COMMITTEE ON THE COSTS OF MEDICAL CARE

Meanwhile, attempts at health care reform were being pushed. The question of payment was only one of the many complex problems of medical care addressed in 1927 by the Committee on the Costs of Medical Care, a group of representative physicians, public health officers, social scientists, and laymen representing the public. With the financial support of eight foundations, the committee undertook a

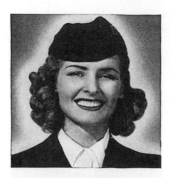

Careers In the Air for Registered Nurses

• American Airlines, Inc., plans to employ and train 100 additional registered nurses for stewardess positions within the next few months. Graduates are assigned to regular service on the Flagships of American's nation-wide air transportation system. The basic requirements are: (1) Registered nurse. (2) Age: 21-26 (inclusive). (3) Weight: not to exceed 125 pounds. (4) Height: not to exceed 5′6″. (5) Pleasing appearance. For complete information address: Personnel Department, American Airlines, Inc., New York Municipal Airport, New York, N. Y.

AMERICAN AIRLINES *Inc.*
ROUTE OF THE FLAGSHIPS

Thousands of nurses sought work in the new occupational health nursing role of nurse-stewardess.

5-year study to determine how to provide "adequate, scientific medical care to all the people, rich and poor, at a cost which could be reasonably met by them in their respective stations in life."[5] Dr. Ray Lyman Wilbur, president of Stanford University and former president of the American Medical Association (AMA), was chairman of this distinguished committee, which included 24 physicians, 3 dentists, and 2 nurses.

The committee revealed the results of its extensive studies in December 1932. The nation's annual medical bill was found to be approximately $3.5 billion, 30% of this amount going to physicians, 24% to hospitals, 12% to dentists, 19% for medicines, 5% for private-duty nurses, 3% for public health work, and 7% for all other purposes. For the whole population, payments by private individuals for medical care were found to average $24 per person, or about $108 per family.

A special study of 9000 families over 12 months showed that although the need for medical care was approximately the same regardless of economic status, only one seventh of the wealthy went without medical attention during the year, whereas the proportion was one fourth among the middle class and one half among the poor. Neither rich nor poor were receiving the care they needed. The committee also found that the incomes of medical practitioners—physicians, dentists, and nurses—were not excessive and in many cases were even inadequate. Unrestricted specialization, uncoordinated establishment of facilities, and uneconomical distribution of personnel were declared responsible for extensive waste.

The chief difficulty appeared to be that the individual family could not budget medical costs because of the unpredictability of sickness. To meet this difficulty, the committee pointed to a variety of experiments in organized medical service that had been developing in recent years under the sponsorship of hospitals and public health, industrial, or medical agencies. These included low-rate hospital services, pay clinics, public health nursing, organized service by trained nurse-midwives, government hospitals, tax-supported physicians in rural areas, state aid for local medical service, and university medical services. Several plans had been put into operation under commercial sponsorship, such as installment payment for medical care through loan companies and medical benefit corporations operating for profit—practices strongly disapproved by the professional groups in general. These businesses sold insurance services provided through contracts with individual practitioners and hospitals.

The committee's five basic recommendations were condensed as follows:

> That medical care be furnished largely by organized groups of physicians, dentists, nurses, pharmacists, and other associated personnel, centered around a hospital, and rendering home, office, and hospital care.
>
> That all the basic public health services be extended until they are available to the entire population, according to its needs.
>
> That the cost of medical care be placed on a group payment basis through the use of insurance, taxation, or both methods, without precluding the continuation of the individual fee basis for those who prefer it.
>
> That a specific organization be formed in every community or state for the "study, evaluation, and coordination of medical services."
>
> That the professional education of physicians, dentists, pharmacists, and nurses be reoriented to accord more closely with present needs, and that educational facilities be provided to train three new types of workers in the fields of health; namely, nursing attendants, nurse-midwives, and trained hospital and clinical administrators.[6]

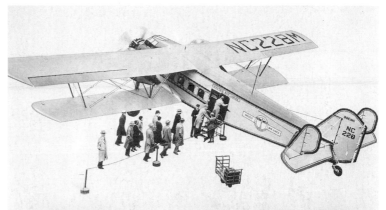

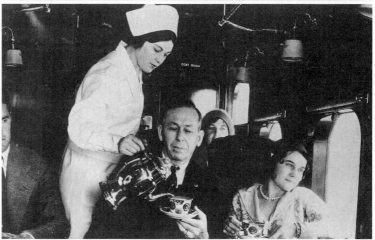

A Boeing 80 passenger plane and nurse-stewardess in the early 1930s.

ATTACK BY THE AMA

Few physicians were impressed by these findings. R. G. Leland, M.D., director of the Bureau of Medical Economics of the AMA, spearheaded the AMA's

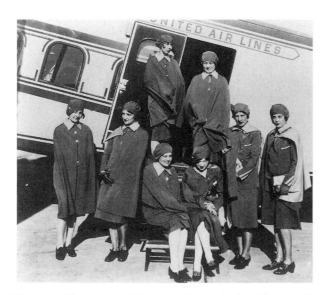

The tens of thousands of flight attendants who fly airlines worldwide owe their careers to the pioneer work of these registered nurses, hired by United Airlines in May 1930.

attack on the group-hospitalization idea. He charged that such schemes were being suggested largely as a result of "tactics of desperation" in which hard-pressed hospitals sought "any port in a storm." He warned that all such plans tended to lessen the control of county medical societies over medical practice, thus decreasing the effectiveness of the most important form of professional control of standards and ethics while increasing the influence of lay commercial interests.

According to Leland, group hospital insurance plans tended also to extend hospital care beyond its proper scope: Patients who would ordinarily be cared for at home by a family physician would more often insist on going to the hospital, where they thought they had already paid for care. The broad effect of all such plans would be to shift the burden of hospital support from philanthropy to taxation of low-paid workers. Leland asked, "Does the public need at the present time an increased amount of hospital care, or will it benefit more from a greater amount of medical care in the home?"[7]

In December 1932, the editor of the *Journal of the American Medical Association*, Dr. Morris Fishbein, wrote an emotional denunciation of the report of the Committee on the Costs of Medical Care. Although this committee had been chaired by a former president of the AMA, who had been a member of

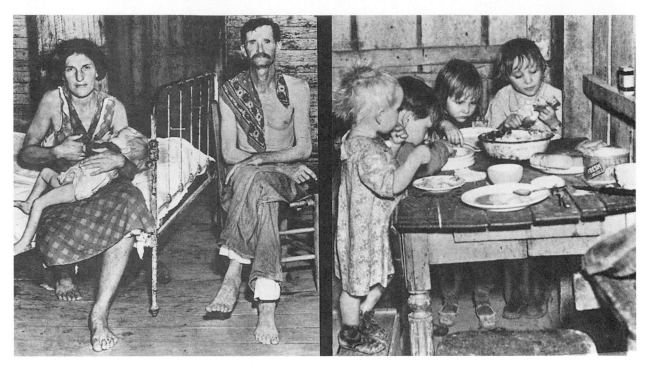

Poor people simply did without health care in the early 1930s.

President Hoover's cabinet, its report was declared to be "socialism and communism—inciting to revolution." [8] The studies and health demonstrations of several foundations—especially the Milbank Memorial Fund, the Julius Rosenwald Fund, and the Twentieth Century Fund—were criticized in a similar vein. Fishbein soon began the policy of issuing "research reports" that omitted facts unfavorable to AMA views and personally attacked persons who disagreed with AMA policy, rather than dealing with the issues they had raised. Fishbein's innumerable speeches, editorials, and articles were effective in unifying opinion on medical economic questions among most physicians.

Graduate nurses were much less agitated than their brothers in medicine over the dangers of socialized medicine, probably because they had long been accustomed to viewing their work as a service rather than as a business. Many nurses were becoming aware of their own need for financial security, and they were beginning to consider health insurance and other plans for illness and retirement more seriously.

EMPTY HOSPITAL BEDS AND SICK PEOPLE

During the early 1930s, about 1 in every 18 people entered hospitals in the course of each year, and the ills of as many more were diagnosed and treated in hospital outpatient departments. There were 6437 registered hospitals in the country in 1933, and hospital bed capacities had mounted steadily. The

so-called general hospitals—for patients having general or acute diseases—operated mainly under private or nongovernmental auspices. The average government hospital, however, was much larger, containing 162 beds, in contrast to the 72 beds in the average nongovernment hospital. In the Pacific Coast states, a considerably larger proportion of care was delivered through governmental facilities—43% in terms of bed capacity compared with 32% for the country as a whole.

According to an unpublished study by the Julius Rosenwald Fund, 42% of the counties in the United

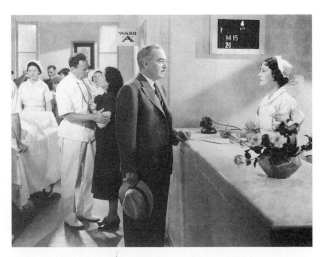

The average hospital occupancy rate fell to 55% in 1933.

States were without hospitals. These were mostly rural or sparsely settled areas, but in certain southern sections they included from 25% to 38% of the state populations. In a still larger group of counties, with a population of 44 million, there were plenty of beds in private general hospitals but no government general hospitals at all. In a smaller group, representing 5% of the counties and 3% of the population, general hospital care was entirely under government auspices.

Low occupancy was perhaps the greatest problem faced by nongovernmental hospitals. The average occupancy, which in 1923 was 62.8% of all available beds, had fallen by 1933 to 55.3%—the lowest being in hospitals owned by individuals or partnerships, which were running at 41.1% capacity. Industrial hospitals were operating with 44.4% of their beds filled and church hospitals at 54.9% capacity. During the same period, however, the rate of occupancy for governmental hospitals advanced from 79.4% to 90.1%. The relatively low occupancy of nongovernmental hospitals had existed before the Depression and had only been accentuated by it; probably there had already been an oversupply of hospital beds in some communities, whereas others had no hospitals at all.

Unlike other bills in the family budget, medical bills fell unevenly and unexpectedly. During the 1930s, in any given year, about half the people were healthy and had very low medical bills, about one third had moderate medical bills, and the remaining one sixth had very high bills. This unlucky one sixth paid half the total medical bills each year. No one could tell in advance whether his family, during the next year, would finish in the lucky half, the moderately fortunate third, or the unlucky sixth. Low income was a major cause of insufficient medical care, but the unpredictable incidence of sickness and the wider range of its costs meant a financial problem even for families far above the poverty level. In proportion, too, as people found it hard or impossible to pay medical bills, the incomes of physicians, dentists, hospitals, and private-duty nurses were unstable and often insufficient.

THE HOSPITAL INSURANCE IDEA

Hospital insurance plans in the United States have a longer history than many people realize. As far back as 1880, hospital-service insurance plans for the benefit of lumbermen had been in operation in northern Minnesota. In other parts of the country, particularly in remote communities such as mining and lumber camps, hospital and medical-service plans were common. In 1912, the Rockford Association was organized in Rockford, Illinois. Set up as a nonprofit Illinois corporation with membership open to any community resident older than age 15 and free from chronic illness, it included 6 weeks of hospital room and board and all operating room fees. In

1921, a hospital in Grinnell, Iowa, developed a plan covering the costs of room, board, and nursing for up to 3 weeks, exclusive of special services. Six years later, the Thompson Benefit Association for hospital service, organized in Brattleboro, Vermont, covered hospitalization expenses up to a maximum of $300, including surgeon's fees.

The plan generally considered to be the nearest prototype of modern hospital insurance systems was organized in 1929 by the schoolteachers of Dallas. In conjunction with Baylor University Hospital, approximately 1500 teachers were insured for hospital care at the rate of $6 per person per year. The plan provided for nursing care in rooms, board, operating room service, anesthesia charges, laboratory fees, routine medicines, surgical dressings, and hypodermics. Full coverage was provided for up to 3 weeks, with a 33% discount for longer periods. Each participant in the plan carried a card that entitled him or her to be admitted to Baylor University Hospital.

Under the leadership of Dr. Justin Ford Kimball, vice-president of Baylor University, the program was soon expanded and enrollment was opened to people other than schoolteachers. In 1929, the Baylor plan began with 1400 teachers; by 1933 the plan had 9388 group subscribers and had helped to cover the cost of 1832 patients with 20,500 patient-days. Members continued to be charged 50 cents per month. Various organizations, such as schools, businesses, and manufacturing plants, collected the monthly payments and submitted a list of participants along with the dues. The service, which brought in about $60,000 per year, was run at a slight deficit of 6% to 7%. This was not nearly as great a deficit as would have been experienced if some of the same patients had been hospitalized as free patients.

Hospitals, running around 50% occupancy, were desperately short of funds, and if they were to keep from going bankrupt, they needed to help devise a system that would not only enable sick people to pay their hospital bills but also encourage them to come to the hospital for care without fear of personal bankruptcy. Kimball pointed out that his new approach served the people when they needed hospitalization at a rate that they could pay. It was also beneficial to the physician in that it left funds for patients to meet their bills. Most important, it helped the hospital financially by guaranteeing the collection of its bills.

The recommendations of the Committee on the Cost of Medical Care gave individual hospital prepayment plans a great impetus for expansion. All these plans constituted a form of social insurance in which individuals or families, usually in employee groups, made equal and regular payments into a common fund used to provide service at a given hospital when required. In some communities, more than one local hospital set up its own plan, resulting in competition. By the end of 1934, nonprofit

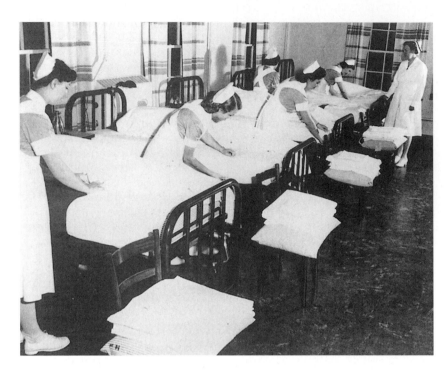

Hospital insurance was invented to fill empty beds.

community hospital service plans had begun to be established so rapidly that they were termed a national movement. In that year, the multihospital Associated Hospital Service Plan of New York (City) was organized under a special enabling act. The passage of this unique legislation was a landmark in the development of the movement. The state

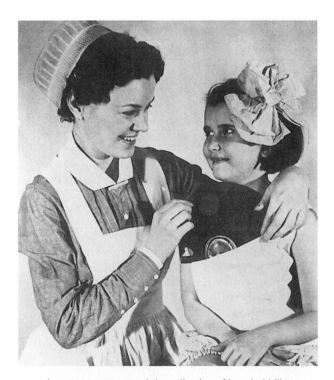

Insurance guaranteed the collection of hospital bills.

superintendent of insurance had ruled that the proposed hospital service plan was a form of insurance. Previously, in the other states where hospital plans had been set up, their sponsors had assumed that rather than operating insurance plans, they were merely selling hospital service on a prepayment basis. When the attorneys general or insurance departments of those states had been asked for a ruling, they had ruled to that effect, holding that the plans were exempt from the regulations covering stock and mutual insurance companies. This exemption was important in that it meant that subscribers did not have to be liable for assessments and that the plans could start without the large capital required of stock companies.

When the New York superintendent of insurance ruled that the proposed New York City plan constituted insurance, local civic leaders, hospital officials, and physicians drafted and sponsored a bill for a special enabling act, which was passed and became law on May 16, 1934. That act stated that any corporation organized for the purpose of operating a nonprofit hospital service plan should be exempt from all other provisions of the insurance law. It also stipulated that rates charged subscribers be subject to review by the insurance department and that the rates of payment to hospitals be subject to the approval of the welfare department. The operatives of such health insurance plans were declared to be charitable and benevolent institutions and exempt from state or local taxes other than taxes on real estate and office equipment. Thenceforth, in virtually all the remaining states, the passage of similar legislation was a prerequisite for the initiation of such plans.

BLUE CROSS

The American Hospital Association provided leadership in the development and coordination of hospital insurance plans. Those that were approved were allowed to use the name "Blue Cross." Such plans were sponsored locally by hospitals, the medical profession, and the general public. The principal initiative in the formation of a plan usually came from the county or state hospital association. Initial working capital was often provided not only by the hospitals but also by local community chests, business and civic organizations, foundations, and individual civic leaders. A Blue Cross plan was a nonprofit corporation organized under community and professional sponsorship and approved by the American Hospital Association for the purpose of enabling the public to defray the cost of hospital care on a prepayment, group basis. Benefits were paid in terms of hospital service rather than cash indemnity and were guaranteed by the participating hospital through contractual arrangements between the hospitals and the plan. An agreement between the subscriber and the plan listed the benefits to which the subscriber was entitled.

During the late 1930s, the annual cost of membership in Blue Cross plans ranged from $5 to $12 per subscriber, depending on the cost levels of the area, the kind of room accommodation received, the types of sickness covered, and the scope of services offered. A subscriber was admitted to any of the participating hospitals when necessary, but only under the care of a private physician selected by the patient. The typical subscriber paid his or her own physician's fee, but without charge received up to 21 days' care in the hospital, including a semiprivate room, nursing service, meals, the operating room, and x-ray and laboratory services.

The growth in enrollment of Blue Cross plans in the United States and Canada proceeded at a phenomenal rate. On July 1, 1938, the total enrollment was 1,949,294; 40 years later it would reach 85,000,000 Americans. Medical insurance, after a slower start owing to the conservatism of the AMA, soon expanded at a similar rate, much of it under the medical profession's Blue Shield emblem.

Some of the private life and casualty insurance companies had offered hospital and medical insurance for many years, but no widespread demand was built up until the Blue Cross and Blue Shield plans began to achieve national popularity by virtue of their service benefit feature and the low operating cost resulting from nonprofit operation. Moreover, as the American public became increasingly conscious of the advantages of medical care insurance, the commercial companies profited by the related publicity and sold their own health and medical policies more extensively than ever before.

Meanwhile, nurses, physicians, and hospital administrators began to note that the health of a large proportion of the population was being affected unfavorably by the Depression. The rate of disabling sickness was found to be 48% higher among families having no employed wage earners in 1932 than among families having full-time workers. The group of workers that had dropped from fairly comfortable circumstances to relief roles during the Depression showed a rate of disabling illness 73% higher than that of their more fortunate neighbors who had remained in the comfortable class.

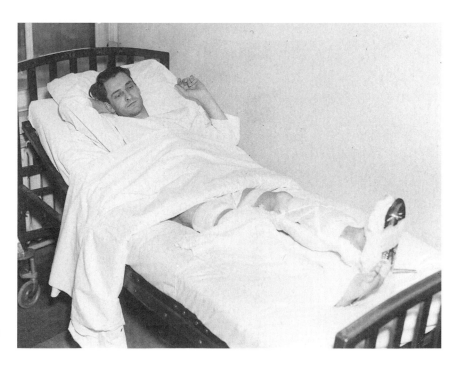

Blue Cross allowed patients to receive hospital service through insurance.

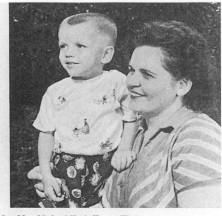

"Pneumonia put little Johnny in the hospital—but we didn't have to worry about the bills!"

"I'm sure glad we belong to BLUE CROSS!"

Says Mrs. Michael Krol, *Harvey, Illinois*

Blue Cross plans grew rapidly and enrollment skyrocketed.

In 1934, for the first time in many decades, the annual death rate in large cities was increasing despite the absence of any serious epidemics. Concurrently, with this evidence of increased need, local appropriations for public health had decreased 20% since 1930. The per capita expenditure from tax funds for public health in 53 cities in 1934 was only 77.5 cents compared with 93.8 cents in 1931.

FEDERAL HEALTH ACTION UNDER THE FEDERAL EMERGENCY RELIEF ADMINISTRATION

Public medical care had been provided by state or local governments to the indigent since colonial days. Nongovernmental agencies, especially local charity hospitals and dispensaries, had also given free care to the needy, but the treatment of the indigent had become more and more a task of government. Over the years, state and local governments had developed varying patterns of administration of public medical care, with a wide range in standards. As the Depression hit bottom in 1931 and 1932, these programs were threatened with disaster because of the great increase in the relief population and the corresponding fall in tax receipts. Accordingly, in 1933, the federal government entered the picture of medical care for the needy through the famous Regulation 7 of the Federal Emergency Relief Administration (FERA).

This administrative regulation stated that health care was a legitimate form of relief and that the regular federal program of grants-in-aid to the states for relief would also cover state programs for medical care in the home. The federal grants were to be confined to severe emergency sicknesses and were not to be used for hospitalization. By September 1934, 20 states had programs.

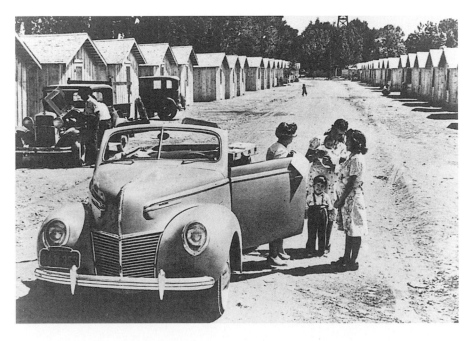

Federal Emergency Relief Administration funds brought jobs for nurses and nursing care for families on relief.

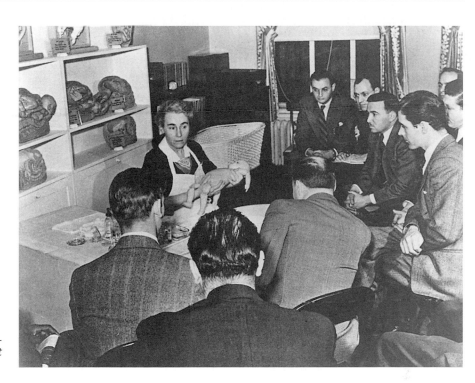

Relief nurses taught classes in prenatal and baby care to expectant mothers and fathers.

Payment for nursing care as well as for medical care of the sick in their homes was increasingly recognized as a legitimate relief expenditure. Under FERA, relief funds were allotted for bedside care to the indigent, and nursing services for patients receiving federal relief were purchased from private agencies with federal funds. The U.S. Public Health Service was consulted by FERA in planning this program and was called into vigorous action by many states and communities in helping to put projects into operation. Provision was made in the rules and regulations for setting up state advisory committees for nursing projects. Because the federal plan was permissive rather than mandatory, there was much variation state by state, but the principles involved were effectively carried out in many communities.

In West Virginia, for example, the Relief Nursing Service was inaugurated in February 1933 to meet the needs of nurses for employment and the needs of families on relief for nursing care. It was essentially a visiting nurse program. One hundred sixty-eight full-time registered nurses were employed in 55 counties under the direction of six district supervising nurses.

Most of these nurses had had no special training or experience in public health nursing. At the beginning of the program, the nurse had to be placed as quickly as possible. Typed instructions based on the principles and techniques of the National Organization for Public Health Nursing manual were given to each nurse by the state director of Relief Nursing. Within 2 months, an advisory committee of physicians was appointed, along with six supervising nurses. These supervising nurses were trained and experienced public health nurses. With the advice of the physicians' committee and the State Health

Department, the nursing service was organized in the various counties, and 1-day institutes were arranged in each district.

The nurses carried on four fundamental services for families on relief: (1) bedside nursing care and health supervision for the family in the home; (2) arranging for medical and hospital care for emergency and obstetric cases; (3) supervising the health of children in emergency relief nursery schools; and (4) caring for patients with tuberculosis. A special effort was made to secure physical examinations of all contacts in the home, and isolation of the patient was made possible in many counties through the construction of portable porches.

Nurses were also responsible for making arrangements for the family physician to attend relief patients needing their care. They saved the physicians many unnecessary calls by making first visits to all patients except in extreme emergencies. Immediate report was made to the physician on cases requiring his or her care, and nursing care was continued under the physician's direction.

Standing orders based on the National Organization for Public Health Nursing manual were given to the nurses of each county, to the physicians composing the county medical relief committee, and to the medical association. These orders, as approved, were carried out by the nurses until a physician gave other specific orders. Sick patients were not cared for by the nurses unless the case was directed by a physician. Emphasis was given to early, complete examination of prenatal cases and adequate provision for delivery and postpartum care of all mothers, no matter how inaccessible their homes might be. In many counties, the relief nurses organized classes for mothers and fathers in prenatal and baby care and for adults and children in personal hygiene, home nursing, and first aid.

NURSES UNDER CIVIL WORKS ADMINISTRATION PROGRAMS

With the conviction that because of the rapidly increasing volume of relief the winter of 1933 would be one of great hardship, Congress created an additional relief program, the Civil Works Administration (CWA), in November 1933. Jobs were provided to 4 million unemployed people on temporary projects submitted by local and state authorities or conducted directly by the federal government.

More than 10,000 unemployed nurses were put to work under the CWA. Nurses were employed in numerous settings: in public hospitals, institutions, and clinics; on public health staffs; in bedside nursing; in immunization campaigns and making surveys; and in many other health services. Health and nursing services were often carried to remote sections for the first time. In the state of Washington, for example, the public health departments had long been hampered in their work because of the necessity of cutting back expenditures. CWA gave them an opportunity to employ 300 needy nurses. Some of these nurses were so destitute that they had to be given clothing and shoes before they could accept work. With the corps of 300 additional nurses supervised by the public health nurses, from December 8, 1933, to March 15, 1934, thousands of Washington children were immunized against diphtheria and

were given smallpox vaccinations. In an area of the state inundated by floods, hundreds were given typhoid vaccine. The results summarized below were amazing, considering that only 300 nurses accomplished all this work within 3 months:

Number having bedside or nursing care	4668
Number of visits to TB patients	1830
Number of maternal care visits	3907
Number of pupils inspected in schools	286,193
Number of defects found	40,943
Number of corrections made	6048
Number of pupils excluded	3337
Number of conferences with parents	3447
Number of lectures or talks given	454

Data collected from more than 500 CWA nurses in New York about themselves showed the following characteristics:

Age: from 19 to 64 years; largest number from 23 to 26 years.

Preliminary education: 47% were high-school graduates; 3% had some college work.

Professional education: out of nurse training for 3 to 38 years; largest number less than 5 years.

Postgraduate courses: taken by 51 of them (9%).

Amount of employment in the year preceding FERA service: less than 6 months, 503; of these, 357 had less than 3 months.

Reasons for unemployment (sometimes a combination): unavailability of work, 476; housewife or other responsibilities, 99; illness, 47.

Average number of months on FERA: 8¼.

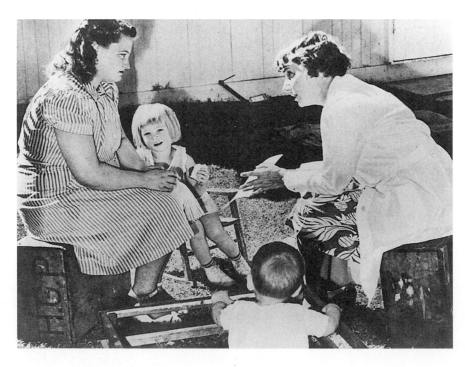

More than 10,000 unemployed nurses were hired by the Civil Works Administration to bring nursing services to needy families.

Duties to Which Assigned:

General public health	401
School	42
Dispensaries and clinics	36
Hospitals	25
Tuberculosis	23
Nutrition survey	18
Communicable disease	18
Records	8
Social hygiene	6
Camp	3
Preschool cardiac	1
Dental work	1
Swimming pool	1
Social service	1
Laboratory	1
Stockroom	1

Cost of transportation, weekly: city, $1.78; rural district, $5.21; town, $4.41; village, $1.40; county, $5.60. Average, $2.95 per week.

Transportation paid by: self, 236; public funds, 135; Visiting Nurses Association, 25; industrial firms, 3; friends, 3.

Reaction to work: very enthusiastic, 425; like it, 138; no remarks, 20; did not like it, 5.

Employment under the CWA program began on November 16, 1933, and the peak was reached on January 18, 1934, when more than 4,260,000 people were at work. It was considerably more costly than anticipated; nearly $1 billion was spent in wages and materials between November 1933 and April 1934, when the program was finally discontinued. Most of the 10,000 nurses it had carried were faced with unemployment again.

CWA marked the introduction of new principles in the relief of unemployment in the United States. It emphasized the claim that the unemployed wanted work and that the abstract right to a job should be supplemented by a public policy and program that provided a job. Furthermore, the right to a job was extended not only to the destitute unemployed but also to other jobless persons. Weekly wages paid on these projects were not related to family budgets but were based on prevailing rates in the community, and employment was provided for a fixed number of hours per week. The nursing projects were more substantial in character than those that had prevailed under FERA. CWA served well in priming the pump while it was operating. It set up standards for work-relief projects: all work had to have social and economic value, it could be performed only on public property, and projects could not include work normally performed by the state or localities.

THE WORKS PROGRESS ADMINISTRATION AND NURSES

The Works Program, established by the Emergency Relief Appropriation Act of 1935, was intended to "provide relief, work relief, and to increase employment by providing useful projects." As originally set up, it contemplated that a considerable amount of work would be directed by established government agencies whose activities could be expanded through employment of relief workers. But to give direction to the relief employment of these agencies and to provide many additional jobs, the Works Progress Administration (WPA) was established. This soon became the most important single unit in the Works Program. Projects to be approved by WPA, according to the original plan, had to be useful. They were to be of such a nature that a considerable proportion of the money spent would go into wages. Self-liquidating projects that promised ultimate returns to the federal treasury of a considerable proportion of the costs were to be sought. In all cases, projects had to be of a character to give employment to those on the relief rolls, and they were to be noncompetitive, if possible.

All WPA projects were sponsored by tax-supported bodies of states, counties, or towns and represented what the various communities desired and requested. The nursing and public health projects in all cases were sponsored by state or local departments of public health or similar public bodies or agencies. Office space and office and nursing equipment were contributed by the sponsor or by some community agency. The WPA paid the salaries of nurses, technicians, and assistants as required to render services that regular staffs of public health departments, because of their heavy burdens, were unable to provide.

Under many of the nursing projects, needy registered nurses, on the recommendation of physicians, went into underprivileged homes to assist with antepartum and postpartum care and also to render nursing service in cases of illness. They performed all types of duties generally listed under the heading of bedside nursing, such as bathing and caring for patients and preparing proper foods for the sick. WPA nurses were employed on projects to promote physical and oral hygiene. They assisted in a program to examine children for physical and dental defects and in immunization campaigns against whooping cough, typhoid fever, diphtheria, smallpox, and other diseases. On projects in some localities, WPA nurses assisted physicians in administering the Mantoux test.

During fiscal year 1936, approximately 6000 graduate nurses were employed on WPA projects of one type or another. WPA nursing and public health projects were operating in 37 states plus the District of Columbia. Up to September 15, 1936, WPA nurses had extended services to millions of people through 9 million visits, examinations, or treatments.

A nursing project under way in New Jersey was typical of WPA projects. In 45 school districts, the WPA project was supplying public health nurses in public schools where no such service previously existed, and in several other districts the project was supplementing inadequate regular service. As a result of this activity, 16 school districts had assumed full responsibility for nursing services and 10 project nurses had found permanent employment with the schools or with public health nursing organizations. As financial conditions permitted, other school districts proposed to undertake the work as a regular activity.

In Georgia, the WPA public health nursing program had been taken over by the State Department of Public Health and was a regular part of the state program. T. F. Abercrombie, state director of the Department of Public Health, said that the establishment of Georgia's public health nursing division was directly due to the inauguration of the state nursing project operating under the federal program. During the first year of the new state program, all but 46 of the 200 WPA nurses had succeeded in getting permanent work, thus removing them from WPA's rolls. During 1935, WPA nurses had given a half-million immunizations in Georgia. More than 400,000 general home nursing visits had been made, and 30,000 infants and preschool children had benefited from the health supervision of the WPA nursing project. Before the government projects were put into operation, there had been no public health nursing programs in the state.

In one county in Wyoming, a WPA nurse established a tonsil clinic that would admit any child in the county whose family was unable to employ a private physician. It had sometimes been necessary to transport patients more than 100 miles to obtain treatment from physicians who donated their services to the clinic. In the same county, the nurse had taken more than 40 persons with eye conditions to one of the leading eye specialists in the state.

Many other examples could be cited. In New York City, 6317 WPA physicians, nurses, research and clerical workers, scientists, and technicians fought against disease. Through project clinics, physicians on one project alone treated more than 18,000 victims of venereal disease between December 20, 1936, and January 20, 1937. Concurrently, 30,000 schoolchildren were treated in dental clinics. As a result of a drive in Charleston County, South Carolina, made possible by federal assistance, diphtheria had been reduced to a minimum. Within 12 months, graduate nurses visited 27,408 homes to persuade parents to protect their children from diphtheria by toxoid immunization.

Dr. J. Moss Beeler, county health commissioner and superintendent of the Spartanburg (South Carolina) County Hospital—which consisted of a general hospital, a hospital for blacks and outpatient and social service departments, an isolation unit, a nurses' home, a laboratory and other service units, and a tuberculosis department 2 miles away—declared, "We would have accomplished about a third of what we have actually accomplished during the past two years if it had not been for the services rendered by WPA nurses." Dr. Beeler was soon able to place 30 WPA nurses on the regular hospital payroll.

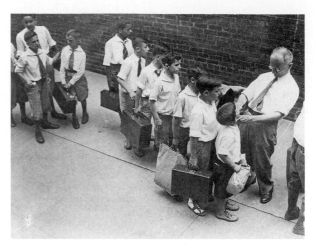

Schoolboys in New York City being examined before departing for a summer camp upstate for "the improvement of the poor."

THE SOCIAL SECURITY ACT OF 1935

To deal with the fundamental problems of economic insecurity, Congress passed the Social Security Act of 1935. This was the one New Deal measure clearly inspired by foreign example. Social security measures, first tried in Germany in the 1880s, had spread through western Europe as well as to Australia and New Zealand. They had also been tried in the United States by state governments and private employers.

The Social Security Act, as approved by the president on August 14, 1935, provided for (1) federal

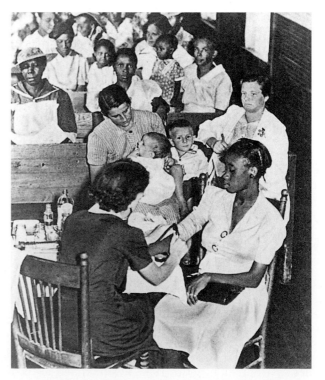

WPA funds allowed the expansion of prenatal care.

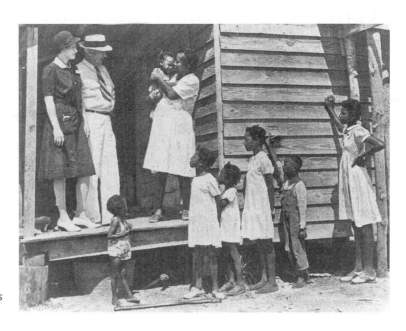

WPA projects brought public health nursing services to poor rural areas.

old-age benefits; (2) grants to the states for old-age assistance, vocational rehabilitation, and unemployment compensation administration; (3) aid to dependent and/or crippled children, aid to the blind, and maternal and child welfare; (4) public health work, including the authorization of grants to states for aid in the development and maintenance of state and local health services; and (5) an annual appropriation to the Public Health Service for additional research and training activities.

It was significant that Title VI of the Social Security Act authorized use of federal funds for the training of public health personnel. When the funds authorized by the act became available early in 1936, about one third of the states had a functioning public health nursing unit in their state health departments. Many young nurses who had become involved in public health nursing activities through the work-relief projects were eager to acquire formal public health training, and during the first year of the Social Security program about 1000 nurses received scholarship stipends through Social Security funds for study at universities offering public health nursing programs approved by the National Organization for Public Health Nursing. No other professional group in the health care field could recruit so many qualified candidates for training in so short a time. Most of the states that had established public health nursing units through work relief retained the same supervisory staff and used grant-in-aid funds provided

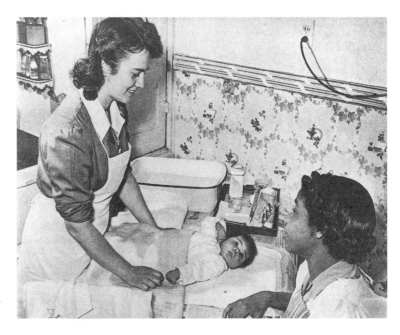

Disease prevention activities constituted a large part of many WPA-funded nursing programs.

under the Social Security Act to establish permanent divisions or bureaus of public health nursing.

The success of the training program for public health nurses under the Social Security Act exemplified the soundness of the plan and the effectiveness of the method of cooperation between the states and the federal government. In 1934, only 7% of the public health nurses then employed had completed an approved course of study in public health nursing at one of the accredited institutions in the United States, although many of the courses of study at those institutions had been in existence for 10 to 20 years. Within the 2 years immediately following implementation of the Social Security Act, 2304 nurses (about 10% of all the public health nurses in the United States) received some postgraduate training at approved schools on training stipends. Almost 15% of those receiving training stipends attended school for a full academic year or more.

NURSING EDUCATION IN THE MID-1930s

While nursing education was not experiencing such a dramatic advance, progress had been achieved. A study of the hospital nursing schools in the late 1930s showed that nursing schools were conducted in hospitals with a daily average patient census ranging from 7 to 6880 and that nursing school enrollment varied from 6 to 350 students. By 1936, 70 so-called collegiate programs in nursing existed, nearly all of which represented 2 years of general education either before or after a conventional 3-year hospital diploma program. More than half of these had been established between 1930 and 1936. Meanwhile, the number of hospital diploma programs had decreased from more than 2286 in 1929 to 1472 state-accredited schools in 1936.

This attrition was attributed to the evaluation studies of the 1920s and the national economic depression. Another major factor in the decrease was the fact that as the Depression had deepened and private patients became scarce, hospitals permitted their graduates to remain at work, often with little more pay than they had received as students. Those without nursing schools could hire graduate nurses for lower wages than they had been paying their untrained "attendants." By 1937, therefore, the number of graduate nurses in hospitals had risen 700%, from 4000 in 1929 to 28,000 in 1937.

THE 1937 CURRICULUM GUIDE

Toward the end of the 1930s, massive unemployment, maldistribution of nursing service, the problems of Depression-stricken hospitals, and many other factors called for a change in school-of-nursing curricula. The third and last revision of the National League for Nursing Education's *Curriculum Guide for Schools of Nursing* appeared in 1937. It was in line with the democratic belief that such a plan could best be put into operation if all concerned contributed to its compilation. Thousands of nurses all over the country were involved in the revision, either creatively or critically.

Two innovative assumptions were made in the guide. One was that the primary function of the nursing school should be education of the nurse. This represented a change from the assumption operating during an earlier period, which held that the function of the school was to provide nursing service for hospital patients. This assumption was not intended to repudiate the nursing profession's responsibility for the care of the sick, but rather was meant to remind the community that the preparation of the

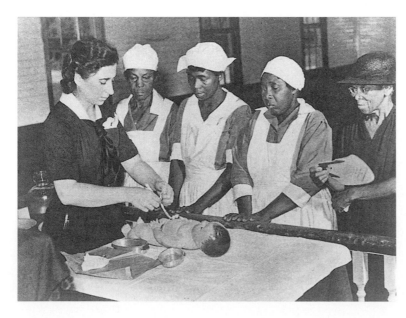

The Social Security Act of 1935 provided scholarship stipends to allow nurses to receive formal public health training.

nurse to care for future patients should not be sacrificed to provision of care in the present. The second assumption underlying revision of the guide was the concept of the nurse serving the total community, rather than just a skewed example of the community—the hospital. Public health nursing, mental health nursing, and understanding of the social setting of health problems and of the economic aspects of health care were all aspects of this concept.

The curriculum covered 2½ to 3 years. It was set up on a plan of either three terms of 16 weeks or four terms of 12 weeks each, both with 4 weeks' vacation every year. To hospital administrators, the nursing practice time was of special interest. The suggested length of the school week was 5½ days, or 44 to 48 hours, with 1 or 1½ days off per week. This ideal program included all regularly scheduled classes and nursing practice and provided sufficient time for study, recreation, and rest. In the first 4 months of the first year, classes and laboratory periods took up 20 to 22 hours per week and did not include any nursing practice. The class hours were decreased to 14 hours in the second term, at which time nursing

practice of 18 hours per week was begun. In the third term, class hours were held to 14 hours and practice was increased to 22 hours. In the second and third years, classes averaged 5 or 6 hours every week; nursing practice, 38 to 42 hours.

The proposed 3-year course required about 1200 to 1300 hours of class and laboratory work and about 4800 hours of nursing practice, compared with 825 hours of class, 200 hours of ward teaching, and approximately 6000 hours of nursing service in the 1927 version. Curriculum courses fell into three categories. The first included basic courses, such as anatomy, physiology, chemistry, microbiology, materia medica, psychology and sociology, and the history and ethics of nursing. These courses supplied a body of principles, facts, methods of study, and laboratory techniques that gave a good background for clinical practice. There was little new or different in this group except that possibly more emphasis was placed on psychology and sociology.

The two other categories of courses contained several new approaches. The major professional and technical courses were concerned with the "art" of

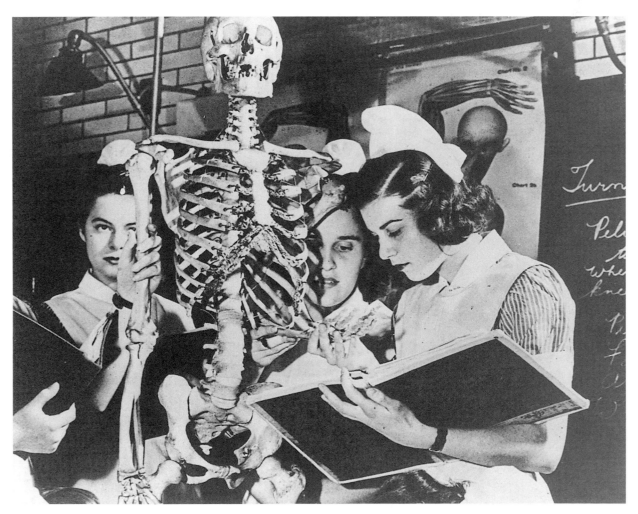

The ideal nursing program of the late 1930s involved 20 to 22 hours per week of class and laboratory time during the first 4 months.

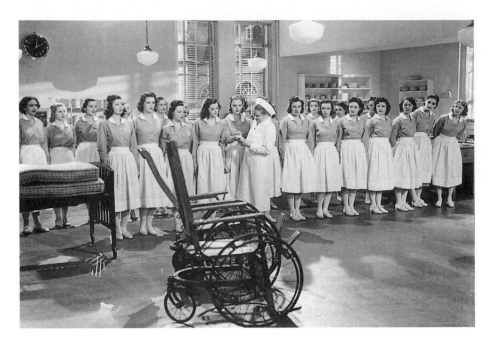

Education versus service for nursing students created conflicts.

nursing and included nursing arts, nutrition and cookery, medical nursing (including nursing in communicable disease), and surgical, pediatric, obstetric, psychiatric, and home nursing. The practical application in actual nursing situations allowed for integration of the basic science courses. A reorientation from sick nursing to health care was proposed. Discussion topics, with content drawn from the nursing content, were a new development and would lead, it was hoped, to a better integration of all the subjects offered to students.

Several other new features were significant. The psychological aspects of nursing were emphasized, and the sequence culminated in a suggested required program in psychiatry in the third year. In the course

on pediatrics, the physical and mental development of the well child was stressed as much as the care of the sick child. Public health and health teaching were incorporated throughout the course. Suggested programs of study and practice included applied sociology, social and professional discussion groups, and sessions on the health-promotion aspects of nursing in the introduction to the nursing arts course.

NURSES ON THE SCREEN

Student nurses of the 1930s—those with the time, energy, and money—began to see Hollywood motion pictures that depicted the nurse in all aspects of her life.

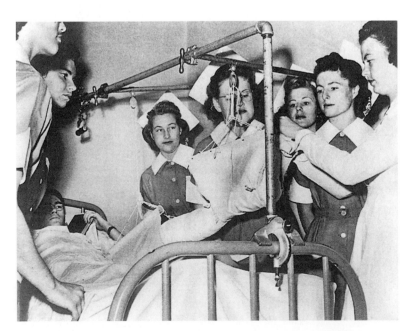

The 1937 Curriculum Guide recommended about 1200 to 1300 hours of class and laboratory work along with 4800 hours of nursing practice.

With the collapse of the American economy in 1929, the effervescent, youthful spirits of flapper heroines vanished, and new models for working women emerged. In the more serious, realistic atmosphere of the 1930s, the nurse character received considerable positive attention. Nursing was generally portrayed as a worthy, important profession that enabled women to earn a respectable living. Nurses were featured in crime and detective movies, war films, hospital and medical dramas, adventure films about aviation and ocean liners, and motion pictures about the nursing profession itself.

The only feature-length films ever produced that focused entirely on the nursing profession were released in the 1930s. *War Nurse* (1930), *Night Nurse* (1931), *Once to Every Woman* (1934), *The White Parade* (1934), *Four Girls in White* (1939), *Registered Nurse* (1934), *Wife, Doctor and Nurse* (1937), and *Vigil in the Night* (1939) all used nursing as the central theme and nurses as the major characters. Some, such as *The White Parade, Four Girls in White*, and *Vigil in the Night*, revealed much about the education and work of professional nurses. In these films, attractive young women put the demands of their profession before personal desires.

One of the most popular, *The White Parade*, starring Loretta Young, gave a realistic, sympathetic portrayal of the difficulties of nurse training in a large hospital school. The story emphasized that not every woman was cut out to be a nurse, and those that were could expect a life of hard work and little monetary reward, but with enormous personal satisfaction. The heroine of the film turned down a proposal of marriage by a millionaire to continue her work as a nurse.

In the Depression years of the 1930s, such idealism and self-sacrifice made an especially strong impression. More important, the viewing public came to understand that the nursing profession espoused high ideals and demanded rigorous self-discipline from its students and practitioners. No longer did Hollywood present nursing as a temporary pastime for rich girls interested in a little humanitarian work before marriage.

Some film biographies, a popular Hollywood product of the 1930s, were about nursing heroines: *The White Angel* (1936), *Nurse Edith Cavell* (1939), and *Sister Kenny* (1946). Kay Francis starred as Florence Nightingale in Warner Brothers' 1936 tribute to the founder of modern nursing, *The White Angel*. It told Nightingale's story, from her early attempts to free herself from her parents' loving restrictions to her triumph over the horrors of the British medical establishment in Scutari during the Crimean War. *Nurse Edith Cavell* retold the inspiring story of the World War I heroine. Rosalind Russell, who had taken a personal interest in Elizabeth Kenny's work in rehabilitating polio victims, played the Australian nurse in the film version. Sister Kenny's greatest foes were the medical men who refused to believe that a nurse "without the benefit of a medical education" could possibly do more for polio patients than orthopedic surgeons. These three nursing heroines demonstrated nobility, self-sacrifice, and relentless determination to pursue the right course of action despite enormous opposition.

The birth of the Dionne quintuplets in 1934 prompted a series of films about the physician who delivered them. *Country Doctor* (1936), *Reunion* (1936), and *Five of a Kind* (1938) actually featured

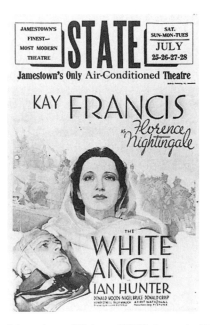

War Nurse *played at the 107-seat Star Theater in Concord, NH, January 1930.*

Residents of Jamestown, ND (pop. 6627), learned of the heroics of Florence Nightingale in The White Angel, *which played at the 800-seat State Theater.*

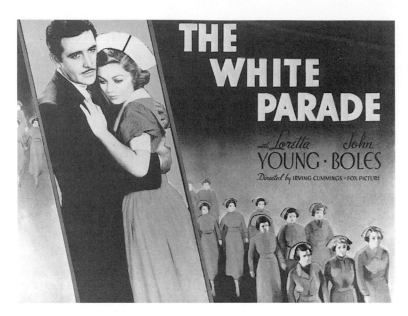

The White Parade was nominated for the Academy Award for Best Picture of 1934.

the quints and their nurses. Jean Hersholt, who played the kindly country doctor who delivered and cared for the quints (based on the actual physician, Dr. Roy DaFoe), tried to buy DaFoe's rights to *Country Doctor*. When he failed, Hersholt simply changed the name and continued the series as Dr. Christian and made six more films between 1939 and 1941. In all the *Doctor Christian* films, nurse Judy Price served Dr. Christian with filial loyalty. This nurse shared in Dr. Christian's concerns and enjoyed a warm and mutually respectful friendship with him. Although the nurse never challenged her boss's wisdom or knowledge, the audience recognized her as a valuable ally for the physician.

Between 1937 and 1947, MGM made 15 *Dr. Kildare/ Dr. Gillespie* movies that centered on the heroic, idealistic efforts of young Jim Kildare, the eternal neophyte, and his superior, Dr. Leonard Gillespie, played by Lionel Barrymore. Three nurse characters recurred in these films: Molly Byrd, the nursing director of Blair General; Mary Lamont, a young staff nurse; and occasionally, Nurse Parker. The image of nursing in this very popular series was mixed. The most important character, Mary Lamont (played by Laraine Day), enjoyed Kildare's admiration and thus stood as a sympathetic, admirable young woman. As a nurse she was docile, never showing much initiative or ambition. She and Kildare became engaged soon into the series, with Mary happily promising to wait 5 years for her doctor. Although a supporting character, Molly Byrd held a stronger professional position than Mary. As supervisor of nurses, she appeared to be authoritative, competent, and vastly skilled—and temperamentally matched to the grouchy, bossy character of Leonard Gillespie. Despite surface conflict between Byrd and Gillespie, their mutual admiration and trust were apparent. Nurse Parker, often nicknamed "Nosy," served as comic relief. An older spinster, she enjoyed gossip and seemed awestruck

with Dr. Gillespie. In all, the nurses paled in comparison with the omniscient, aggressive physicians.

Nurses were most often featured as major characters in detective and crime stories, in which the nurse helped to solve a mystery or vindicate a falsely accused man with whom she had fallen in love. The Mary Roberts Rinehart character, Miss Pinkerton, and Mignon Eberhardt's Sarah Keate—nurse-detectives working as private-duty nurses for wealthy patients—became popular screen characters. Although these films usually ended with the nurse in the arms of her boyfriend, often a police detective, they were not primarily romantic stories. The nurse often displayed great wit, mental acuity, and courage. These worldly wise nurse-detectives were not easily taken in by outward appearance, yet they were sympathetic and kind. Actual nursing care was not emphasized in these stories; however, by portraying nurses as sleuths in complicated mysteries, Hollywood offered examples of nurses being appreciated for their intelligence, logic, and bravery. None of these films was particularly memorable, yet they were popular; titles included *Miss Pinkerton* (1932), *The Nurse's Secret* (1941), *Murder by an Aristocrat* (1936), *While the Patient Slept* (1935), *The Great Hospital Mystery* (1937), *Mystery House* (1938), *The Patient in Room 18* (1938), and *The Murder of Dr. Harrigan* (1936).

Nurses also lent their support to innocent men or reformed criminals embroiled with the law. In *Mayor of Hell* (1933), a nurse not only worked to improve conditions in a boys' reformatory, but also inspired a borderline gangster to reject the underworld. In *Fight to the Finish* (1937), a nurse in love with a cab driver involved in gang warfare encouraged him to stop fighting and prove his innocence to the police. *Secrets of a Nurse* (1938) was about a nurse who fell in love with a prizefighter framed for the murder of a hoodlum; she was responsible for the fighter's leaving the ring for good, and she saved him from execution by securing a deathbed confession from the real killer. In *Nurse From Brooklyn* (1938), a hospital nurse worked to clear the name of her deceased brother who was framed and then killed. In *Prison Nurse* (1938), the heroine helped clear an inmate falsely accused of shooting a guard and also discovered the killer. In all these gangster and prison films, the nurses were portrayed as noble women who bore no prejudice against men who had been in prison or had dabbled with the underworld—as long as they demonstrated a desire to reform. The nurse as an inspiration for moral reform drew some of its strength from the legacy of World War I nurse characters.

Adventurous aviation and ocean-liner films, also prevalent in the 1930s, routinely climaxed with characters adrift and faced with the need to resolve overwhelming problems with their own limited resources. Because many seagoing vessels had included a nurse among the crew and the airlines, during the early days of commercial flying, had wanted only registered nurses as stewardesses, quite naturally the nurse could play an important role. Nurses would have to perform emergency surgery with only wire-

less instructions (*King of Alcatraz*, 1938; *The Storm*, 1938), assist with the birth of a baby (*Luxury Liner*, 1933), fight a raging cholera epidemic aboard ship (*Pacific Liner*, 1939), subdue a pain-driven passenger (*Man Who Found Himself*, 1937), or land a plane by wireless instructions when the pilot and co-pilot were killed or incapacitated (*Flying Hostess*, 1936; *Without Orders*, 1936). Although often the characters did little nursing, they routinely emerged as intrepid women, willing and able to perform critical tasks under pressure. It made little difference that the action in these films, as viewed by more than 85 million people each week, was not totally realistic. What mattered was the enlivening of the public image of the nurse in a relatively positive way.

THE PUBLIC WORKS ADMINISTRATION BUILDS HOSPITALS

Hospitals were also looking better, thanks to massive federal expenditures and low construction costs. The new Public Works Administration (PWA),

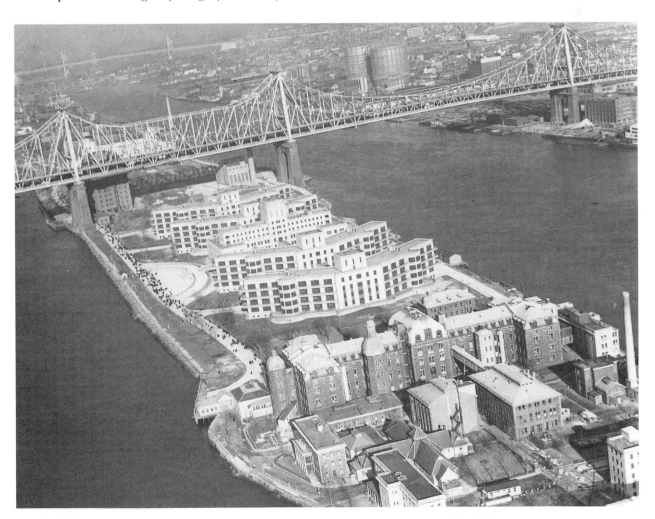

PWA funds helped build the new $7 million Hospital for Chronic Diseases on Welfare Island, New York City, which opened in July 1939.

a Depression-inspired "pump-priming" device conceived by President Roosevelt to stimulate heavy industry through construction projects using basic industrial output such as steel, cement, and lumber, was set up in June 1933. The PWA received an initial appropriation of $3.3 billion and was placed under the direction of the secretary of the interior. It was authorized to start its own construction projects, to support those administered by other federal units, and to make loans and matching grants sponsored by state and local public agencies. The PWA's total achievement between 1933 and 1939 was impressive. During that time it spent $6 billion, created jobs for about 4 million people in more than 34,000 projects, and helped build about 70% of the new educational buildings and about 35% of the new hospitals and public health facilities in the United States. Tremendous skyscraper hospitals in large cities and smaller facilities in rural areas were constructed with the aid of PWA funds.

AN IMPROVED WORKING ENVIRONMENT FOR THE NURSE

During the early part of the 20th century, nearly all hospital equipment had been constructed of cast iron and sheet metal and was generally finished in white enamel or porcelain. In place of crude castings, the new hospitals had streamlined, electrically welded equipment of noncorrosive or corrosion-resistant metal. Such metals were used to construct operating room furniture, laboratory equipment, sterilizing equipment, kitchen and laundry equipment, and elevator cabs and even in utensils such as basins, jars, and trays. Wood furniture with stain-resistant finishes was also widely used in patients' rooms, waiting rooms, solariums, and offices. Hospitals made extensive use of sound-absorbent materials, and acoustic installations were found in corridors, patients' rooms, preparation and serving kitchens, utility rooms, offices, and other areas.

Improved casters facilitated the introduction of mobile equipment. In the rare instances when it was necessary to move older stationary beds, a bed conveyor was used. In new hospitals, all beds were equipped with casters, and many nurses moved the patient directly to surgery, the x-ray department, the physiotherapy department, or the solarium in his or her own bed, without first transferring the patient from bed to wheelchair or stretcher. New mobile equipment included stretcher carts, wheelchairs, food conveyors, linen trucks and linen hampers, and two- and four-wheel trucks for the delivery of supplies. Also equipped with casters were bedside tables, overbed tables, metabolism and oxygen-therapy apparatus, therapeutic and examining lamps, and operating room and instrument tables. Stretcher carts and the various types of easily storable folding trucks were also available. Some of the larger hospitals used

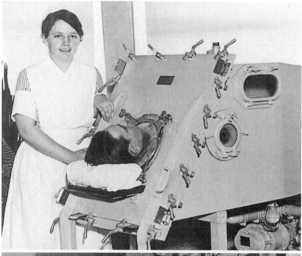

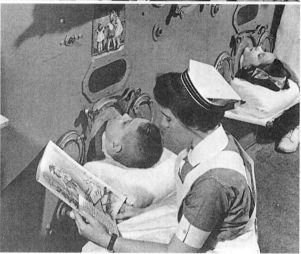

Iron lung machines of the late 1930s.

electrically operated tractors, which made it possible to haul a number of trucks at one time.

The progress in hospital service, made possible partly through the use of modern equipment, could also be seen in the great number of mechanical devices, many of them electrically operated, that had been developed during the 1920s and 1930s. Such equipment was used in every department, from the operating room and x-ray suites to the offices, kitchens, and laundry. Fever therapy apparatus, respiratory and oxygen-therapy machines, iron lungs, electrically heated blankets, stupe and inhalation kettles, incubators, electrically operated breast pumps, suction pressure apparatus, electrically heated ranges, food machines and conveyers, electric locks, bedside deodorizers, floor-scrubbing machines, check protectors and check signers, bill machines, and photographic equipment—virtually thousands of mechanical devices had been developed for the use of the nurse as well as of other hospital workers.

Nurses working in new buildings noted improved illumination. Modern hospitals installed emergency

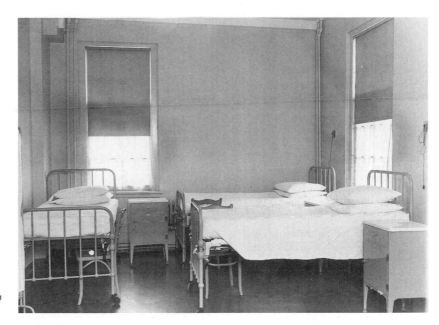

New beds were equipped with casters to facilitate movement.

lighting systems, operated by storage batteries or by steam- or gasoline-driven generators, in operating and delivery rooms, corridors, stairwells, and elevator cabs. Operating room fixtures could light the operating field without casting a shadow and were constructed to create minimal heat, thereby adding to the comfort of the surgical staff. Lighting of patients' rooms had been improved in several ways. Ceiling and wall-bracket fixtures enabled the night nurse to observe the patient without disturbing him or her, and illuminated directional signs were used extensively.

Communication devices had been adopted for hospital use. More and more hospitals were equipped with some type of signaling device that enabled the patient to call the nurse. The type generally used was operated at the patient's bedside by a push button that flashed a light in the corridor, over the doorway to the patient's room, and in other areas where the nurse was likely to be. A few hospitals installed communications equipment between the patient's bedside and the nurses' office, which enabled the patient to speak directly to the nurse. Some hospitals used standard telephone equipment with satisfactory results. The air conditioner was a popular new luxury. Air conditioning was usually limited to operating room and delivery room suites and nurseries, although a few institutions had installed individual units in a few private rooms, and several hospitals had air-conditioned rooms for the care of premature infants.

In the newer hospitals, every effort was being made to make patients' rooms as attractive and homelike as possible. Overbed tables had been installed to accommodate food trays, and bedsprings with adjustable, built-in backrests facilitated sitting up in bed and added to the patient's comfort. Many

hospitals had replaced the cotton mattress with a comfortable innerspring or sponge-rubber version. Special beds had been designed for cardiac and fracture cases, and many beds featured a special built-in bedpan. Removable side rails, attached to hospital beds to protect the semiconscious patient, were available. Occasionally, carpeting and attractive window

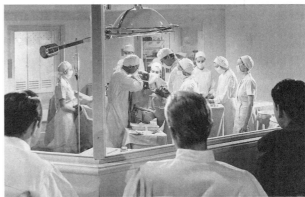

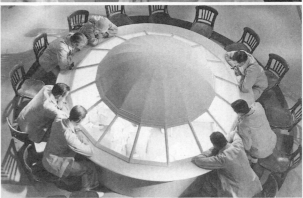

A modern operating room of the late 1930s.

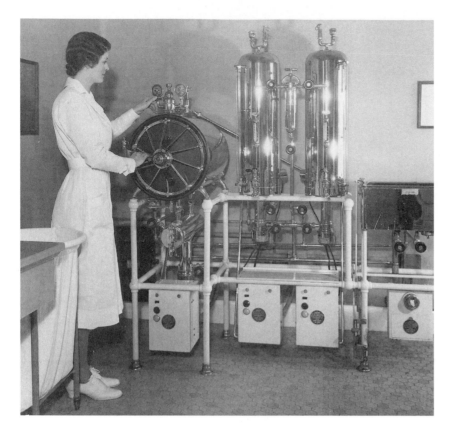

The latest in sterilizing equipment.

draperies were used in private and semiprivate rooms. Some hospitals used cubicle screening in accommodations for two or more patients to ensure privacy; this screening consisted of a metal rod, suspended from the ceiling and extending around the patient's bed, on which curtains were fastened.

Despite the Depression and with the assistance of hospital insurance plans and medical advances, by 1939 the hospital had become accepted as a necessary institution in every American community. The 40 million people inhabiting the United States in 1870 had had fewer than 50,000 hospital beds available for their use; the 133 million people in 1939 had 1,200,000 beds. During the 70 years in which the population of the nation had more than tripled, the number of hospital beds had multiplied 24-fold. Health care was increasingly being associated with hospitalization, and graduate nurses were a part of this movement.

REFERENCES

1. *New York Times*, March 5, 1933.
2. "Binghamton Is Over-Crowded, So Is Birmingham, So Is Colorado Springs," *American Journal of Nursing*, vol. 30 (January 1930):97.
3. "Too Many Nurses in These Localities," *American Journal of Nursing*, vol. 30 (March 1930):344.
4. J. A. Diekmann, "Nursing Schools in Hospitals Under 100 Beds Should Close," *Hospital Management*, vol. 37 (March 1934):29–30.
5. Michael M. Davis, "The Committee on Costs of Medical Care Makes Its Report," *Modern Hospital*, vol. 39 (December 1932):41–46.
6. Committee on the Costs of Medical Care, *Medical Care for the American People: The Final Report of the Committee on the Costs of Medical Care* (Chicago: The University of Chicago Press, 1932), pp. 1–10.
7. R. G. Leland, "Seventeen Defects or Objections to Group Hospitalization," *Hospital Management*, vol. 35 (April 1933):25–26.
8. Morris Fishbein, "The Committee on the Costs of Medical Care," *Journal of the American Medical Association*, vol. 99 (December 3, 1932):1950–1952.

NURSING IN THE WAR FOR THE WORLD

In the spring of 1939, an issue of the *American Journal of Nursing* carried a perceptive editorial entitled "To the Graduates of '39," which alluded to the extraordinary demands looming on the horizon.

> We salute you, graduates of '39. We wish you well. The world has need for more nursing.
>
> If such a thing were possible, and all the graduates of '39 could be massed in one great stadium, what a heart-stirring sight it would be.
>
> We don't know what our hypothetical speaker would say to you, you thousands of young and eager American nurses on so great an occasion. Probably he (or she) would begin with some description of the shattering fears of the world we live in, of the undeclared wars, of changing national boundaries, of problems of migration, and of the health problems created by all of them.
>
> Nurses of '39, the world has need of you. If war should come, we have faith to believe that you will fulfill the traditional role of the nurse.[1]

A reduction in working hours for undergraduate and graduate staffs had resulted in increased nursing school enrollments from 67,000 students in 1935 to more than 82,000 4 years later. When enrollment increased by 8000 from 1938 to 1939, many nurse educators began to fear that an overproduction of graduate nurses would lead to a corresponding decline in their quality, as it had in the 1920s. Patients in American hospitals were receiving over 60 million more days of care in 1939 than in 1934; the number of hospital beds had increased by 14%.

THE OUTBREAK OF WAR

The 1501 nurses who registered at the 45th Annual Convention of the National League of Nursing Education (NLNE) in New Orleans in April 1939 were unaware of the worsening international situation in Europe. Because New Orleans offered a variety of unsurpassed tourist attractions, the delegates explored the quaint streets and fascinating shops of the Vieux Carré, visited the wharves, and dined in exotic restaurants.

Meanwhile, international relations in Europe were steadily deteriorating. Since the Treaty of Versailles, which had ended World War I, Germany had been denouncing, among other things, the so-called Polish Corridor, a strip of territory 120 miles long and 60 miles wide separating East Prussia from the rest of Germany. The Treaty of Versailles had awarded this territory to the newly formed state of Poland and had placed the German city of Danzig under the control of the League of Nations. In late August 1939, the German dictator Adolf Hitler demanded that Danzig be returned to the Reich and that Poland grant him the right to build a road across the corridor. He also accused Poland of fostering atrocities against its citizens of German ancestry. To eliminate the danger of a war on two fronts, Hitler negotiated a 10-year nonaggression pact with the Soviet Union in August 1939. By demarcating German and Russian spheres of influence in Poland, this pact cleared the way for a joint invasion of the unfortunate country by the new allies. Several days later, Hitler delivered an ultimatum to the Polish government, but before it even had time to reply, German troops invaded Poland without formally declaring war.

The Poles expected to offer resistance until at least winter, when bad weather would come to their aid by slowing the progress of the invaders. Long before winter, however, the new German armies won a complete victory. Their rapid, lightning-like movements even caused a new word to be invented—*blitzkrieg*, or "lightning war." While German armored divisions encircled Polish defenders, the Luftwaffe, which had already destroyed the Polish air force on the ground, ruthlessly bombed cities and fleeing refugees in a deliberate

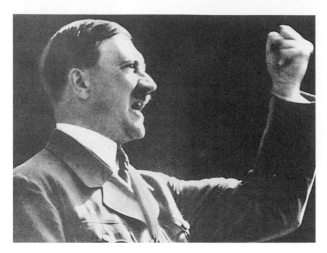

Talk of European war and Adolf Hitler dominated the May 1940 ANA convention.

attempt to terrorize civilians. Warsaw fell within 3 weeks, and in little more than a month all Polish resistance to the Germans had collapsed. Meanwhile, the Soviet Union, in accordance with their terms of the nonaggression pact, occupied eastern Poland. Two days after Hitler's armies invaded Poland, Great Britain and France declared war on Germany. Their lack of military preparedness, however, prevented them from coming to the aid of the Poles.

The 6 months following the Russo-German conquest of Poland were quiet, as Hitler paused before assaulting the other European nations. Only Stalin's invasion of Finland excited the American public during this *sitzkrieg*, or "phony war," which took place during the winter of 1939–1940. This Soviet move to secure the Baltic front against the Germans was fiercely resisted by the Finns and aroused the indignation of most Americans.

Nurses were becoming increasingly aware of the international crisis. In the February 1940 *American Journal of Nursing*, editor Mary Roberts wrote:

> Congress, as this is written, has been in session only ten days. The very air is supercharged with tragedy. The wars of other countries are profoundly influencing life in our own, and the Congress is concerned with such matters as neutrality, reciprocal trade agreements, and armaments for defense.[2]

Four months later, at the May 1940 convention of the American Nurses Association (ANA) in Philadelphia, Roberts noted that, day by day, the agonies of Europe were growing more acute and that the convention theme, "Nursing in a Democracy," was daily becoming more appropriate in view of the grave war news.

In April 1940, Hitler's armies suddenly struck in Norway and Denmark. A month later, German troops began storming across the Dutch and Belgian borders in the now-familiar blitzkrieg fashion. This lightning thrust caught Great Britain and France unprepared as German dive-bombers wrought havoc behind the Allied lines and massed tanks broke through their defenses. As Belgium neared collapse, German forces penetrated the rugged Ardennes country, avoiding the awesome fortifications of the Maginot Line, and moved across northern France. Veering toward the English channel, the onrushing Germans pinned a half-million British and French troops into an ever-narrowing salient around Dunkerque. The near-miraculous escape of the bulk of the British armies from that trap between May 26 and June 3, 1940, could not minimize the catastrophe of the Allied defeat.

NURSES PREPARE FOR THE DEMANDS OF WAR

During one session of the 1940 ANA convention, the radio carried President Roosevelt's announcement of national preparedness. Although many delegates immediately asked what preparations were being made for nursing service in case of war, no general plans had yet been formulated. A nurse from Finland spoke at the closing business session. She had come, she said, to express the gratitude of the Finnish people for the material aid and moral support of American nurses. "More than ever I am impressed by our internationalism in the field of nursing," she declared.[3] She vividly described how many of Finland's nurses had lost their lives in their response to the call of duty. Finland, which knew the full meaning of "nursing in a democracy," was painfully recovering from the effects of the Soviet attack. A resolution endorsed by the NLNE and the ANA was passed, offering President Roosevelt "the support and strength of our organizations in any nursing activity in which we can be of service to the country." On that high note, the convention closed.[4]

Meanwhile, the alumnae of the Army School of Nursing also met. Stimulated by preparations for national defense, this small group discussed reopening the army school. Although Annie Goodrich was enthusiastic about this suggestion, Julia Stimson, chief of the Army Nurse Corps and president of the ANA, reacted unfavorably. Despite her 11 years as dean and administrator of the school and her stout resistance to closing it, she now considered the expense of reopening it unjustifiable if other adequate training schools were available.

After the ANA had failed to support reopening the army school, Goodrich decided to act individually. At her suggestion, Frances Payne Bolton, a member of Congress and a staunch friend of nursing, appealed directly to Secretary of War Harry B. Woodring. Because of insufficient military appropriations, however, he

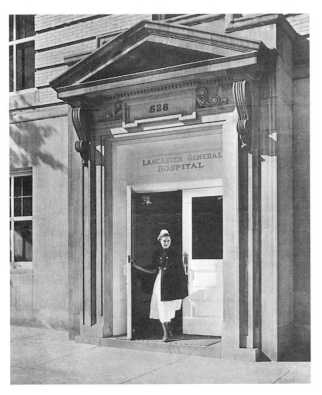

In 1939, nursing school graduates faced an uncertain future.

FORMATION OF THE NURSING COUNCIL FOR NATIONAL DEFENSE

Five top officials of the nursing profession—Julia C. Stimson, Stella Goostray, Grace Ross, Mary Beard, and Mary Roberts—gathered for a cheerless meeting in the conference room of ANA's New York headquarters on July 29, 1940. The main issue was how to prepare nursing for the war that was almost certain to come. Years later, Stella Goostray recalled the events that had precipitated this meeting:

> On July 10, 1940, Isabel Stewart, as the newly-elected president of the NLNE, wrote me regarding "the need of some official nursing committee or commission to think through the position that nurses should take with respect to national defense and the many adjustments that may be called for within the next few months. . . . I believe we should have such a commission or board that is representative of the nursing profession as a whole and that it should be at work now, and not wait until Miss Beard calls on us to do something in connection with the American Red Cross." I wrote [to Julia Stimson] on July 9, 1940. . . . Julia Stimson lost no time, and on July 29, just short of three weeks from the date of Miss Stewart's first letter to me, representatives of five national nursing organizations—ANA, NOPHN, NLNE, NACGN, ACSN, and representatives of several Federal agencies—Army Nurse Corps, Navy Nurse Corps, Children's Bureau, USPHS, Divisions of State Relations and of Hospitals, Nursing Service, Veterans Administration Nursing Service, Department of Indian Affairs, and the ARCNS met in New York. By the end of that day, the Nursing Council on National Defense was on its way.[6]

could not assure her that the school would be reopened.

Nor did Congresswoman Bolton limit her appeals on behalf of the Army School of Nursing to the secretary of war. Together with Mary Beard, Annie Goodrich, and other alumnae, she called on the surgeon general of the army, who told them firmly that the Medical Department had no intention of training personnel for its various technical branches. Bolton later recalled that she had kept

> some correspondence with the then Acting Secretary of War to the effect that all of the skeleton framework [for the Army School] would be most carefully kept and if we ever needed it, it would immediately be opened up again. So, in the innocence and naivete, I can't say of youth, when things became embroiled this time, Miss Byrd and Miss Goodrich and Sister Olivia and Miss Hoherty and one other, and myself, called upon the Surgeon General. We thought that all we had to do was to remind him of the skeleton framework [for the Army School] that was there and he would immediately start moving. But not Surgeon General Magee! We were told most definitely that the Army was not going to teach all these various branches, he was too busy with the Army, and that it was up to the civilian hospitals to furnish the nurses.[5]

While the Nursing Council on National Defense was being formed, the news of the war in Europe continued to be bleak. By June 22, 1940, all resistance to Hitler in western Europe had ceased. France had already fallen and Britain stood in mortal danger. Apparently, only a miracle could prevent Hitler from total victory. Many Americans thought that the fall of France might be followed by that of England—which would bring Hitler's forces within conceivable striking distance of America.

On September 16, 1940, the president signed the first peacetime conscription measure ever enacted in American history: the Selective Training and Service Act of 1940. This law, which reflected an awareness of imminent danger, was an attempt to satisfy the exigencies of modern warfare, which could no longer be waged on a voluntary basis but required instead the total mobilization and disposition of manpower through a system at once compulsory and selective. The Selective Service System provided for the registration, first of all men between the ages of 21 and 36, and subsequently of those between 18 and 64.

Six months later, on March 1, 1941, an emergency health and sanitation bill was passed, which provided funds to supplement public health nursing services for the families of workers in major defense industries. The funds for this program, which were administered by the U.S. Public Health Service, mandated the recruitment of 115 public health nurses. In addition, 90 more were needed at once by the Public Health Service.

DEFENSE SPENDING AFFECTS HEALTH FACILITIES AND NURSING EDUCATION

On June 28, 1941, President Roosevelt signed the Community Facilities Act, which was popularly known as the Lanham Bill. Under the terms of this act, nonprofit private agencies received grants from the federal government for the equipment and

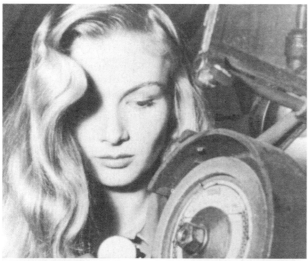

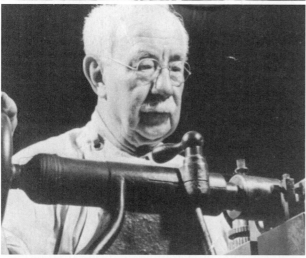

Full mobilization of manpower brought women and elderly into the workforce.

operation of community service facilities in defense areas, including schools, hospitals, and clinics. Within 6 weeks after the bill's passage, President Roosevelt had approved federal grants for a number of health projects, including hospitals, clinics, and nurses' homes.

To ensure an adequate supply of well-trained nurses for military and civilian nursing services, Congress passed the Labor-Federal Security Appropriation Act, which the president signed on July 1, 1941. An initial appropriation of $1,800,000 was earmarked for nursing education. Specifically, funds were allocated for refresher courses to prepare retired nurses in modern methods, for supplementary courses in special fields, and for aid to basic nursing schools to increase the number of students in regular undergraduate classes. Letters specifying the conditions under which funds could be allocated and the procedure to be followed in requesting such funds were sent to all 1400 state-accredited nursing schools and to universities offering programs of study in nursing education. Soon, 88 of the 300 nursing schools that applied were selected to receive this federal aid to train additional student nurses. Sixty-seven schools in 32 states offered refresher courses to 3000 graduate nurses, and 26 other schools enrolled 500 graduate nurses for postgraduate study.

CRASH PROGRAM TO TRAIN NURSES' AIDES

In August 1941, 800 nursing schools were invited by New York mayor Fiorello H. LaGuardia, director of civilian defense, to participate in a nationwide program to augment the nursing services of hospitals, clinics, and public health and field nursing agencies. Mayor LaGuardia urged these institutions to cooperate with the American Red Cross and the Office of Civilian Defense in training 100,000 volunteer nurses' aides so that each hospital nurse might have at least one trained aide to help her extend her services to many more patients. "The deficiency in nursing personnel will be overwhelmingly accentuated if this country becomes actively involved in defensive combat," Mayor LaGuardia predicted in extending his invitation to the schools.[7]

The Office of Civilian Defense, which urged hospitals and nursing schools to cooperate in training aides, listed five requirements for the effective use of volunteer nurses' aides: (1) they had to be intensively trained; (2) throughout the period of national emergency they had to continue serving an adequate number of hours in a hospital or clinic or in field service; (3) they had to be prepared to conform to the discipline of the organization in which they were to work; (4) they were to render service without pay; and (5) they were not to replace paid hospital personnel but were to serve specifically as nurses' assistants.

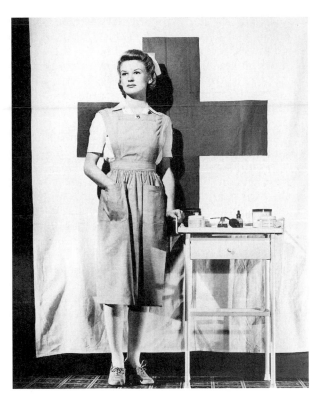

A program to train 100,000 volunteer nurses' aides was started.

THE DRIFT TOWARD WAR

As the nation continued to prepare for war, figures indicated that state-accredited schools had admitted 41,397 students for the 1940–41 academic year, approximately 5000 short of the estimated need. These figures provided clear evidence of the additional need for federal aid. At the same time on the international scene, two ships carrying nurses of the London-bound Red Cross–Harvard Unit were torpedoed and five nurses and the house mother died. Soon afterward, President Roosevelt decided to furnish naval escorts to merchant ships crossing the North Atlantic.

The incident that finally brought America into conflict with the Axis powers did not occur in Europe, however, but in the Pacific. During the long months when American relations with Germany were growing increasingly tense, Secretary of State Cordell Hull was conducting complicated negotiations with the Japanese. Since the invasion of Manchuria, Americans had observed with growing apprehension the advance of Japanese imperialism in Asia. As December began, hopes for peace were faint.

Although it was known that the Japanese were preparing to mount an offensive, most military experts expected them to attack the British and Dutch possessions in Southeast Asia. Hardly anyone suspected that Hawaii would be the target of a Japanese strike. American commanders had received routine warnings but had taken few precautions. At Pearl Harbor, the double row of American war ships, most in port for the first time since July 4, presented perfect targets to the first wave of Japanese bombers that burst unexpectedly out of the skies at 7:55 a.m. on December 7, 1941. The Japanese sank five battleships, severely damaged three others, and hit numerous lesser vessels. Of the 2403 Americans killed during this surprise air raid, nearly half lost their lives when the battleship *Arizona* exploded. Military and civilian nurses at Pearl Harbor rendered heroic service in caring for the many casualties.

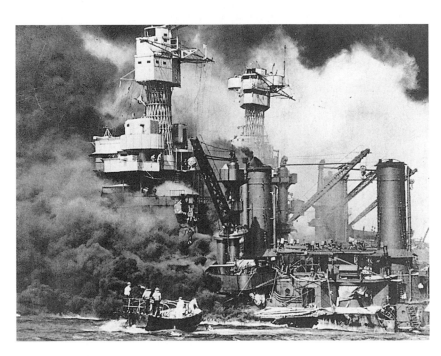

The attack at Pearl Harbor brought America into the war.

More than 16 million women, a third of the nation's work force, played a significant role in the record-breaking production of 1941–1945. Increasingly, the nation had come to recognize its skilled womanpower. At the time of Pearl Harbor, 12 million women were in the labor force, but by 1945, only 4 years later, there were more than 18 million. In 1940, 22% of all women were employed outside their homes. In 1944, 31.5% of the female population older than age 14 was in the labor force outside the home.

PERSONNEL POSSIBILITIES OF THE MILITARY NURSE SERVICES

During the early years of World War II, nurses were in a quandary as to whether they should join one of the military nursing services or remain in their civilian positions. To help hospitals and other employing agencies as well as individual nurses, the National Nursing Council for War Service established guidelines for two categories of service. These guidelines were approved by the health and medical committee and the nursing subcommittee of the Office of

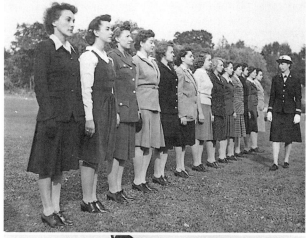

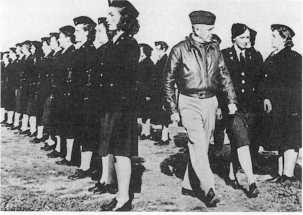

As more nurses entered the Navy Nurse Corps and Army Nurse Corps, the civilian sector was depleted.

Defense Health and Welfare Service and by the American Red Cross. A nurse should serve with the armed forces, according to the council, if she was single and younger than age 40 and (1) doing private duty; (2) on a hospital's general staff; (3) a head nurse not essential for teaching or supervision; (4) a public health nurse not essential for maintaining minimum civilian health service in any given community; (5) in a non-nursing position; or (6) an office nurse.

Conversely, a nurse should serve at home if she had a position as (1) an administrator, instructor, supervisor, or head nurse in a hospital having a nursing school; (2) an administrator or supervisor in a hospital without a nursing school; or (3) an administrator, teacher, supervisor, or staff nurse in a public health agency essential for maintaining minimum civilian health services in any given community.

Nurses who joined the military at the beginning of the war received few benefits. The army offered nurses "relative rank," which amounted to an officer's title and uniform without an officer's commission, retirement privileges, dependents' allowances, or pay. Similarly, the navy offered only vague "officer's privileges" until this disparity was partially corrected by Congress in July 1942, when members of the Navy Nurse Corps were also given "relative rank." Even then, the injustice of less pay for the same rank prevailed: The nurse ensign received a base pay of $90 a month, compared with $150 for a male ensign.

On December 1, 1943, Frances Payne Bolton introduced in the House of Representatives a bill to remedy this injustice. It would have provided full military rank for members of the Army Nurse Corps. After considering this bill for 4 months, the War Department reported adversely on it, primarily because it authorized permanent officer's rank for nurses. Meanwhile, the sad plight of the army nurse with mere relative rank was highlighted by a reporter in a March 1944 column in the *Rocky Mountain News*:

> Here is the case of Sue—consider it, and reach your own conclusions.
>
> Sue is a college graduate. After an arts degree, she studied nursing and after graduation taught nursing in a university. Early in 1941, believing war was imminent, she volunteered as an Army Nurse. She was at Pearl Harbor when the attack came. She was under fire, and cared for wounded men during long weeks of agony. Exposure, fatigue, the strain of intense and exciting work, shattered her health. She was sent to Fitzsimons Hospital to be treated for tuberculosis. After a year's treatment she was found to be totally and permanently disabled.
>
> Her discharge pay, as an Army nurse, second lieutenant, is $60 a month.
>
> Had she held the same rank as WAC or WAVE or a Navy nurse, her pay would be $112.50 a month.
>
> "We are proud to be Army nurses," several young women whose situation is similar to that of

Sue told me. "But we don't like to be treated as stepchildren."

At this moment there are more than 100 nurse patients at Fitzsimons Hospital who are facing the same sort of discrimination.[8]

After referring to several other cases of blatant injustice to disabled military nurses, the columnist went on to say:

Maybe they will recover, and be able to return to active duty. They hope so, of course. But if they don't—well, they'll be subject to the same sort of discrimination that worked to the detriment of Sue.

Why isn't the Army nurse given a square deal? Because, from some strange quirk—or perhaps from plain neglect—the Army nurse, although she belongs to the oldest service women's corps, holds only what is called "relative rank." A Navy nurse is entitled to the same benefits and privileges of any other officer of her grade; so is an officer of the WACs or WAVEs. But, whereas any of the other second lieutenants is allowed under a permanent disability three-fourths of a base pay of $150 a month, the Army nurse is given an allowance on a base pay of $90 a month.

Why? Because the rank of the others is permanent, the rank of the Army Nurse is relative.[9]

Finally, on June 22, 1944, Congress enacted a law providing members of the Army Nurse Corps and the Navy Nurse Corps with temporary officer's rank. For the duration of the war and for 6 months

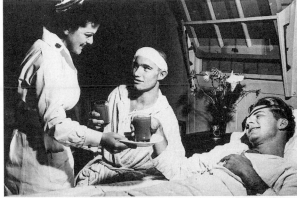
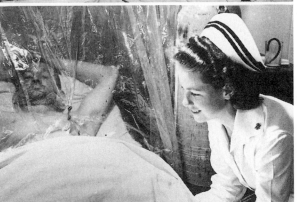

Navy nurses caring for patients.

thereafter they were entitled to the same initial pay, allowances, rights, benefits, and privileges as prescribed by law for commissioned officers.

NURSES IN NORTH AFRICA

Meanwhile, after invading North Africa, the Allies waged a seesaw struggle across the desert with the German forces, which were finally defeated at Bizerte in Tunisia in May 1943. A note written by Lieutenant Charlotte Jean Webber of the army's Thirty-eighth Evacuation Hospital contained a description of the new African base of operations.

We live in tents somewhere in Northwest Africa and love it. Only we don't take baths, wash our hair, shave, or wash clothes—just one big, dirty, happy family. It's cold at night. I sleep on an Army cot in my sleeping bag with my wool robe on and four Army blankets over me and my fur coat in my little field hospital. Worked like blazes to get it set up these first few trying days—and now we have something to be proud of.

We've named all our little streets in the field—my ward tent is on the corner of Kentucky Ave. and Second St. Our mess tent's called "New York Hotel" and my tent is named "My Old Kentucky Home."

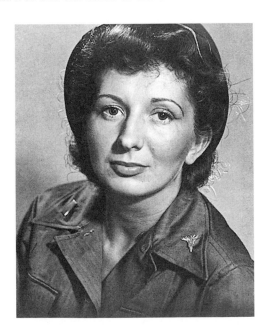

In June 1944, nurses received temporary officer's rank and benefits for the duration of the war.

I certainly have a time trying to talk French with these French people. Those two years I had in French in Cynthiana High do come in handy. When I was in town I went to a shop to buy some pins; the French shopkeepers kept jabbering to us and we couldn't understand a thing they said. Finally, I gathered they wanted us to go with them for a drink of wine. Well, they left their shop wide open and took us down to their house, sat us down, and brought out three bottles, and finally FDR's picture, and we all drank a toast to Roosevelt.[10]

The evacuation hospital was an intermediate link in the medical chain that extended from the battlefield to general hospitals in the United States. Badly wounded men were treated in field hospitals close to the front, but they began actual recovery in the evacuation hospital, located from 5 to 50 miles farther to the rear. Less serious casualties were sometimes sent directly to the evacuation hospital from frontline medical clearing stations. When patients who needed treatment were strong enough to travel, they were transported to larger, more specialized hospitals far from the battle zone. Those who required more than 30 days to recover were evacuated to hospitals in Sicily and North Africa, and those who required at least 120 days were returned to the United States. Although evacuation hospitals lacked the tiled neatness of peacetime facilities, they were nonetheless complete and efficient medical units. Many of their patients could be discharged without further treatment. At the evacuation hospital, the sick and the wounded enjoyed the luxury of warm baths, clean pajamas, and soft bathrobes for the first time since leaving home. There they also often received medical attention from nurses for the first time.

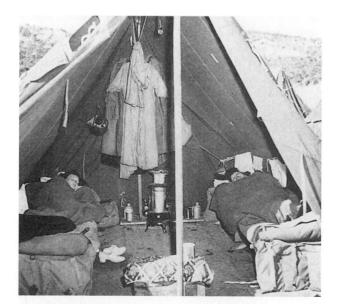

Army nurses rest in between battles in Tunisia during the North African campaign.

Ernie Pyle was one of an estimated 1600 American war correspondents, but probably no other combat journalist will be as long remembered. Reporting from the European and Pacific theaters, he captured a devoted following of Americans at home and overseas. His simple style, his directness, and his admiration for the frontline soldier seemed to satisfy the public's appetite for humanized war reporting. Beginning in November 1942, Pyle followed American fighting men and women from North Africa to Sicily and then to Italy. He made the following comments about the Thirty-eighth Evacuation Hospital's nurses:

The officers and nurses live two in a tent on two sides of a company street—nurses on one side, officers on the other. The street has a neat sign at the end on which is painted "Carolina Avenue." Some Yankee has painted under this "Rebel Street." . . . The 300 men who do the non-medical work live in their little shelter tents just on beyond. They're mostly from New England. They've built a little wall of whitewashed rocks between the two areas and put up a sign saying "Mason-Dixon Line." . . . The nurses wear khaki overalls because of the mud and dust. Doctors go around tieless and with knit brown caps on their heads. Pink female panties fly from a line among the brown warlike tents. On the flagpole is a Red Cross flag, made from a bed sheet and a French soldier's red sash.[11]

The American nurses—and there were lots of them—turned out just as you would expect: wonderfully. Army doctors, and patients, too, were unanimous in their praise of them. Doctors told me that in the first rush of casualties they were calmer than the men.

The Carolina nurses, too, took it like soldiers. For the first ten days they had to live like animals, even using open ditches for toilets, but they never complained.

One nurse was always on duty in each tentful of 20 men. She had medical orderlies to help her. Most of the time the nurses wore army coveralls, but Colonel Bauchspies [commanding officer] wanted them to put on dresses once in a while, for he said the effect on the men was astounding. The touch of femininity, the knowledge that a woman was around, gave the wounded man courage and confidence and a feeling of security. And the more feminine, the better.[12]

NURSING UNDER FIRE IN ITALY

The Allies followed up their victory over the Germans in North Africa by landing first in Sicily and then in Italy. In September 1943, American troops landed at Salerno and began a long, arduous campaign up the mountainous Italian peninsula. On September 15, the first American army nurses to set foot on European soil since 1918 landed in the Salerno sector of Italy and immediately went to work in a field hospital. Wearing GI helmets and fatigues with long trousers, these 57 nurses dug in like regular soldiers to take cover during air raids to remain with the wounded men.

Only 100 miles separated Naples from Rome, but despite their numerical superiority on land and in the air and their control of the adjacent seas, the Allied troops needed 8 months to cover this distance. Some of the most mountainous terrain in Europe barred the way to Rome, the objective of the winter campaign of 1943–1944. In an attempt to break the stalemate, the Allies made an amphibious landing in the rear of the Germans, at Anzio, 37 miles south of Rome, on January 23, 1944. Even though this landing caught the Germans by surprise, they reacted swiftly. Luftwaffe bombers sank numerous Allied transports and warships, and the Allied troops along with the hospital units had to dig in on an open plain, where they were subjected to constant air and ground attacks by the enemy. Instead of becoming the spearhead for an Allied military thrust, the Anzio beachhead became a beleaguered fort.

Six nurses, five of them members of the Army Nurse Corps, the other serving as a Red Cross worker, were the first American women killed in the war as a direct result of enemy action. They died of wounds received on the Anzio beachhead on February 7 and February 10, 1944. The nurses included First Lieutenant Blanche F. Sigman, a graduate of Bellevue Hospital, New York; First Lieutenant Marjorie Morrow, a graduate of Iowa Methodist Hospital School of Nursing, Des Moines; First Lieutenant Glenda Spelhaug, a graduate of St. Luke's Hospital School of Nursing, Saint Paul, Minnesota; and Second Lieutenant La Verne Farquhar, graduate of King's Daughters Hospital, Temple, Texas.

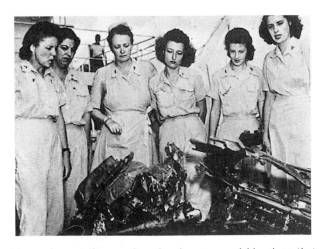

Nurses inspect the remains of a Japanese suicide plane that crashed into the hospital ship USS Comfort *near Okinawa, killing 29 and wounding 33 patients, nurses, and medical personnel.*

Once again, military nurses witnessed dreadful suffering. One young University of Minnesota graduate wrote to a relative:

> It is now 3 A.M. Most of my patients are asleep so I have a chance to write a few words. . . . Oh, aunt, I feel so tired lately, my stomach feels to be upside down. When I am asleep I wake up constantly and can't get a rest. . . . Recently we are getting very bad casualties. It makes me shiver to just look at them. You can't imagine, aunt, what we see over here. I will never forget it—it is heart-breaking.
>
> One of my patients, only 24, has a piece of shrapnel in his heart, another 29 and married, has both legs off—his hips are broken, his intestines exposed. Another, 19, was shot through the abdomen, and after the Germans found him lying, they kicked him and shot him into the head, to finish him. . . . He suffers much. His eyes are gone. I have also two patients who were shot through the brain. They lost their eyesight and are crazy. This is just a little part of what we see.[13]

THE BIRTH OF FLIGHT NURSING

One of the most exciting innovations in military nursing was the development of flight nursing. Lauretta M. Schimmoler, who as early as 1932 established an Aerial Nurse Corps of America, is credited with the original idea of the flight nurse. By 1940, the Army Nurse Corps and the Red Cross Nursing Service were receiving many requests for information about flight nursing. Answers to these inquiries revealed official opposition to such an organization and a lack of imagination concerning the possibility of using aircraft to evacuate the wounded.

When the war began, it was thought that cargo or bomber-type aircraft would be used to transport ill or injured army personnel. It was not deemed necessary to assign nurses to the Air Corps, inasmuch as enlisted men in the Medical Department were taught first aid. After the war began, however, this policy was sharply reversed by the establishment of a Nursing Division in the Air Surgeon's Office in September 1942.

Nurses clamored for admittance to the new Flight Nursing School organized at Bowman Field, Kentucky. There the flight nurse was trained to perform a variety of duties in connection with air evacuation of the sick, wounded, and injured as well as at ground medical installations. After applying for a commission in the Army Nurse Corps, a graduate nurse had to serve a minimum of 6 months in an Army Air Force unit hospital before applying for admittance to the Flight Nursing School. In addition, she had to fulfill the following physical qualifications: between 62 and 72 inches tall, between 105 and 135 pounds, and between 21 and 36 years of age.

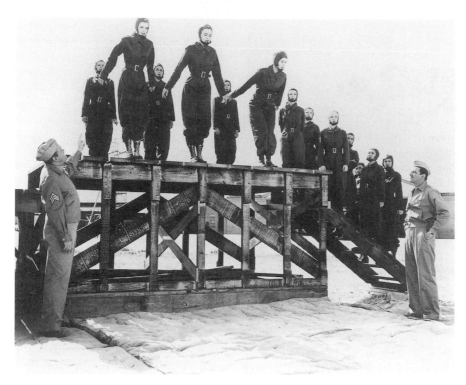

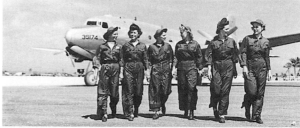

Flight nurse candidates were young, physically fit, and eager to fly.

These qualifications limited flight nurse candidates mainly to the young and physically fit who were anxious to fly and to practice their profession close to a combat area. They performed most of their duties at flight altitudes of 5000 to 10,000 feet in aircraft without pressurized cabins. Because work under such conditions was extremely strenuous, it was important for the nurses to be in excellent health.

In February 1943, the first class of flight nurses graduated at the Bowman Field chapel. The 39 members of this group, which included many former airline hostesses, had been poorly housed and had completed a program of instruction still in the experimental stage. The 4-week course had included class work in air evacuation nursing, air evacuation tactics, survival, aeromedical physiology, and flight-related mental hygiene. In addition, the nurses had received training in plane-loading procedures and military indoctrination and had participated in a 1-day bivouac.

The School of Air Evacuation, the first of its kind, exerted worldwide influence. In November 1943, the course of instruction for flight nurses was increased from 4 weeks to 8 weeks. Anatomy, physiology, ward management, operating-room technique, nursing, first-aid hygiene, and sanitation were emphasized courses of study. Two weeks of the course were devoted to specialized training at cooperating hospitals in Louisville, Kentucky.

A nurse did not automatically receive the designation of "flight nurse." After completing the course, she had to submit a request to the commanding general of the Army Air Forces, who had the au-

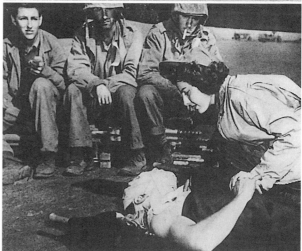

Flight nurses at work.

thority to grant such a designation. On certification, the nurse was permitted to wear the flight nurse's wings. From December 1942 to October 1944, 1079 flight nurses graduated from the AAF School of Air Evacuation.

ADVENTURES OF FLIGHT NURSES

The work of the flight nurse was extremely dangerous, because the aircraft in which she flew, usually C-46 Commandos, acted in a dual capacity. After transporting cargo and troops to the battle fronts, they were unloaded and rapidly converted into ambulance planes for the return trip. Because of their dual function, C-46s were not marked with the Geneva Red Cross or other noncombatant designation; consequently, even though loaded with sick and wounded on return trips, they were fair game for enemy fighters. For this reason, all flight nurses were volunteers.

An adventurous life awaited the flight nurse. Second Lieutenant Mary Louise Hawkins of Redwood City, California, had charge of 24 litter patients en route to Guadalcanal when the plane began running low on fuel. As the pilot was passing over a tiny island, he spotted a 150-foot-square clearing fringed by tall coconut palms. Rather than ditch the plane at sea, he decided to attempt a crash landing. During the landing, a propeller tore a hole in the side of the fuselage, but the patients and crew escaped injury except for one man whose windpipe was severed by a severe cut that fortunately missed the jugular vein. By devising a suction tube from a syringe, a colonic tube, and the inflation tubes from a "Mae West" life jacket, Lieutenant Hawkins was able to keep the man's throat clear of blood until help arrived 19 hours later. After establishing radio contact and receiving supplies of glucose and plasma by parachute, the stranded passengers were picked up by a navy destroyer and brought to Guadalcanal.

Lucy I. Wilson, one of the nurses who had escaped from Corregidor, later returned to the Philippines as a flight nurse. On its first flight from Leyte, her plane evacuated 15 soldiers. "After watching men suffer and die on Bataan and Corregidor because of lack of medical facilities," she said, "it gave me the greatest satisfaction to realize that these men were being flown to the finest hospital care within a few hours." Elsewhere in the European theater, the Distinguished Flying Cross was awarded posthumously to Lieutenant Aleda E. Lutz of Saginaw, Michigan, who was killed after flying more than 190 missions to evacuate wounded personnel from combat areas. Lieutenant Lutz also received the Air Medal with four oak leaf clusters.

Not to be outdone, the navy instituted a flight nurse training program that included lectures, demonstrations, and practice of skills, such as loading patients into planes, the various phases of inflight nursing care, preparation for emergency abandonment of the plane in flight, and maintenance and use of medical equipment. The nurse was also trained to use oxygen in flight and to administer it to her patients. Survival training prepared her to discharge her responsibilities to preserve life and health in any given situation.

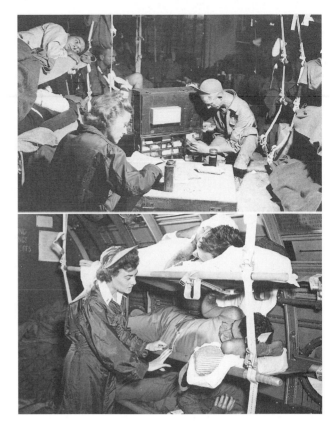
Providing care on board an evacuation plane.

The navy flight nurse and a pharmacist's mate worked as a team. They evacuated patients from forward naval stations to base hospitals or to larger hospitals where patients received more prolonged treatment. The pharmacist's mates assigned to this service received their training with the nurses in naval air transport squadrons. After completing this training, they flew with the nurses aboard hospital planes in the continental United States and thereby gained practical experience on regular hospital flights of the Naval Air Transport Service.

On completion of this training, the nurse and the pharmacist's mate were ready for assignment to the navy's new air evacuation service. One of the major goals was to equalize the patient load of naval hospitals in the United States so that those nearest the Pacific combat zones were not overfilled while beds in hospitals farther from the front remained empty. Another objective was to give the sick or wounded men specialized treatment at hospitals that concentrated on certain types of cases. Finally, whenever feasible, an attempt was made to place the men in hospitals as near their homes as possible. Two-engine Douglas Skytrains served as flying ambulances for the navy. Marked with a large red cross on each side of the fuselage, the planes could accommodate 24 litter patients or 27 walking wounded. If the plane was not filled, regular passengers could be carried, provided there were no patients aboard with contagious diseases.

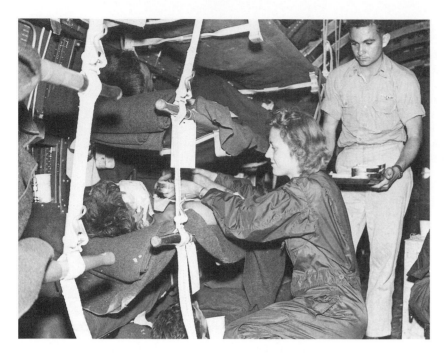

The navy flight nurse and the pharmacist's mate worked as a team.

The medical kit for each flight contained equipment similar to that kept in a medicine cabinet on a ward. There were bedpans and urinals for the litter cases, first-aid articles, and sterile supplies such as needles, syringes, catheters, Levin tubes, and dressings. Because this medical kit also contained stimulants, narcotics, blood plasma, and intravenous fluids, the flight nurse kept the key at all times. Thus equipped, an aircraft was ready to carry any type of patient for any distance.

Ensign Jane Kendleigh, one of the early navy flight nurses, was the first navy nurse to fly to Iwo Jima to evacuate casualties. Landing at the airfield under heavy mortar fire, she and the crew took cover in foxholes while planes dispatched by an aircraft carrier wiped out enemy positions north of the field. Later, Ensign Kendleigh became the first navy nurse to land on Okinawa, where her plane evacuated 20 wounded men on its first flight back to Guam.

INDUSTRIAL NURSING BOOMS

Meanwhile, back on the civilian front, nurses were aware of the massive boom in the defense industry that had developed to support the war effort. One of the more striking effects of the war on the nursing profession was a 100% increase in employment of public health nurses in industry, from 5512 in 1941 to 11,200 by the end of 1943. The nurse was usually employed by a company to carry out a nursing program of preventive medicine and health education among the employees. Small plants were purchasing increasing amounts of part-time service from visiting nurse associations.

After Pearl Harbor, the Committee on Duties of Nurses in Industry recommended that one industrial nurse be provided for up to 300 employees, two or more nurses for up to 600 employees, three or more for up to 1000 employees, one nurse for each additional 1000 employees up to 5000, and one for each additional 2000 employees above that point. The small plant was the most deficient in health care services. Approximately 26 million workers in the United States were employed in plants with fewer than 500 workers each, and 13 million worked in plants with fewer than 100 workers. Part-time service by a voluntary or official public health nursing group represented the only feasible way of satisfying the health care needs of these small plants.

In March 1941, a public health nursing consultant had been assigned to the staff of the division of industrial hygiene at the National Institutes of Health in Bethesda, Maryland. Her activity did much to stimulate the progress of industrial nursing on a national scale through her many contacts as well as through the various industrial hygiene departments. The number of state health departments employing nursing consultants in the field of industrial hygiene grew steadily, and by the end of 1942, 18 of these consultants were located in various states.

The nurses were employed in all types of manufacturing plants. As the war progressed, data issued by the Office of War Information revealed that 65,000 people had been killed in industry in the 2 years from December 7, 1941, to December 31, 1943—more than the military casualties for the same period. The 210,000 workers injured during the same period greatly exceeded the number wounded in battle. According to the same agency, about 50,000 workers were absent every day from industrial

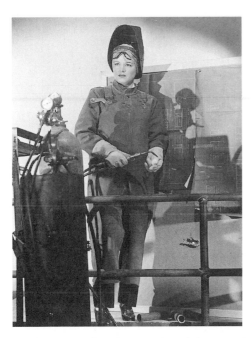

Industrial accidents to workers threatened war industry productivity.

jobs because of accidents or injuries. Deaths and injuries on the job resulted in the loss of 270 million workdays per year—equivalent to a loss of 900,000 workers from production lines.

By analyzing the data collected in 1943 from industrial establishments throughout the nation, one investigator concluded that a nurse on 8-hour dispensary duty should be able to attend to and record from 50 to 115 problems per day. These figures were averages for nurses whose full time was spent in the dispensary; the higher number of visits per day per nurse were found in the larger industrial medical units, where nursing service was more specialized. A caseload as high as 600 for one nurse in 1 day was boasted by one company during a successful immunization program. Apparently, all nurses who had an average caseload of at least 75 per day were limited to the routine changing of dressings on minor injuries and to the dispensing of medications. Conversely, it is interesting to note that all industrial medical departments surveyed expected a nurse to see at least 50 cases if she stayed in the dispensary all day.

The war-induced employment of millions of women, especially in small plants, presented numerous problems, among which was the legal restriction on work hours for women. Another problem was the new Federal Contracts Act, which stipulated that no work should be performed in surroundings that were unsanitary, hazardous, or dangerous to the health of either women or men. Employers were usually willing to cooperate with these regulations, which nurses helped to enforce. This assistance, however, represented only one aspect of the nurse's usefulness to the tens of thousands of new women workers in industrial plants. Nurses appreciated the special

concerns of women, such as rest periods following strenuous activity, facilities to ensure cleanliness, the availability of nutritious foods, relief from some of the emotional and physical demands made by children at home, and reactions to the work environment. For example, safe clothing for women presented a problem. Because long hair was fashionable for women at that time, female workers covered their hair with the greatest reluctance.

The government requested actress Veronica Lake to pose for photographs illustrating the dangers of wearing long hair while operating machines and circulated these pictures widely.

THE NATION'S HEALTH IN 1943

When the nation completed its first year of war in early 1943, concern for civilian health had not decreased. Under wartime conditions, weaknesses in health care would rapidly show in statistics. The general death rate in the United States for 1918 had been 18.1 per 1000 population. For 1942, it was estimated at 10.4. This gratifying reduction had been achieved very slowly.

It is interesting to contrast the 10 leading causes of death in 1918 with those in 1943. In 1918 they were heart disease, pneumonia, tuberculosis, kidney disease, cerebral hemorrhage, birth injuries and other diseases associated with early infancy, cancer, accidents, diarrhea, and diabetes. In the few short years since 1936, the new sulfonamide drugs had revolutionized the treatment of a long list of infections: blood poisoning, puerperal fever, septic sore throat, scarlet fever, and pneumonia. Certain threats to the nation's health had been effectively eradicated and no longer caused great concern; however, others had not been reduced, and still others had actually increased.

The 1918 death rate from typhoid, for example, had been at least 15 times higher than in 1943, and the diphtheria rate for 1918 had been 25 times higher. Despite the disruption of civilian life due to the war, typhoid fever and diphtheria had continued to decline since 1941. Physicians and nurses knew how to prevent these diseases and how to control their spread at minimum expense to communities and individual families. State and local health departments maintained close supervision of water, milk, and food supplies; vulnerable groups were vaccinated against typhoid; and a higher proportion of children and young people had been protected against diphtheria than at any time in the past.

In 1918, tuberculosis had been the third highest cause of death. By 1943 it had dropped to seventh place, claiming about 4 lives in every 10,000. Yet tuberculosis of the lungs remained the leading cause of death among people 20 to 45 years of age—the young men and women on whom the nation heavily

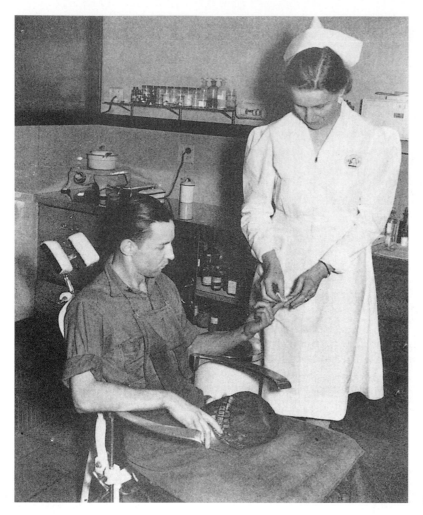

Wartime production greatly increased the need for industrial nurses.

relied for building the army and navy and for producing the weapons of war.

Pneumonia had been the second most frequent cause of death in 1918 and not entirely because of the influenza epidemic. It continued to rank third among the leading causes of death until 1938, when the widespread use of sulfa drugs began to reduce drastically the number of deaths from this disease. The actual number of cases, however, had not substantially decreased, because there still existed no preventive medicine for mass application.

Although malaria had not been listed among the great killers in the United States during World War I, it was among the 10 highest causes of death in many southern states. It was estimated during the early 1930s that approximately 2 million cases occurred each year. No concerted effort was made to eradicate the malaria mosquito in the South until 1935, when federal funds were allotted for work projects in 17 states for ditching, draining, dusting, and oiling the breeding waters of *Anopheles quadrimaculatus*, the principal malaria-carrying mosquito.

By 1943, most of the diseases affecting infants no longer ranked among the leading causes of death. Conversely, diseases associated with old age had

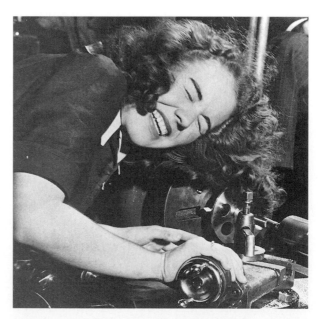

The government warned women workers of the dangers of leaving long hair uncovered while operating machinery.

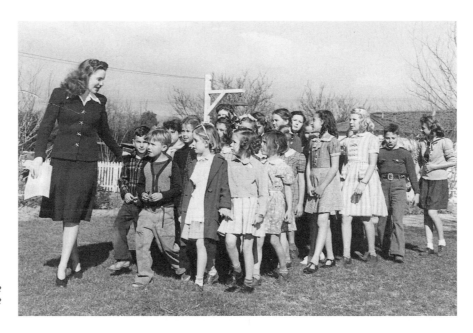

Immunization against communicable diseases had greatly improved the health of children by 1943.

become more prevalent since 1918. Cancer, seventh on the 1918 list, had risen to second place in 1943. The mortality rate for heart disease, the number one killer in 1918 and still number one in 1943, had actually increased. Cerebral hemorrhage, kidney disease, and diabetes, which had all moved up a notch or two on the list since 1918, now caused a larger proportion of deaths than they had 25 years earlier.

This shift among the leading causes of death occurred primarily because a significant reduction in deaths from childhood diseases had enabled a greater proportion of the population to reach an age at which they were vulnerable to cancer, heart disease, and diabetes. Moreover, medical knowledge about communicable diseases was still inadequate, and methods of preventing and treating adult diseases had not yet been developed. The little knowledge physicians and nurses had acquired concerning the chronic diseases of middle and late life had not been applied on a wide enough scale to alter the death rates resulting from these diseases.

The first attempts to improve civilian health on a large scale had occurred in the 1920s and thereafter began to yield considerable results. Between 1923 and 1943, the average life expectancy in the United States increased from about 55 to 65 years. The average newborn baby in 1943 could expect to live a decade longer than children who had been born during the First World War. This increase was all the more significant when one considers that during the first 20 years of the century the gain had been only 5 years.

INDICATORS OF HEALTH PROBLEMS

Despite these achievements in combating the effects of disease, the results of examinations conducted by local selective service boards and military induction centers indicated that the health of the nation's young men was no better at the start of World War II than at the time of the World War I draft. A report of physical examinations from 21 selected states, issued by National Headquarters, Selective Service System, on August 1, 1943, in *Medical Statistics Bulletin No. 2*, summarized the findings for approximately 121,700 registrants. This publication was a valuable information source for nurses and other hospital personnel on the incidence of many diseases. The report analyzed the number of draft rejections, which were classified as follows: In a typical group of 1000 registrants examined by local boards, 438 (43.8%) were rejected; 90 (16.0%) of the remaining 562 were then rejected at induction stations.

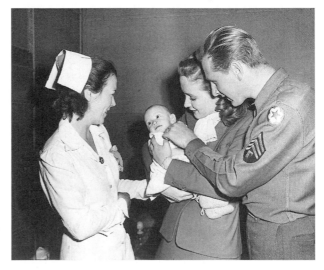

By 1943, control of diseases affecting infants and children had increased the average life expectancy dramatically.

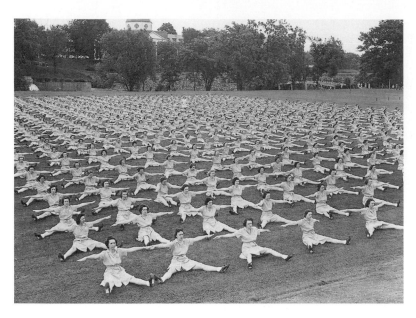

The war effort focused new attention on the health and fitness of Americans.

Rejection rates increased steadily with age. For example, 41.6% of the 22-year-old registrants were rejected at either local boards or induction stations, whereas 80.3% of the 36-year-old registrants were rejected.

Tooth defects were the leading cause of rejection, accounting for 16.5% of all rejections at local boards and induction stations. Other causes of rejection and the percentages they constituted of all rejections were as follows: eye defects, 11.7%; mental and nervous defects, 10.4%; cardiovascular defects, 10.0%; musculoskeletal defects, 8.9%; hernia, 5.9%; venereal diseases, 5.9%; ear, nose, and throat defects, 5.5%; tuberculosis and other lung diseases, 3.8%; educational deficiency, 3.8%; defects of the feet, 3.0%; underweight, 2.9%; other causes, 11.7%.

NEEDS ON THE HOME FRONT

Although the emotional appeal of the military service attracted many nurses, the needs of the home front, though less dramatic, were no less real. Dr. William P. Shepard, a public health physician on the West Coast, wrote a letter containing a vivid description of these needs. Health officers in many other parts of the country could recount similar stories:

> Increasing pressure for public health nurses to enlist is becoming apparent on the West Coast. It is the public health nurses who are conscious of community needs and, therefore, more prompt in responding to a national appeal.
>
> Knowing what I do of nurses' duties in the Army and Navy, I cannot but feel that this is an unwarranted waste of woman power when public health needs of the civilian population are becoming so urgent and complex. These needs

are particularly acute in the many war production areas of this Coast. Out here, industry was less important than mining and agriculture until now.

Almost overnight, great cities of industrial workers have suddenly sprung up where there was little population before. Many small towns have doubled their populations, and I can name 10 or 15 in which the population has been tripled or quadrupled.

Until you see it, you cannot conceive of the serious public health problems this entails. In some of these areas, sewer manholes are overflowing into the streets; rat population, always a serious plague menace on this Coast, has even outstripped human population increases; sanitation of public eating places has broken down; immunization is being neglected. Hospitalization is at a premium in all places and actually unobtainable in many. Remaining physicians are so overworked they must refuse all house calls. One doctor told me the other day a frantic mother phoned that her child had been lying on his head and heels, unconscious, with a high fever, since four that afternoon. He was the fifth doctor she had called and all had been unable to come. He, too, was obliged to decline the call. Deliveries are taking place in homes without even a midwife, let alone a physician, and mothers are being discharged from the hospitals three days postpartum.

For the first time in my memory, organized medical groups, such as county societies and the California Physician's Service, Inc., are appealing for bedside nursing programs. Despite all this, somewhere in the nursing profession there is coercion of public health nurses to join the armed forces. With the winter upon us, which on this Coast means wet clothes and wet feet, and with the overcrowding and migratory problems described above, I am deeply concerned lest this war might be lost on the home front because of lack of wisdom in using trained people where they can do the most good.[14]

The quality of service to hospital patients was much poorer in 1943 than in 1938 because patients were receiving fewer hours of care from graduate nurses. Whereas either graduate or student nurses had provided all bedside care in 1938, nonprofessional workers had assumed an appreciable part of this burden by 1943. Full-time personnel had dispensed all bedside care in 1938, whereas in 1943 part-time personnel were responsible for many services in some hospitals. In addition, the scarcity of physicians had forced the nursing staff to assume duties formerly performed by physicians. Even worse, the shortage of auxiliary workers—orderlies, ward helpers, and kitchen maids—had compelled the bedside nurses to perform duties for which these workers had formerly been responsible.

HOSPITALS IN NEED OF HELP

Because of the obvious need of civilian hospitals to bolster their nursing services, they turned to the federal government for help. At the beginning of

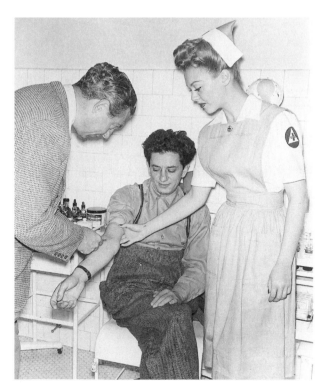

Nurses' aides could not fully replace the more than 75,000 graduate nurses in military service.

federal fiscal year 1942–1943, Congress appropriated a sum of $3,500,000 for nursing education, almost double the $1,800,000 that it had voted for the fiscal year 1941–1942. The goals for which these funds had been appropriated, however, were limited. About 3700 inactive graduate nurses had returned to active duty after taking refresher courses. About 4300 graduate nurses had profited from advanced study of such specialties as teaching in nursing schools, nursing in public health, and supervision. Admissions to basic nursing schools had increased about 12,000 over the first-year enrollments in these same schools during baseline year 1940–1941. Under this program, a school could not receive federal aid, except for tuition scholarships, unless it could demonstrate an increase in admissions over the year 1940–1941.

Despite the need for student nurses, federally aided schools achieved only 80% of their projected spring 1943 admissions. At the same time, only 67% of the expected spring enrollments at all schools materialized. Admission to federally aided nursing schools declined 10.4% in February 1943 compared with February 1942. The nursing schools' difficulty in attracting an adequate number of student nurses could be explained by the increasingly acute competition for womanpower in 1943. Many young women who would ordinarily have entered nursing schools were instead joining the women's auxiliaries of the military forces and war industries. Employment statistics for December 1942 indicated that 2 to 2½ million women were needed for war industries, 1 million for nonwar industries, and 200,000 for the women's armed forces auxiliaries.

Although there were an estimated 7 million women in the United States available for full-time work, potential candidates for nurse training were limited largely to young women between 18 and 21 years of age who had graduated from high school and who were physically fit for this strenuous career. An estimated 95% of all students admitted to nursing schools were high-school graduates. In 1940, 643,793 young women graduated from high school, of whom a mere 10% could be expected to complete a college education.

Employers in other types of war-related work engaged in fierce competition for the services of this tiny group of high-school and college graduates. In peacetime, many young women had been willing to undergo the rigors of nurse training only because of the lack of more attractive employment options. Under the competitive conditions fostered by the war, however, they could not be expected to limit themselves to nursing when there were opportunities for other types of war service, many of which included paid training. Unless nursing schools immediately adopted a comprehensive plan for aiding their students, enrollments for 1943 were certain to drop below prewar levels.

Because the armed forces enjoyed the highest priority for receiving nursing care, it was difficult to maintain high standards for nursing services on the home front at the same time. Indeed, the war accentuated the truth of the words of Surgeon General Thomas L. Parran of the U.S. Public Health Service. "The strength of any nation does not exceed the strength and health of its people." During an all-out war, an unchecked epidemic was the ablest ally of the enemy. When for a time armies were being raised faster than ships could be built to transport them, the health of civilian shipbuilders became as important as the health of the army and navy. The most obvious solution to this health problem was to educate more nurses. Because a student nurse's potential for service was roughly 60% to 80% of that of a graduate nurse, a rapid increase in student nurse enrollments was regarded as the fastest way of enlarging the hospital nurse service force.

THE U.S. CADET NURSE CORPS

To deal with this crisis, the Federal Security Agency arranged a series of conferences to explore possible solutions to the acute nursing shortage. Attended by representatives from all the major professional nursing and hospital associations, these conferences resulted in a bill introduced into the House of Representatives by Frances Payne Bolton, congresswoman from Ohio. Widely endorsed by educational groups and professional associations, the bill that created the U.S. Cadet Nurse Corps became law on June 15, 1943.

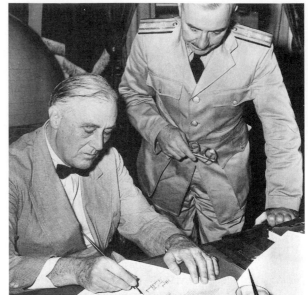

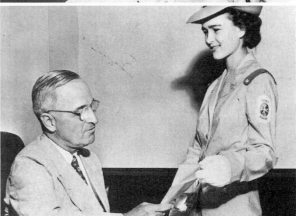

President Roosevelt signed the Cadet Nurse Corps Bill; President Truman extended it until 1948.

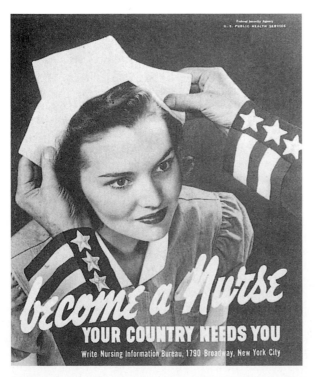

An appeal to the nation's young women to become nurses during World War II.

Under the provisions of the Bolton Act, the U.S. Public Health Service subsidized the entire education of nursing students—tuition, fees, books, uniforms, maintenance, and monthly stipends. To obtain the benefits of the U.S. Cadet Nurse Corps, a student was not required to prove actual need of funds, but she did have to promise to engage in essential *military* or *civilian* nursing for the duration of the war. Candidates were to be between the ages of 17 and 35 and fulfill minimum admission requirements, which included good health and graduation, with a good scholastic record, from an accredited high school.

To accelerate the period of nurse education, the Bolton Act stipulated that it be reduced from the normal 36 months to 30 months or fewer. Because state boards of nursing required a 3-year program, a compromise establishing three levels of cadets was worked out: pre-cadets, junior cadets, and senior cadets. Pre-cadet was the designation given the student during her first 9 months in the school, when she was studying the basic sciences and fundamentals of nursing. Junior cadets were nursing students enrolled for the next 15 to 21 months of their training. Senior cadets had actually completed their basic educational requirements. The state boards, however, demanded an additional 6 months' experience. During this period, students undertook an important practice assignment either in their home school or in another civilian, military, or government institution.

Immediately after passage of the Bolton Act, the Division of Nurse Education was established within the U.S. Public Health Service and made directly responsible to the surgeon general. Lucile Petry, who had been on the nurse education staff of the Public Health Service for 2 years and had recently been named dean of Cornell University–New York Hospital School of Nursing, New York, was appointed as its director. Federal Security Administrator Paul V. McNutt promptly appointed an advisory committee on the training of nurses to assist in implementing the act.

After national nursing needs were carefully considered, enrollment quotas were established for the Cadet Nurse Corps: 125,000 for the first 2 years of the program, 65,000 to be recruited during the first 12 months, and 60,000 the following year, ending June 20, 1945. Under the efficient direction of Petry and her staff, along with major assistance from the War Advertising Council, both quotas were exceeded, a performance that established the nurse recruitment program as the most successful of the war.

CHARACTERISTICS OF MILITARY NURSES

An examination of the detailed American Red Cross tabulation of the qualifications of the 75,029 nurses in the service—12,239 in the navy and 62,790 in the

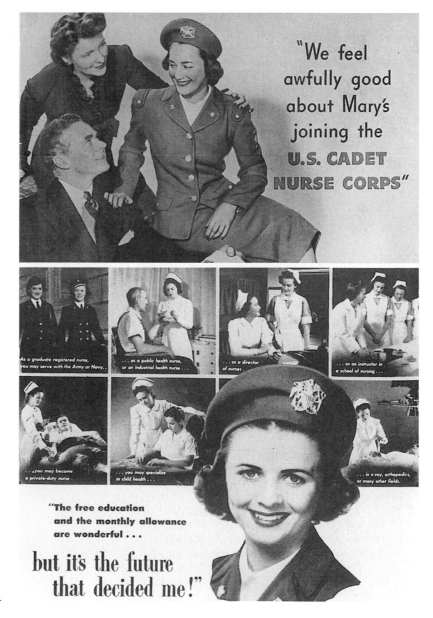

Cadet Nurse Corps recruitment advertisements.

TABLE 14-1	Ages of Army and Navy Nurses in 1945 (In Percentages)		
AGE (Y)	NAVY	ARMY	TOTAL
21–25	34.6	26.8	28.1
26–30	40.0	34.6	35.5
31–35	15.6	18.2	17.8
36–40	6.9	11.4	10.6
41–45	1.8	6.3	5.5
46 and older	1.1	2.6	2.4
No record	—	0.1	0.1

army—reveals several interesting facts. For example, a much larger percentage of younger nurses served with the navy (Table 14-1).[15]

Regarding educational background, 97% of the navy nurses were high-school graduates, compared with 94% of the army nurses. Of the 75,000 nurses, 20% had had some college education, either before or after their nursing education. Almost 90% had received their nursing education after 1931, and 72% had graduated from hospitals having a daily average of more than 100 patients. Only 16% had undergone any undergraduate training in psychiatry, either in their home school or through affiliation. The breakdown of the 7% of nurses who had postgraduate training was as follows: 1%, communicable diseases; 1.3%, operating room technique; 0.7%, anesthesia; and 4.1%, public health. A sample of 5000 nurses revealed that only 10% had done any other type of work, most of it clerical.

IMAGE OF THE MILITARY NURSE

How did servicemen regard the female military nurses? Male veterans often remarked that the so-called weaker sex was often cooler under fire. Coming from wounded men who had recently been in the thick of combat, this was a high compliment. Accustomed to the suffering of patients in peacetime, the nurses tended to take the horrors of war in stride. Death and wounds had been a part of their routine in civilian life. Even so, the kind of death and suffering that the nurses witnessed in war was something new.

An editorial in *America* magazine perceptively analyzed the role of the military nurse:

> Nurses do not receive the publicity of Four Jills and a Jeep. Their pictures do not fill the papers, for there is nothing pictorially pretty about a grimy-faced young girl sponging dirt and blood from the face and body of a wounded soldier. They are not at all glamorous, our nurses, for their profession is not glamorous. There is nothing glamorous in caked blood and torn arms and legs and faces half blown away. There is nothing glamorous in a hospital just behind the

lines when the wounded come pouring in, nothing glamorous in the long night's watch at the bedsides of boys in pain, delirious, afraid, crazed, some of them. Nothing glamorous in the washing and the scrubbing and the cleaning. Their days and nights are full of work and sights that strong men could not stand.

> Their great glory is that they have offered themselves to service, calmly, almost casually. It is their vocation to tend the sick. Their place is wherever the sick and wounded happen to be. Their task is to be composed in disaster, smiling in the face of suffering, cheerful in the blackest moments, beautiful in the midst of horror.

> Their reward is in their giving and in the grateful memory of those to whom they give. Long after the soldiers shall have forgotten the entertainers and come to blush a bit at their silly devotion to pin-up girls, they will remember with a warm, cleansing glow of gratitude the nurse who smiled at their irritable demands, the nurse who helped them to walk again, the nurse who mothered them in the ugliness of their illness.[16]

Scores of movies with nurses as leading characters were made during the war. In late 1943, a movie dramatized the heroism of the 100 army and navy nurses who served with the embattled American forces in the Philippines during the opening months of the struggle against Japan. Entitled *So Proudly We Hail* and starring Claudette Colbert, Paulette Goddard, Veronica Lake, and Barbara Britton, the

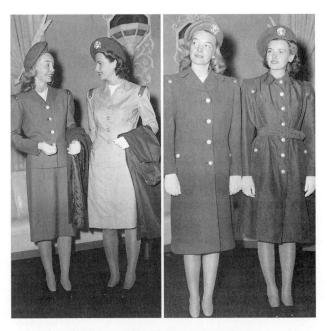

Uniforms of the U.S. Cadet Nurse Corps.

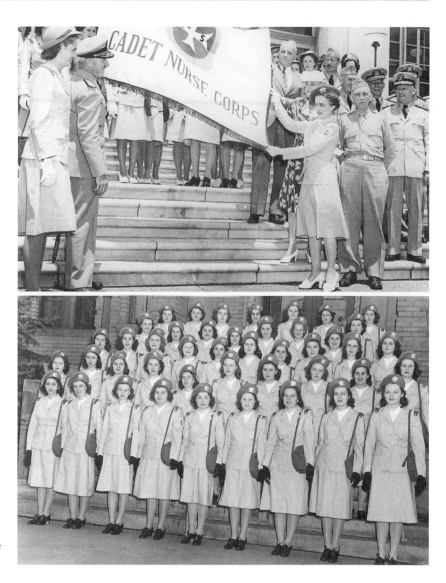

Lucile Petry with Cadet Nurse Corps flag; cadets at Carbondale Hospital School of Nursing in Pennsylvania.

film received great acclaim. According to a review in *Life*,

> *So Proudly We Hail* is one of the most terrifying war films to come from Hollywood this year. The reason for this is the authenticity and grim realism of the movie. For 126 minutes audiences see the next best thing to an actual pictorial record of the last bloody days of Bataan and Corregidor. Almost documentary in form, the story tells of the heroic part played by the small band of Army nurses in the Philippines.[17]

Photographs of the nurses and their surroundings taken by a war correspondent who had escaped from Corregidor in the last days lent an air of technical authenticity to the film. These pictures were used to reproduce the jungle background and the hospital facilities where the nurses worked.

Another unusual film, *Cry Havoc*, presented a somewhat harsher version of the nurses' story. In this movie, which starred Margaret Sullavan, Ann Sothern, Joan Blondell, and Fay Bainter, male roles served only as background cases for the nurses to care for. These two films provided a rare opportunity to display the work of nurses to the public, helped satisfy the public demand for information about the epic battles of Bataan and Corregidor, and improved morale on the home front by depicting the heroism of American nurses in battle.

THE NURSE SHORTAGE BECOMES ACUTE

The last Allied offensive in Europe began in early November 1944, when seven Allied armies pushed forward. It might have been more successful had the weather been better and had the lines of supply been able to keep pace with the advancing troops. On December 16, 1944, the Germans launched a sudden counterattack. For a time it appeared that the enemy, who overran 700 square miles of Belgium and Luxembourg, might actually stem the tide of the Allied advance. As American troops suffered

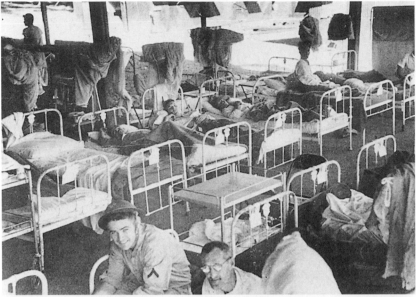

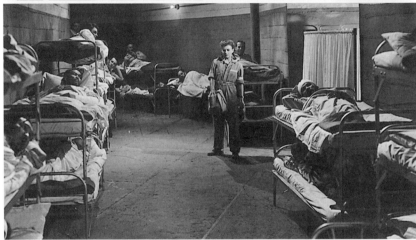

Corregidor and Bataan hospital scenes.

their heaviest casualties of the war, more than 1750 per day, the need for nurses quickly became acute. One of the initial reactions to this sudden reversal in the fortunes of war was, "Give us nurses—10,000 overnight."

At the same time, a serious shortage of professional and nonprofessional personnel in America's civilian hospitals coincided with an all-time demand for hospital care. According to a survey conducted by the American Hospital Association, certain beds, wards, and operating rooms in 23% of the nation's hospitals were not being used because of insufficient personnel. This situation, were it allowed to continue, would adversely affect the nation's physical and mental health.

The acute shortage of nursing personnel during the winter of 1944–1945 occurred for several reasons. The army and navy had enrolled more than 65,000 registered nurses, most of whom had volunteered from civilian hospitals. Approximately 13,800 nurses were employed in industry—nearly twice as many as before the war—and they proved

their worth in maintaining workers' health throughout wartime production. In an attempt to fill this vacuum, student nurses carried about 80% of the work of the 1300 hospital-affiliated nursing schools.

THE NURSE DRAFT BILL

Gradually, Washington began to understand how vital nurses were to the war effort. On December 19, 1944, newspapers across the nation carried an article by columnist Walter Lippmann, who charged the army with gross neglect of wounded soldiers by not having provided an adequate number of nurses to care for them:

> The last thing our people will put up with is that sick and wounded American soldiers should suffer because the Army cannot find enough women to nurse them. Yet, I am reporting only the stark truth, which is well known to the Army

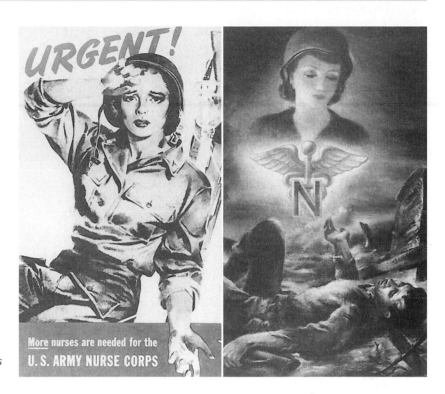

By late 1944, the need for military nurses was desperate.

and to the leaders of the medical profession, when I say that in military hospitals at home and abroad our men are not receiving the nursing care they must have, and that with casualties increasing in number and in seriousness, this will mean for many of the men brought in from the battlefields that their recovery is delayed, and even jeopardized.[18]

Lippmann maintained that there were already plenty of trained nurses and nurses' aides in the United States. In addition, there were many women being trained as nurses and more who could be trained as nurses' aides. He further pointed out that, about 2 months before, approximately 27,000 nurses had been declared to be engaged in nonessential nursing in civilian life and were therefore eligible for the army, pending examination.

In his State of the Union message on January 6, 1945, President Roosevelt startled the nation with the unprecedented request for a draft of women nurses:

Since volunteering has not produced the number of nurses required, I urge that the Selective Service Act be amended to provide for induction of nurses into the armed forces. The need is too pressing to await the outcome of further efforts at recruiting.[19]

Many congressmen were also alarmed by the nursing shortage in the army and navy as well as by reports of 11 army units being sent overseas without a single nurse, when each should have had 80 or 90. Considerable debate took place, both in and out of Congress. Because nurses were not volunteering in sufficient numbers, some congressmen supported the president's proposal for conscription as the only practical solution to this problem.

Editor Janet Giester of *Trained Nurse and Hospital Review* wrote that "the story of the 11 hospital units that sailed without nurses had been told to me apprehensively by elevator men, bus drivers, and the cleaning women, all of whom have kin in the services. . . . Another woman told me the nurses' actions in 'letting our boys die' was a national scandal." Congresswoman Clare Boothe Luce, socialite, playwright, and member of the powerful House Committee on Military Affairs, told the press: "Perhaps there is something wrong with our method of training and recruiting nurses, but in this phase American women have not been doing their part as well as the British. American women have done wonderfully, though, in industry."

On February 2, 1945, the Gallup poll posed the following question to a cross section of Americans: Do you approve or disapprove of the proposal to draft nurses to serve with the army and navy? The results of this poll showed that 73% approved, 19% disapproved, and 8% had no opinion. Three weeks later, another group was polled on a similar question: Do you think that single nurses 20 to 45 years of age should be drafted for service with the armed forces? This time 65% answered yes, 28% said no, and 7 percent had no opinion.

Reports on conditions in a cross section of civilian hospitals revealed that, far from hoarding nurses, these institutions were serving their communities under extreme hardship and privation. The following examples served to illustrate this problem:

A 475-bed West Virginia tuberculosis hospital. On duty were 20 nurses, 10 of whom had had tuberculosis; 5 of these served part-time and 5 full-time on light work only. Two of the 10 healthy nurses were threatening to enter the Army Nurse Corps, lest they be considered slackers.

A New York State hospital of 106 beds. In 1941 it had 32 full-time staff nurses and 4 part-time on a 48-hour week. In 1945 it had 19 full-time and 22 part-time on a 60-hour week.

A Missouri state mental hospital. For 2600 patients there were 9 graduate nurses.

A South Dakota hospital of 125 beds and 30 bassinets. Daily census for 1944 of 150; for early 1945 it had increased to 187. It had already released 50 graduate nurses to the armed services, and 10 others had filed applications. No general duty nurses were employed.

After quickly passing the House of Representatives, the bill to draft nurses into the armed forces became bogged down in the Senate. Because of the military successes of the Allied armies on both the eastern and western fronts of Europe, Congress began to question the need for additional manpower legislation. On March 24, 1945, the Allied armies succeeded in crossing the Rhine, and 5 days later General Patton captured Frankfurt. Just as V-E Day was approaching, all the drastic attempts short of conscription to recruit nurses became embarrassingly successful. Stimulated by the threat of the draft, the nursing profession had responded with an overwhelming mass of applications for commissions, 10,000 of which were filed between January 8 and January 29, 1945, alone. Similarly, the pressure of possible conscription had induced 60% of the senior cadets to choose the army instead of civilian employment.

When Colonel Florence A. Blanchfield, superintendent of the Army Nurse Corps, returned from Europe, she found that there were actually too many nurses. By late April 1945, the Medical Department was in an embarrassing position. Too many of its 54,000 graduate nurses were idle, while the number of senior cadet nurses in military hospitals had more than doubled, to a total of 6000. This excess of nurses posed a serious problem, because the overstaffing of hospitals had caused a plunge in morale. In view of this overabundance, Colonel Blanchfield recommended that 2000 civilian nurses be released and that Congress cease efforts to pass the proposed draft legislation.

THE WAR ENDS

The last days of the Third Reich were a nightmare. As the Allies overran Germany, they encountered indescribable examples of Nazi barbarism in the

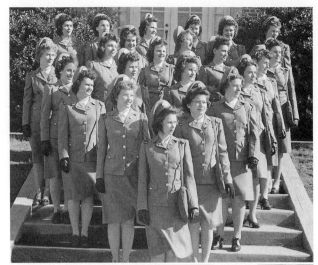
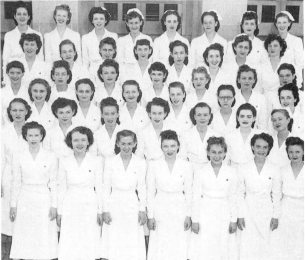

Cadet and civilian nurses enlisted in droves in response to the threat of being drafted.

concentration camps of Belsen, Buchenwald, Gotha, Auschwitz, and Dachau, where more than 10 million civilians had been executed in gas chambers and in "scientific experiments." About 6 million of these victims were Jews, including children; most of the others were eastern Europeans and political prisoners. Army nurses in Germany had a rare opportunity to observe the effects of starvation on the human body and to learn how survivors recovered from such a grim ordeal. The physical abuse suffered by prisoners in German concentration camps was worse than anything they had ever seen.

The invasion of Japan, scheduled for autumn 1945, was expected to encounter stubborn resistance and to exact a heavy toll on American and British lives, because the Imperial Japanese Army, unlike the navy and air force, was still relatively intact. Its strength was estimated at 5 million—2 million on the islands of Japan and an additional 3 million in Manchuria, China, and Formosa. In view of such a

SEVENTY-NINTH CONGRESS

JANUARY 3, 1945, TO JANUARY 3, 1947

H. R. 1284. Mr. May; January 9, 1945 (Military Affairs).

Registered female nurses between 18 and 44 years of age are subject to registration and induction, under the Selective Training and Service Act of 1940, for medical duty.

H. R. 1666. Mrs. Rogers; January 22, 1945 (Military Affairs).

Female graduate nurses between the ages of 20 and 45 must register and shall be liable to induction into the armed forces. Persons inducted shall be commissioned in the Army at a grade not lower than that of second lieutenant or in the United States Naval Reserve (or appointed to a relative rank in the Navy Nurse Corps) at a grade not lower than that of ensign. Classes of persons deferred or exempted, etc., are listed. Bounties, substitutes, and purchases for release are prohibited. Provisions shall be administered by the President through the Selective Service System. The penalty for evasion, interference, etc. shall be imprisonment for not more than 5 years or a fine of not more than $10,000 or both.

H. R. 2277. Reported in Senate March 28, 1945.

Nurses' Selective Service Act of 1945—Every woman between 20 and 45 years of age who is (1) a registered nurse, or (2) a graduate nurse, or eligible to apply for examination as a registered nurse, is subject to registration and induction in accordance with procedures under the Selective Training and Service Act. No person registered with a selective-service local board under this act shall be ordered to report for induction until after all qualified graduates of the United States Cadet Nurse Corps registered with such board, who are not deferred, have been ordered to report for induction. A graduate of the United States Cadet Nurse Corps may be deferred from service in the armed forces under this act only on grounds of dependency or physical defects, etc. Except as to graduates of the United States Cadet Nurse Corps, no person shall be classified as available for induction if she has been declared by the Procurement and Assignment Service to be engaged in essential services and not available for induction, and no nurse in a Veterans' Administration hospital facility shall be so classified unless she is released by the Administrator of Veterans' Affairs. Persons who have consecrated their lives to religious service or, who are taking theological training for the purpose of so doing, and those who have volunteered for such service are exempt. Provisions cover male as well as female nurses.

After President Roosevelt's State of the Union speech, bills to draft female nurses began moving through Congress.

formidable military obstacle, it had been calculated that the war could drag on until late 1946 and that the assault on Japan would cost between 500,000 and 1 million American casualties.

The atomic bomb brought the war to a sudden and dramatic end. On August 6, 1945, an American B-29 flew over Hiroshima and at 9:15 a.m. dropped an atomic bomb over the center of the city. Hiroshima had been selected as the target because it was the headquarters of the Japanese army in southern Japan and a key military assembly and supply point. This atomic bomb, the first ever used for military purposes, plummeted 5 miles before exploding with a destructive force equal to 20,000 tons of TNT. The explosion blotted out the sky in a blinding flash. In that instant, thousands died. A mushroom-shaped cloud of dust and smoke swiftly rose to a height of 40,000 feet. More than 78,000 people perished in this holocaust, 37,000 were injured, and about 13,900 were reported missing. Japanese nurses played a heroic role in the terrifying chaos that followed.

Despite the horrible destruction of Hiroshima, Japanese militarists refused to surrender. On August 8, the Soviet Union declared war on Japan, and on August 9 a second atomic bomb leveled Nagasaki, another major railroad junction, supply depot, and industrial center in southern Japan. After this second blow, Japan could endure no more and petitioned for peace on August 10, 1945. On August 14, President Truman announced that Japan had accepted the Allied terms of surrender. The formal end of World War II came on September 2, 1945, when General MacArthur conducted the official ceremonies of surrender on the battleship *Missouri* in Tokyo Bay.

THE CONTRIBUTION OF NURSES

"There has been a larger number of war-service volunteers from nursing than from any other American profession," stated the *American Journal of Nursing* in evaluating the performance of nurses in the war. Almost half of the 240,000 active registered nurses in the United States, many of whom could not meet the physical requirements, had volunteered for military service. As of June 30, 1945, about 29% of all active nurses (65,377) were on duty with the armed services.

In the nation's nursing schools, the total student nurse enrollment had increased 30% since 1943,

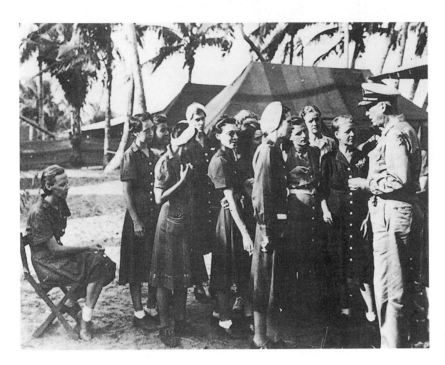

Army and Navy nurses liberated from Santo Tomas Japanese prison camp in Manila.

thanks largely to the 179,000 young women who joined the Cadet Nurse Corps and pledged to engage in essential civilian or military nursing for the duration of the war. To comply with President Truman's request for an orderly termination of this massive educational program, the U.S. Public Health Service established October 15, 1945, as the final date for new admissions to the corps. By permitting students admitted before this date to graduate, the federal government temporarily cushioned the effect of the withdrawal of its funds from the schools.

When the Cadet Nurse Corps program finally terminated in 1948, it had received over $160 million in federal appropriations and had graduated 125,000 students. In addition, approximately 15,000 graduate nurses had received federal funds for advanced study before the grants were discontinued on October 15, 1945. Of this group, about 5000 took intensive courses designed for nurses who could not leave their jobs. The importance of nursing within the U.S. Public Health Service reached an all-time high in fiscal year 1945, when the appropriation for the Cadet Nurse Corps amounted to $62,140,760, more than one half the total Public Health Service budget of $120 million.

As a result of these federal aid programs, hospital nursing schools obtained more students and better qualified instructors and head nurses. In addition, over $17 million worth of Lanham Act building funds were allotted to schools in the cadet nurse program for the construction of nurses' residences and instructional facilities. During the senior cadet period of instruction, 73% of the senior cadets remained in their home hospitals, whereas the other 27% served in the army, navy, Veterans Administration, Public Health Service, Indian Service, or other civilian hospitals or public health agencies.

The price of America's victory in World War II had been high. Some 16,300,000 Americans had served in the armed forces, of whom 292,131 were killed and 671,000 were wounded. The excellent record of lives saved—96 of each 100 wounded—had been

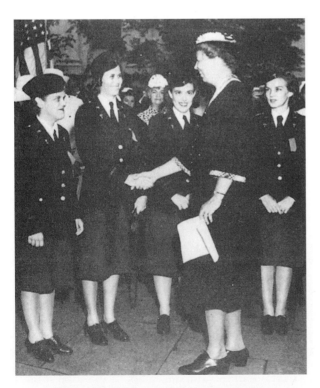

Eleanor Roosevelt congratulates army nurses.

achieved because of nursing care, effective first-aid treatment, frontline surgery, the availability of blood plasma, chemotherapy, and early evacuation from battle areas. Had it not been for these essential factors, the number of deaths would have been far greater.

REFERENCES

1. "To the Graduate of '39," *American Journal of Nursing*, vol. 39 (May 1939):529–530.
2. "Federal Legislation—and the World We Live in," *American Journal of Nursing*, vol. 40 (February 1940):176.
3. "The Philadelphia Biennial: Nursing in a Democracy," *American Journal of Nursing*, vol. 40 (June 1940):673.
4. Ibid.
5. U.S. Public Health Service, "Minutes, First Meeting of the Advisory Committee on Rules and Regulations of the Surgeon General," Federal Record Center, Suitland, Maryland, RG 90, p. 8.
6. Stella Goostray, *Memoirs: Half a Century in Nursing* (Boston: Boston Nursing Archives, Boston University Mugar Memorial Library, 1969), pp. 116–117.
7. "Training Program Announced for 100,000 Nurses' Aides," *Hospital Management*, vol. 52 (September 1941):44–45.
8. Quoted in the U.S. Congress, House, Committee on Military Affairs, *Army Nurse Corps, Hearings on H.R. 3718* (Washington, DC: Government Printing Office, 1944), pp. 28–30.
9. Ibid., p. 30.
10. Legette Blythe, *38th Evac: The Story of the Men and Women Who Served with the 38th Evacuation Hospital in North Africa and Italy* (Charlotte, NC: Heritage Printers, Inc., 1966), pp. 43–45.
11. Ernie Pyle, *Here Is Your War: The Story of G.I. Joe* (Cleveland: World Publishing Co., 1944), pp. 71–84.
12. Ibid., pp. 82–83.
13. Personal letter, copy in Katherine Densford Papers, University of Minnesota Archives, Minneapolis.
14. "When Does the Home Front Have Priority?" *Public Health Nursing*, vol. 35 (February 1943):77–78.
15. Unpublished document, Records of the War Manpower Commission, National Archives, Washington, DC.
16. "The Nurse," *America*, vol. 41 (January 15, 1944):407.
17. "So Proudly We Hail: Realistic Story of Nurses in the Philippines," *Life*, vol. 15 (October 4, 1943):69.
18. "American Women and Our Wounded Men," *Washington Post*, December 19, 1944.
19. U.S. Congress, House, *Message from the President of the United States Transmitting a Message on the State of the Union* (Washington, DC: Government Printing Office, 1945), Document No. 1, p. 7.

POSTWAR REAPPRAISAL, 1945–1950

The end of World War II did not ease the demand for nurses. The greatest turnover ever known among American nurses began with the war and received new impetus with V-J Day. The coming of peace affected not only the 76,000 graduate nurses who had served at some time with the armed forces but also the more than 164,000 who had carried on their own jobs and also filled in for those away in the armed services. All through the war, nursing staffs at home had been weakened to supply the imperative needs of military service hospitals. Under these conditions, hospitals welcomed any help they could obtain, and practical nurses, volunteer aides, and orderlies had played an important part in the nursing of patients. In such an atmosphere, it was understandable that the home-front nurse eagerly anticipated the return of the military nurse.

THE CASE OF THE MISSING RNs

Although the war had ended, the surrender of the Axis powers did not bring the civilian hospitals relief. Instead, it shattered illusions about the supply of nurses. While millions of men and women returned to civilian life, the anxiously awaited nurse reinforcements failed to reach overburdened hospitals. Questionnaires returned by 31,000 members of the Army Nurse Corps and tabulated by the American Red Cross revealed that only one army nurse in six expected to return to her prewar position. Although 69% planned to remain active in nursing, their interests were varied. Specifically, when one realized that 64% of army nurses had come from posts in hospital nursing, the finding that only 26% planned to return to civilian hospital nursing and 4% to teaching in hospital nursing schools portended disastrous consequences for hospitals. Many military nurses claimed that the reason they did not wish to return to general-duty hospital positions was that they had carried considerable responsibility in the army or navy and

had found real satisfaction in more flexible, autonomous roles.

The extent to which civilian hospitals were short of nursing and non-nursing personnel was evident in the 1060 responses to a questionnaire sent to institutional members of the American Hospital Association by the Council on Professional Practice. Administrators of member hospitals were asked to estimate the number of employees needed in the different categories. Their replies produced the following figures on unfilled positions in late 1945:

Registered nurses	65,000
Nurses' aides	90,000
Non-nursing personnel	90,000
Untrained volunteers	45,000

Sixty-five percent of the hospitals reported that they were acutely short of nursing personnel. These hospitals had an average census of 220 patients per day, whereas the group not acutely short had an average census of 125 patients per day. The former reported a 379% increase in part-time employment of nurses; the latter, a 150% increase.

Nearly 6000 vacancies on the nursing staffs of hospitals and health agencies in New York City made it necessary to close 1200 beds during a time of unprecedented demand for hospital facilities. No solution was in sight, and nursing and hospital officials predicted that the situation would worsen with the increasing incidence of illness in fall and winter. Factors contributing to the shortage of nurses were, according to a *New York Times* survey, the poor pay for hospital nurses compared with the pay for nurses in industry and in physicians' offices and for non-nursing jobs; the shorter hours in nonhospital jobs; the increase in retirement and marriage of nurses; the opportunities for advanced education under the GI Bill; and the housing shortage. The report said that volunteer help in New York hospitals had also declined since the end of the war.

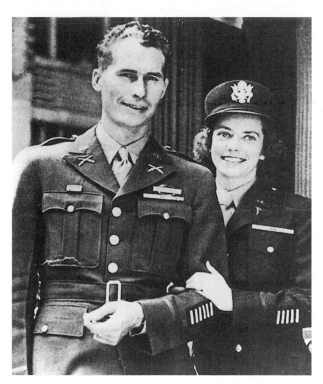

Millions of men and women returned to civilian life when the war ended, and many women chose to start families rather than continue careers in nursing. (Trained Nurse, June 1945.)

POOR WAGES AND BAD WORKING CONDITIONS

In a 1946 national salary survey, the American Hospital Association found that the average starting salary for a staff nurse was $35.75 a week. The average work week was 48 hours, yielding a pay rate of 74 cents per hour. Most nurses wanted the work week cut to 40 hours and the pay increased to at least $40. In sharp contrast, typists were averaging 97 cents an hour; bookkeepers, $1.11; and seamstresses, $1.33. Sue Z. McCracken, general secretary of District No. 4 of the Ohio State Nurses' Association, told of hospitals in her area that paid their regular nurses $30 per week and hired "extras" at $60 weekly to tide them over acute nurse-shortage periods. Two nurses might be working side by side, one knowing that the other was getting twice as much pay for doing exactly the same work. As one superintendent explained, "When the Depression comes, we'll just fire the $60 ones."[1]

Such practices were common in hospitals across the nation. In many hospitals, salaries had to be kept secret or dismissal was risked. But the facts leaked out and the head nurse went in to ask a few questions. "We'll raise you to $45 if you promise not to say a word to the others," she was told. Nurses wanted to see the end of such outmoded personnel arrangements and, in their place, the establishment of uniform, above-board salary scales.[2]

Although the registered nurse had achieved a status of "professional," she often was not treated accordingly by physicians, administrators, or the public. Few nurses thought of hospital nursing service in

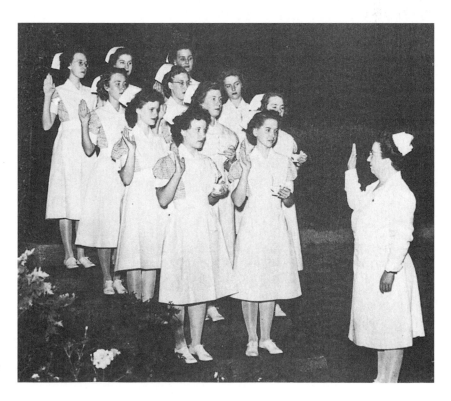

Interest in entering the nursing profession rapidly declined in the late 1940s.

terms of professional career work. In one postwar study of 500 registered nurses, only 12.2% reported that they looked forward to making a career out of hospital nursing. About 5.2% planned on careers in nursing education, and 6.2% were planning careers in nursing administration. The remaining 76.4% planned either to use nursing as a desirable "pin-money" job supplementing the husband's income or to stop nursing altogether after marriage. Nearly 20% of the hospital nurses sampled reported that they planned to switch to another line of work or study. Such data generally reflected the low level of job satisfaction and a lower esteem for hospital nursing.

Hospital nurses saw themselves as working under more rigid discipline than women in other occupations. They believed that they had fewer social activities but followed more rules and orders. Moreover, there was a preponderant feeling among nurses that their work required greater precision than was required of women in other lines of work. According to most nurses' appraisals of their work, satisfaction in a profession was associated with independence of action and self-direction along with opportunity for social activity and recreation. Nurses sought recognition as professionals worthy of trust and responsibility. They were unhappy at being held to a studentlike status entailing blind obedience and uncomplaining acceptance of criticism rather than being accorded a status involving cooperative effort and participation in planning and decision making.

In 1941, the hospital nurse had generally worked a 48-hour week; in 1946 she worked 46 hours. These figures did not tell the entire story. In 1940, approximately 70% of all hospitals had required their nurses to work "split shifts," which meant that the nurse's working day consisted of two segments of duty hours with an intervening period of time off without pay. Because it was difficult to make effective use of 3 to 4 hours of leisure time between assignments, the split shift was exceptionally burdensome. By 1946, one of every four hospital nurses was still working a split shift. Without the split shift, it took three or more nurses working a 7- or 8-hour day to do the work that formerly required two persons, each paid for 9 or 10 hours a day.

Another 1946 survey reported that one of five hospital nurses was critical of her job as a whole. In addition to the conditions that were major grievances in almost all branches of nursing, hospital nurses frequently objected to the unevenness of their workload, the number and arduousness of their duties, the proportion of time spent on nonprofessional work, the quality of supervision, the lack of educational opportunities, and the long hours. Half of all hospital nurses who expressed opinions on any aspect of their job were dissatisfied with the quality and quantity of nonprofessional help, provision for retirement, and employment security.

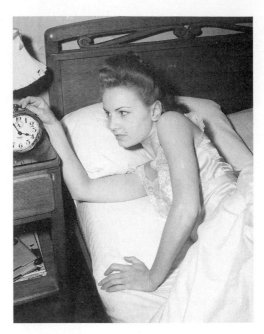

A 40-hour work week at $35.75 was insufficient incentive to retain many hospital staff nurses.

The complaints regarding the arduousness of the work referred to heavy workloads and to the general physical strain associated with nursing assignments. Examples were numerous:

> At times it requires a strong, large nurse to lift the heavy patients—and the transporting of heavy equipment and oxygen tanks. It is hard work and there are never people available to

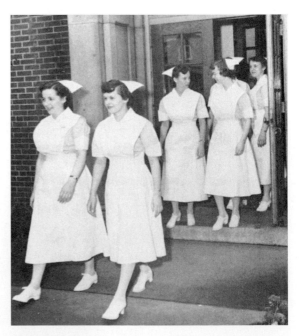

Working split shifts was hard on staff nurses but efficient for hospitals.

lift these things. It is much easier to turn to a different position than to suffer these strains.

Work is very heavy everywhere. Everyone leaves the floor with the feeling that his work is incomplete—if one stayed two hours longer the feeling would still be the same.

You work like a demon, wondering why you couldn't be an octopus and a centipede at the same time. You stay on duty until everything is completed, and if you punch the clock an hour or more late, it apparently is your own fault for not being able to plan your work better. Our time clock seemed to be installed as a means of checking on the time we reported for duty, but the payroll department blindfolded their eyes and their conscience to any overtime.

I feel a little more understanding and a little more kindness and consideration from doctors, hospital executives, and also from private individuals would have prevented the present shortage of nurses. Don't get me wrong, in my quarter of a century of nursing I have had more good than bad but surely hope [that the nurse of the future has] a life with more time for fun and play and normal living, that she won't be considered a queer duck because she works nights, etc.

The daily load carried by each nurse is so heavy that of necessity minor details are neglected that the important things might be done for the patient. Instead of receiving the slightest bit of encouragement from the people that sit in the office and make rounds very infrequently, these small things are criticized, and the nurse, who is overworked physically [and] as a result, tense mentally, is made to feel that she is doing nothing.

People expect nurses to be more or less like a high-class servant, instead of giving them the status of an actual professional.[3]

THE AMERICAN NURSES ASSOCIATION BECOMES AGGRESSIVE

With the theme "Nursing in the Nation's Plans for Health," 12,000 nurses from all parts of the United States gathered in Atlantic City during the last week of September 1946, as the American Nurses Association (ANA), the National League for Nursing Education (NLNE), and the National Organization for Public Health Nursing met for the fourteenth time in a joint biennial session. The convention also marked the golden anniversary of the ANA.

The convention concerned itself primarily with the adoption of a series of resolutions known as the platform of the American Nurses Association. The 1946 platform contained the following 10 points:

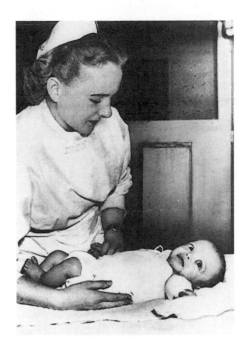

Demanding work, such as nursing this battered child back to health in April 1948, received little recognition by employers.

1. Improvement in hours and living conditions for nurses so that they may live a normal personal and professional life. Specifically, action toward: (a) wider acceptance of the 40-hour week with no decrease in salary, thus applying to post-war conditions the principle of the 8-hour day adopted by the American Nurses Association in 1934; (b) minimum salaries adequate to attract nurses of quality and to enable them to maintain standards of living comparable with other professions.

2. Provision for optimal nursing care for all, and the furtherance of a positive health program in all communities.

3. Increased participation by nurses in the actual planning and in the administration of nursing service in hospitals and other types of employment.

4. Greater development of nurses' professional associations as exclusive spokesmen for nurses in all questions affecting their employment and economic security. Such a development should be based on past successful experience of professional nurses' organizations in collective bargaining and negotiation.

5. Removal, as rapidly as possible, of barriers that prevent the full employment and professional development of nurses belonging to minority racial groups.

6. Employment of well-qualified practical nurses and other auxiliary workers under state licensure, thus protecting both the patient and the worker.

7. Continuing improvement in the placement and counseling of nurses, to give greater stability and job satisfaction to the profession and to facilitate a better distribution of nursing service to the public.
8. Further development of nursing in prepayment health and medical care plans, in order to spread the cost of nursing service to the public.
9. Maintenance of educational standards, and development of educational resources, that nursing may keep abreast of the rapid advances in medicine and other sciences. Such a development may well require federal subsidies and contribution from foundations and other educational philanthropies.
10. Appraisal of our own national organizations through the report of the Structure Study and fearless action based upon such appraisal to make sure that the nursing profession will be organized and equipped to deal most effectively with its problems and its opportunities.[4]

In an obvious step to counter union organizers who had begun efforts to unionize nurses, the ANA adopted a carefully worded resolution in which it went on record as endorsing the qualifications of the several state and district associations to act as the exclusive agents of their respective memberships in the field of economic security and collective bargaining. The resolution continued:

The association commends the excellent progress already made and urges all state and district associations to push such a program vigorously and expeditiously. Since it is the established policy of other groups, including unions, to permit membership in only one collective bargaining group, the association believes such policy to be sound for the state and district nurses' associations.[5]

It was emphasized that adoption of this policy by any state association would be optional and that the individual nurse had free choice whether she wished to join her professional organization or a union.

Under the NLNE's sponsorship, the convention delegates held a panel discussion on the general subject, "Who shall pay for nursing education?" The panel concerned itself with whether student nurses were serving primarily as labor in caring for patients or as students acquiring a professional education. The group argued whether the prevailing system of nursing education—carried on largely by hospitals, which were primarily service institutions and only secondarily educational institutions—was adequate to meet national nursing needs.

The panel generally agreed that it would be wise to foster the establishment of nursing schools in universities and colleges, because 91% of the nursing schools were being operated by hospitals as diploma programs. Senator Claude Pepper of Florida, one of the participants in this discussion, abhorred the fact that, under the current hospital nursing system, the patient was paying for what Senator Pepper called a "deterioration in nursing service" by reason of increased fees for medical care accompanied by a nursing shortage and a relative decline of enrollments in nursing schools. He stated that adequate nursing care for all could come about only when conditions in the nursing field were such as to attract sufficient numbers of high-quality personnel. According to the senator, nursing education, like other forms of professional education, should be directly financed by the individual or the student's family and by tuition grants, loans, scholarships, and fellowships paid from private and government sources.

CONTINUED PEACETIME NURSE SHORTAGES

The postwar shortage of registered professional nurses in the United States was due primarily to a decline in enrollment of nursing students at a time of rising demand for nursing care and heavy losses of graduate nurses through marriage. The lag in student enrollment seemed related to problems of student training and to competition from fields of employment that required less specialized education and thus provided almost immediate earnings. Workers in industry generally had shorter hours and fared better with respect to overtime pay and retirement pensions, although nurses typically received more liberal vacations and sick-leave benefits.

By midsummer 1948, there were 380,500 active registered nurses in the United States. They were distributed among the major fields of nursing as follows: 167,400 in institutions, including 4400 full-time instructors in nursing schools; 22,100 in public health; 52,800 in private duty; 12,700 in industry; and 25,500 in other areas, including physicians' offices. The better hospitals were slowly learning that efficiency and productivity in the nursing service was far less a matter of the amount of hard work done by each individual than of the engineering of the job, the kind of mechanical equipment used by the nurse, the size and flexibility of the institution, the layout of work space, and the relationship of jobs to one another.

In 1948, in a report from the Bureau of Employment Security of the Social Security Administration to Federal Security Administrator Oscar R. Ewing, the national nurse shortage was estimated to be approximately 40,000. This report examined nursing needs in hospitals, physicians' offices, schools, industry, and public health agencies. It was estimated that there was also a "potential demand" for an additional 40,000 nurses to staff new hospital facilities and to meet

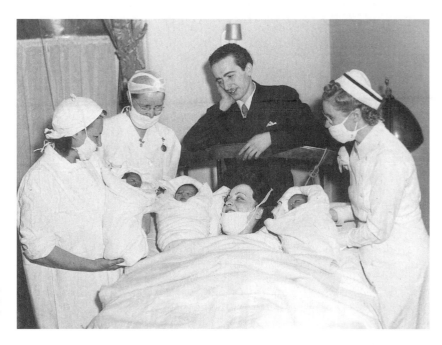

The United States had about 380,000 registered nurses in 1948, three of whom care for these triplets at Swedish Hospital in Brooklyn, NY.

other nursing requirements during the next 3 to 5 years. The report said the nursing shortage was still acute, with thousands of vacant beds in hospitals attributable to lack of nursing personnel. The estimated shortage of 40,000 was broken down as follows: hospitals and clinics, 20,000; public health, 6000; private duty, 4000; nursing schools, 3000; physicians' offices, 3000; industry, 2000; and miscellaneous, 2000.

The Cadet Nurse Corps Program had exerted a marked effect on the number of young women applying for admission to nursing schools. During the war years, these classes gradually increased, not only because of the patriotic urge that prompted applications but also because of the financial program inaugurated and carried out by the government. After graduation of large cadet nurse classes came a dearth of student nurses in many schools. In 1941 there had been 93,977 students enrolled in accredited nursing schools. In 1945 there were 130,909. In 1947 there was a marked decrease in enrollment to 94,133 students.

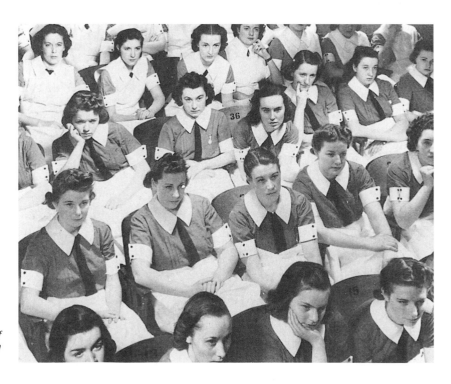

Enrollments plummeted after graduation of the last Cadet Nurse Corps students in 1948.

FALLING POPULARITY OF NURSING AS A PROFESSION

Fewer young women were choosing a nursing education. In 1910, the number of American women who entered nursing approximated 1.5% of those eligible. This proportion had passed 3% by 1940, and wartime enrollment rates averaged almost 5%. The first few postwar years brought a sharp drop. An all-time-high withdrawal rate of student nurses, 30%, was reported during 1947 in a statistical survey of graduating classes from state-accredited nursing schools. The national graduating class total reached a new high of 40,744, but this reflected the war-swollen admission figures of 1944. Only 1779 students, or 4% of the total graduated, received university degrees. A mere 42 nursing graduates of 1947 were men. The 582 black graduates constituted an increase of 50 over the previous year.

Nursing schools were having great difficulty filling their classes. There was no telling, of course, how many prospective nurses were scared away from nursing by Clarence Woodbury's critical article entitled "Student Nurse—Could You Take It?" in the June 1949 *Woman's Home Companion*.[6] Commenting on the piece, administrator John F. Latcham of Trumbull Memorial Hospital in Warren, Ohio, believed that the article was a "pincer movement" in the government's plan to socialize medicine. Latcham noted that "at the Trumbull Memorial Hospital we know that our students are properly housed and fed. The Nurses' Home is a modern building, with attractive rooms, a parlor, a good library, adequate classrooms and excellent bath facilities." He noted that "some religious schools of nursing were noted for harsh discipline, but, as far as the majority of schools go, I would believe that lack of discipline would be the more proper charge." He emphasized that "no apprentice ever learned a trade from theory. Our nurses work a 44-hour week, with classroom time included."[7]

Another hospital executive believed that "nurses should either get off their high horses and do the physical work they started out to do or move over and let others do it. There is too much talk about 'high professional standards' and not enough about taking care of the sick." A third hospital administrator did not think that there was any use in castigating the *Woman's Home Companion* over the article. He thought the real fault for declining interest in nursing was the small but highly vocal lunatic fringe, the current vogue group in high nursing circles.[8]

THE ANTICOLLEGIATE NURSING FACTION

The big controversy was whether nursing education should go the collegiate route. Dr. Frank Lahey, former president of the American Medical Association

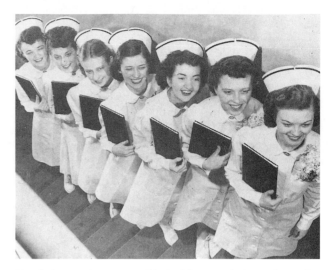

Hospital executives were critical of "too much theory in nursing curricula."

(AMA), charged that nurses were "legislating and educating themselves out of jobs." Conversely, nurses like Eunice D. Johnson, director of the nursing school of St. Luke's Hospital, New Bedford, Massachusetts, maintained that "you can never overeducate a nurse."[9] The editors of *Hospital Management* submitted this dispute to a panel of hospital administrators. Hundreds of different views were expressed, making it difficult to tabulate the results accurately. Still, an attempt was made to set down some figures in response to the question of whether nurses were pushing for too much education. Forty-eight percent said no, 30% said yes, and 22% were undecided.

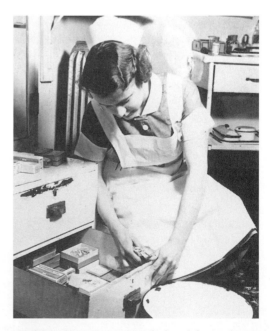

Some physicians favored more practical work for nursing students.

Edith W. Bailey, administrator of the Canonsburg General Hospital in Canonsburg, Pennsylvania, commented:

> The nurses attending universities and colleges insist only on supervising—no physical work. . . . Not everyone is fitted for supervising—and strangely enough, a sick person doesn't give a hang whether his nurse possesses a B.A. or B.S. The root question is "Can she make him comfortable?"[10]

Another comment along this line came from A.M. Frank, M.D., chairman of the staff at Lutheran Hospital, St. Louis. He predicted that practical nurses would be in greater demand than those with degrees and added that "one definitely does not need a Ph.D. degree to carry a bedpan. The patients are only interested in whether it is hot or cold. Student nurses are spending too much time in the lecture halls and too little time on the floor so that we are getting too many desk models and insufficient floor models."[11]

According to a postwar survey made by the American College of Surgeons (ACS), less expensive nursing care was needed. The survey revealed that the quantity of nursing was 50% of the total need and that the quality had deteriorated about equally. Eighty-four percent of the replies stated that, with few exceptions, the needs of the sick could be met by auxiliary help.

The ACS held that such requirements were incompatible with the expensive developments in nursing education over the years. The professional nursing associations had been concerned with elevating their professional status and advocating more years of education. Actual nurse training had been relegated to a place of secondary importance behind general educational aspects. It was agreed that, as nurses, such graduates had been less well prepared. The immediate need to initiate action independent of the control of nursing organizations was apparent and urgent. The board of regents of the ACS adopted the following resolution on December 20, 1946, during its annual meeting at the time of the Clinical Congress in Cleveland: "The American College of Surgeons advises hospitals to admit and utilize the assistance of auxiliary nursing aides. In addition, approved hospitals should provide training for such vocational nurses by means of short courses."[12]

STAFFING DILEMMAS

During the war, four types of nurse staffing were common: (1) graduate registered nurses only, (2) graduate registered nurses and paid auxiliary workers, (3) graduate registered nurses and student nurses, and (4) graduate registered nurses, student nurses, and paid auxiliary workers. In 1943, the most important facts established about the variation in hours of care per patient per day by different types of personnel were:

Students gave almost two thirds of the hours of care in the hospitals with nursing schools.

The total hours of care per patient per day decreased consistently as the size of the hospital increased.

The hours of care per patient per day given by general staff nurses in hospitals without schools decreased as the size of the hospital increased.

The hours of care given by students decreased as the size of the hospital increased.

The hours of care given by paid auxiliary workers in hospitals without schools decreased as the size of the hospital increased; by contrast, in hospitals with schools, such hours of care increased as the size of the hospital increased.

The hours of care given by general staff nurses ranged from an average of 2.1 hours of care per patient per day in hospitals without nursing schools and without paid auxiliaries to only 0.6 hours in the hospitals with schools and without paid auxiliaries.

During World War II, in the average hospital, the proportion of direct nursing care supplied by registered nurses dropped drastically; an estimated 3100 of the total 4200 general and related special hospitals throughout the United States employed paid auxiliary nursing workers in 1944. The practice of employing paid auxiliary nursing workers was considerably more prevalent among hospitals without nursing schools than among hospitals with them—81% versus 58%. In the hospitals without nursing schools, 42% of the total nursing care was given by paid auxiliaries. The remainder of the care was provided by the only other group of workers giving nursing care—the general staff nurses. In the hospitals with nursing schools, only 17% of the care was given by the paid auxiliaries. The remainder of the care in these hospitals was provided by the general staff nurses and the students.

WIDESPREAD INTRODUCTION OF NURSES' AIDES AND PRACTICAL NURSES

Many believed that the registered nurse represented too large an investment in education for some of the tasks she was given to perform. One study showed that of 150 practices and procedures involved in nursing care, only 35% needed to be done by a registered nurse, whereas 65% could be performed by a practical nurse. During the war, approximately 150,000 volunteer nurses' aides had been trained and had served in wartime hospitals. They had literally "saved the day" in many hospitals. Additionally, they had been prepared to care for family members with mild illnesses in their own homes. Another group of volunteers, the more than 500,000 certificate holders from the Red Cross home nursing classes, were also urged

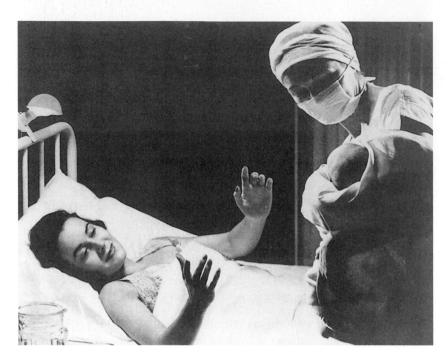

During the war the proportion of RN-direct care had sharply declined.

to offer their services to hospitals in nonprofessional capacities. Many members of these two groups gave voluntary service of no fewer than 150 hours a year in more than 100 army hospitals, more than 25 veterans' hospitals, and more than 2000 civilian hospitals. Others undertook this work at a rate of pay approaching that of the graduate nurse.

Those who received this training had at first been asked not to use their preparation in any paid capacity. Later, to relieve a serious personnel shortage in army hospitals, the Civil Service Commission, through its regional offices, recruited nurses' aides who had taken the Red Cross course for jobs paying $1440 a year, with overtime. This was close to the professional nurse's salary and was considered to infringe on the professional nurses who had helped to train the aides.

Owing to the recruitment of nurses by the armed services, the limited number of student nurses, and the increased patient-load of civilian hospitals, it became increasingly necessary to pay auxiliary nursing workers to perform many of the more routine and less technical nursing duties previously performed by graduate registered nurses. An auxiliary worker was defined by the three major national nursing organizations to include "all persons other than graduate registered nurses: attendants, trained attendants, licensed attendants, licensed undergraduate nurses, licensed practical nurses, ward helpers and orderlies, nurses' aides, nursing aides, etc."[13]

SCHOOLS OF PRACTICAL NURSING PROLIFERATE

The term *practical nurse* had been approved by the ANA, the NLNE, and the National Organization for Public Health Nursing joint board of directors. A practical nurse was defined as a person trained to care for subacute, convalescent, and chronic patients requiring nursing services at home or in institutions. She worked under the direction of a licensed physician or a registered professional nurse and gave household assistance when necessary. A practical nurse might be employed by physicians, hospitals, custodial homes, public health agencies, industries, or the public. This definition suggested specific controls and limitations on practical-nurse activities as well as a specified relationship with physicians and professional nurses.

If the preceding functions of the practical nurse were used as a criterion, during the 1940s thousands of self-styled practical nurses lacked the range of training and the supervised experience necessary to qualify them to use the title. In many states, anyone who assisted in homes or institutions where illness prevailed might designate herself a practical nurse, although her qualifying experience might have consisted only of raising a family in her own home or serving in a limited capacity as a hospital aide.

There were comparatively few standards governing the practice of practical nursing. As of December 1945, only 19 states and 1 territory had any legislation dealing with practical nurses, and licensure of practical nurses was mandatory in only 1 state. Many titles were used to describe workers in the field of practical nursing. There was also considerable variation in the interpretation of the range of duties of the practical nurse and her requisite training.

The first school for training practical nurses had been organized in 1897. By 1930, only 11 schools had been established, but between 1930 and 1947, 25 more were opened. In contrast to the 36 schools established over a half-century, there was an increase of 260 between 1948 and 1954. Most of the early practical-nurse schools were attached to hospitals and to institutions for chronic, crippled, aged, or mentally ill patients. Some training programs had been organized under the auspices of YWCAs and other private institutions and agencies. In a few states, practical-nurse training was offered in publicly supported vocational education programs.

Under the provisions of the federal vocational education acts, funds to support the training of practical nurses could be provided only as part of a program of trade and industrial education. The federally aided classes, conducted by local public schools, included practical experience in cooperating hospitals. In 1949, federal money went to 50 classes operating in 22 states and graduating approximately 1100 practical nurses per year. The classes averaged about 20 students each, and the duration of the courses ranged from 9 months to 1 year. The greater proportion of time spent in the first part of the course involved class work. The latter part was devoted largely to practical hospital experience gained under immediate medical and nursing supervision. Graduate nurses were used as instructors and supervisors.

Practical-nurse programs in the public schools generally did not charge tuition unless the student resided outside the school district. Elsewhere, however, a fee might be charged, and in some schools it was as much as $200. Without any strong professional association to police the programs, some schools resembled exploitative trade schools. In some there were no provisions for a maintenance allowance, but a few cooperating hospitals paid the students as much as $1820 for the service portion of their training.

DUTIES OF THE LICENSED PRACTICAL NURSE

At midcentury, there were more than 144,000 practical nurses, 95% of them women. This was a 35% increase over 1940. Many hospitals gradually expanded the range of duties assigned to practical nurses; for example, they were increasingly being trained for service in the operating room. In effect, the practical nurse was repeating the history of the registered nurse, who had inherited tasks from the physician. She was broadening her work spectrum by piecemeal accumulation of activities that the registered nurse lacked time to complete. Once the practical nurse had begun to undertake a certain task, she was likely to think of it as being within her domain. Some professional nurses worried that, as the salary of the diploma-holding nurse was raised higher, every purchaser—hospital administrator, clinic administrator, nursing-home administrator—would seek protection through substitution. Each would try to get the job done by using less expensive personnel.

By 1952, the nonprofessional group employed in nursing service accounted for 56% of professional and nonprofessional personnel combined. Although it was apparent that acceptable nursing care could be provided by people with less training, refusal to acknowledge that in the future most nursing personnel would be other than registered nurses created some bitterness among RNs. In addition to the general criticism of the quality and quantity of nonprofessional help, there was resentment about the status, privileges, and responsibilities granted to practical nurses. Objection was also voiced that uniforms of

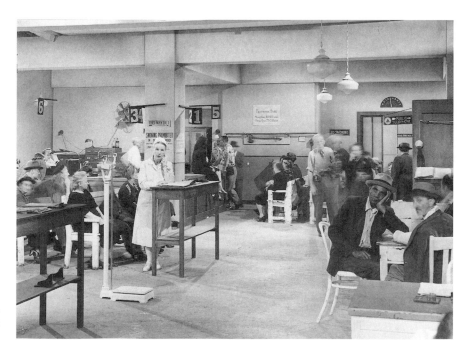

The number of practical nurses increased, as did the range of tasks they performed.

practical nurses did not adequately distinguish them from professional nurses. Comment elicited in one study included the following:

> Nonprofessional help are literally treated with kid gloves at the expense of the nurses. They refuse to do their work, do it slovenly, are openly abusive, and when such situations are reported, the nurse is invariably held at fault.
>
> The once "thrill" of being "capped" is gone. We find a few months' course and we can become a "trained" nurse, cap and all, and practically receive the same salary as an RN. Many of our public do not know the difference. We once had something to look forward to at the end of our three- or five-year course, a cap and that wonderful distinction of being an RN, an honor we wanted the whole world to know; we were a little different than others. Now we even take orders from nonprofessionals, instead of doing what we know is best, and like it.
>
> I believe that where there is a shortage of registered nurses, there is a need for nurses' aides. There are many things which nurses' aides can be trained to do, but I feel that the administration of medicines and assisting with operations, etc., should be done only by those trained professional nurses who are fit for the responsibility involved.
>
> This hospital allows these practical nurses to do medications, intravenous, and all procedures in general; however, you hear complaints from patients continuously about poor treatment. This hospital also calls practical nurses to do private duty when there are registered nurses available.
>
> I really don't blame girls for not taking up nurses' training when they can get positions in the profession without a moment's training of any sort, right out of high school, are requested to wear white caps, white uniforms . . . and receive a higher wage than RNs working in an MD's office. The nurses' white uniform is worn by anyone who wishes to don it and it certainly burns [us] up.[14]

THE BROWN REPORT

About this time, far-reaching changes in nursing practice and nursing education were recommended in a 1948 report, *Nursing for the Future*, by Esther Lucille Brown, Ph.D., of the research staff of the Russell Sage Foundation. "Today the nurse probably ranks close to the teacher as a social necessity," observed Brown. Nevertheless, society did not assist nursing education as it did teacher training, and other conditions within and outside the profession had alarmingly reduced the number of applicants available for training. Nursing was fighting a losing battle in attracting the needed numbers of young women. "Many thoughtful persons," remarked Brown, "are beginning to wonder why young women in any large numbers would want to enter nursing as practiced, or schools of nursing as operated today." The report also pointed to "authoritarianism" in the hospitals, where the nurse was caught between the dictates of the medical administration and those of the hospital

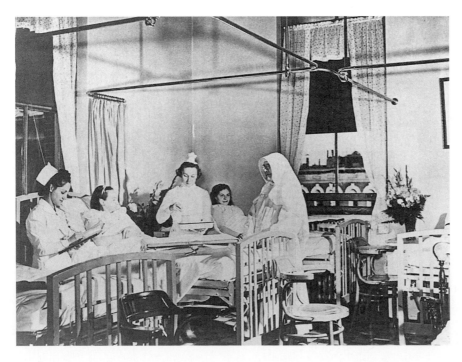

By 1952, practical nurses and nurses' aides provided most nursing services.

administration; it pleaded for more freedom for nurses and a larger share in policy determination.[15]

Conditions in nursing education were regarded as central to the whole problem of the profession. "By no stretch of the imagination," the report charged, "can the education provided in the vast majority of some 1,250 schools be conceived of as professional education." Brown perceived that many hundreds of hospitals still operated schools to avail themselves of the services of student nurses. She recommended "that effort be directed to building basic schools of nursing in universities and colleges, comparable in number to existing medical schools, that are sound in organizational and financial structure, adequate in facilities and faculty, and well-distributed to serve the needs of the entire country."[16]

Without giving approval even to the best hospital schools for the indefinite future, the report stated that "the continued existence of a considerable number is essential for an interim period until adequate other facilities have been established and are sufficiently patronized to guarantee a steady flow of personnel into nursing." But the report added that there had long been "consensus that an undetermined number of weak schools—running certainly into several hundreds—should be closed." The smaller schools, in particular, had rendered a poor performance record. Brown pointed to a 1945 evaluation by the Division of

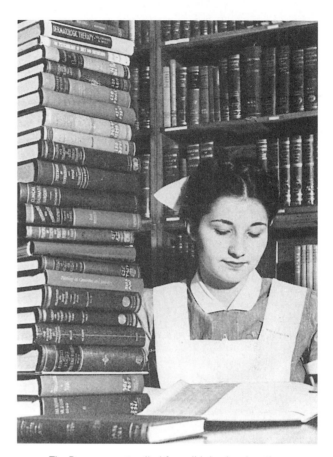

The Brown report called for solid, basic education.

Nursing of the U.S. Public Health Service of 602 schools of fewer than 100 students that rated only 4% as excellent or good, 50% as fair, and 46% as poor or very poor. Brown's report recommended the following:

That nursing make one of its first matters of important business the long overdue official examination of every school.

That lists of accredited schools be published and distributed, with a statement to the effect that any school not named had failed to meet minimum requirements for accreditation or had refused to permit examination.

That a nationwide educational campaign be conducted for the purpose of rallying broad public support for accredited schools and for subjecting slow-moving state boards and nonaccredited schools to strong social pressure.

That provision be made for periodic re-examination of all schools listed or others requesting it, as well as for first examination of new schools, and for publication and distribution of the revised list.

That, if organized nursing committed itself to this undertaking of major social significance, the public assume responsibility for a substantial part of the financial burden.[17]

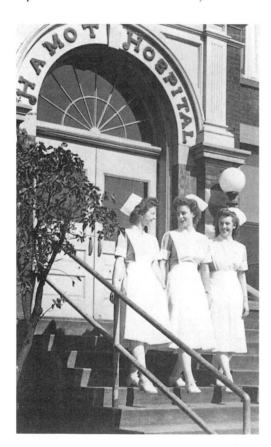

The Brown report called for far-reaching changes in nursing practice and nursing education.

The Brown report was predicated on the assumption that a solid basic education is essential for every citizen of a free and self-governing nation, particularly for every nurse, regardless of her work. Formerly a system of apprenticeship, nursing education was slowly becoming a well-planned program of preparation for a calling that could rank as the equal of other professions. In making this transition, nursing education was moving unmistakably into colleges and universities. Like other professions, it was finding in colleges the proper intellectual climate for the preparation of the professional worker. Nurse educators with vision were strongly impressed with the need for better teaching and for better resources in libraries, laboratories, and other physical facilities for education available in colleges and universities. They were beginning to realize the need for developing research in nursing and for professional writing and publication if nursing were to be brought abreast of its associated professions. Alert nurses, because of new insights into the advantages of higher education, were also anxious to associate with stimulating persons in other fields within higher education.

REACTIONARY ATTACK ON THE BROWN REPORT

Many physicians and hospital administrators were hostile to these aspirations. In his final appearance as president of the American Hospital Association, Graham Davis of Battle Creek, Michigan, told the 1948 AMA convention in Atlantic City that Esther Lucille Brown's report ignored the facts of life. "Nurses 20 years from now will not look back with pride on this period in their history," Davis said, referring to what he termed the "trade unionism element" in nursing. "There is a better way to seek economic security," he declared. Davis pointed out that Brown was not a

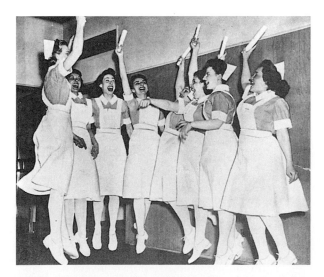

Nursing education built on a collegiate basis on par with other professions became an exciting prospect.

nurse and that the survey on which the report was based covered a comparatively small number of nursing schools. He was especially critical of her characterization of many small hospital nursing schools as "socially undesirable." He defended these schools, pointing out that they had made it possible for hospitals to provide nursing service throughout the wartime and postwar shortages.[18]

ACCREDITATION FINALLY BECOMES A REALITY

To strengthen schools to meet the new needs for better-prepared nurses, the nursing organizations began to establish their long-discussed accreditation program, through the Committee to Implement the Brown Report, soon renamed the National Committee for the Improvement of Nursing Services. It was recognized that some classification method was necessary to focus attention on the need for more rapid improvement in basic nursing programs. Accordingly, the Subcommittee on School Data Analysis was appointed to study all nursing schools in the United States. Although participation was voluntary, 96% of the schools returned the subcommittee questionnaire.

Statistical procedures were used to analyze information submitted on the questionnaires, and each school was evaluated in terms of long-accepted criteria by the profession. Schools were classified according to their total score on a 100-point scale based on standards of nursing recommended by the professional organizations. The weight given to various criteria and the maximum scores assigned to them were as follows:[19]

Administrative policies	3
Financial organization	3
Faculty	22
Curriculum	16
Clinical field	22
Library	6
Student selection and provisions for student welfare	13
Student performance on state board examinations	15
Total score	100

When ranked according to general, overall excellence, schools in the upper 25% were classified as Group I, those in the middle 50% as Group II, and those in the lowest 25% as Group III. The schools reporting to the subcommittee (1150 of 1190 state-accredited schools) were classified as follows:[20]

	NUMBER OF SCHOOLS	NUMBER OF STUDENTS
Group I	301	36,436
Group II	567	46,483
Group III	282	13,779

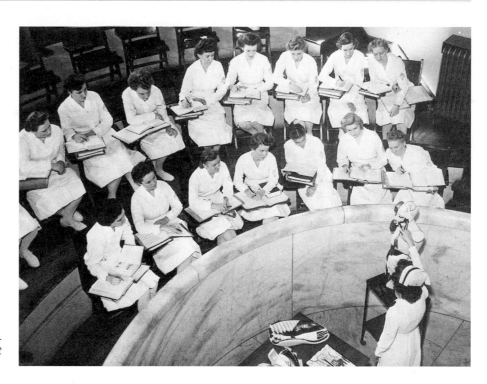

Nursing schools controlled by colleges and universities had the best programs.

All of the 114 college-controlled schools participated and were classified in Group I or Group II. The findings were published in a report entitled *Nursing Schools at the Mid-century.*

THE NATIONAL ORGANIZATION OF HOSPITAL SCHOOLS OF NURSING FIGHTS BACK

In reaction to the classification project as well as to the general thrust toward nursing in higher education, the National Organization of Hospital Schools of Nursing (NOHSN), headquartered in Atlanta, was formed to aid hospital nursing schools in what was termed a "struggle for existence." The new association protested that approximately 240 schools of nursing had been omitted from the list "accredited" by the National Committee for the Improvement of Nursing Service. The NOHSN believed that too many "good schools of nursing which have served their communities well do not appear on this list" and that all "present schools are needed and should continue." It claimed that accreditation had been arbitrary, because the classification had been based on a survey questionnaire that the schools had not known would be used for this purpose, and no visits to the unaccredited schools had been made.[21]

Because the Brown report had advocated the movement of nursing education into a collegiate setting and the NLNE had urged that hospital schools "give early consideration to the transfer of control and administration to educational institutions," the NOHSN believed that a new organization was justified to aid

existing hospital nursing schools. According to Lucy I. Mace, secretary-treasurer, "the incorporators believe that all hospital nursing schools approved by State Boards of Nurse Examiners should be accepted for membership. We will publish our own list of approved schools and conduct a general public relations program which will be favorable to the hospital schools."[22]

"Confusion, discouragement, and even despair exist among nurses, physicians, and hospital administrators today," said one NOHSN release. It also mentioned that "it is well known that the described conditions furnish fertile fields for the seeds of ideologies contrary to Americanism." It was also charged that the accreditation and collegiate nursing movements were "contingent upon use of federal subsidy and therefore inevitable federal control." To accept such programs knowingly was characterized as a step "to aid and abet the enemies of free enterprise and freedom."[23]

CONTROVERSY OVER NATIONAL HEALTH INSURANCE

The postwar crusade to upgrade nursing education carried over into the emotionalism and controversy about national health insurance. On November 19, 1945, President Truman submitted to Congress his recommendation for a comprehensive, modern national health program, which consisted of five parts:

Federal grants for construction of hospitals and related facilities

Expansion of public health, maternity, and child health services

Federal grants for medical education, nursing education, and research

Establishment of a national social insurance system for the prepayment of medical costs

Expansion of present social insurance systems to furnish protection against loss of wages from sickness and disability

The same day, Senator Robert F. Wagner of New York introduced, with Senator James E. Murray of Montana, a bill to establish such a plan. Representative John Dingell of Michigan introduced a companion bill in the House. The Wagner-Murray Bill, S. 1606, was the subject of extensive hearings between April and July of 1946. Chances of passage looked poor at the outset, when Senator Robert A. Taft of Ohio got involved in a heated argument with committee chairman Murray after declaring that the bill was "the most socialistic measure that this Congress has ever had before it, seriously."[24]

The medical provisions were the most controversial part of the bill, which provided for a single payroll deduction of 6% on annual incomes up to $3000, with employers paying a like amount. Self-employed persons, such as grocers, farmers, and physicians, would pay 7%. One quarter of the total funds would be applied to medical care costs, the balance going to insurance against old age, unemployment, maternity, temporary illness, and permanent disability. For the employed person, complete medical care for oneself and dependents would cost 1.5% of his or her income, up to $3000, or not more than $3.75 a month. An average middle-income family in 1946 paid 4% of their income on medical bills alone, or about $120 annually on $3000. Of course, most families would not pay the maximum $3.75 monthly or $45 annually for medical and hospital care, because three fourths of them made less than $3000 a year.

Opponents charged that the bill was "communistic," "un-American," "a stab at free enterprise," and a scheme to provide an inferior kind of "political medicine" to the people. Led by the AMA, the opposition included several large national drug chains, some private insurance companies, a group of patent medicine and drug manufacturers, the American Bar Association, and the American Hospital Association.

Those in favor of the bill argued that tax-supported medicine was no more un-American than tax-supported education. They were led by sponsoring senators and congressmen and by a minority of physicians within the AMA. Other backers included organized labor (the AFL and the CIO), some farm groups, the National Lawyers' Guild, the Association of Interns and Medical Students, and the American Public Health Association.

The opposition forces insisted that the bill (1) would rob patients of their right to choose their own physician; (2) would lower standards of medical care; (3) would make physicians "slaves" to bureaucrats; (4) would cut physicians' incomes by ending the fee-

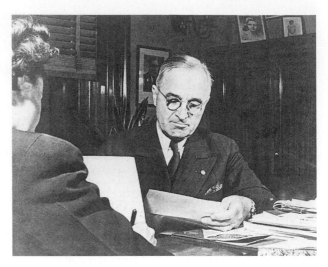

President Truman's proposed national health program was bitterly opposed by the medical profession.

for-service system; and (5) was unnecessary because anyone could get the medical care he or she needed, either privately or through voluntary insurance or charity.

Those who favored the bill replied that (1) the bill did not limit free choice of physicians but rather extended the privilege to those who had not had much choice before; (2) standards of care would be raised, because a physician would be able to make free use of costly equipment, specialists' services, and laboratory tests that were often beyond the financial means of patients; (3) physicians would still be independent, and under National Health Insurance they would be sure of getting paid; (4) most physicians' incomes would be raised, and those who wished to keep on with private practice could do so; and (5) many people who were not getting adequate care would at last gain access to its benefits.

Although results differed from poll to poll, public opinion seemed to favor some federal assistance for medical care payments. One poll, commissioned by the California Medical Association to determine how physicians could meet the "threat of federal medicine," found that 50% of California's citizens favored federally supported medicine. They noted:

> Among upper-income groups, federal medicine is desired because of the poor. Among the poor it is desired because they want proper care themselves. . . . If it were to come up on the ballot today . . . it seems abundantly clear that you [the California Medical Association] would lose the issue—perhaps by a landslide.[25]

Organized nursing produced two witnesses at the congressional hearings. Katherine J. Densford testified for the ANA before a Senate Committee on April 24, 1946, but could only state that the 181,000-member ANA had taken no action regarding S. 1606, because the House of Delegates would not be meeting until September 1946. Ruth Sleeper, president of the NLNE, submitted a statement that favored the bill. She emphasized that to meet current and future demands of the health care system it was essential that federal grants be provided to nursing schools to improve clinical courses in undergraduate nursing education and to improve, expand, and develop new programs for graduate nurses preparing to become teachers or administrators in nursing schools and administrators or supervisors in all types of nursing services. According to Sleeper, the NLNE favored federal aid to nursing education on a direct basis, from Washington, rather than through individual state health departments.

Because congressional support for national health insurance was insufficient to bring about passage of the program, President Truman convened a National Health Assembly in May 1948, attended by 800 professional and community leaders, including several prominent nurses. Using this assembly as a publicity springboard, Federal Security Administrator Oscar Ewing prepared a report to the president entitled *The Nation's Health: A Ten Year Program*, outlining a plan for comprehensive, federally sponsored, compulsory health insurance. The leaders of the AMA regarded this report as a danger signal. They were frightened by its attractive format almost as much as by its content. They decided that a grave danger had arrived, to be forcefully attacked if Truman won his second term.

THE AMA "EDUCATES" THE PUBLIC

In December 1948, shortly after the election, the AMA assessed its members $25 each for a nationwide plan of "education," and during the next 3½ years it spent more than $4.5 million in informing the American people about the hazards of "socialized medicine." A public relations firm managed the campaign, which on the whole allied organized medicine with the Republican party and with Senator Robert A. Taft of Ohio.

Rhetorically, they asked, "Does the report on the nation's health give a factual picture of the people's health in America?" They answered: "No. This widely publicized report is a hoax. It is a propagandist treatment of a subject far too important for such loose handling by political experimenters." They asked, "Who is for Compulsory Health Insurance?" and answered, "The Federal Security Administration. The President. All who seriously believe in a Socialistic State. Every left-wing organization in America . . . the Communist Party." The plan to improve the nation's health was dismissed as part of a trend toward complete socialization of American life: "The Government proposes to assume control not only of the medical profession, but of hospitals—both public and private—and drug and appliance industries,

dentistry, pharmacy, nursing and allied professions."[26]

In terms of money spent, the heart of the AMA's national education campaign was the production and distribution of pamphlets. Literature was produced by the national office and distributed by physicians, through cooperating organizations, and by direct mail. In the first year of the campaign alone, the total distribution of literature was more than 54 million pieces, at a cost of more than $1 million. The principal distribution agents were physicians and physicians' organizations; however, dentists, druggists, the insurance industry, and other groups made substantial contributions.

Clem Whitaker and Leone Baxter, directors of the campaign, addressed the Conference of State Medical Societies in Chicago on February 12, 1949:

> Mr. Chairman and ladies and gentlemen; every minister preaches from a text—and every campaign, if it is a successful campaign, has to have a theme! The theme, if it is geared to reach more than 100 million people, as we must in this campaign, should have simplicity and clarity. Most of all, it must high-point the major issues of the campaign with great brevity—in language that paints a picture understandable to people in all circumstances. That's one of the reasons we have a large blown-up color reproduction of the famous Fildes painting, *The Doctor*, on exhibit here today, with the simple caption under it: "Keep politics out of this picture!" The picture and the caption, even without elaboration, focus attention on one of the most important arguments against government-controlled medicine. Smaller color reproductions of this famous painting soon will go up in doctors' offices all over America as one of the first steps in dramatizing our case to the American people—and more important—as the first step in making doctors campaigners in their own behalf. For this purpose we have added a hundred words of text which help to establish the theme of this campaign.

The public relations experts then read the 100-word text that accompanied the painting:

> "Keep Politics out of this Picture!"
> When the life—or health—of a loved one is at stake, hope lies in the devoted service of your doctor.
> Would you change this picture?
> Compulsory health insurance is political medicine.
> It would bring a third party—a politician—between you and your doctor. It would bind up your family's health in red tape. It would result in heavy payroll taxes—and inferior medical care for you and your family. Don't let that happen here.

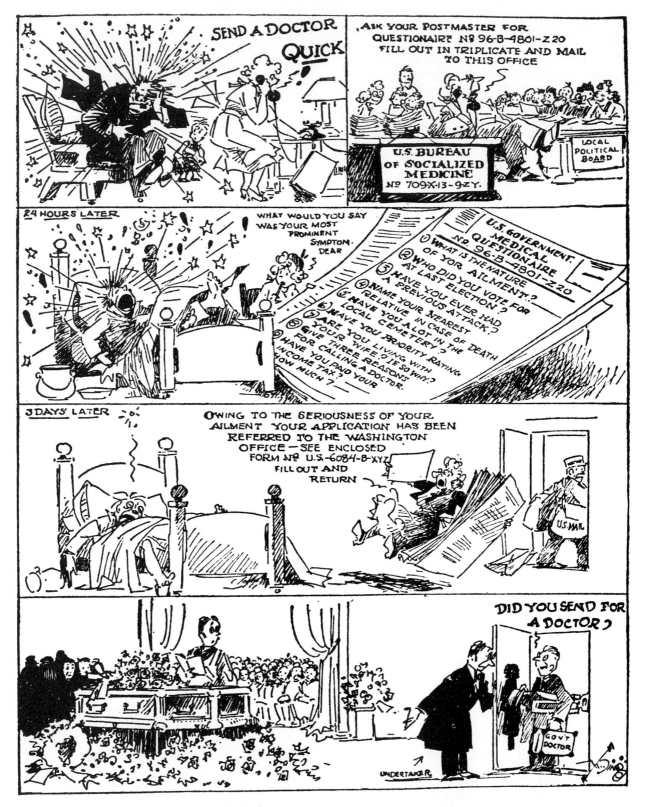

Cartoon opposing national health insurance (c. 1948).

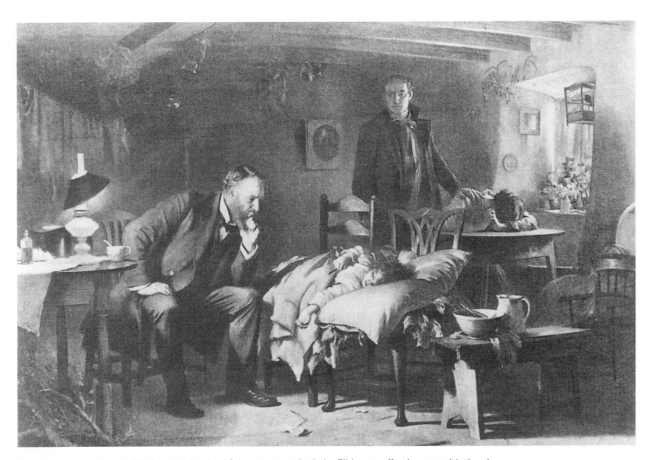

The AMA campaign put The Doctor, *by the 19th-century artist Luke Fildes, to effective use with the slogan, "Keep Politics out of this Picture!"*

> You have a right to prepaid medical care—of your own choice. Ask your doctor, or your insurance man, about budget-basis health protection.
> This is signed: American Medical Association.[27]

Physicians at the state and local levels nearly abandoned their professional ethics to engage in political arm twisting. One letter to the patients of a number of New York physicians appealed frankly to the patients' sense of gratitude for services rendered. "You and I have been friends for some time," it said. "I believe I have served you faithfully and well with sympathy and understanding in your hours of need. There are evil forces creeping into this country which would destroy this personal relationship. They would deny you my services and would deny me the freedom of exercising my skill in serving you." The letter went on at length and closed with the request that "as a service to yourself and to me and to America, that you, your family, and your friends vote in this coming election" for John Foster Dulles, described earlier in the same letter as "thoroughly opposed to socialized medicine and all other European 'isms.'" [28]

FEDERAL AID TO NURSING STYMIED

Aware that the controversial national health legislation package was effectively blocked by a coalition of conservative Republicans and southern Democrats, Senator Elbert D. Thomas of Utah, in June 1949, extracted the Title I health manpower provisions out of a pending national health insurance measure and introduced them as a separate bill. This proposal envisioned a 5-year program of aid for nursing education ranging from $13 million in fiscal year 1950 to $20 million in fiscal year 1954. Eligibility for federal aid for nursing schools was to be determined by an agency designated by the surgeon general of the Public Health Service.

Under the management of Senator Claude Pepper of Florida, the Emergency Professional Health Training Act of 1949 passed the Senate unanimously on September 23. Hopes for passage were high as the House Committee on Interstate and Foreign Commerce reported favorably on the accompanying House version of the bill, sponsored by Representative Andrew Biemiller, on October 11, 1949, but now the new NOHSN flexed its muscles. According to the NOHSN, the bill was aimed at "regimentation or nationalization of the medical, dental, and nursing professions." It would enable the surgeon general of the United States Public Health Service to control hospital nursing schools, because it would give him the power to select the body or bodies approving schools eligible to receive federal funds.

The bill bogged down in the House Rules Committee as a result of the efforts of some Georgia and North Carolina nurses:

> A small group of insurgent members of the nurses' organization in Georgia and North Carolina, and the owner of a private hospital in the latter state, got the impression that the measure would somehow set up the American Nurses' Association as an accrediting body for all nursing schools—and thus force the closing down, for lack of accreditation, of some of the less qualified schools in the Southern States. On behalf of this group, Representative Robert L. (Muley) Doughton of North Carolina protested to the Rules Committee. The sponsors of the Bill offered to amend the measure to overcome the objection. This satisfied Doughton and he withdrew his protest. But the Biemiller bill had, by then, become "controversial." The Rules Committee, fearful of setting a precedent that would throw a host of other controversial measures on the House Floor in the last two weeks of the session, withheld its approval. The bill was held up until Congress could meet again.[29]

Although reintroduced in the next Congress, the bill failed even to pass the Senate, because supporters such as Claude Pepper, Elbert Thomas, and Frank Graham of North Carolina had met with defeat in the 1950 congressional elections, a defeat due partly to the efforts of the AMA lobby. The postwar phenomenon of an acute shortage of graduate nurses brought entirely new demands on a profession formerly faced with perennial oversupply. As preparation for nursing began shifting from a process of apprenticeship and training to one of education, the student labor component was accordingly diminished as general hospitals were expanding. Many nursing leaders looked to the federal government for a solution to the nurse shortage, but the mood of the country was growing conservative, and plans for federal assistance were successfully blocked.

REFERENCES

1. Howard Whitman and Douglas J. Ingalls, "Don't Curse the Nurse," *Colliers*, vol. 119 (May 31, 1947), pp. 26, 67–69.
2. Ibid., p. 67.
3. U.S. Department of Labor, Bureau of Labor Statistics, *The Economic Status of Registered Professional Nurses, 1946–1947* (Washington, DC: Government Printing Office, 1948), pp. 42–43.
4. "The Biennial," *American Journal of Nursing*, vol. 46 (November 1946):728–746.
5. Ibid., pp. 728–729.
6. Clarence Woodbury, "Student Nurse: Could You Take It?" *Woman's Home Companion*, vol. 76 (June 1949):36.
7. "What's All This About the Deplorable State of Nursing Schools?" *Hospital Management*, vol. 67 (June 1949):31.
8. Ibid., pp. 31–32.
9. Kenneth A. Brent, "Are Nurses Getting Too Much Education?" *Hospital Management*, vol. 67 (April 1949):68.
10. Ibid., pp. 68–70.
11. Ibid., p. 70.
12. "College of Surgeons Surveys the Nursing Situation," *Modern Hospital*, vol. 69 (August 1947):59.
13. Joint Committee on Auxiliary Nursing Service, "Annual Report to the NLNE," *Proceedings of the Fiftieth Annual Convention of the National League of Nursing Education*, vol. 50 (September 1946):239–250.
14. Bureau of Labor Statistics, op. cit., p. 46.
15. Esther Lucille Brown, *Nursing for the Future* (New York: Russell Sage Foundation, 1948), pp. 45–46, 165–166.
16. Ibid., pp. 48, 178.
17. Ibid., pp. 132–170.
18. "Graham Davis Attacks Brown Report on 'Nursing for the Future,'" *Modern Hospital*, vol. 71 (October 1948):138.
19. M. West and C. Hawkins, *Nursing Schools at the Mid-century* (New York: National Committee for the Improvement of Nursing Services, 1950), p. 56.
20. Ibid., pp. 81–85.
21. "New Group Will Combat Legislation Unfavorable to Unclassified Nursing Schools," *Modern Hospital*, vol. 74 (February 1950):128.
22. "Survival of Hospital Nursing Schools Called Matter of Utmost Urgency," *Hospital Management*, vol. 69 (January 1950):30.
23. Ibid.
24. U.S. Congress, Senate, Committee on Education and Labor, *National Health Program. Hearings before the Committee*, Part 2 (Washington, DC: Government Printing Office, 1946), pp. 46–47.
25. N. Adams, "Why Opinion Polls on Socialized Medicine Don't Agree," *Medical Economics*, vol. 24 (February 1947):72–74.
26. James G. Burrow, *AMA: Voice of American Medicine* (Baltimore: Johns Hopkins Press, 1963), pp. 368–369.
27. U.S. Congress, House, Committee on Interstate and Foreign Commerce, *National Health Plan. Hearings Before the Committee* (Washington, DC: Government Printing Office, 1949), pp. 28–31.
28. R. M. Cunningham, "Can Political Means Gain Professional Ends?" *Modern Hospital*, vol. 77 (December 1951):51–56.
29. *Congressional Record*, October 3, 1951.

16

NURSING AT MIDCENTURY

Approximately 390,000 professional registered nurses were employed in 1950 in the United States and its territories. About half of the active professional nurses were now working in hospitals and other health institutions, whereas in 1928 less than one fourth of the active RNs had been so employed. In the period after World War II, some had feared that the release of nurses from military service would create a civilian oversupply, but the opposite occurred.

PERSISTENCE OF AN ACUTE NURSING SHORTAGE

In 1950, the American Hospital Association stated that 22,486 vacancies for graduate nurses existed in 2677 of the 4830 hospitals that reported on the nurse shortage. More registered nurses were working than ever before in the nation's history, yet a critical shortage of nursing service existed in almost every city and rural area. Reports from all over the country described the shortage as "critical," "severe," "serious," "acute," and "pressing." What was meant was that hospitals had been forced to shut wards, new units could not be opened, and new programs for health services could not be started.

In Birmingham, Alabama, many hospitals were working nurses on 12-hour shifts instead of on the normal 8, with some nurses performing double-shift duty. Many hospitals were using practical nurses to cover situations where professional nurses were needed. The Alabama Nurses' Association and the Alabama Hospital Association pooled $5000 and appointed a full-time nurse recruiter for the state. Although many young women were recruited during the year this drive took place, the funds were exhausted and the drive had to be closed.

In Boston, the Massachusetts General Hospital affiliated with a school of practical nursing, giving students from that institution 13 months of bedside training out of a 15-month program. The practical-nursing students helped to free professional nurses for other duties, as did the aides the hospital hired and trained in a 6-week course. These persons were replacing the volunteers of the war years. The hospitals operated on a team plan, whereby a graduate nurse served as team leader and was assisted by aides and practical nurses to care for a group of patients. The auxiliary workers took morning temperatures, got breakfast trays passed, and then received instructions for the day's assignments from the team leader. Nursing students and occasionally other graduate nurses were also assigned to these teams and carried out selected aspects of patient care. The team leader received her instructions from the head nurse.

In Chicago, the Illinois Hospital Association and the Blue Cross Plan for hospital care were entering the third year of a joint drive to increase enrollment in nursing schools and reduce the nursing student withdrawal rate. The group's goal was 3500 admissions each year and 2250 graduations. Cooperating in the drive were the Illinois State Nurses' Association, the Illinois League of Nursing Education, and the Illinois Medical Society. A feature of the campaign was Student Nurses' Week, which was to be proclaimed annually by the governor. Before the week's opening, sponsors of the drive got their message to the public through the newspapers, television, radio, church sermons, hospital-sponsored poster contests in schools (with scholarships awarded to the winner), hospital equipment exhibits in department stores, open houses at hospitals for high-school students, and teas for prospective nurses. Also supporting the drive were civic and fraternity organizations and women's groups. Meanwhile, the Chicago Council on Community Nurses had assumed leadership in educating practical nurses as one approach to easing the shortage. Working with the Board of Education and aided by several grants, the council had training branches in two Chicago schools.

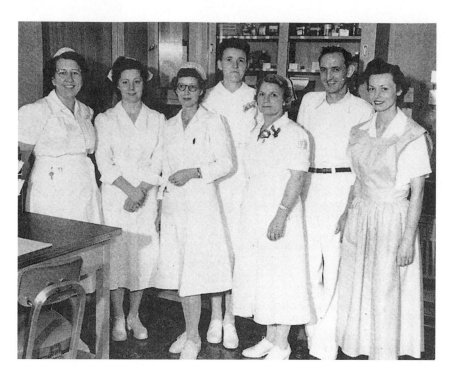

Team nursing was the most common response to the mid-century nurse shortage.

Cleveland hospitals, in a desperate attempt to obtain qualified nurses, had adopted a general 40-hour work week, increased wages, and improved working conditions. One hospital opened an adjacent nursery in an effort to attract nurses who had married and left the work force. Ten nurses with young children took advantage of the project and returned to active nursing. Several hospitals experimented briefly with nurseries for the children of hospital personnel but abandoned the plan, fearing an epidemic of childhood diseases. Other hospitals did not initiate nurseries because of the high cost of operations. In the emergency shortage of registered nurses, hospitals had been employing students as nursing assistants, and many interns were also earning spending money by working extra hours as nurses.

In Los Angeles, the nurse shortage had caused a mushrooming of hit-and-run commercial schools advertising that, for less than $200 tuition and in as little as 24 hours of instruction, they could prepare practical nurses who could earn "big money." Such schools actually did not even have nurse's aide training, much less a practical-nurse course, but they gave graduates a cap and a pin and turned them loose. Several such schools were transplanted eastern enterprises, one of them having taught air conditioning and television repair in Baltimore.

In Seattle, the legislature had passed a law providing for the licensing of practical nurses with only 450 hours of special preparation and 5 months of on-the-job training. The University of Washington School of Nursing planned to announce a working agreement with the Virginia Mason Hospital, Seattle, to conduct a training program tied in with the nursing school. Hospitals in Seattle were using more practical nurses and nurses' aides than ever before. Practical nurses were assigned by the Professional Nurses Registry for duty both in private homes and in hospitals under supervision. The King County Nurses' Association voted against the use of practical nurses for private duty in hospitals, believing that enough responsibility had been delegated to practical nurses already.

The nationwide shortage of nurses hit New York harder than any other large U.S. city. Nurses were leaving the city hospitals faster than replacements could be found. Those remaining could not care for patients adequately because of their increased workload in already overcrowded facilities. As a result, the city's department of hospitals was operating with only 53% of the registered nurses it needed. The shortage in the hospitals was paralleled in the Department of Health. To maintain its public health services, it needed at least 1600 nurses; the department, however, had an authorization for 1071 but employed only 795.

Why was the shortage so great if there were more nurses than ever? Nursing and other health groups generally agreed that, although there was a need for more nursing service because of the tremendous expansion of health and medical services emphasized by the mobilization program, the following factors had changed the pattern of medical and nursing care: the rising average age of the population; the growth of population and its urbanization; the growth of hospitalization and group health insurance plans; the change in the techniques of medicine, such as the use of "miracle" drugs that kept patients alive who formerly would have died; the spread of nurses out of hospitals and into industry and public health services; and the large increase in the number of mothers who had their babies in hospitals.

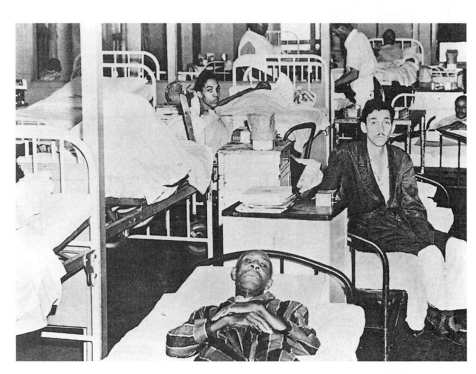

Overcrowded hospitals and too few nurses created havoc in many cities.

CHARACTERISTICS OF THE LABOR FORCE PERTAINING TO NURSING

In 1940, the number of women 15 to 19 years old in the population was 6,153,370, but in 1950 the number was only 5,431,000. According to census figures, in 1950 there were about 300,000 fewer women 18 and 19 years of age than in 1940. Not until 1960 would the declining trend in the number of young women in the population be reversed. Meanwhile, the general population increased in the decade 1940–1950 among the youngest and the oldest age groups. The lowest point in the nation's recorded national birthrate had been in 1933. From 1933 to 1940, the birthrate had increased only 8%, whereas from 1940 to 1947 it rose 45%. The number of young women available to enter a nurse preparation program was less than in former years, because the high school graduates of the 1950s were born in the Depression, when the nation's birthrate was at its lowest ebb.

Also of importance was that in 1950, 54% of all women 18 to 24 years of age were married (with husbands at home rather than away in the military), compared with 39.8% in 1940. The birthrate per 1000 female population aged 15 to 19 increased from 48.9 to 79.7 by 1950, and the number of children younger than 5 years of age increased by 54.7% from 1940 to 1950. The increase in the number of marriages among young women was reflected in the accelerated withdrawal rate of nurses from the work force, estimated at 6.5% per year.

In the 1950s, the birthrate astonished all the experts by maintaining the rise it had shown just after World War II. Despite the insecurities of the postwar world and the apparent degree of relaxation in the family structure, most young American married couples wanted several children. Another shift in family patterns was the marked tendency toward earlier marriages and the consequent necessity that many wives support their husbands until they had finished preparing for professional careers.

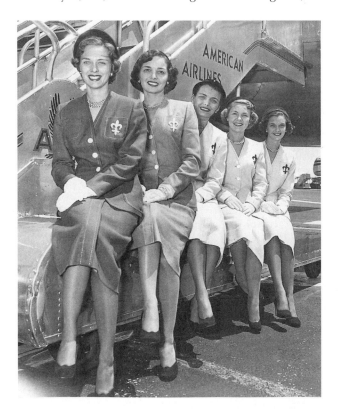

Fewer nurses worked as stewardesses as air travel became safer.

In most professions, the majority of new graduates immediately began working and in many cases stayed in the profession until death or retirement. This was not the case with nurses. Although most new graduates began work at once, a substantial proportion dropped out of their profession within the first 3 years after graduation and did not re-enter the labor force until they were 45 or older, if indeed they ever returned. In other words, nurses tended to withdraw from the labor force in order to marry and raise families.

Married women generally were not accepted as students by most nursing schools due to the conflict between living in the hospital and maintaining an outside home. Most hospitals and institutions and some public health agencies also preferred single nurses (although the married nurse had briefly become popular during the wartime shortage). Married nurses, particularly those with children, tended to be strongly committed to their families. For most student and graduate nurses, marriage and children seemed more important than nursing, and although the motivation for nursing was higher than for any alternative occupation, it could not equal the attraction of marriage and family. Even among nurses who remained active, turnover was high: The nurse shortage was conducive to a high degree of job mobility, and in some hospitals, annual turnover exceeded 66%.

THE ORIGIN AND DEVELOPMENT OF THE STATE BOARD TEST POOL

A postwar movement in nursing that greatly improved standards in nursing schools was the development of the State Board Test Pool. During the late 1930s, state board examinations had generally been poorly constructed and unreliable. Questions such as the following were asked in a test on hygiene:[1]

> Name the six essentials for personal hygiene.
> What is the peculiar opportunity of the nurse in public health education?
> How often should a schoolchild be given a physical examination?
> Lacking an instrument, what is the natural guide for humidity of a room?
> Name two health essentials for a student nurse.
> Name two organizations which guard public health.

The outbreak of World War II had increased the pressure on licensing authorities to license eligible candidates immediately after they had completed their basic programs. Schools quickly found that preparing students to meet the minimum standards for their own state board licensing examinations was no longer adequate; the national norms of competence in nursing had to be taken into consideration. As graduates joined the Army or Navy Nurse Corps and many senior cadets served in federal hospitals, individual schools were compared informally with schools of nursing in other states.

In December 1942 at an emergency conference on state boards, the Subcommittee on Tests of the Committee on State Board Problems of the National League of Nursing Education had met and recommended that the league assist states in adopting machine-scored examination questions and implement the proposed plan of developing prepared state board examinations "for the use of all states in order

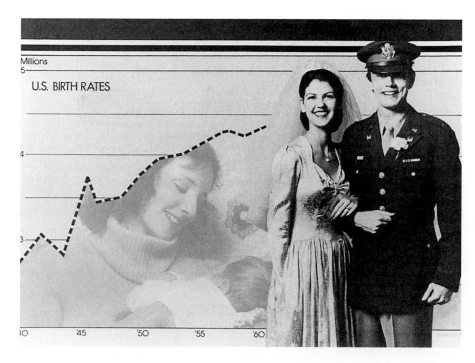

Early marriages and a soaring birthrate characterized the 1950s. (United States Census Bureau.)

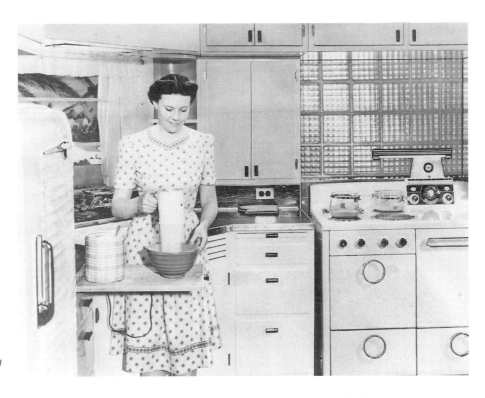

Married nurses with children rarely worked outside of the home.

to have more valid and reliable sets of examination questions and to have these available for more frequent examinations."

The objectives that the committee set up and that the state boards of nurse examiners approved for the State Board Test Pool were as follows:

> To provide objective tests of nursing competency which will enable each state board of nurse examiners to discover the level of ability of each candidate and the average for each school in the state, and for the state as a whole, in comparison with the level of all other candidates tested, and the average for each other school and state.
>
> To develop improved tests of nursing ability and work towards a comprehensive test battery of high validity and reliability.
>
> To study nursing ability, as revealed in the examinations, in order to arrive at a clearer concept of the minimum level of competency as well as the average level of expectancy of professional nurses.
>
> To secure data which will be of help to the state boards of nurse examiners and the schools of nursing in improving the level of nursing preparation.
>
> To lighten the burden of busy state boards of nurse examiners by serving as their agent in preparing and scoring the licensing examinations.[2]

State boards were asked to submit sample questions to the Committee on Nursing Tests, which selected those judged most suitable. The examinations were then set up for machine scoring. Within 1 year, by January 1944, the pool was in operation and six states had agreed to use the examinations.

During the first complete year of operation, 15 states administered these examinations. Licensing authorities in other states were quick to recognize the values to be derived through such a cooperative effort, and soon the State Board Test Pool became well established. The pool simplified the administration of state licensing examinations for nurses and provided participating members with a comparable

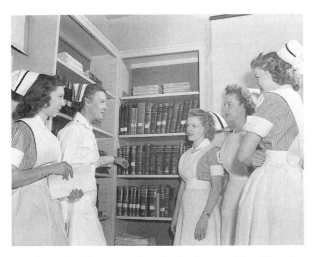

As senior cadets from a number of schools served in military hospitals, variations in state licensing examinations became more apparent.

system of measures for evaluating nursing ability. Participation in the test pool program saved time for busy state boards of nurse examiners in correcting papers, speeded up the issuance of licenses to newly graduated nurses, and simplified registration of nurses who moved from one state to another in which the same tests were used.

When the pool was initiated in 1944, the licensing examination had included 13 tests: anatomy and physiology, chemistry, microbiology, nutrition and diet therapy, pharmacology and therapeutics, nursing arts, communicable disease nursing, medical nursing, nursing of children, obstetric and gynecologic nursing, psychiatric nursing, surgical nursing, and social foundations of nursing. The number of tests used varied among states: some used all of them, whereas others used only one. By 1949, the number of tests had been reduced to six: medical nursing, surgical nursing, obstetric nursing, nursing of children, communicable disease nursing, and psychiatric nursing.

Each test included questions designed to evaluate the candidate's understanding of principles of physical, biologic, and social sciences considered important, as well as questions designed to test nursing skills and abilities in a given clinical area. A concerted effort was made to center most of the test questions around nursing care in given situations. The questions were also designed to test candidates' abilities to apply knowledge gained through classroom and clinical experience. Some faculty members had long criticized the mechanical acquisition of factual data required by state board examinations. Because the pool tests emphasized principles rather than facts, instructors could now concentrate on the

mastery of working theories and thus better prepare their graduates for nursing.

Although each state determined its own passing score, the basic fund of knowledge required for licensure as a registered nurse was the same nationally. Only the degree of knowledge required for licensure varied. The members of the conference of state boards of nurse examiners occasionally considered the feasibility of establishing a common score on each test, which they would accept as the minimum level of performance for licensure of professional nurses. In 1951, the conference recommended that a standard score of 350 be used as the passing score in as many states as possible for purposes of interstate registration or for registration by reciprocal agreement. As a result of this action, state boards of nurse examiners in many states accepted this standard for each test as the minimum level of performance acceptable for licensure.

Growth of and participation in the State Board Test Pool was rapid. Within 5 years, from January 1944 to March 1, 1949, this service expanded from the original 6 states to 41 states. During 1950, the last of the 48 states joined the State Board Test Pool, and nursing became the first profession for which the same licensing examination was used throughout the nation, the District of Columbia, and Hawaii. In addition, the Canadian provinces of British Columbia and Alberta were members of the test pool. The development of the State Board Test Pool broadened each school's concept of its goals.

PSYCHIATRIC HOSPITALS

A significant postwar social phenomenon was the increase in psychiatric disorders in society as a whole. By 1948, there were 540,000 inmates in American mental institutions, representing a ratio of 3.7 for every 1000 people, in contrast to only 1.1 per 1000 in 1910. Among young men of draft age during World War II, 1,825,000 were rejected and 600,000 were discharged because of psychoneurotic disturbances. This high figure was widely interpreted as an indication that the pressures of modern living increased feelings of anxiety and insecurity. But this increase was perhaps more apparent than real, inasmuch as people had now acquired a better understanding of what constituted emotional and mental disorders. Many people who in the 19th century would have been considered a little strange but in no need of medical attention were now diagnosed as having neurotic tendencies. The emergence of psychiatry was one of the major scientific developments of the 20th century, and most educated Americans acquired some understanding of its basic concepts.

Karl Menninger defined mental health at midcentury as "the adjustment of human beings to the world and to each other with a maximum of effectiveness and happiness."[3] He added that this definition did

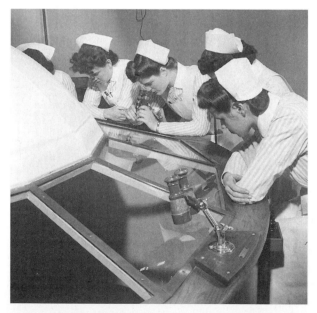

The State Board Test Pool in 1944 included an examination in surgical nursing. Students observe surgery through binoculars into an amphitheater below.

not mean only the attainment of contentment or the grace of obeying the rules of the game cheerfully; rather, it was a combination of both these states—the ability to maintain an even temper, an alert intelligence, socially considerate behavior, and a happy disposition. Mental health, like physical health, varied greatly in form and degree among individuals.

Government agencies spent $250 million a year on institutions for the mentally ill, compared with less than $1 million allocated annually for research into mental and nervous diseases. Although such disorders caused most chronic disability in the United States, they represented one of the least-explored fields of investigation. The problem of mental disease illustrated the nation's deficiencies in medical knowledge and in the application of knowledge already acquired. Since the founding of the first psychiatric hospitals in the United States in the 18th century, mental illness had gradually come to be accepted as a public responsibility. Unfortunately, this concept of public responsibility for the mentally ill had not expanded beyond the original idea that persons whose abnormal behavior could no longer be tolerated should be placed in institutions.

The quality of care given to patients in public mental institutions varied in different parts of the country. A few state institutions provided a reasonably high standard of care, including specialized treatment and medical and hospital care for physical illness. However, surveys made by the Public Health Service revealed deficiencies in patient care that could not be attributed solely to lack of funds, personnel, beds, and facilities. The average public mental health institution did not deserve the name *hospital*; rather, it was a storehouse for human wreckage that had to be removed from the sight of the more fortunate members of society. States, communities, and the nation as a whole needed to reappraise their services for the growing numbers of patients with mental illness.

PSYCHIATRIC NURSING

In 1940, there had been only 4252 graduate nurses employed in state mental hospitals. In one of the West Coast states, for example, there were seven state hospitals, with a patient population of approximately 27,000, yet a total of only 18 graduate nurses were

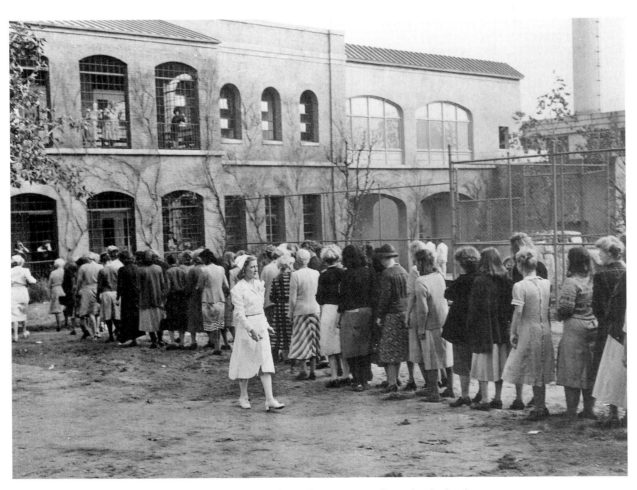

The average public mental health institution was a storehouse for human wreckage that had to be removed from the sight of more fortunate members of society.

employed. In January 1944, there were 14 states in which no psychiatric nursing courses had ever been given, yet each of these states had hospitals for the care of psychiatric patients as well as general hospital schools of nursing. Often, nursing schools operated by psychiatric hospitals did not deserve their official status: One school visited had been in operation for many years, yet never in its history had an instructor been employed on the staff.

Graduate nurses in psychiatric hospitals represented several different types of preparation. Some were graduates of general hospital schools who had moved into psychiatric nursing either by taking a postgraduate course in it or by learning through experience in a psychiatric hospital. Others, graduates of psychiatric hospital schools of nursing, had acquired in their 3 years of preparation some knowledge of general nursing and a special knowledge of psychiatric nursing. Still others were older graduates of 2-year courses who, for various reasons, had not pursued work in other schools to qualify themselves for registration under the requirements of state boards of licensure.

The duties of psychiatric hospital nursing personnel included much more than the care and treatment of the physically ill. Most psychiatric patients were ambulatory rather than bedfast and presented complex social needs. Olga Weiss, in the March 1947 issue of the *American Journal of Nursing*, effectively described the psychiatric nurse's role:

> She must learn to respect her patients as fellow human beings. The person who develops a wholesome respect for other persons as individuals with the same rights and privileges as himself has taken great strides toward reaching understanding.
>
> This is perhaps the most difficult lesson for the nurse to learn, as it means giving up some of the "privileges" of being a nurse, an authoritative creature in a white uniform whose word is law. Because nurses are trained so rigidly, they tend to become rigid, and it is not easy for them to give up some of the precepts learned so painfully. It is difficult to substitute skillful conversation for manual dexterity; the former actually demands more of the nurse. The psychiatric nurse must learn to give much of herself to the patient: her time, patience, and understanding. By understanding we do not mean the useless, sweet, blanket understanding of the willing, but untrained volunteer who pats the head of a withdrawn schizophrenic and speaks condescendingly to him. The nurse working with such patients must have a true scientific knowledge of the illness and its symptoms and must recognize that these people, no matter how withdrawn they seem, are acutely aware of what goes on around them and that condescension is as infuriating to them as to any well person.[4]

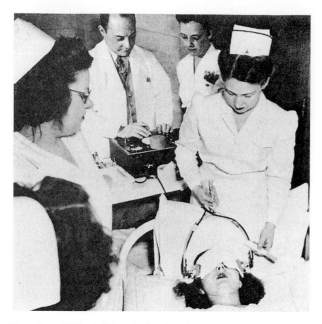

More than 50% of all hospitalized patients in the United States in the early 1950s were mentally ill, but nurses received little training in psychiatric nursing.

Although more than 50% of all patients in the United States in the early 1950s were mentally ill, nurses were taught primarily to care for the other 50%, and nurses' education usually did not cover psychiatric nursing. Progressives of the era pointed out that a psychiatric nurse should have all the education and ability of a general hospital nurse and much additional experience in the psychological aspects of mental illness. It was not generally recognized at this time that psychiatric nursing content was helpful for all aspects of nursing practice.

THE NATIONAL MENTAL HEALTH ACT

The federal government launched an attack on the deficiencies in the care and treatment of the mentally ill in July 1946 with the passage of the National Mental Health Act. The purpose of the act was to provide a method for financing research and training programs and to assist the states in establishing community mental health services. The National Institute of Mental Health (NIMH) of the U.S. Public Health Service was responsible for administering the program. The act provided for the establishment of a National Advisory Mental Health Council composed of six outstanding civilian mental health authorities. This council made recommendations to the Public Health Service on all matters relating to mental health and formed committees on community services, research, and training. The training committee consisted of four subcommittees set up to evaluate training projects in psychiatry, psychiatric social work, psychology, and psychiatric nursing. The council's approval was necessary to obtain a grant for research or training.

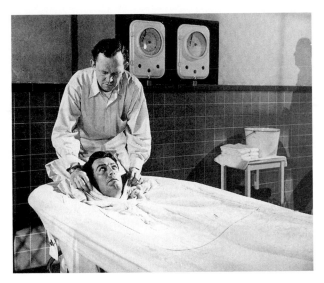

Hydro-therapy was a common treatment in 1947.

Soon research grants were awarded for the investigation of child personality and development, psychosomatic disorders, neurosurgery, epilepsy, schizophrenia, marital counseling, social factors in mental illness, and a number of other related areas. Research fellowships were granted to psychiatrists, psychologists, neurophysiologists, neurologists, anatomists, pediatricians, sociologists, and biologists.

In 1949, graduate-training grants totaling about $2.5 million were made to 28 schools of psychiatric social work, 18 collegiate nursing schools, 46 clinical psychology training institutions, and 56 psychiatric centers. Training stipends were awarded to 471 people through these graduate training centers. The

NIMH traineeship program, which began in 1948 (at the same time that the U.S. Cadet Corps program was in final phaseout), kept alive the principle of federal aid to nursing education.

State grants-in-aid to community services programs provided $3.5 million in 1949. The amount granted to each state depended on its population, its financial need, and the extent of its administrative problem. Annual grants varied from $20,000 to $283,000. Each state designated a particular agency as its state mental health authority, empowered to administer the federal funds that became available. These designated agencies had to prepare a plan and a budget for approval by the Public Health Service, in which $1 of state or local public funds was to be matched by $2 in federal funds. The federal funds could be used to finance mental health activities other than those pertaining strictly to the care and treatment of hospital patients. By 1950, all but one of the states and territories had initiated or expanded their mental hygiene program by using the grant-in-aid funds made available under the National Mental Health Act along with new or increased state appropriations.

THE HILL-BURTON ACT AND HOSPITAL-BUILDING PROGRAMS

On another front, passage of the Hospital Survey and Construction Act of 1946 laid the foundation for development of an integrated, balanced system of hospitals throughout the country, for coordination of hospitals and public health centers, for ultimate organization of all personal health services to the

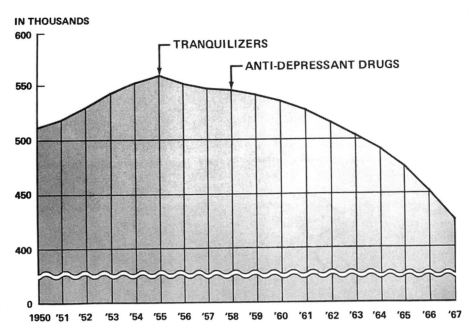

The use of new pharmaceutical interventions led to a decline in state mental hospital populations.

DECLINE IN STATE MENTAL HOSPITAL POPULATION

states, and for construction of additional facilities. This act applied to all types of nonprofit (voluntary as well as public) hospitals and established quantitative and qualitative standards for facilities eligible for aid. General tax funds were allotted to the states on the basis of a special schedule. The total cost of approved projects was borne jointly by federal and state governments, the federal share ranging from one third to two thirds. During its first 6 years, the program, which allocated funds mainly to general hospitals in rural areas, resulted in the total addition of approximately 88,000 beds.

Although priority had been given to the construction of hospitals and public health centers in badly undersupplied areas, the few states with high per capita incomes continued to have much larger proportionate numbers of hospital beds and more public health centers than did many states with comparatively low per capita incomes. Most of the hospitals meeting high standards were in large cities, and the new hospital movement was slow to reach sparsely settled rural areas. Because rural people had been unable to establish tax-supported hospitals in their communities, the burden of initiating building programs fell to local physicians as personal ventures, undertaken chiefly to provide places where surgery might be performed. Thus, rural hospitals were frequently proprietary institutions.

The rural proprietary hospital was fast proving to be an economic impossibility. Rural populations were constantly declining, and the relatively low earnings of the physicians who owned rural hospitals did not allow for institutional operation in accordance with acceptable standards. Improved roads enabled rural people to go to larger towns for better hospital care. Nevertheless, an estimated 20 million people still lived in sparsely settled areas beyond the range of satisfactory hospital care. Rural people were also losing their physicians and nurses to the cities. Authoritative studies of this trend revealed a declining ratio of nurses and physicians to population, an increasing average age of nurses and physicians, and a negligible number of new graduates settling in rural communities.

THE RISE IN NURSING HOMES

The early 1950s saw many changes in nonhospital institutions for the chronically ill. The Social Security Act of 1935 and its amendments of 1950 led to the closing of public homes for the aged and resulted in a tremendous growth in the number of proprietary nursing homes. The number of public homes had declined from 2350 in 1929 to 1260 in 1949. The number of private nonprofit homes had increased from 1270 to 1500, and the commercial nursing homes had shot up from a negligible number to a total of about 8500. The population of the proprietary homes had increased to an estimated 111,000.

The greatly increased number of private nursing homes made it difficult to enforce acceptable standards through inspection and licensure. The 1950 amendments to the Social Security Act required that states claiming matching funds for the costs of care of individuals residing in medical institutions establish and maintain adequate standards for them, and by mid-1953 only four states—Arizona, Florida, Mississippi, and Wyoming—had no statutes regarding such standards. Few public-assistance programs provided sufficient funds to help pay for adequate private nursing home care, and most homes lacked organized affiliation with other medical care facilities. Despite these serious deficiencies, the demand for beds was so urgent that substandard care was sometimes tolerated. Many state and local groups recommended that religious, fraternal, and government organizations undertake more construction and operation of nonprofit nursing homes.

RESTRUCTURING THE PROFESSIONAL ORGANIZATIONS

Meanwhile, regarding a revision of the organizational structure of nursing, the initial move was taken at the biennial convention of the American Nurses Association in 1950, when delegates approved the division of the profession into two large organizations to replace existing operating associations. Under the reorganization plan, the American Nurses Association and the National Association of Colored Graduate Nurses merged, while the National League of Nursing Education, the National Organization of Public Health Nurses, and the Association of Collegiate Schools of Nursing formed another group, the National League for Nursing.

The convention also tabled a resolution opposing compulsory health insurance. The convention thus ignored a telegraphed appeal from the American Medical Association to join the "fight against socialization of medicine." During a discussion of a resolution that the association formally declare its opposition to compulsory health insurance, representatives of the New York, Florida, and Georgia associations spoke in favor of the resolution, claiming that compulsory health insurance had caused a decline in national health and a deterioration of medical standards and facilities wherever it had been introduced. Speakers opposing the resolution urged the nurses to avoid becoming a "pressure group" and maintained that the ANA had not studied the problem of health insurance sufficiently to take any position.

In reaffirming the "principles relating to organization, control, and administration of nursing education" adopted in 1947, the ANA again asserted that nursing education, "in common with other types of education, should be the charge of the educational institutions of the country." The ANA further declared that the education of professional nurses should be an integral part of an institution of higher education, managed according to approved principles, and the basic professional nursing program "should include or be built upon at least two years of general collegiate education."[5]

WAR AGAIN

The peacetime complacency of nurses was suddenly shattered on June 25, 1950, when the Korean War broke out. At the beginning of the action, the total strength of the Army Nurse Corps was below 3500 and that of the Navy Nurse Corps below 2000. The Army Nurse Corps could draw from only 6300 inactive reservists. Many nurse leaders, anticipating a major war, had predicted dire consequences for nursing service in civilian hospitals. Alice Clarke, editor of *R.N.* magazine, thought it a foregone conclusion that, in case of full-scale war, there would be "a general exodus from these hospitals—for nurses in large numbers will always volunteer for military service when they are needed."[6]

Aware that the civilian and military needs for nurses required cooperative planning, the special Joint Committee on Nursing in National Security recommended that the mobilization of nurses be guided by several basic assumptions. First, it was thought that military needs for nurses should receive highest priority, provided that the military set reasonable quotas, recruit personnel according to functional category and field of nursing, and make full use of male nurses and auxiliary workers. It was predicted that in the event of a full-scale war, civilians as well as soldiers might serve on the battlefront; thus, nursing service would be as essential for civilians as for the armed forces. It was thus important to maintain a reasonable distribution of nurses throughout the country for both civilian and defense requirements.

The six national nursing organizations represented on the Joint Committee on Nursing in National Security recommended the following:

That all possible means be developed for recruiting more students for schools of nursing.
That a program be instituted immediately for encouraging inactive nurses to return to practice.
That as many practical nurses be trained and employed to help professional nurses as hospitals and other community agencies could utilize to good advantage.
That nurses be withdrawn systematically from the civilian services for military duty according to a plan that ensured their employment at the highest level of skill for which they were prepared.
That state and local advisory boards of nurses be organized and be given the authority by the

government to review assignment of nurses to the armed forces and to civilian agencies.
That, if there was total mobilization, nurses be redistributed within the fields of nursing and within community agencies so that the most essential civilian needs would be taken care of first.
That major effort be directed to improving sound basic nursing education and to increase enrollment in schools of nursing that offered effective programs.
That selected nurses be encouraged to prepare for responsibilities as teachers, supervisors, and administrators, as well as for the special fields, in order to safeguard essential nursing service.
That administration of nursing services be improved so that nursing skills would be used to the best advantage and their full value would reach more people.
That nursing service be stabilized as much as possible and turnover of staff held to a minimum through the adoption and application of sound personnel policies for nurses and allied workers.[7]

Despite these fears of an acute nursing shortage, military nursing services experienced only a limited

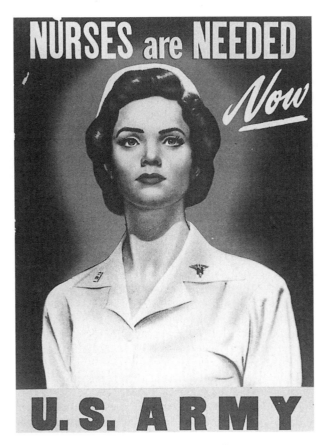

A Korean War Army Nurse Corps recruitment poster.

buildup during the Korean War. During the 3 years of fighting, 2000 nurses volunteered or were recalled for service with the Army Nurse Corps, which reached a peak strength of 5500. Only 10%, or about 500 members, however, received assignments in Korea.

Similarly, in June 1950, there were 1950 regular and reserve Navy Nurse Corps officers on active duty assigned to 26 naval hospitals and dispensaries in and outside the continental United States—three hospital corps schools, two hospital ships, and eight Military Sea Transport Service ships. The Navy Nurse Corps attained its peak strength during the Korean War on June 30, 1951, when 3238 corps officers were on active duty. Three hospital ships, *Consolation*, *Repose*, and *Haven*, rotated as station hospitals in Korean waters during the hostilities.

Before the war, on July 1, 1949, 1199 army nurses had been transferred from the Department of the Army to the new Department of the Air Force. As the Air Force Nurse Corps prepared to celebrate its first anniversary in July 1950, it faced the grim but essential task of supplying, within a period of 48 hours, a large number of nurses to assist in the air evacuation of battle casualties from the Korean area. By mid-July 1950, 200 air force nurses were actively engaged in the air evacuation of patients.

NURSING IN THE MOBILE ARMY SURGICAL HOSPITALS

There were periods in the Korean campaign when battle casualties ran exceedingly high. The difficulties in rescue and treatment of the wounded and injured were heightened by the extremes of weather and the mountainous terrain, but the fatality rates among these patients were surprisingly low. The major reasons for the decrease in fatalities were the availability of prompt and effective first-aid treatment, rapid evacuation, and surgical treatment near the scene of action. A steady supply of whole blood and antibiotics also played a vital role. The use of air force and marine corps helicopters represented a significant advance in the evacuation procedure.

World War II had demonstrated to the military the need for a new type of hospital as an adjunct to the existing methods for treating casualties in the field. Thus the Mobile Army Surgical Hospital (MASH) was organized and integrated into the line of evacuation of battle casualties. Designed to be highly mobile, this hospital provided expert care by physicians and nurses. It was to be located as close to the front line as was safely practicable—approximately 8 to 20 miles.

Korea provided the first test for these mobile units, six of which supported frontline divisions throughout the Korean campaign. A typical MASH unit was set up in tents; buildings were used, however, when available. Patients were first admitted to the receiving ward, where the medical officer and nurses surveyed the

extent of the wounds and determined the presence or absence of shock. Immediately afterward, they began resuscitative measures, ordered x-rays, and decided on the course of therapy. This therapy usually included the administration of blood or oxygen or both and general supportive measures designed to prepare the patient for surgery.

The typical MASH unit comprised approximately 156 personnel. There were about 15 medical officers, specializing in general surgery, thoracic surgery, orthopedic surgery, internal medicine, and anesthesiology. The nursing staff consisted of approximately 16: 5 nurses each for the preoperative and postoperative wards, 4 for the operating room, and 2 nurse-anesthetists. The remaining hospital complement consisted of about 4 administrative officers and 120 enlisted personnel who performed the various tasks necessary for the hospital to function smoothly.

Attached to each MASH unit was an army helicopter detachment whose mission was to provide immediate means of evacuation for critically injured battle casualties or seriously ill medical patients. Rapid helicopter evacuation of the wounded contributed greatly to the marked decrease in mortality from wounds. When conditions were not suitable for air evacuation, patients were brought to the hospital from the battalion aid stations by ambulances, which were attached to all combat units. Evacuation from this hospital, in turn, might again be by helicopter or ambulance, depending on the patient's condition.

The MASH unit was the first hospital to which the wounded man was sent on evacuation to the rear.

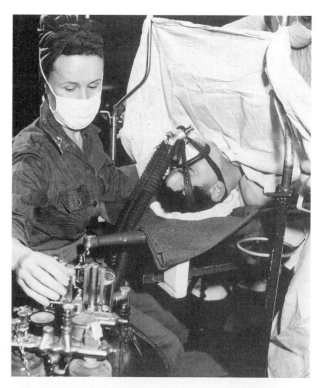

An army nurse administers anesthetic at a MASH hospital.

Because the soldiers liked the security that nearness could provide, MASH units were a great factor in maintaining morale. The proximity of the unit to the front, its trained personnel, its adequate supply of whole blood, and its rapid helicopter and ambulance evacuation services all contributed greatly to the reduction of mortality rates in Korea compared with those during World War II: the mortality rate among wounded soldiers who reached hospitals in Korea was half the corresponding rate during World War II.

FLIGHT NURSING MATURES

Along with advances in antibiotics and medical techniques, one of the major factors in reducing fatalities was the quick air delivery of patients to hospitals. Air evacuation of the wounded from the battlefields of Korea to military medical centers in Japan was the responsibility of the Military Air Transport Service and a unified air force–navy complement of medical technicians and flight nurses. One flight nurse was assigned to each plane carrying ambulatory and litter patients. Flight nurses and medics worked around the clock, sometimes as long as 72 hours without a break, getting their only rest while en route to Korea with a load of cargo. Nurses saved many lives during the summer of 1950 by supplying prompt medical attention and by advising pilots of the cruising altitudes suited to the individual requirements of seriously ill patients. Sometimes speed of delivery was vital; at other times a smooth flight was more important.

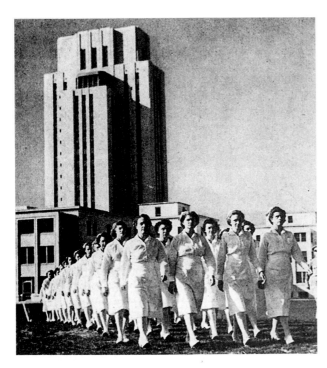

Navy nurses at Bethesda Naval Hospital ready to receive patients from Korea.

Wounded soldiers, direct from combat, dirty, and disheveled, were happy to talk to American women again and proud of the bravery of the nurses who flew repeatedly into dangerous areas. One flight nurse and a medic were killed when a C-54 took off from Kimpo, near Seoul, crash-landing at night on the Sea of Japan not far from the Japanese coast. Another flight nurse was later awarded the Distinguished Flying Cross for helping other passengers on the plane to escape, even though she was severely injured herself.

Airlifting the wounded became an international venture as Australian, British, Turkish, and Filipino soldiers joined the fighting in Korea. Nurses learned an informal and international sign language of sorts that enabled them to help patients whose languages they could not understand. There were usually people on board who could help interpret a little. When the Chinese crossed the Yalu River and struck hard at American troops, air evacuation of the wounded stepped up considerably, reaching a high point in early December, when C-47s air-evacuated 4700 wounded and frostbitten Marines in 4 days. On December 5, 1950, flight nurses air-evacuated a record high of 3925 patients in a single day. At that time, it looked as though the Chinese might overrun all of Korea, and Eighth Army medical officers decided to empty all Korean hospitals for safety's sake.

Sometimes the medical flight personnel included wounded Korean physicians and nurses who, disregarding their own disabilities, helped with the patients. On the hurried and hazardous flights out of Wonju, flight nurses had little or no time to examine patients or give them serious medical attention. Because the enemy was generally lurking nearby, it seemed more important to rush the loading and get the patients out fast. The C-47s were often incredibly crowded, with patients sitting or lying in the aisle.

Flight nurses assumed all the risks of the aircrews, taking their chances with the rugged terrain and weather, inadequate landing strips, possible enemy air attacks, frequent ground fire, and possible sabotage by patients. Nurses checking wounded prisoners on board one plane found that a North Korean had a live hand grenade stowed away in his clothes; they took away the grenade and let the POW fly with the other patients.

Gradually, a systematic air-evacuation pattern evolved. Wounded men whose total hospitalization was likely to require 30 days or less, with subsequent return to duty, were air-evacuated to southern Korea. Patients expected to be hospitalized for 6 months or less were moved by C-54s to Japan and returned to Korea to finish their tour of duty on recovery. Patients whose probable recovery would take more than 6 months were airlifted back to the United States by the Military Air Transport Service to clear the hospitals in Japan for other patients. The general policy was to move the wounded as quickly as possible from the front lines to a rear-area hospital. Many of those airlifted to Korean bases were later evacuated to

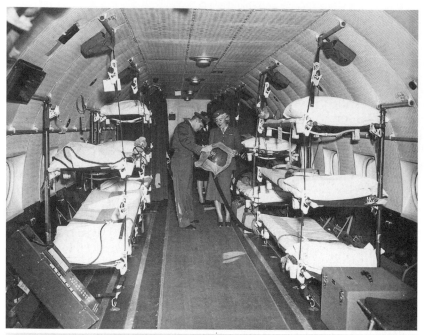

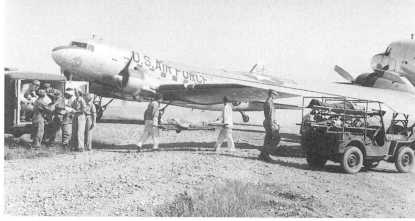

Interior and exterior views of C-47 Air Evacuation aircraft.

Japan and perhaps moved once more for eventual airlift home.

One result of air evacuation in the Korean War was the virtual elimination of the hospital ship as a means of transporting the wounded. During the early days of the war, army medical officers were inclined to regard the hospital ship as the safest way to move large numbers of wounded. Gradually, they came to agree with the air force that air evacuation of the wounded was the cheapest, most efficient, and most sensible method of transportation. Navy hospital ships off the Korean coast were used mainly as floating hospitals and were assigned to transport patients only when en route to Japan for overhaul or refitting.

A DAY IN THE LIFE OF A FLIGHT NURSE

A typical trip into and out of Korea on a flight leaving from Japan was vividly described by Captain Janice Albert of the Air Force Nurse Corps:

Your alarm goes off at 0100. You are to be picked up at 0130 for a 0300 take-off. You're wide awake because you have a lot to do before your transportation arrives. You go about getting ready quietly while your roommate sleeps (she didn't get back from her flight until late that evening and is not scheduled for take-off until much later). Before you went to bed, you checked and rechecked your medical supplies—ready for any emergency, since you do not know what type of wounded you'll be caring for until you load your patients aboard. You've slept in your "longjohns," so all you do is put on your flight suit and make-up, pick up your jacket and pocket-book, and you are on your way. Transportation arrives with your aeromedical technician. Together, you recheck your supplies—oxygen, medical kit, extra dressing, blankets, straps—they are all there and you proceed to the airplane that will take you to Korea. The plane is loaded with cargo. This time it is mail, but it could have been anything from blood plasma, whole blood, or medical supplies to ammunition, gasoline, airplane parts, jeeps, rifles—tools for waging war or preserving life—perishable foods, propaganda leaflets, or personnel returning or reporting to the fighting zone.[8]

On arrival and unloading in Korea, the aircraft was swept out, litter straps were unrolled, and the cargo plane became a hospital ward. Patients began to arrive from the MASH units, and the nurse made out her report of patients to be evacuated. The loading ramp—a converted jeep—pulled up to the plane, and one by one the wounded were gently carried aboard on litters and secured to their proper spot. Albert continued her story:

> You and your aeromedical technician scarcely realize that you are 7,000 feet above the ground as you go about your job. And though there is a language barrier, compassion serves as a universal tongue to bring understanding between you and your patients. You reassure a frightened private, redress the colostomy, give oxygen to the Turk with the penetrating chest wound, administer a narcotic to the boy who is still not fully aware of the absence of his left leg—a smile here, a gentle hand there, and soon the tension of the cabin is lessened, at least for the moment. The Frenchman shows you pictures of his wife and baby, and soon the rest want you to look at their pictures too. You light a cigarette for the Greek whose right arm is in a cast, you pass sandwiches, tuck in a blanket here, readjust the position of the man with a fractured leg, and check on the drainage bottle of the patient with a gunshot wound in his back.

Time passes rapidly and so far the trip has gone off smoothly. Suddenly, you become anxious about the Turk with the penetrating chest wound. After stepping up the oxygen, you consult with the pilot as to the position of the aircraft and find you are still an hour from your destination. You decide that the patient may not be able to stand that long a flight, so you ask the pilot to call the nearest airfield to have a doctor meet the plane. At your request he makes an emergency landing. The injured man is off-loaded and the plane continues its scheduled trip.

About an hour later, the plane had landed. Ambulances were waiting and the remaining patients were off-loaded. Albert further related:

> Though your nose is shiny and you need lipstick, to these patients you look beautiful—you are the girl they left home, the one they expect to see soon.

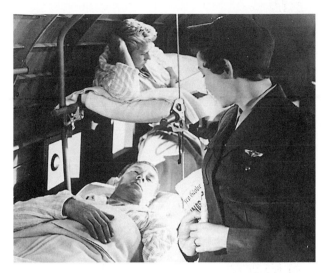

Wounded soldiers on their way home from Korea.

> Your trip is ended! You gather your medical supplies and head towards quarters. You have been on duty almost 16 hours. Tired? Yes, but a hot shower, a few hours sleep, and you are ready to do it again tomorrow if necessary. (Many times it is.)
>
> As you reach the nurses' quarters, you feel a warm sense of spiritual satisfaction. You have once again contributed your small share toward easing and erasing the pains and anxieties of war's combat casualties.[9]

THE END OF THE WAR

In April and May of 1951, American and United Nations forces in Korea repelled two Chinese offensives, during which the attackers suffered staggering losses estimated in excess of 1 million casualties. On June 23, 1951, the head of the Russian delegation at the United Nations indicated that the war could be ended if both sides began discussions that would lead to "a cease-fire and an armistice providing for a mutual withdrawal of forces from the thirty-eighth parallel."[10] Two years of negotiations, during which the fighting continued, took place before an armistice agreement was accepted. All fighting stopped on July 27, 1953. When the final casualty report for the 37 months of war was prepared, American losses totaled 142,091, of whom 33,629 were killed, 103,284 were wounded, and 5178 were missing or captured. The bulk of these casualties occurred during the first year of fighting. The war had witnessed great advances in medical care provision to the wounded, and nurses had made a tremendous contribution to this effort.

ACCREDITATION ADVANCES

Meanwhile, the National League for Nursing's accreditation program was beginning to have a

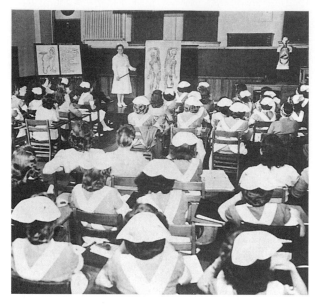

The temporary accreditation program helped many schools improve their educational standards.

noticeable effect on nursing educational standards. Helen Nahm described the "poorer" school of 1952 as those having some or all of these characteristics:[11]

> Very few full-time faculty members.
> Unstable faculty.
> High workload for faculty and students.
> Much evening and night duty for students.
> Little or no planned clinical or ward instruction.
> Low service hours carried by graduate staff nurse or nonprofessional workers or both.
> High withdrawal rates.
> Low daily average patient census in one or more clinical areas.
> Low score on state board examinations.

The temporary accreditation program in effect from 1952 to 1957 was geared toward helping the inferior schools find ways of improving themselves. Under this program, many special meetings were held, self-evaluation guides prepared, and consultations arranged. The purposes of these conferences were:

> To learn more about the needs and problems of nursing schools throughout the country so that the professional nursing organizations could take steps to provide assistance in improving education programs.
> To assist nursing schools in interpreting information presented on the school profiles as well as other information sent to them following the meetings of the boards of review.
> To discuss the criteria which were used by the boards of review in evaluating programs for temporary accreditation.

> To discuss other criteria which probably should be used in evaluating nursing school programs.
> To discuss steps which individual schools could take to improve their own programs.
> To discuss measures which could be taken to help schools offering programs not approved for temporary accreditation.
> To discuss whether a consultant service should be set up by the National League for Nursing through which schools of nursing could obtain individual assistance.[12]

When this program ended in 1957, the number of fully accredited schools had increased by 72.4%. In the meantime, the total number of nursing schools dropped from 1139 to 1115, but schools offering degree programs increased by 37 between 1952 and 1957, and 18 associate degree programs, representing an entirely new development, were established. In the same 5-year period, the total number of diploma-granting schools was reduced to 936, or 79 fewer than in 1952.

Evidence of the positive effect of the temporary accreditation program was contained in the National League for Nursing publication *Report on Hospital Schools of Nursing, 1957.* Based on data collected in the last year of the program, the report revealed the progress made by hospital schools and identified areas still presenting problems:

> The hospital school of nursing of 1957 in most instances has come a long way toward achieving the characteristics of a truly educational institution. Although its students are to some extent still used for staffing the nursing services, its major concern is the development of its student. Preparation for nursing practice is . . . its primary aim . . . but its offerings extend beyond those required for technical or vocational training into those which provide the type of broad educational background that makes for personal as well as professional development.[13]

Concrete evidence of improvement appeared in many areas. Schools had more and better qualified full-time faculty members than in 1949. The 4-week annual vacation had become universal. Three fourths of the schools reported students on a 40-hour week and with better planning of evening and night assignments. However, the report particularly emphasized the need for redefinition of clinical learning experiences, the area least influenced by school improvement. Finance was another area in which relatively little progress was noted: "In most schools of nursing . . . the curriculum is developed as an income-producing as well as a 'learning-producing' operation."[14]

As professional nursing celebrated its 78th birthday (1873 marked the founding of the first three

American nurse training schools—Bellevue, Connecticut, and Boston) and moved into the 1950s, prevailing feminine values strongly affected nurse career patterns. The high turnover among registered nurses helped to perpetuate a nurse shortage aggravated by the demands of the Korean War and the greater involvement of nurses in the psychiatric nursing field. Minimal qualifications demanded of nurses were significantly increased by the development and implementation of a common state board test pool throughout the United States. Educational standards were further upgraded by the launching of an aggressive school accreditation program.

REFERENCES

1. Florida State Board of Nursing, "Registered Nurse Examination for 1939," Jackson Memorial Hospital School of Nursing Archives, Miami.
2. "The State Board Test Pool Examination," *American Journal of Nursing*, vol. 52 (May 1952):613–615.
3. Karl Menninger, "The Future of Psychiatric Care in Hospitals," *Modern Hospital*, vol. 64 (May 1945):43–45.
4. M. O. Weiss, "The Skills of Psychiatric Nursing," *American Journal of Nursing*, vol. 47 (March 1947):174–176.
5. V. A. Turner, "American Nurses' Association Settles Important Issues," *Trained Nurse and Hospital Review*, vol. 124 (June 1950):260.
6. Alice Clarke, "Draft Nurses . . . A New War and Old Theme," *R.N.*, vol. 14 (March 1951):24–25.
7. Joint Committee on Nursing in National Security, "Mobilization of Nurses for National Security," *American Journal of Nursing*, vol. 51 (February 1951):78–79.
8. Janice Albert, "Air Evacuation from Korea—A Typical Flight," *Military Surgeon*, vol. 112 (April 1953):256–258.
9. Ibid., pp. 257–258.
10. *New York Times*, June 24, 1951.
11. Helen Nahm, "Temporary Accreditation," *American Journal of Nursing*, vol. 52 (August 1952):997–1001.
12. National League for Nursing, Division of Nursing Education, "Report on the Program of Temporary Accreditation of the National Nursing Accrediting Service: Part I, Study of Basic Programs Offered by Schools of Nursing, 1952" (mimeographed).
13. National League for Nursing, *Report on Hospital Schools of Nursing, 1957* (New York: The League, 1959), p. 5.
14. Ibid., p. 30.

MINORITIES IN NURSING STRIVE FOR RECOGNITION

In 1953, when births in the United States reached 4 million for the first time and filled hospital nurseries to the overflow level, business periodicals happily predicted prosperity. Americans were growing older, with the over-65 bracket increasing more rapidly than any other age group, largely because the death rate had been cut in half since 1900. Life expectancy, which had been 63 years in 1940, had jumped to 67 in 1950, although it remained at 60 for nonwhites. For the first time, a magazine was published exclusively for those preparing to retire. At the other end of the age scale, school enrollment boomed to an all-time high of 30 million and continued to climb.

But quite another story was buried under these cheering national averages. Nearly 3% of Americans older than age 14 were illiterate, and among non-whites the figure was four times higher. Despite wartime prosperity, black Americans were much worse off than whites with respect to level of education, life expectancy, housing, percentage of children who survived birth, and, most visibly, average annual income—$2000 for black workers in general and $815 for black women, compared with $3500 for whites.

OUTLAWING RACIAL SEGREGATION

One of the most important and difficult domestic issues in America during the mid-1950s arose out of the Supreme Court ruling in *Brown* v. *Board of Education of Topeka* on May 17, 1954, which outlawed racial segregation in public schools. Despite improvements in the political, economic, and, to a lesser degree, social conditions among northern blacks, no comparable progress had taken place for those living in the South, where rigid social barriers limited their opportunities and denied them the equality to which they were entitled under the Constitution and federal law. Nowhere was this more apparent than in the public school system, which adhered to the "separate

but equal" doctrine set down by the Supreme Court in *Plessy* v. *Ferguson* in 1896.

In *Brown* v. *Board of Education*, by unanimous decision, the court overturned its old "separate but equal" doctrine by asserting that "separate educational facilities are inherently unequal," that "segregation in public education" denied the black students "equal protection of the law," and that separating black children "from others of similar age and qualifications solely because of their race generates a feeling of inferiority as to their status in the community that may affect their hearts and minds in a way unlikely ever to be undone."[1]

The editor of the *Nursing Outlook* noted this momentous court case in a vigorous editorial:

> We rejoiced with others when the Supreme Court of the United States handed down its decision on May 17. We were glad that the National League for Nursing had been a bit ahead of the times in its decision, reaffirmed by the Board of Directors in January, 1953, "that all activities [of the National League for Nursing] shall include all groups regardless of race, color, religion, sex. . . ."
>
> But the satisfaction we feel in the "rightness" of this step is only a beginning. We know that Negro nurses are employed by many hospitals and health agencies. We know that Negro nurses hold commissions in the armed services, that they receive all the benefits and carry all the responsibilities which go with those commissions. We know that 710 of our 1,148 accredited schools of nursing accept qualified Negro students. We know, too, that some, although not many, Negro nurses hold administrative positions in hospitals and health agencies.
>
> No, this is not enough. Is participation on the board, on committees, and on staffs of all service groups extended on an equitable basis? Are all nurses free to take part in our organizations'

360

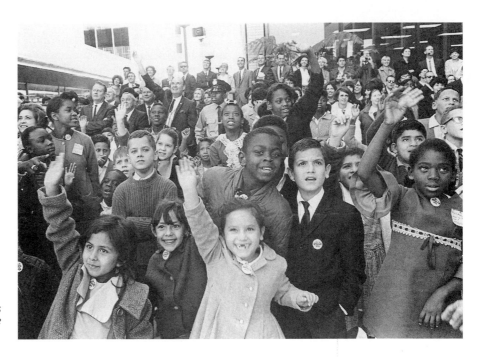

Racial integration in public schools was accelerated by the Supreme Court ruling in 1954.

programs, policy decisions, and conferences? There is much yet to be done. And we shall do it—slowly and quietly. What is most important just now is to look to the future and determine what this ruling will mean in the next few decades.[2]

SLOW DEVELOPMENT OF BLACK NURSING

In 1950, about 6% of all graduate and student nurses in the United States were black. Seventy-one years earlier, in 1879, the first black trained nurse, Mary E.P. Mahoney, had received a diploma in nursing from the School of Nursing of the New England Hospital for Women and Children in Boston. The first school for black nurses, at the Provident Hospital, Chicago, had been organized in 1891. Advancement for the black nurse came slowly, because she was caught between two evolving processes in the social order. Racially, she was a member of an emerging group that had not been fully recognized on a merit basis by other groups; professionally, she was part of an emerging group whose worth to society had not been fully recognized.

Until after World War II, black nurses could secure membership in the American Nurses Association (ANA) only through membership in the state nurses' associations in those states where black nurses were eligible for membership. Obviously, in certain southern states where black nurses were barred from admission to the state nurses' association, they were unable to belong to the ANA, although they qualified for membership in every other respect. Partly as a result of this discrimination, the National Association of Colored Graduate Nurses

was organized in 1908. At the first annual convention of the association held in Boston in 1910, there were 26 charter members present, representing 10 states. From this nucleus, the association grew to a mem-

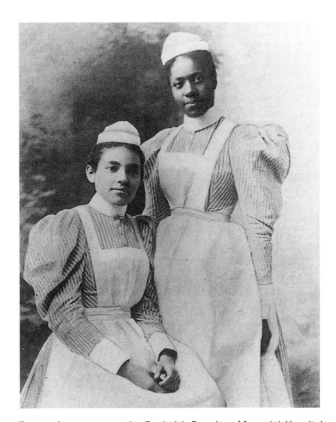

Two student nurses at the Frederick Douglass Memorial Hospital Training School for Nurses, Philadelphia, circa 1896. (Pennsylvania Auditor General's report 1898.)

bership of more than 1200 nurses by 1940, drawn from practically every state in the Union.

According to information in a report published in 1924 by the Hospital and Service Bureau of the American Conference on Hospital Service, only 58 state-accredited schools of nursing admitted black students, and most of these schools were located in black hospitals or in departments for the care of black patients in municipal hospitals. Twenty-eight states were found to offer no opportunity for education in nursing to the black woman. Of the 58 accredited schools, 39 (77%) were located in the South. This distribution closely followed the distribution of the black population of that time, 80% of which was in the South.

BLACK NURSING IN THE SOUTH

A report entitled "Observations on Negro Nursing in the South" by Nina D. Gage, executive secretary of the National League for Nursing Education, and Alma Haupt, associate director of the National Organization for Public Health Nursing, in 1932, made the following comments about some of these schools:

> In the six states visited (Alabama, Georgia, Louisiana, Mississippi, Tennessee, and Texas) there are 23 Negro schools of nursing which are accredited by their respective Boards of Nurse Examiners. . . . The schools of nursing themselves are of many varieties—some so poor

as to make one question how they can possibly meet the standards of a State Board of Medical Examiners. Others are pioneering in the field of education with great success. [In one poor school] two shabby houses were used as a hospital of thirty-five beds and a nurses' home for twelve students. A colored nurse is superintendent of nurses and the sole member of the faculty. A three-year course is given, every subject being taught by the one nurse. With a wide range of subjects now necessary for the preparation of the nurse to meet the demands of the field, it is manifestly impossible, both physically and mentally, for one person to carry the entire teaching program of a school. Without some specialization of the faculty, the student cannot get the variety and different points of view needed to prepare her adequately for her future work. No public health subjects are included in the curriculum of this school, but the students are frequently sent out to homes as private duty nurses, and the wages thus earned help to run the hospital.[3]

The critical lack of opportunities for preliminary education among black youth in the South was highlighted in 1931 in *Brown America*, by Edwin R. Embree:

> The inadequacy of the schools and the low level of literacy and activity in the South are such that not only Negroes but the whole population is retarded. . . . To the visitor, colored schools seem

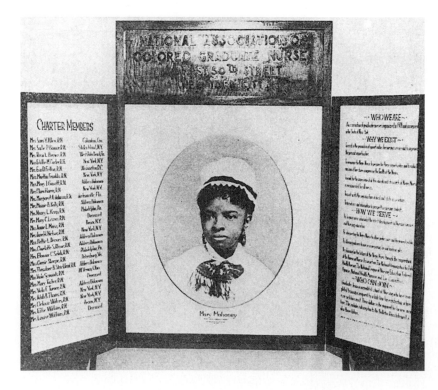

The founding of the National Association of Colored Graduate Nurses in 1908 was an important milestone in the development of black nursing.

not a system, but a series of incidents: bizarre, heroic, pathetic, romantic . . . many of the schools run for only three or four months, with teachers paid but $25 to $30 a month for these short terms. Studies of eight Southern states show an average expenditure of $44.31 per capita for whites and only $12.50 for Negroes. In certain states with huge black populations, the discrepancies are even greater. Georgia spends on the average $35.42 per white child and $6.38 per colored child. The figures of Mississippi are $45.34 against $5.45. The inadequacy of these provisions for either race is seen when one compares them with the average expenditure throughout the United States as a whole, which is $87.22 per child.[4]

Black women from better homes were not readily attracted to nursing. They seemed to be more interested in teaching and music, because these careers offered more immediate social prestige than did nursing. Although black nursing schools located in the South were in desperate need of qualified instructors, the black nurse could not take graduate work in nursing in any university or college in the South. This pointed to the need for the establishment of a graduate department in nursing education in one of the universities that would admit blacks. Such lack of opportunity was especially unfortunate, because there were in the South approximately 23,000 black midwives wholly unprepared by training for the work they were doing. If the midwife could be replaced by the well-educated nurse who would combine midwifery with public health nursing, one of the outstanding health needs of southern blacks could be met.

The U.S. census for 1930 listed 5728 graduate, registered black nurses in a total black population of 11,891,143. Before World War II, the principal places of employment for black nurses had been black hospitals and institutions, large public hospitals in the North, and local official and voluntary public health agencies serving large numbers of black patients. Sixty-three percent of active black nurses in 1941 were in hospital and institutional work, and 28% were in public health, compared with 47% and 10%, respectively, of all active nurses. Private practice and industrial work offered little opportunity, judging by the 6% of black nurses in private duty and 1% in industrial nursing, compared with 27% and 3%, respectively, for all nurses. Many opportunities in teaching and supervisory work required graduate training—all but unavailable to black nurses.

HEALTH AMONG BLACK AMERICANS

Although authorities pointed to a remarkable decline in mortality among blacks, the black morbidity rate in 1930 was 18 per 1000 of the population,

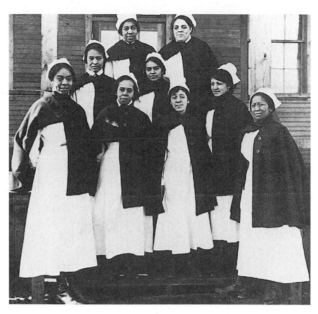

Black nurses served in special hospital facilities for black troops in World War I.

whereas that of whites was 9.9. The urban black death rate was 95% higher than that of the urban white population. This fact assumed increasing importance as blacks migrated to cities. As a result of tuberculosis, heart disease, pneumonia, syphilis, and other preventable diseases, the death rates of blacks ranged from 1½ to 8 times that of whites. Unhealthy living and working conditions, perpetuated by racial discrimination, and fewer available health care providers combined to increase health hazards for blacks.

Health facilities for blacks lagged far behind demonstrated needs, which were rapidly increasing. Julius Rosenwald Fund administrators pointed out that although the black death rate had receded from an estimated 32 deaths per 1000 in 1890 to about 15 in 1940, the rate still exceeded the national average of 11.2. The inadequacy of hospital services for blacks in most states and the nonexistence of such services in some southern rural areas accounted for much of this problem. The fund reported that in some predominantly black rural areas, as few as 75 hospital beds were set aside for the use of 1 million blacks. In many cities, black patients were treated only through clinics. Even those able to pay for adequate hospital care encountered difficulty in obtaining it and were seldom permitted free choice of physicians. Restrictive hospital policies limited the number of black physicians and nurses and excluded them from important postgraduate experience.

The 110 black hospitals in the United States in 1940 had a total of only about 10,000 beds, and more than 70% of these hospitals were privately owned and depended on the patients' ability to pay. Only 22 black hospitals were fully approved by the American

TABLE 17-1 Nursing Schools for Black Students in 1940

NURSING SCHOOL	LOCATION
Fraternal	Montgomery, AL
Tuskegee	Tuskegee, AL
Freedman's	Washington, DC
Brewster	Jacksonville, FL
Grady Hospital–Municipal Training School	Atlanta, GA
University Hospital–Lamar School	Augusta, GA
City–School for Colored Nurses	Columbus, GA
Provident	Chicago, IL
Red Cross	Louisville, KY
Provident	Baltimore, MD
Afro–American	Yazoo City, MS
General Hospital Number 2	Kansas City, MO
Saint Louis City Number 2	St. Louis, MO
Harlem	New York, NY
Lincoln	New York, NY
Good Samaritan	Charlotte, NC
Lincoln	Durham, NC
L. Richardson Memorial	Greensboro, NC
St. Agnes	Raleigh, NC
Mercy	Philadelphia, PA
Good Samaritan	Columbia, SC
Jane Terrell	Memphis, TN
Hubbard	Nashville, TN
Prairie View	Prairie View, TX
Hampton Institute	Hampton, VA
St. Philip	Richmond, VA

College of Surgeons, with 5 others provisionally approved. Only 26 black nursing schools existed, and few others, governmental or voluntary, admitted black students (Table 17-1). Even in northern cities, hospital accommodations were limited because of the restrictive policies of private institutions and segregationist practices in many public hospitals.

AN AMERICAN DILEMMA

In 1937, the Carnegie Corporation of New York decided to sponsor "a comprehensive study of the Negro in the United States, to be undertaken in a wholly objective and dispassionate way as a social phenomenon."[5] For nearly a century, the whole question had been so emotionally charged that it appeared wise to seek as the responsible head of the undertaking someone who could approach the task as freshly as possible, uninfluenced by traditional attitudes or by earlier conclusions. Thus, Gunnar Myrdal, a distinguished Swedish scholar, was chosen to direct the study.

The "dilemma" analyzed and described by Myrdal was the failure of the American credo as it applied to blacks. In the early 1940s, Myrdal had suggested that numerous solidly entrenched beliefs about blacks that were demonstrably false and loaded with emotion were used to excuse white mistreatment of blacks. As summarized by Myrdal, a caste system had been rationalized and defended by whites on the grounds that black people belonged to a separate race of mankind and were inferior in all important respects.[6]

Myrdal conceded that there were inherent differences between the races, but he attributed these to environmental conditions. "When we approach these problems on the hypothesis that differences in behavior are to be explained largely in terms of social and cultural factors, we are on scientifically safe ground. If we should, however, approach them on the hypothesis that they are to be explained primarily in terms of heredity, we do not have any scientific basis for our assumption."[7]

Since first brought to this country as slaves, the black population had been heavily concentrated in the South. It was a curious phenomenon that, since the Revolution, each of the major wars had resulted in large black migrations. The movement did not reach a flood tide, however, until World War I. "The Great Migration," as Myrdal called it, starting in 1915 and continuing in waves since then, had dramatically changed the black distribution in the United States. World War II, in progress when Myrdal was writing, vastly accelerated the steady drift toward the North and the West. The problems encountered by blacks were no longer wholly southern but had become national in scope. Furthermore, the shift from a rural to an urban environment had added to black unrest. In any case, Myrdal believed that "migration to the North and West is a tremendous force in the general amelioration of the Negro's position," but, at the same time, he stressed that a "solution" to blacks' problems was much too complicated to be effected by migration."[8]

FEDERAL EFFORTS AID BLACK NURSES

Blacks attained an impressive advance on June 25, 1941, when President Roosevelt issued Executive Order 8802, which declared:

> The policy of the United States is to encourage full participation in the national defense program by all citizens of the United States, regardless of race, creed, color or national origin, in the firm belief that the democratic way of life within the Nation can be defended successfully only with the help and support of all groups within its borders.[9]

Although verbal affirmations of this principle had been made before, Roosevelt went much further and appointed the Fair Employment Practices Committee to investigate complaints and to take steps to redress

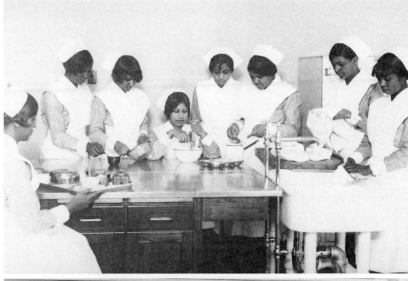

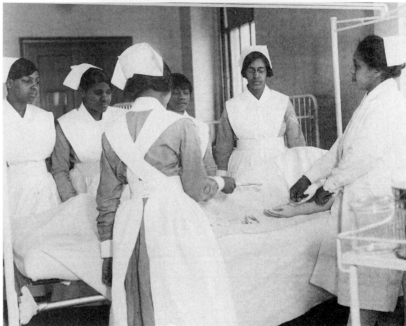

In 1940 there were 26 black schools of nursing.

grievances. The Fair Employment Practices Committee conducted public hearings and focused adverse publicity on discriminatory employers and unions. The effort to open up new areas of employment for blacks was well timed, because war production provided an almost unlimited demand for labor of all kinds. Between 1940 and 1944, the number of blacks employed in manufacturing and processing grew from 500,000 to around 1.2 million, and the number of blacks in government service increased from 60,000 to 200,000.

During the war, a special staff member, Estelle Massey Riddle, supported by a grant from the General Education Board of the Rockefeller Foundation, was added to the National Nursing Council for War Service and was authorized to hold institutes and to visit

nursing schools and colleges to improve the preparation and use of black nurses in the war effort. The objective of this unit was to help integrate nursing school enrollments as well as the military nursing services. Previously, the program had been run largely by the National Association of Colored Graduate Nurses, under the leadership of Mabel Staupers, but its staff and budget had been steadily overburdened.

The subsidized program of the Cadet Nurse Corps proved a boon to black students, and by September 1944 there were approximately 2000 black nursing cadets, representing all but 500 to 600 of the total number of black students enrolled in all nursing schools. Of the nursing schools accepting black students, 20 were all-black schools enrolling 1600 of the

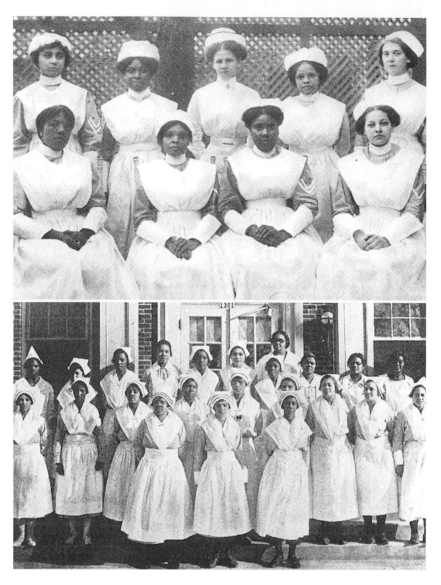

Employment opportunities were very limited for black graduates.

2000 students, and the remaining 400 black students were distributed among 22 integrated schools.

Opportunities for black women to obtain a nursing education increased greatly during the war, first through scholarships made available through Public Health Service funds and later through the Cadet Nurse Corps. National Nursing Council consultants continually strove to break educational barriers for black women who wanted to become nurses. A list of schools admitting black nurses was prepared for use in the council's clearing bureau, which answered letters from persons wanting to become nurses. It contained the names of 32 black and 14 racially mixed schools.

In 1943, the 32 black schools approved by the National League of Nursing Education admitted 1918 black students, but the bed capacity, patient census, and clinical facilities available in those 32 black hospitals with nursing schools presented a bleak picture. Obviously, there were not enough schools to educate black nurses, and the existing schools had insufficient clinical facilities, a lack of prepared instructors, and poor housing.

Seventeen of the schools for black nurses listed by the league were situated in the South. Many of the black applicants were graduates of nonaccredited or poor high schools. Consultants reported that black educators and vocational counselors in high schools and colleges generally did not see nursing as a profession worthy of attracting their better students, an attitude attributed to these educators' experience with poor nursing schools. A most helpful move was to include black colleges in the college field program set up jointly by the National Nursing Council for War Service and the Division of Nurse Education of the U.S. Public Health Service. Orieanne Collins and Pauline Butler visited 82 campuses and talked with thousands of black female students about the leadership positions awaiting the college-prepared nurse and about the free education offered through membership in the Cadet Nurse Corps.

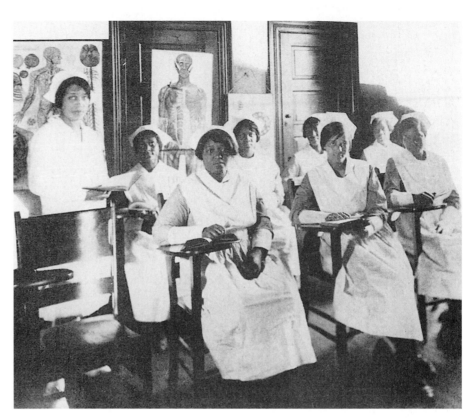

Anatomy class at the Harlem School of Nursing, New York City.

RACIAL AND ETHNIC PREJUDICE

In November 1942, high-school students representing a national cross-section were asked to respond to a survey of prevailing racial opinion among American teenagers (Table 17-2); the results highlighted the special problems of blacks.[10]

In May 1944 and again in May 1946, a cross-section of Americans were asked, "If you were sick in a hospital, would it be all right with you if you had a Negro nurse, or wouldn't you like it?" The results are shown in Table 17-3.[11]

EFFORTS TO PROMOTE INTEGRATION

In 1944, fighting such discrimination, 49 nursing schools with black and mixed enrollments had admitted black students, compared with 29 in 1941. Among those with mixed student bodies were some known to offer a variety of experience, such as the Philadelphia General Hospital and the Bellevue Hospital in New York. Gradually, the list of mixed schools increased. By 1945, about 2600 black students were enrolled in nursing schools, a 135% increase over that of 1939.

TABLE 17-2 Results of a 1942 Poll Indentifying Racial and Ethnic Prejudice Among Teenagers

	PERCENT		
ETHNIC GROUP	Last Choice Roommate	Would Not Work With	Would Not Marry
Swedes	5	—	9
Protestants	4	—	9
Negroes	78	21	92
Catholics	9	1	16
Jews	45	7	51
Irish	3	—	5
Chinese	38	5	73
Makes no difference	5	69	1
Don't know	3	3	2
Total*	190	10	25

*Because the respondents were asked to name more than one group if they wished, the percentages add up to more than 100.

TABLE 17-3 Public Reaction to Being Cared for by a Black Nurse

YEAR	ALL RIGHT	WOULDN'T LIKE IT	DON'T KNOW	QUALIFIED ANSWERS
1944	53%	42%	1%	4%
1946	52%	47%	1%	—
1946 RESULTS BY RACE				
White	47%	51%	2%	—
Black	97%	3%	—	—

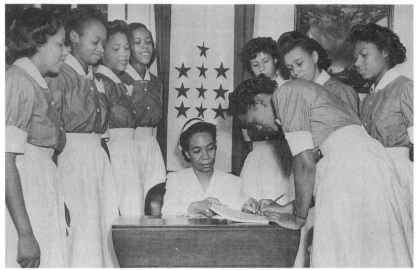

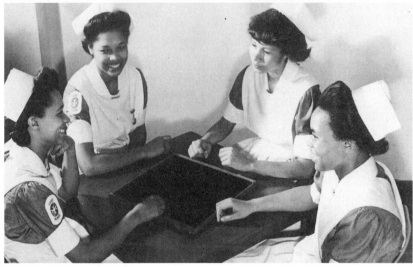

Cadet Nurse Corps students at Freedman's Hospital.

Enrollment in the all-black nursing school of Freedman's Hospital, Washington, DC, dramatically increased from 77 nursing students in 1939 to 166 students in 1944. This rapid expansion of the student

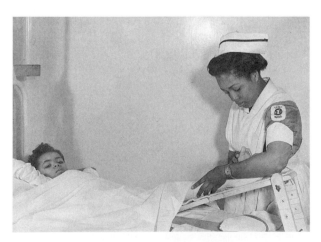

Caring for a pediatric patient.

body was repeated in other black nursing schools throughout the country. Only the wartime difficulties of securing adequately prepared instructors and supervisors as well as housing and clinical facilities prevented black enrollment from climbing still higher.

Executives of state boards of nurse examiners were slowly becoming aware that lower standards in nursing schools for blacks were neither desirable nor profitable in terms of health service. Standards set by black educators discouraged acceptance of lower standards for black educational institutions. Although there were signs of improvement, there was still a pronounced tendency to approve schools connected with hospitals that lacked the essential ingredients for a sound program. In a national survey of black nursing schools and black nurses conducted for the Public Health Service in 1944, Estelle Massey Riddle reported:

> In talking with several executives, it was obvious that political pressure, real or imagined, has deterred positive action. For instance, in one school the State Board of Nurse Examiners had

made some very important recommendations repeatedly about conditions which affected the welfare and education of the students, none of which have been complied with to date. The officials of the school have effective connections with the state politicians and seem to have no fear of disregarding the recommendations made by the State Board of Nurse Examiners.

In another instance, a state board executive asked for a recommendation from the National Nursing Council that a certain school for Negro nurses be closed. This was complied with. Within six weeks after the letter was sent, another visit was made to the school. The consultant was shocked at being told by the administrator that the state nursing executive had visited the school during the interim, at which time she expressed her displeasure at the "audacity" of the consultant for making a recommendation for closing the school. The school was moved from the tentatively approved to the fully approved list before any of the improvements had been made.[12]

On the list of black nursing schools distributed by the National Nursing Council for War Service, 12 of the 26 academic directors were white. Riddle also observed that white directors of black nursing schools, with few exceptions, seemed indifferent or even hostile to their students. These attitudes were reflected in the nursing programs and in community reaction to the students. According to Riddle, there was evidence of subtle and overt diversion of black nurses with leadership abilities from the teaching and administrative fields. In the North, prejudice took the more subtle form of advancing the nurses who were least aggressive. In the South, the overt lack of respect for the students and graduate nurses brought forth such expressions as "That's my school, but I would do anything before I would go back there to work," or "The instructor punished us for addressing our own Negro patients as Mr., Mrs., or Miss, even though some of these people are most-highly respected citizens of our community." As a consultant on official visits, Riddle reported that she encountered the same lack of respect.[13]

THE ARMED FORCES BALK

By 1944, the number of black graduate nurses was estimated at 8000. The greatest gains for blacks in civilian service were reported to have been made in the hospitals of New York City, where in 1942 more than 1250 black nurses were serving under the Department of Hospitals. On the whole, nursing staffs in black hospitals were scarcely affected by the withdrawal of a few nurses who had been accepted into the Army Nurse Corps, even though the Procurement

and Assignment Service had rated these hospitals as being overstaffed by hundreds of graduate nurses, according to established wartime standards.

The National Nursing Council for War Service urged that physically and professionally qualified graduate registered nurses, regardless of race, be appointed to military vacancies. Thus, as additional black cadets graduated, they were not only willing but also encouraged to apply for commissions. Hundreds of cadets and other black nurses received the following form letter from the army:[14]

Dear Miss:

I am directed by the Surgeon General . . . to inform you that your application for enrollment in the Army Nurse Corps cannot be given favorable consideration because the quota of colored nurses required by the Corps has been filled.

The policy regarding the assignment for colored nurses is outlined by the War Department Planning Board and colored nurses are authorized for assignment only to those stations where colored troops predominate.

Your offered service is appreciated . . . will be given consideration at such time as vacancies occur.

Very truly yours

Before Pearl Harbor, Surgeon General James C. Magee of the U.S. Army Medical Corps stated that black nurses would not be used in the Army Nurse Corps. The American Red Cross and other leading nursing organizations, however, joined the National Association of Colored Graduate Nurses in protesting this situation. Partly as a result of this effort, a small number of black nurses was assigned to duty at Fort Huachuca, Arizona; Fort Bragg, North Carolina; Camp Livingston, Louisiana; and Maxwell Field, Alabama. Although the Army Nurse Corps gradually increased the number of black nurses to 217, all but 1 were confined to segregated areas in the South.

National nursing groups and friends of the National Association of Colored Graduate Nurses repeatedly tried to force a change regarding the restrictions pertaining to black nurses. Although Surgeon General Magee adamantly opposed appeals for increased use of black nurses, Surgeon General Norman T. Kirk, named to succeed Magee in June 1943, was thought to be more flexible. On June 14, 1943, he received a strong protest from the National Nursing Council for War Service, to which he replied on June 28, stating that military policies were not unlike those used in civilian hospitals. As a result, the council sent a carefully worded questionnaire to hospitals employing both black and white nurses to produce convincing evidence for the new surgeon general. This effort resulted in the compilation of data covering 17 situations where black and white nurses worked together. The survey showed that working relations were harmonious even where integrated living and eating accommodations were provided.

Despite the persuasive information on civilian use of integrated personnel provided for the surgeon general in the early summer of 1943, no immediate revision of Medical Department policy was made. Although the results of the survey were sent to army and navy officials concerned with nursing personnel, neither service acknowledged receipt of this report. In response to a pointed communication from the council, the navy sent the following letter to Executive Secretary Elmira Wickenden:[15]

My Dear Mrs. Wickenden:

Your letter of 1 March 1944 is hereby acknowledged.

Up to the present time there are no established billets for the appointment of Negro nurses in the Navy Nurse Corps.

Sincerely yours,
Ross T. McIntire
Vice-Admiral, USN
Chief of Bureau

Meanwhile, Surgeon General Norman Kirk had told Eleanor Roosevelt that the Army Nurse Corps' personnel difficulties lay not in professional use of black nurses on the wards but in the many social complications related to quartering them and providing their off-duty subsistence allowances. As standing policy, the War Department accepted approximately 10% of the total troop strength in blacks, but this quota was impractical as applied to physicians, dentists, and nurses, he continued. The black population could not provide that proportion of fully qualified professionals, nor could that number be removed from civilian services without jeopardizing black health. Kirk explained that the army had adopted the policy of assigning black physicians and nurses only to those stations having a large complement of black troops. He thought that this arrangement provided reasonable workloads and believed that it solved recreation and off-duty entertainment problems.

At the beginning of 1945, acceptance of more black nurses by the army and navy was urged as an immediate step toward meeting increased nurse shortages. In a joint statement by the National Nursing Council for War Service and the National Association of Colored Graduate Nurses, Elmira Wickenden and Mabel Staupers, the executive secretaries of the two organizations, emphasized that the 330 nurses then in the Army Nurse Corps represented less than one tenth of the proportion of black soldiers in the army. Rejections, and the fear of rejection, had kept down the number, they stated, although it had been estimated that at least 2000 of the total of 8000 or more black graduate nurses then active in nursing might have been eligible for the military.

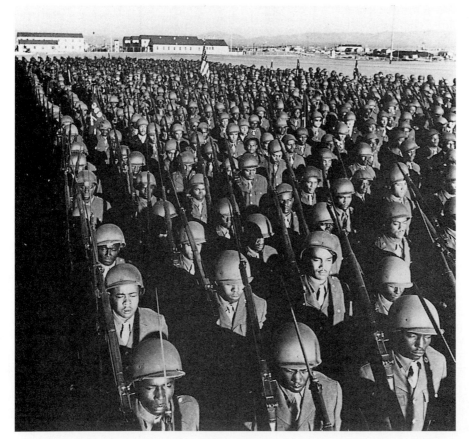

Black nurses were generally assigned only military installations with black soldiers, like this one at Fort Huachuca, AZ.

Assignment of more black nurses to the army and actual admission of black nurses into the navy were urged on the following grounds, among others:

> It would add materially to military nursing resources in the present emergency.
>
> It would demonstrate that as American men, regardless of race, creed, or color, are fighting for democracy, American women are being given the opportunity, equally without discrimination, to care for them when ill or wounded.
>
> It would, if administered without segregation, carry over into military life the policy of integrating professional services, regardless of color, now being increasingly practiced in civilian life.
>
> It would demonstrate to young Negro women who are considering nursing as a career the fact that opportunities to serve will not be denied them, thus paving the way for a greater contribution by Negro nurses after the war to the health not only of Negroes but of the whole population.[16]

Although the Navy Nurse Corps had never accepted black nurses on the grounds that there were no "billets" provided for them, on January 31, 1945, the following statement was authorized by the surgeon general of the navy:

> There is no policy in the Navy which discriminates against the utilization of Negro Nurses. Each and every application for appointment in the Navy Nurse Corps or the Navy Nurse Corps Reserve is given full consideration provided the applicant meets the physical and other requirements for appointment.[17]

Shortly thereafter, the first black nurse was sworn into the Navy Nurse Corps.

GAINING ACCEPTANCE FOR BLACK STUDENTS

In 1950, slightly more than 200 nursing schools had at least one black student enrolled. Within the group of schools having no black students were some that indicated a willingness to admit blacks, although they further stated that they had never had any black applicants or that black applicants did not meet entrance requirements. Also in this group were schools reporting that their policy prevented admission of blacks. Others stated that no policy existed. There had been a steady increase in the number of schools reporting that they would admit qualified blacks and

a decrease in the number of schools reporting that their policy prevented such admissions.

Schools that had changed admission policies between 1948 and 1952 included a number located in Kansas, Kentucky, Maryland, Oklahoma, and West Virginia. Of the few schools that reported that their policies prohibited black enrollment, most were located *outside* the southern states. Some schools were forbidden by state law to admit blacks, and there were a few instances where city regulations made the admission of blacks impossible. Some schools, although willing to admit blacks, were located in areas not conducive to the welfare of the individual black student. In a locale where segregation was enforced, the black student could not be housed in the nurses' residence and could not use the cafeteria.

Other directors reported that acceptance of blacks had presented a difficulty only in scheduling social affairs for the students or in planning recreational activities. Schools in Wisconsin, Washington, Pennsylvania, Illinois, and Ohio found this to be true, as did schools in Kansas and Kentucky. In some areas, if a mixed group entered a restaurant, no one was served. One school found it necessary to plan for a picnic at a private residence because the black students were not permitted in the public park where the activity was customarily scheduled.

Two schools reported difficulty in having black students accepted by agencies used for affiliation. A few schools found individual members of the medical staff reluctant to accept black students in the operating room or at their patients' bedsides. In one incident, a registered nurse refused to stay on duty with a black student. The director related that "although we needed nurses, we let her [the RN] go rather than give in, and there has been no further difficulty." This attitude probably reflected the way many of the isolated incidents had been handled. There were also encouraging reports of black students being selected "campus queen," holding class offices, and being accepted into the nurses' homes with no difficulty. One director related that the parents of black students were given a somewhat indifferent reception at meetings of the parents' association of the school, but the attitude of the students themselves would probably help to break down prejudice in the parent group.

Nursing school directors repeatedly made the comment that success in the admission of blacks depended primarily on careful selection, a factor considered important in the admission of any student. A few schools had secured the support of their student bodies before accepting their first black students. Some had let it be known well in advance that blacks would be admitted. In contrast, other schools had made no effort to prepare any particular group for the first black student, believing that the more matter-of-fact the attitude of the faculty, the less difficulty would be encountered. Unfortunately, not all integration efforts in nursing went smoothly among

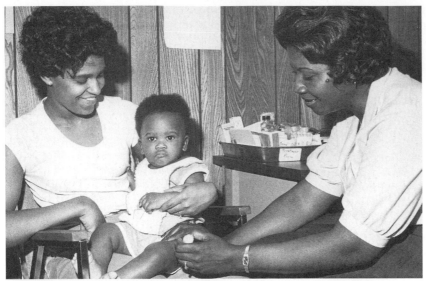

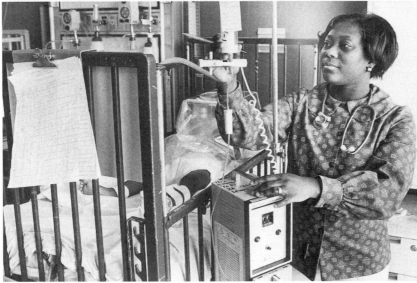

Since the outlawing of segregation, black nurses have entered all health care settings.

students. In one border state, hospital service was carried on uninterruptedly, although a group of graduate staff nurses walked out because the hospital refused to discharge three black nurses in the early 1950s.

In January 1951, the 42-year-old National Association of Colored Graduate Nurses was dissolved to merge with the ANA. The dissolution, described as an "act of faith," created new responsibilities for the ANA, which it attempted to meet through its Intergroup Relations Program. One of the primary goals of this program was the removal of membership barriers in district and state associations.

Substantial progress was made quickly. Although before WWII 15 state nursing associations had not admitted blacks, only the Georgia association retained race restrictions in 1954. Similarly, although in 1941 only 42 nursing schools admitted blacks, by 1954 the number had risen to at least 710, including

some of the nation's most outstanding hospital schools and collegiate programs.

The two decades after *Brown* v. *Board of Education of Topeka* saw black nurses fully integrated into virtually all U.S. health care settings. A much larger percentage of blacks entered nursing under the stimulus of federal programs to redress the underrepresentation of this group in the profession.

A NURSING SCHOOL FOR NATIVE AMERICANS

The one school of nursing for Native Americans during the 1940s and 1950s was located on a remote plateau in northeastern Arizona, at Ganado, 56 miles northwest of Gallup, New Mexico, in the heart of the Navajo Indian Reservation. Sage Memorial Hospital was the largest Native American hospital in the

Southwest, with beds and ample clinical experience for the needs of the nursing school. The operating room, x-ray and clinical laboratories, and dietetic department were well equipped. Sage Memorial Hospital, built in 1929 by the Board of National Missions of the Presbyterian Church, was owned and operated by that organization primarily for the benefit of the Navajo Indians, although other tribes and white patients were cared for as well. This medium-sized hospital, although remotely located, was modern and had been approved by the American College of Surgeons.

The School of Nursing had been established in 1930, the first class graduating in 1933. The school's purpose was to provide young Native American women with an opportunity to become nurses, so that this profession could be open to them and so that they would be able to render a much-needed nursing service to their people. From its beginning in 1930, the school had grown, until in 1945, 40 young women were enrolled, representing 25 tribes from 12 states.

THE HARASSED MALE NURSE

The male nurse also suffered minority status. That this condition was long-standing is borne out by a quotation from a 1914 manual on hospital administration:

> Those of us who practiced medicine, or directed the affairs of hospitals, under the old regime, when the trained woman nurse was unknown, and when the male nurse was a composite of drunkenness and genius, wonder whether the change that has wholly eliminated the trained male nurse is for the best. There is no doubt that there is something more virile, more substantial, and certainly less finicky in the male nurse than in the female.

Conversely, the authors insisted that the male nurse

> has usually some overpowering failing, some inherent weakness that forbids his success in any permanent line of human endeavor. In other words, the male nurse has been nearly always "a failure." Many times he has become a periodical drunkard. Sometimes he has been a bright young businessman or mechanic or clerk whose intemperate habits have brought him to the hospital, and, after repeated trials and repeated failures, he has found that his only safety lies in shutting himself out from the world, and subjecting himself to the discipline of the hospital or the eleemosynary institution. The most competent and reliable male nurse will oftentimes go along for weeks or months, attending conscientiously to his duties, taking most efficient care of patients, until in some

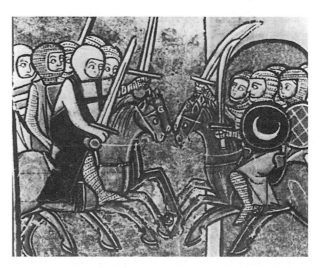

The image of the male nurse had deteriorated enormously since the 13th century, when military nursing orders such as the Knights Hospitalers had both battled for the Holy Land and supplied excellent nursing care.

> unlucky moment he finds the whiskey bottle in the medicine cabinet and takes "just a drop to steady his nerves." The rest of the story is easily imagined. It has become a maxim that a trained nurse would not be a nurse if he were fit for any other occupation, and that is probably true.[18]

Forgotten was that half the nursing of medieval times had been done by men and that the Knights Hospitalers, Teutonic Knights, Franciscans, and many other male nursing orders had supplied excellent nursing care. It was St. Vincent de Paul who had first conceived the idea of social service. Similarly, John Howard, Pastor Theodor Fliedner, Dr. Thomas Bond, Benjamin Franklin, and Henri Dunant had recognized the value of men in nursing.

In World War I, a large percentage of qualified male nurses had volunteered for military service. Many capable male nurses were absorbed into army divisions, where there was no opportunity for them to contribute effectively to the nursing needs of the service. For instance, some male nurses who were especially knowledgeable about psychiatric nursing had been used by National Guard units and assigned to a variety of menial tasks. They had not been made available to help in the tremendous task of caring for the thousands of psychiatric cases generated by the war.

During the 1930s, Helen G. McClelland, director of nursing at the Pennsylvania Hospital, Philadelphia, commented on the effectiveness of male nurses:

> It was with definite misgivings on the part of the medical staff and a number of the nursing staff that the project of giving a year of training to the men studying nursing at the Department for Mental and Nervous Diseases was started in the General Hospital.

However, it was only a short time before there was a realization on the part of all concerned that there was a decided improvement in the service given to the men patients when they were cared for by well-prepared men nurses.

It was also found that the men seemed to have a better understanding of the psychology of men patients and, due to their previous psychiatric training, were better able to solve the problems of the patients during their period of adjustment to the various hospital routines. While this was true in all services to which they were assigned, the most marked improvements in nursing service to the men patients was noted in the genitourinary wards.[19]

According to the Department of Commerce, Bureau of the Census, in April 1940 there were 7509 male nurses and students employed and 563 seeking employment. For the academic year 1939–40 there were four accredited schools of nursing in the United States that admitted only male students. The total enrollment in these four schools was 212. At the same time, there were 63 coeducational schools of nursing, with 710 male and 3798 female students enrolled. The schools admitting men were geographically distributed approximately as follows: in the eastern states, 50%; in the southern states, 25%; in the midwestern states, 15%; and in the western states, 10% (Table 17-4).

The tentative program for the new Men Nurses' Section of the ANA, as approved by the ANA board of directors in January 1941, was as follows:

> With few exceptions, men nurses have taken little part in nursing education, especially in the teaching of nursing arts and sciences and acting in the capacity of officers in the schools

TABLE 17-4 Nursing Schools for Men in 1940

SCHOOL	LOCATION	SCHOOL	LOCATION
SCHOOLS FOR MALE STUDENTS ONLY		*SCHOOLS THAT ACCEPTED BOTH MALE AND FEMALE STUDENTS (CONTINUED):*	
Alexian Brothers' Hospital	Chicago, IL		
Alexian Brothers' Hospital	St. Louis, MO	St. Mary's Hospital	Rochester, MN
Bellevue Hospital–Mills School	New York, NY	Notre Dame de Lourdes Hospital	Manchester, NH
Pennsylvania Hospital–Department for Mental and Nervous Diseases	Philadelphia, PA	Essex County Hospital	Cedar Grove, NJ
		Jersey City Medical Center	Jersey City, NJ
SCHOOLS THAT ACCEPTED BOTH MALE AND FEMALE STUDENTS		Binghamton State Hospital	Binghamton, NY
Norwood Hospital	Birmingham, AL	Brooklyn State Hospital	Brooklyn, NY
St. Mary's Hospital and Sanatorium	Tucson, AZ	Buffalo State Hospital	Buffalo, NY
St. Edward's Mercy Hospital	Fort Smith, AR	Central Islip State Hospital	Central Islip, NY
Glendale Sanitarium and Hospital	Glendale, CA	Gowanda State Homeopathic Hospital	Helmuth, NY
Los Angeles County General Hospital	Los Angeles, CA	Kings Park State Hospital	Kings Park, NY
Paradise Valley Sanitarium and Hospital	National City, CA	Middletown Homeopathic Hospital	Middletown, NY
St. Joseph's Hospital	San Francisco, CA	Manhattan State Hospital	New York, NY
St. Helena Sanitarium and Hospital	Sanitarium, CA	St. Lawrence State Hospital	Ogdensburg, NY
St. Elizabeth's Hospital	Washington, DC	Rockland State Hospital	Orangeburg, NY
Florida Sanitarium and Hospital	Orlando, FL	Hudson River State Hospital	Poughkeepsie, NY
Samaritan Hospital	Nampa, ID	Creedmoor State Hospital	Queens Village, NY
St. Joseph's Hospital	Alton, IL	Rochester State Hosptial	Rochester, NY
St. Elizabeth's Hospital	Chicago, IL	Craig Colony Hospital	Sonyea, NY
St. Mary of Nazareth Hospital	Chicago, IL	Westchester School–Grasslands Hospital	Valhalla, NY
Hinsdale Sanitarium and Hospital	Hinsdale, IL	Willard State Hospital	Willard, NY
St. Joseph Hospital	Mishawaka, IN	Harlem Valley State Hospital	Wingdale, NY
Lutheran Hospital	Sioux City, IA	Danville State Hospital	Danville, PA
Newman Memorial County Hospital	Emporia, KS	Mercy Hospital	Johnstown, PA
William Mason Memorial Hospital	Murray, KY	St. Joseph's Hospital	Philadelphia, PA
T. E. Schumpert Memorial Hospital	Shreveport, LA	St. John's General Hospital	Pittsburgh, PA
Waldo County General Hospital	Belfast, ME	Madison Rural Sanitarium and Hospital	Madison, TN
Queen's Hospital	Portland, ME	Hendrick Memorial Hospital	Abilene, TX
Sisters' Hospital	Waterville, ME	Hotel Dieu	Beaumont, TX
St. Agnes Hospital	Baltimore, MD	St. Joseph's Infirmary	Houston, TX
Washington Sanitarium and Hospital	Takoma Park, MD	St. Mary's Hospital	Port Arthur, TX
Carney Hospital	Boston, MA	Providence Hospital	Waco, TX
New England Sanitarium and Hospital	Melrose, MA	Bishop De Goesbriand Hospital	Burlington, VT
McLean Hospital	Waverly, MA	St. Ignatius Hospital	Colfax, WA
Worcester City Hospital	Worcester, MA	St. Joseph's Hospital	Tacoma, WA

of nursing which do train men. Better candidates might be chosen if graduate men nurses had some part in selecting them. As a part of our program, we urge them to seek such positions when the opportunity arises.

If men nurses as students were encouraged to take part in all activities which might serve to stimulate the interest of the student in his profession, a continued or greater interest would be shown on graduation.

Men patients would receive much better care if attended by a graduate registered man nurse rather than by an orderly.[20]

MALE NURSES AND MILITARY NURSING

Since 1901, male nurses had been barred from the Army Nurse Corps, because the law that had brought it into being designated it as the "Army Nurse Corps, Female." This fact was brought to the attention of the ANA board of directors in January 1941 by the Men Nurses' Section of the ANA, which sought repeal of this law and enactment of a law to give "men and women nurses equal opportunities in the military service." The board of directors voted that this request of the Men Nurses' Section of the ANA be referred to the surgeon general of the army. On April 7, 1941, the following reply was received from Acting Surgeon General Albert G. Love of the Medical Department:

In the absence of General James C. Magee from the city, I am acknowledging the receipt of your letter of April 2, in which you refer to the desirability of legislation to place male nurses on the same military status as female nurses.

I regret that this office cannot concur in your opinion. It would be impracticable to employ male nurses in times of peace since such employment could complicate unnecessarily the administrative problems. We feel that we have provided a satisfactory and dignified position for such male nurses as may be employed during the military emergency. In addition, we feel sure that the Secretary of War would not approve the legislation suggested by you.[21]

In early 1942, Edith Smith of the Federal Security Agency's Subcommittee on Nursing discussed the problem with Dr. James Crabtree of the Health and Medical Committee. Crabtree thought that unless the army and navy said that they would use these young men as nurses on completion of their courses, there was no justification in requesting that they be granted student deferments. Smith pointed out the need for these men in civilian life, but Crabtree thought that the need was so comparatively small and manpower requirements for the armed forces

were so vast that, if necessary, schools of nursing for male nurses would have to be closed. He thought it a relatively minor problem and said that if draft boards were to exempt all the men who were taking any kind of training, the army would be made up exclusively of boys younger than age 17.

Smith checked on the status of male nurses elsewhere around Washington. Pearl McIver said that she had recommended to the Venereal Disease Control Department of the U.S. Public Health Service that male nurses be employed in connection with government-sponsored venereal disease investigations. She persuaded that department to employ 10 men, but when 3 had been secured whose qualifications were satisfactory, the men were drafted.

A great need for male nurses had been reported at St. Elizabeth's Hospital in Washington, DC. This psychiatric hospital had employed 13 male nurses but had quickly lost 7 to the military services. In June 1942, the hospital had seven male nursing students but was not accepting any more, because it could not be certain that the men would not be drafted. The Veterans Administration thought that St. Elizabeth's had about 10 men employed in the genitourinary wards. However, those men were not satisfactory. "They get drunk," said Superintendent of Nurses Mary Hickey, "and the doctors do not like them. They do not find them as good as female nurses in the psychiatric wards."[22]

To fight such biases, the following resolution was adopted at a meeting of the ANA House of Delegates held in Chicago in May 1942:

Whereas, the Army and Navy are in great need of the services of graduate, registered professional nurses; and whereas, the graduate, registered professional men nurses, members of the American Nurses' Association, are prepared to render this service; therefore, be it resolved: that the American Nurses' Association in convention assembled in Chicago, May 17–22, 1942, address a communication to the Surgeons General of the Army and of the Navy, respectfully requesting that graduate, registered professional men nurses, members of the American Nurses' Association, be given the opportunity to serve as nurses as soon as possible after induction or enlistment into the armed forces of the country.[23]

MALE NURSES SEEK RECOGNITION

Despite these appeals, arrangements continued to call for the induction of registered male nurses into the armed forces as privates in the army or as pharmacist's mates third class in the navy. The result was that male nurses who were employed in military service had no official status. They received no recognition as a professional group, no authority, and no distinctive marking to identify them to the wounded or to other health workers. Reports from male nurses in the army showed that their services as nurses were not used. Others revealed that although they were serving as nurses, they were doing it without nursing rank.

Several nursing groups appealed to the War Department to secure rank for male nurses, but such requests were consistently opposed by the Army Nurse Corps. One male nurse wrote in response to this attitude:

> Ever since Pearl Harbor, we men nurses have been striving for recognition as nurses in the armed forces. We are not seeking glory; rather, we wish to serve in a capacity in which we sincerely believe the greatest value would be gained from our highly specialized training and experience.
>
> We have intensified our efforts recently because of the critical shortage of nurses in the services. We want our fighting men to have the best care that medical science can give. We have received favorable replies from many Congressmen and other interested officials, yet the Army and Navy Medical Departments continue to offer the same objections to our recognition.[24]

In an account of his personal experiences, Private Jacob Rose, RN, asked that, if the army needed nurses, what difference did it make if they were men or women as long as they were equally trained for a specific job? He recalled how the army "cried for nurses, spent huge sums in advertising that urged nurses to volunteer, threatened a draft of all nurses, but a registered male nurse didn't merit recognition in the Medical Department. Instead, we continued to hear lectures from a non-medical officer on first aid, whose lectures made little sense." Rose related that during his basic training at Camp Barkley, Texas, there were five registered male nurses in two training companies alone, and four were Bellevue graduates. He did not know how many others whose nursing skill was going to utter waste were scattered throughout this tremendous training camp.[25]

After almost 20 weeks of basic training, these male nurses were separated and Rose went to the India–Burma theater. There he learned to drive a 12-ton bulldozer and leveled out a baseball field. He also filled in all the potholes in the road leading past the Twentieth General Hospital at Ledo. Such experiences were probably duplicated by hundreds of male nurses in the armed forces.

The effect of the war and of selective service was practically to wipe out the enrollment of men in nursing schools. Male nurses believed that the prevailing policy was a serious error. It markedly affected the quality of nursing service, especially in psychiatric hospitals, and contributed to the later shortages of male nurses.

THE DILEMMA OF SEX STEREOTYPING

After the war, male nurses urgently recommended that the ANA Committee on Federal Legislation continue its efforts to obtain appropriate regulations under selective service for the deferment of male nursing students. Male nurse veterans strongly urged that legislation be obtained to provide commissions for male nurses. They reiterated that their services had not been used effectively during the war. In 1946, Leroy N. Craig claimed that the ANA had been and remained fully supportive of military status for male nurses, but the proposed legislation was blocked because the surgeons general of the army and navy believed that male nurses should not be allowed commissions in the Nurse Corps.

A 1946 survey showed that 27 states had a total of 68 schools that admitted men to the basic course, but that 13 states had only 1 school each. New York topped the list with 22 schools. Eighteen of them were in state mental hospitals, which admitted men and women. From 1938 to 1946, 24 of the reporting schools admitted 853 men, of whom 633 went on to graduate. Lack of appropriate housing facilities was the primary obstacle to the admission of men to more schools. This was true also of affiliated institutions, and it tended to prevent male students from securing preparation in fields such as tuberculosis, communicable disease, and cancer nursing.

Existing barriers to the employment of male nurses appeared to be due more to sentiment and tradition than to any actual ineptitude based on sex. About 1950, Ruth Sleeper noted that at Massachusetts General Hospital there had been objection to male nurses from the medical staff, perhaps because physicians had found them a little more difficult to work with than female nurses. She also said that there had been some question as to whether the relation of the male nurse to the patient had always been "right," and she had been requested in some instances not to employ a man as head nurse. Conversely, Katherine Densford related that she had employed male nurses in many capacities, including that of faculty member on her teaching staff, without any difficulty whatever. Two male nurses who had received their preparation for faculty positions in Minnesota had been able to use their education as a stepping stone to hospital administration. Densford did not believe that the men's education was lost when applied later in hospital administration.

The male nurse would have a difficult road ahead in the coming decades, and the battle against feminine stereotyping of nurses would never really get off the ground until a massive effort could be launched at resocializing the general public. The strength of the link between women and nursing was

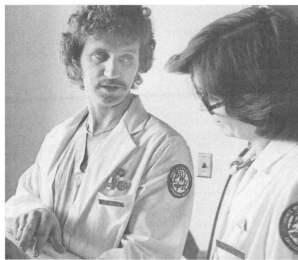

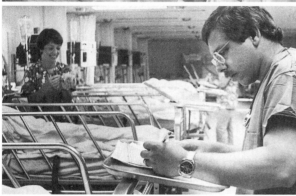

Men in nursing still face stereotyping that defines nursing as a woman's profession.

perhaps one of the strongest in any occupation and would only be overcome slowly as increasing numbers of men underwent the unique interpersonal and social demands of all phases of nursing education and service.

The war enhanced opportunities for black women in nursing while militating against male nurses. Perhaps this dichotomy is best explained in terms of professional and lay pressure. The cause of black women had adherents in the National Nursing Council for War Service and all the way to the White House and Eleanor Roosevelt. By contrast, the movement for fair treatment of men desiring a nursing education and male nurses entering the armed forces never

really got started. Most nurses and the general public seemed to adhere to the view that the man's place in wartime was on the battlefield and that, at all times, women alone should take care of the nursing. Consequently, men continued to constitute the smallest minority in nursing, amounting to only 1% of the 440,000 active nurses in 1960.

REFERENCES

1. *New York Times*, May 18, 1954.
2. "The Long View," *Nursing Outlook*, vol. 2 (August 1954):403.
3. Nina D. Gage and Alma C. Haupt, "Some Observations on Negro Nursing in the South," *Public Health Nursing*, vol. 24 (December 1932):674–680.
4. Edwin R. Embree, *Brown America: The Story of a New Race* (New York: Viking Press, 1931), pp. 88–104.
5. Gunnar Myrdal et al. *An American Dilemma: The Negro Problem and Modern Democracy* (New York: Harper & Brothers, 1944), p. ix.
6. Ibid., pp. 137–153.
7. Ibid., pp. 175–181.
8. Ibid., pp. 191–201.
9. *New York Times*, June 26, 1941.
10. Hadley Cantril, *Public Opinion, 1935–1946* (Princeton: Princeton University Press, 1951), p. 477.
11. Ibid.
12. Estelle Massey Riddle, "National Report of Negro Nursing Schools and Nurses, May, 1945," Federal Records Center, Suitland, Maryland, Cadet Nurse Corps Files, RG 90.
13. Ibid., p. 510.
14. Ida W. Danielson to Negro nurse applicants to the Army Nurse Corps, undated, Records of the War Manpower Commission, National Archives, Washington, DC, RG 211.
15. Ross T. McIntire to Elmira B. Wickenden, March 7, 1944, copy in Katherine Densford Papers, University of Minnesota Archives, Minneapolis.
16. "Minutes, Meeting of the National Nursing Council for War Service, February 21, 1945, New York City," Densford Papers.
17. Ibid.
18. J. A. Hornsby and R. E. Schmidt, *The Modern Hospital: Its Inspiration, Its Architecture, Its Equipment, Its Operation* (Philadelphia: W. B. Saunders Co., 1914), p. 335.
19. Leroy N. Craig, "Opportunities for Men Nurses," *American Journal of Nursing*, vol. 40 (June 1940):669.
20. "Report of Men Nurses' Section of the American Nurses' Association, May, 1942." National Archives, RG 215.
21. Acting Surgeon General Albert G. Love to Leroy Craig, April 7, 1941, National Archives, RG 215.
22. Quoted in memorandum regarding drafting male nurses from Edith Smith to Alma Haupt, July 10, 1942, National Archives, RG 215.
23. American Nurses' Association, Thirty-third Convention, "Men Nurses' Section Reports, June 1, 1942, Chicago, Illinois," National Archives, RG 215.
24. Quoted in the *Congressional Record*, 1945, Appendix, p. 838.
25. Jacob Rose, "Men Nurses in Military Service," *American Journal of Nursing*, vol. 47 (March 1947):146.

18

TOWARD PROFESSIONALISM

As America passed midcentury, fears of Communist infiltration, frustrations over the Korean conflict, and the conservative mood of voters provided the Republicans with a sweeping victory in the 1952 elections. Blessed with Republican control of both the House of Representatives and the Senate, the new president, Dwight D. Eisenhower, recognized that much of the demand for change and reform that had created the social welfare programs and proposals of FDR's New Deal and Truman's Fair Deal had subsided. He did, however, establish the Department of Health, Education, and Welfare on April 11, 1953, an action that culminated more than 30 years' effort by citizens who believed that the federal government needed an agency of cabinet status to carry out effectively its constitutional responsibility for "promoting the general welfare." Only by such action could the health, education, and welfare interests of the American people receive their due consideration at the policymaking level.

WONDER DRUGS

Before the 1940s, few people had heard of antibiotics. In the 1950s, these drugs, even with their short clinical history, had helped erase many infectious diseases from prominence. Mortality rates for tuberculosis, syphilis, whooping cough, and gastritis were at an all-time low, and the mortality rate for pneumonia was more than 40% below the average for the 1940s. Much of the credit for this belonged to antibiotics.

Although penicillin, in 1943, was the first to be given wide clinical use, antibiotics had been known long before then. Louis Pasteur, for example, had hinted that such substances might have medical value, and in 1928 English scientist Alexander Fleming discovered that a certain type of microorganism was somehow able to halt the growth of certain disease organisms. By 1939, hundreds of scientists, their scientific curiosity ignited by an apparent paradox, were concentrating on these drugs; they noted that while disease organisms fell constantly on the earth's soil, soil was often relatively free of disease bacteria.

The reason for this was found when researchers uncovered signs of a battle for survival being waged in the soil by millions of microorganisms, some of which engaged in a kind of chemical warfare, emitting a potent substance to kill or weaken neighboring organisms. Once these and other microscopic "battles" were understood, scientists turned their attention to the next logical question. What would happen if one of these chemicals were given to a human being suffering from one of these diseases? Certain chemicals obviously destroyed certain microorganisms, including some that caused human disease. Would the chemical still destroy, or help to destroy, the responsible agent? Would it also destroy the patient?

Answers to these questions were found in the amazing clinical record of antibiotics, or "wonder drugs," including penicillin, streptomycin, chlortetracycline, chloramphenicol, and oxytetracycline. Although no antibiotic proved to be entirely free of side effects or adverse reactions when given to people who were found to be abnormally sensitive to them, the relatively few patients so affected were outnumbered by countless millions of others whose health benefited or whose lives were saved. The use of antibiotics altered nursing care requirements for some patients. The importance of supportive nursing care measures diminished.

HOSPITALS IN TRANSITION

More than 6600 hospitals with over 1.5 million beds were listed in the American Medical Association census of 1952. In that year, hospitals admitted nearly 19 million patients and cared for an average of 1.3 million inpatients each day. Approximately 1000 of these hospitals, with more than half of all hospital beds and

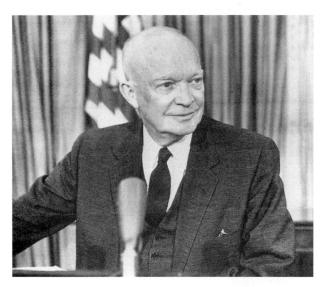

President Dwight D. Eisenhower.

60% of hospital patient-days, provided care exclusively for tuberculosis or psychiatric patients. Because the length of stay in mental and tuberculosis hospitals had to be measured in months or years, care in such institutions was beyond the financial resources of most people and had to be provided almost entirely through taxation. Ninety-six percent of the beds in these hospitals were supported by tax dollars.

Approximately 5600 hospitals provided general services or a special type of service usually associated with the general hospital. Although general hospitals and allied special hospitals contained fewer than half of all hospital beds and accounted for only 40% of patient-days, 98% of all hospital admissions were made by this group. In 1952, 55% of the general hos-

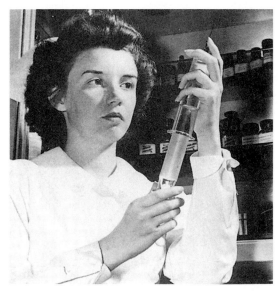

New "wonder drugs" altered nursing care requirements for some patients.

pitals were owned and operated by churches, fraternal organizations, and other voluntary groups on a nonprofit basis, and 20% were proprietary hospitals operated by individuals or corporations on a profit basis. The remaining 25% were government hospitals: 16% municipal, 3% state, and 6% federal.

Typically, the patient entered the hospital expecting care from professional nurses. However, instead of finding the familiar figure in the white uniform, the patient instead encountered a succession of nonprofessional workers in blue, gray, and striped uniforms. During the entire stay, the patient would receive on the day shift an average of 54 minutes of direct bedside care, divided as follows: 6 minutes from graduate nurses, 14 minutes from professional students, and 34 minutes from nonprofessional personnel.

In 1946, nursing students had made up 20.9% of the personnel in general hospitals, but by 1952 the percentage had dropped to about 12% nationwide. Relative to the number of patients served, the number of students of professional nursing had decreased markedly, from 40 per 100 patients per day in 1944 to 25 per 100 patients per day in 1952, a drop of nearly 38%. Although the total number of nursing students had increased slightly in the latter years of that period, it did not match the increased number of patients. In addition, the amount of service provided by each student was decreasing. As a result of new standards in nursing education, nursing students were spending a higher proportion of their time in the classroom and laboratory and a lower proportion at the bedside. The growing emphasis on upgrading the educational experience was indicated by the fact that the number of full-time instructors had increased despite the decline in the number of students. In 1944, there were 37 students per instructor; in 1952, there were only 19.

Nearly 390,000 nurses were working in the United States in 1952. The number of hospital nurses, the largest single group, had increased by 15% in the previous 4 years to 231,000. Private-duty nurses, the next largest group, who were also at the bedside, numbered 74,000. Approximately 35,000 nurses working in physicians' offices, 25,300 public health nurses, 14,000 industrial nurses, and 8200 nurse educators in schools of nursing made up the remainder of the total, along with 1900 nurses in a variety of other fields.

The volume of nursing required for modern medical and health service and the expanding range of activities had introduced a large number of auxiliary workers who came to be classified as nursing personnel. In 1946, hospitals throughout the country employed 177,552 auxiliary workers, including maids. In early 1952, they employed 297,310. This resulted in a changing pattern of nursing service. In New York hospitals, for example, registered nurses performed 75% of the nursing care in the early 1940s, but 10 years later they performed 30% of the nursing care. The same thing was happening nationwide.

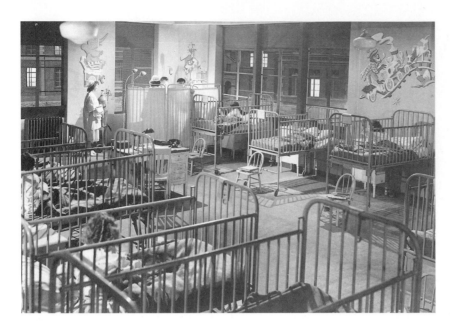

These pediatric beds were among the 1.5 million U.S. hospital beds in 1952.

HOSPITAL STAFFING PATTERNS

An analysis of hospital staffing patterns indicated that in the typical 100-bed general hospital, more than half of all hospital personnel were in the nursing department. The dietary and housekeeping departments each accounted for slightly more than 10% of the personnel. Between 7% and 8% of the personnel were required for administration, business office, record-keeping, and related functions; 6% for laundry; 3% for plant operation and maintenance; and 6% for the laboratory, x-ray, and other professional service departments.

Regarding maximal use, the nursing department personnel were considered by administration to be the most important, not only because they predominated numerically but because they served to coordinate the activities of personnel in other departments providing direct patient care. In many hospitals, the nursing staff assumed responsibility for various activities customarily associated with the attending physicians, the house medical staff, housekeeping, and the dietary, laboratory, business office, and other departments. Increasingly, there was a tendency to shift responsibilities either to or from the nursing department, depending on the relative shortages of

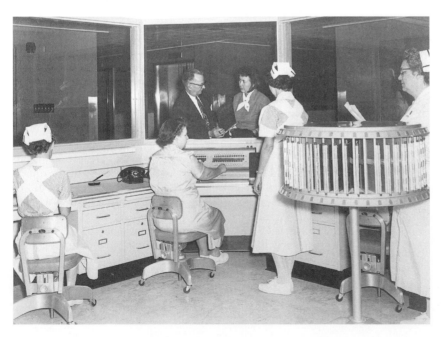

Most RNs now spent more time managing personnel and administrative details.

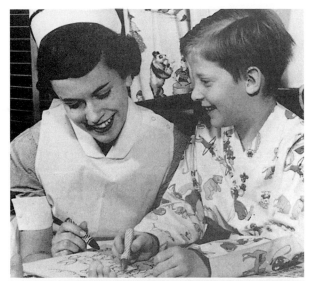

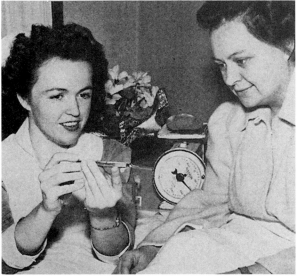

The early 1950s saw major studies of nurses' activities.

different types of personnel and the prevailing theories of organization of hospital service.

The average nurse spent more and more time managing personnel and administrative details. In 1944, there had been approximately one general-duty nurse and three auxiliary nursing workers for each supervising nurse. By 1952, there were approximately two general-duty nurses and four auxiliary workers for each supervisory nurse. Some nurses and employers of nurses were convinced that the professional nurse of the future would have largely supervisory and managerial responsibilities and would delegate patient care to other less extensively prepared members of the nursing team. This view was reflected in the task-oriented philosophies of some schools, whereas others sought to prepare the nurse for more patient-centered activity. Delegation was often praised as a management essential. The primary responsibility of the registered nurse had changed

from direct nursing care and maintenance of the environment to administration of complex systems, supervision of workers with diversified skills, and provision of comprehensive nursing services.

Throughout the field of nursing, the word "utilization" was being used more and more as hospitals conducted studies, aided by engineers in some cases, to find out how many functions of the nurse could be performed safely by others. The number was surprisingly large. In a Division of Nursing Resources, U.S. Public Health Service–assisted study at Harper Hospital in Detroit, for example, it was found that 42% of all treatments could be handled by practical nurses and 30% by nurses' aides. A New York State official estimated that from 30% to 50% of the nurse's time was spent in non-nursing functions. Hospitals everywhere, however, were reassigning such activities to non-nurses as a matter of necessity, not of theory.

A major effort was made to encourage more efficient use of professional nursing skills. The Division of Nursing Resources made hospital studies and developed techniques to determine whether professional nurses were performing clerical, housekeeping, or other routine duties that could be assigned to others. These findings were used as a basis for several handbooks to facilitate written analyses of hospital nursing duties.

A manual, *How to Study Nursing Activities in a Patient Unit*, was developed by the Division of Nursing Resources to help hospitals determine whether nursing time was diverted from nursing care of patients to duties that other employees could perform. The method, which adapted industrial work sampling techniques to the problems of use of hospital personnel, had been tested in three hospitals. Results showed that staff nurses were actually spending about half of their time caring for patients, the remaining time being spent on tasks that could be assigned to clerks, maids, and messengers.

EDUCATIONAL DEFICIENCIES

According to 1954 estimates, about 20% of the positions held by registered nurses entailed responsibilities that could be best fulfilled by persons who were prepared in master's degree programs; for another 30% of these positions, preparation at the baccalaureate level would be adequate. Against this estimate stood the actual situation, in which approximately 1% of all nurses held master's degrees and 7.2% held baccalaureate degrees—not all of which had been conferred in the field of nursing.

According to data on graduate nurse education in colleges and universities collected by the National League for Nursing (NLN), the enrollment in graduate nurse programs had remained about the same from 1947 to 1955. Although there was an increase in the number of students enrolled in advanced nursing programs between 1951 and 1953, there was a

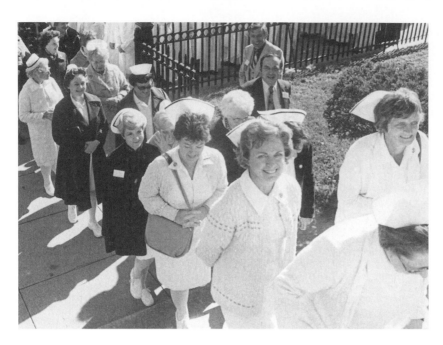

*Fewer nurses were completing postgradu-
ate training in the 1950s.*

sharp decrease—from 1125 to 814—in the number
who were graduated from baccalaureate programs
preparing nurses for the specialty positions of administrator, supervisor, teacher, and consultant. At
the same time, the number of nurses who had
earned their master's degree in the specialty programs was no higher in 1953 than it had been in
1952. This meant that there were proportionately
fewer nurses completing postgraduate training each
year.

Private philanthropy answered this challenge first.
Early in 1955, an NLN fellowship program for nurses
working on master's and doctoral degrees was made
possible through a grant from the Commonwealth
Fund. The fund supported this program to help
overcome a critical shortage of nurses prepared for
administration in nursing service and education,
teaching, and nursing research. The grant provided
opportunities for more than 200 nurses to undertake
master's or doctoral study during the years
1955–1963.

From 1936 through 1955, 14,000 to 15,000 nurses
received government assistance for academic study
in public health nursing under provisions of the
Social Security Act of 1935. Although these grants
had diminished in number in recent years, this aid
allowed nurses to complete programs leading to a
baccalaureate degree; consequently, the percentage
of public health nurses with baccalaureate or post-
baccalaureate preparation was about three times
greater than that of the general nursing population.
In contrast was the small proportion of full-time students enrolled in programs in medical-surgical and
maternal-child nursing. A larger program was desperately needed, and only the federal government
had the sizable resources required to implement it.

THE FEDERAL NURSE TRAINEESHIP PROGRAM

In 1956, the first appreciable step since World War II
toward a major program of renewed federal aid to
nurses was effected. The Health Amendments Act of
1956 was passed by Congress and signed by President
Eisenhower on August 1, 1956. Title II authorized
funds for financial aid to registered nurses for full-
time study to prepare for administration, supervision, and teaching in all fields of nursing. The use of
the funds was limited to tuition and fees, stipends,
and allowances (including travel expenses for
trainees). The law prohibited the federal government or any employee from exercising any direction,
supervision, or control over the personnel or curriculum of the recipient training institutions. From
1957 to 1964, appropriations grew from $2 million to
$7.3 million. A short-term program was initiated in
1960 whereby professional nurses, unable to study
full time but in need of additional skills to maintain
their positions, could be financially supported in the
necessary course work for periods of 5 days to 1
month.

During the first 6 months of the program, long-
term traineeships were awarded to more than 9000
nurses, and nearly half were 30 years of age or
younger. Slightly more than 60% studied at the graduate level, some of these nurses earning a doctoral
degree. Of the total, 55% were preparing for positions in teaching, 24% for supervision, and 21% for
administration. Although data for earlier years are
not available, of the 1447 graduate-level trainees in
1960–1961, 835 completed their programs of study
during their traineeships.

Follow-up on the accomplishments of former trainees was conducted routinely through questionnaires sent 6 months after completion of the program. Replies from nurses who received traineeships during the period from 1957 through 1961 showed that 39% were teachers, 31% were in nursing service positions as head nurses or administrators, and 7% were continuing in school. In the 1960 and 1961 follow-ups, trainees were asked to provide additional information regarding any change in their level of responsibility after traineeship study. Fifty-six percent said that they were holding positions at a higher level. Nursing leaders generally agreed, however, that, even with this new influx of prepared nurses, the demand far exceeded the supply.

The short-term training provisions associated with the Title II program were begun in 1960 with $300,000, an amount that quickly tripled in the following 2 years. During the first 3 years of the short-term program, more than 10,000 nurses had benefited from the courses, 500 of whom had had their training financed by sources other than the federal government. Three hundred seven courses were supported through grants to 73 sponsoring agencies. Because the number of approved applications for grants had exceeded available funds, it had been necessary to make awards on the basis of priority ratings set by a review committee. Most short-term trainees had been supervisors and head nurses in hospitals. Data regarding the educational qualifications of the 10,184 federally aided trainees revealed that 65% had no degree, 26% had baccalaureate degrees, and 9% had master's degrees.

Evaluations of short-term courses by program directors and students showed that the major value of the courses had been in the initiation of new ideas for the improvement of patient care, and subsequent employers reported that former trainees effected

changes in work situations that resulted in improved nursing practices. Instances were also reported of nurses who, after having participated in a short-term course in a university setting, had gone on to enroll for full-time academic study. All but 12 states had at least one school offering traineeships under this program to registered nurses, and many schools had used training funds to support students on two or more academic levels.

BIRTH OF ASSOCIATE-DEGREE NURSING

A project aimed at developing nursing education programs in junior and community colleges was announced in January 1952 by Louise McManus, director of the Division of Nursing Education at Teachers College, Columbia University. She explained that the purpose of the experiment was to determine if a 2-year program, which would prepare bedside nurses for beginning general-duty positions, was feasible. Such an approach would help reduce the critical shortage of nurses throughout the nation by producing more nurses faster; it would also help move nursing education into the overall system of American higher education.

Commenting on the need for the project, McManus asserted that nursing education was largely outside the general system of education in the United States and, unlike education for other professions, had not had the benefit of research. She declared that the current system of nursing education had failed to produce the required number and types of nurses.

Ninety percent of the nation's nursing schools were owned and operated by hospitals, McManus pointed out. Their programs were mainly of the apprentice type, directed primarily at the immediate care of patients, without regard for the community and academic experiences that the modern nurse should receive. She emphasized that the demands of the hospitals, as far as nursing education was concerned, required a 3-year program that included repetitive practices believed to be considerably in excess of that needed for efficient and effective learning. Mildred L. Montag, assistant professor of nursing education at Teachers College, was appointed project coordinator.

Seven community junior colleges were selected for inclusion in the 5-year research project to develop and evaluate associate-degree nursing education. The colleges represented different sections of the country, varied in size, had different sources of support, and had different curriculum patterns. As these programs were established, general education accounted for one third of the total curriculum, whereas nursing courses accounted for about two thirds. Of the nursing portion, 75% was clinical practice. Emphasis was placed on giving the student as much experience as possible through careful planning and instructional

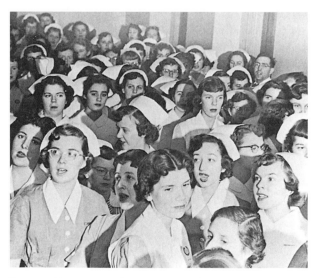

Short- and long-term U.S. Public Health Service traineeships supported additional study for thousands of nurses.

supervision, yielding more effective use of time spent in the clinical area.

Students would qualify for the associate degree and would be eligible for the licensing exam of the state in which the college was located. Eight hundred seven students were admitted to the programs. The dropout rate was about 20%, with reasons resembling the pattern of college education rather than that of hospital schools.

In 1958, the results of the 5-year study indicated that the 2-year curriculum could prepare a registered nurse and that the program could become an integral part of a total college, financed as any other college program. One hundred ninety-two associate-degree graduates had taken state board licensing examinations by then, and 91.7% of these students passed the examinations the first time. In nursing programs of all types, the figure was 90.5%. According to the study findings, associate-degree graduates were found by head nurses to be as good as or better than most of the graduates with whom they worked in 80% of the cases. The graduates themselves were satisfied with their preparation.

Diploma program advocates insisted that graduates of hospital nursing schools were more competent in patient care than were those coming from collegiate schools. Hospital school diploma programs provided learning experiences that were more functionally and realistically related to the competencies, skills, and knowledge involved in patient care. Representatives of this group pointed out that the number of hospital schools had dropped from 1190 to 768 in the previous 8 years. College and university graduates would not be sufficient to staff the hospitals of tomorrow.

The diploma program in the hospital nursing schools had always been, and still was, the backbone of nursing education in the United States, but changes had to be made if this form of nursing education was to survive. Ruth Sleeper of Massachusetts General Hospital was convinced of the value of the

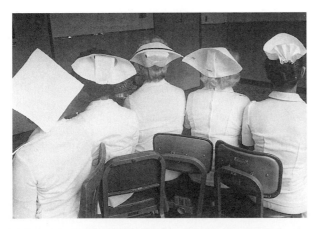

Diploma graduates still remained the backbone of nursing education.

diploma program but warned that those responsible for the 3-year nursing schools must make many changes if the diploma programs were to be respected by the country's educational system. Unless changes were made, she said, "the hospital school will not continue to attract desirable candidates in sufficient numbers and a new system of preparing our nurses will be found."

BIOMEDICAL RESEARCH BOOMS

Public responsibility for biomedical research was assumed on a larger scale in the 1940s. It was now accepted public policy to use tax funds for supporting research in voluntary as well as public institutions, and many laws embodying these principles had been passed. General authority for research grants and fellowships in the entire health field had been given to the Public Health Service of the Federal Security Agency through the Public Health Service Act of 1944 and its amendments. Federal acts dealing with cancer (1937), mental diseases (1946), dental diseases (1948), heart diseases (1948), and hospital construction (1949) contained provisions for research.

In 1947, governmental agencies contributed about 28% of all funds expended on medical research, the federal government carrying by far the largest share; industrial companies were responsible for 45%, foundations for 13%, and other sources for the remainder. Leading among the civilian federal agencies was the Public Health Service, using the National Institutes of Health as its research arm and administering research grants and fellowships to individuals affiliated with voluntary institutions.

The purpose of the Public Health Service Research Grants Program was to support research in medical and allied fields for which funds were inadequate or which could not otherwise be conducted in the grantee institution. The major objectives of the grants program were (1) to expand research activities in universities and other institutions; (2) to stimulate the initiation of research in small colleges where previous research programs had been very limited or nonexistent; (3) to encourage investigators to undertake research in neglected areas; and (4) to provide training for scientific personnel. The vast volume of requests for research grants soon required the establishment of a priority system for determining funding awards. This priority system was established to permit all new applicants to compete for funds equally and to ensure quicker response to an action on the applicant's request.

Medical research in the 1950s concentrated on human bodily responses to the environment. To cope with the problems of chronic disease and other causes of death and disability, science needed to provide medicine and public health with innumerable facts about the growth, aging, and regeneration of living tissues. Research probed into such mysteries as

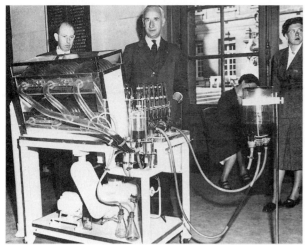

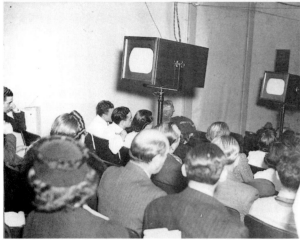

A heart–lung machine of 1951; televised surgery.

the metabolism of cells and the molecular structure of body chemicals. The problems studied required scientists trained in many different fields, working closely with scientists in other institutions, and using a great variety of specialized equipment.

NURSING RESEARCH

Research into the practice of nursing was seen as more and more essential if the health needs of modern society were to be met. Increasingly, extension of health services and developments in medicine without adequate corresponding developments in nursing practice had diminished the quality of nursing. Opportunities for professional nurses to use their special knowledge and skill in generating new knowledge for the profession had not kept pace with the prevention of illness or with the health needs of society. Nursing research was concerned with the systematic study and assessment of nursing problems or phenomena and was aimed at finding ways of improving nursing practice and patient care through creative inquiry. It included studies of nursing practice, nursing

services, nursing service administration, nursing education, and the individual nurse and involved every field of knowledge related to nursing.

In the early 1950s, the scholarly journal *Nursing Research* had been launched, and the first issue went out to approximately 8500 subscribers all across the nation and in 22 other countries. This journal quickly emerged as the leading indicator of nursing's thrust into research and development and became essential reading for the expanding cadre of nurse-researchers.

A research program approved by the American Nurses Association (ANA) House of Delegates in 1950 was designed to enable nurses, with the help of allied groups and social scientists, to study nursing functions in various settings and geographic locations and nurses' relationships with coworkers and associates. The ANA depended entirely on membership dues for the financing of this series of studies. By 1954, research grants had been made to institutions or organizations in 13 states, and nursing had been studied in more than 80 hospitals.

This scholarly look at the profession included surveys, interviews, attitude–role relationship studies, observation or "shadow" studies of nurses on the job, classification of activities, and time analyses revealing proportions of time spent by various personnel on different activities. In the first years of the ANA program, most of the research was done by social scientists of various disciplines; later, many nurses had gained the qualifications to undertake studies as well. Under this program, researchers learned that nurses performed more than 400 functions. Other findings pointed out the extent to which functions

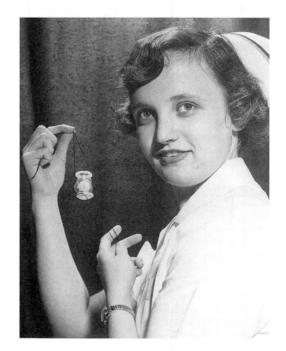

A heart valve was developed in 1952 with the support of a National Institutes of Health research grant.

performed by the different categories of nursing personnel overlapped. Changes in the role of the professional nurse were confirmed by findings that indicated that many of the tasks once considered the sole province of the physician were now being assigned to nurses. The number of these tasks was found to vary among states, with some direction from the state laws governing the practice of nursing and medicine.

In 1955, the ANA formed a membership corporation, the American Nurses' Foundation, organized exclusively for charitable, scientific, and educational purposes. The foundation solicited tax-deductible grants and gifts from the general public and from other charitable organizations. The primary objectives of the foundation were to increase public knowledge and understanding of professional nursing, practical nursing, and the arts and sciences on which the health of the American people depended. The foundation was to conduct studies, surveys, and research; provide research grants to graduate nurses; make grants to public and private nonprofit educational institutions; and publish scientific, educational, and literary work. The ANA board of directors donated $100,000 to the new corporation, to be disbursed during 1955 for studies of nursing functions.

The extramural grants program in nursing research of the U.S. Public Health Service Division of Nursing Resources originated in fiscal year 1956. In contrast to most of the extramural programs of the National Institutes of Health, which were focused on basic disease research, the Division of Nursing Resources program emphasized applied research. During the fiscal year ending June 30, 1956, the Public Health Service awarded nearly $500,000 to qualified researchers for nursing projects. This was the first time that a specific grants program for nursing research had been made available from federal sources. Over the next 2 decades, this program helped to nurture the embryonic growth of nursing research with support for individual research projects, faculty research development projects, and nine special national nursing research conferences held under the auspices of the ANA.

Federal support for research training for nurses was provided in two ways. In 1956, a program of spe-cial predoctoral fellowships was established by the Division of Nursing Resources. This program made individual awards to qualified nurses for training for individual research and collaborative interdisciplinary research and for the stimulation and guidance of research. In 1962, nurse-scientist graduate training grants were initiated to assist the institutions developing nursing research competence as well as to provide stipends for the graduate nursing students who were preparing for research. These grants were made to graduate nursing schools and provided support for full-time students of nursing and anthropology, psychology, sociology, anatomy, physiology, and microbiology.

The first doctoral programs in nursing had originated within the schools of education at Teachers College, Columbia University, in the early 1920s and at New York University in 1934. The growth of the concept was extremely slow: It was 1954 before the University of Pittsburgh added a small maternal-child nursing Ph.D. program and 1960 before Boston University began a Doctor of Nursing Science (D.N.S.) program in psychiatric nursing. The first comprehensive doctoral level movement came in 1964 at the University of California, San Francisco, with the establishment of the D.N.S. degree in several nursing specialties.

CHARACTERISTICS OF THE HEALTH SERVICES INDUSTRY IN 1960

As a new decade began, the 1960 census provided data for an overall look at how nursing fit into the nation's health care picture. The United States Bureau of the Census divided the civilian labor force into 71 separate industries. Between the 1950 and 1960 censuses, the health services industry had gained almost 1 million workers, for a growth rate of 54%. Only 7 of the 71 other industries had experienced a higher growth rate. The health services industry ranked third among these industries, employing more than 2.5 million persons.

From 1927 to 1945, hospital costs per patient-day had increased 25%. The annual increase in patient-day

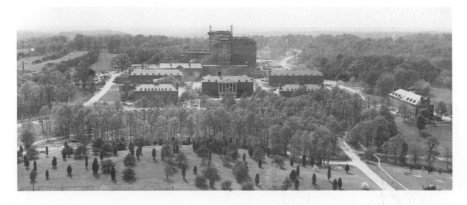

The new medical research and hospital center of the National Institutes of Health opened in 1952 in Bethesda, MD.

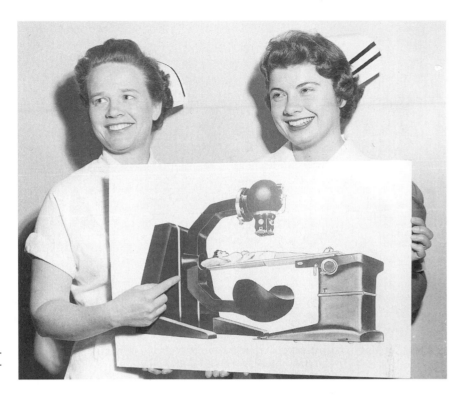

As medical technology grew more complex, the need for nursing research became more apparent.

costs over this period averaged $.10 a day. By comparison, from 1945 to 1960, hospital costs per patient-day had increased by more than 250%, and the annual increase in patient-day costs over this period averaged about $1.65 per day. Through health insurance and through greater use of local, state, and national tax funds, more and more hospital money was coming from healthy people. Healthy people did not pay for hospital care piecemeal as it was delivered to them; rather, they paid for it, in whole or in part, through health insurance plans. By 1960, nongovernmental general hospitals received, on the average, nearly half their total income from insured patients. In many such hospitals, the proportion from insurance was two thirds or more and growing fast.

Growth and diversification were the principal characteristics of the health occupations. In 1940, hospitals had had approximately one professional nurse for every 15 beds and one practical nurse, aide, attendant, or auxiliary for every 10 beds. By 1960, they required one professional nurse for every 5 beds and one auxiliary person for every 3 beds.

A study of 325 hospitals in 1961 showed that about 20% of the positions for professional nurses were vacant, as were 18% of the positions for practical nurses. In New York City, more than half of the positions for professional nurses in the public hospitals were unfilled. In all hospitals in Los Angeles, private as well as public, 25% to 30% of the positions for professional staff nurses were reported as unfilled. In a survey of all general hospitals in the state of Massachusetts, it was found that 20% of the positions for professional staff nurses were not filled.

Because the need for professional and practical nurses was increasing so much faster than the supply, hospitals had employed ever-larger numbers of nursing aides, many of whom were inadequately trained. This pragmatic solution to the problem of shortages had produced an alarming dilution in the quality of service. In some hospitals, the use of auxiliary workers had reached such extreme proportions that nursing aides gave as much as 80% of the direct nursing care.

How was the United States to secure the needed nurse supply when wages were so inordinately low? In 1959, of all professional women who worked from 40 to 49 weeks during the year, nurses had the lowest median income. For secondary school teachers, the median was $5200; for elementary school teachers, it was $4900; for librarians, $4200; for social, welfare, and recreation workers, $3700; and for professional nurses, $3200.

A number of other factors also militated against the probability of a larger proportion of women and men choosing a nursing career. Relative to most of the other predominantly women's professions, particularly teaching, the working conditions and hours in nursing were unfavorable. Teachers worked fewer weeks of the year and had more hours in which to fulfill home and family responsibilities. In addition, the proportion of female high-school graduates who later completed a nursing education was generally declining. From 1957 to 1960, 4% of the female high-school graduates from 3 years previous had completed a program in professional nursing. In 1963, this had dropped to 3.35%.

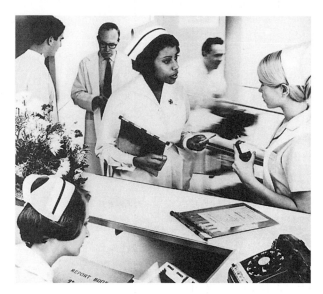

The early 1960s saw no relief from the nursing shortage.

Even hospital administrators, nursing directors, and members of hospital boards of trustees who believed that graduate nurses should be more realistically remunerated for their services had problems finding the money. The cost of nursing care was the hospital's largest single expense and an important factor in determining room and board rates. Medical care was expensive, and its cost was rising at a rate greater than that of the cost of living.

As operating costs increased, hospitals had to pass most of it to consumers in the form of higher daily service charges. The hospital daily service charge was the fee for routine nursing care, room and board, and minor medical and surgical supplies and usually excluded the costs of laboratory work, x-rays, operating rooms, and special nursing services, which were additional charges made on the hospital bill. From 1946 to 1961, hospital daily service charges had risen 228%, over four times as much as the consumer price index for all items.

Several developments had contributed to the rapid rise in hospital costs. Improved medical technology, including new and expensive drugs and equipment, and new medical techniques, such as open heart surgery, had inflated hospital care costs. The most important factor, however, was the increased payroll expense, which accounted for 62% of the total expense of hospital operations in 1961. The payroll expense in short-term hospitals had increased by 521% between 1946 and 1961.

During 1961, an estimated 74,000 new students were admitted to professional and practical nursing schools, compared with 71,297 in 1960. The 1126 professional nursing programs offered in hospitals, colleges, universities, and junior colleges admitted 49,487 new students in 1961, an increase of only 3000 since 1953. Among professional nursing schools, diploma programs in hospitals continued, as in the past, to enroll the largest number of new students, but their enrollment of 38,702, or about 78% of the total, marked the first time in history that diploma schools in the United States had admitted fewer than 80% of all professional nursing students. Both baccalaureate and associate-degree programs showed a rise over previous years. Colleges and universities admitted 8700 nursing students (18%) to study for bachelor's degrees in nursing. Associate-degree programs, usually in junior and community colleges, admitted the remaining 2085 new students (4%).

FINANCIAL DEFICITS OF DIPLOMA SCHOOLS

In the diploma schools, the prevailing pattern of financing had changed very little over the previous half-century. There had been a few modifications and moderately increased charges, but the pattern remained the same: apprentice-type financing, which hospitals had formerly exchanged for apprentice-type training. The real difficulty was that the cheap-labor component of the traditional hospital system had virtually disappeared. Higher standards had pushed almost all diploma programs far into the red. The outdated idea, still almost universally applied to fiscal practice, was that the student should pay for his or her education through service to patients. This conviction was strongly ingrained in the thinking patterns of most people and was not easily altered.

By 1960, few hospital administrators would deny that the operation of a modern school of nursing was an expensive proposition. Significantly, the official reports of 30 hospitals operating schools of nursing

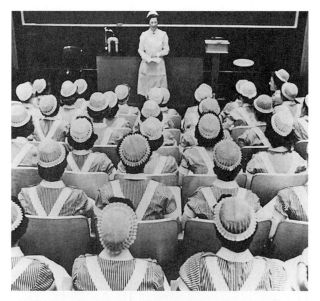

A declining portion of female high school graduates was choosing nursing as an occupation.

in Ohio showed an average net cost per student of $963.21 in 1955. Another hospital had operated its school that same year at a net cost of $1517 per student. Yet another hospital school, with an excellent record of scholastic achievement and a good reputation among nurse educators, had 162 students enrolled and spent $304,000 more than it had received in tuition, fees, value of student service, and other credits.

Only highly reactionary policies by hospital administrators could halt such deficits. In 1960, Dr. Thomas Hales, administrator at Albany Hospital, New York, boasted that he still operated his nursing school on the philosophy of a balanced budget. For hospitals to plan for this type of school operation, however, he insisted that it was necessary for the school and the hospital to agree to a list of basic principles:

Hospital and school must agree that their objective is to turn out a competent bedside nurse.

Hospital and school must believe in the "apprenticeship" philosophy of nurse education—that the student "learns by doing," and that she cannot learn nursing skills by spending most of her time in the classroom and laboratory.

They must agree that "repetitive practice" is valuable in the training of a student nurse, because every patient presents a different challenge.

They must be willing to cut to the minimum the assignment of students that take them away from the service areas where patient care is provided.

Vacation, holiday, and sick leave policies must be kept on a realistic basis. They cannot follow college campus patterns without bankrupting the school.

A work week of no less than 40 hours (preferably 44 hours) of combined classroom and ward experience is essential for the sound financial operation of the school.

A reasonable and fair evaluation of student services must be developed.

Strict accounting must be kept of the student's time on the wards when she is rendering the services to patients that justify the hospital in compensating for these services.[1]

Hospital administrators were now anxious for federal dollars. One noted that federal subsidization was no longer as radical an idea as it had been in the United States over the past 200 years. Nursing was perhaps the only profession for which the government had not taken responsibility for education. There were state universities for the preparation of teachers, lawyers, veterinarians, engineers, pharmacists, physicians, and

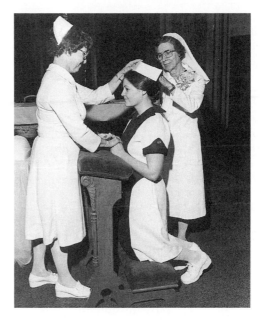

Despite financial difficulties, diploma schools continued to initiate students in the ideals of the nursing profession.

others, but only a few for the education of nurses. A program of federal grants to hospitals sponsoring diploma schools (with additional state matching funds) was proposed in Congress but met with little support.

VARIABLES IN NURSING EDUCATION

Several studies documented the improved quality of diploma programs at the end of the 1950s. The NLN's *Report on Hospital Schools of Nursing, 1957* was designed "to help hospital schools of nursing determine where they stood in relation to their goals and, on the basis of this stock-taking, to plan the emphasis and direction of their continuing efforts to improve their programs."[2] Comparative data pointed out that about one half of all hospital schools had, at the time of the study, demonstrated that they had met the NLN-accrediting criteria. A follow-up study, *Today's Diploma Schools of Nursing*, published in 1963, reported that "the majority of the diploma schools of nursing were full-fledged educational institutions, competent to identify their own problems and to determine for themselves the ways by which they can best meet current criteria for educational excellence."[3]

One of the main obstacles to growth of baccalaureate nursing education during the 1950s could be attributed to the character of many of the so-called baccalaureate programs. These were often standard diploma programs that were offered in a collegiate setting, with a few science and general education courses added to the curriculum. The difference between baccalaureate preparation and diploma preparation was often too obscure to be recognized by the employers of the graduates, and the main difference noted by prospective students was probably financial. Thus, baccaulaureate education for nursing was, in too many instances, of unknown quality.

Nurses for a Growing Nation, published by the NLN in 1957, projected nursing personnel and education needs to 1970 and pointed conclusively to the need for increasing the number of baccalaureate degree graduates and expanding facilities to meet this need. Viewing these programs as providing the foundational knowledge and skills for graduate study (and as the shortest and most economical preparation for teaching, administration, supervision, and clinical specialization), the report estimated that one third of all nursing graduates should be from baccalaureate programs. Yet in 1962, only 14% of nursing's basic students were being graduated from these programs.

During the 6-year period from 1956 to 1962, the number of baccalaureate nursing programs increased from 161 to 178, and the average enrollment in these programs increased from 116 to 132. On the surface, this increase would appear to have been most encouraging, because it came at a time when more students, both men and women, were entering college than ever before. Despite the increase in number and size of baccalaureate programs, however, there had not been a sufficient increase in the number of graduates from master's programs who were preparing for college teaching.

In the fall of 1962, enrollments in master's programs in nursing (of both full- and part-time students) totaled 2472, whereas graduations from these programs totaled 1098 for the academic year

1961–1962. The dearth of candidates qualified for college teaching was reflected in statistics reported in 1962: Only 4% of the nursing faculty members teaching in baccalaureate and higher degree programs held doctoral degrees, 76% held master's degrees, and 20% held baccalaureate degrees. Master's-level preparation was acknowledged as the minimal base for quality instruction.

In addition to the 192 baccalaureate and higher degree programs seeking to attract master's graduates in 1962, there were 874 diploma and 84 associate-degree programs that were also bidding for the potential candidates. In the same year, the budgeted vacancies in these three types of programs totaled 1202. Added to the needs of the schools were the demands for administrative and supervisory personnel of approximately 6000 hospitals and 7800 health agencies and boards of education. It could readily be seen that the nursing administrator had to compete for a scarce supply of well-qualified faculty.

Some of the responsibilities to be undertaken by any college or university that would offer a program in nursing education were identified by Margaret Bridgman in her study, *Collegiate Education for Nursing*:

> Recognition of nursing as a subject comparable to others that are established as college majors and realization that it must be developed in the same way to justify a degree and give students the benefits they have a right to expect from college education for their chosen profession.
>
> Recognition of the need to produce graduates really competent for the functions for which college-educated nurses are so urgently needed.
>
> Establishment of an educational unit in nursing in the institution on a completely equal basis with other units of the institution, with a faculty adequate in number and well qualified in the various special types of nursing to teach all the courses in nursing, including faculty-guided clinical practice. A minimum number of faculty members is six, with specialists, respectively, in medical, surgical, obstetric, pediatric, psychiatric, and public health nursing.
>
> Provision for the necessary facilities for education: classrooms, faculty offices, and library.
>
> Provision of housing and all other student personnel services required for college students.
>
> Provision of available and accessible hospital and other agency facilities for the practice of nursing, since it is here that faculty help students to develop professional skills and to use pertinent knowledge from all preceding academic and professional sources.[4]

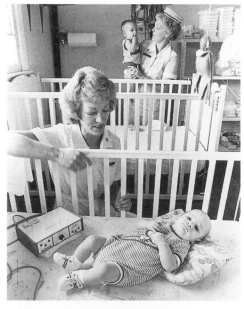

Although aided by electronic equipment, the nurse's abilities remained at the heart of nursing care.

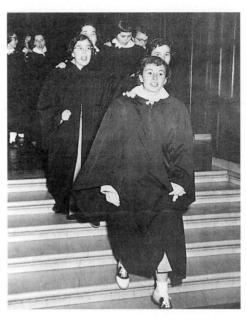

Colleges and universities offering nursing programs needed to provide educational resources of a quality similar to those of preparation programs in other professions.

In other words, the university had to accept the same responsibility for this type of education as for any other in which it undertook to provide the kind, level, and quality of preparation that was characteristic of the institution and represented by its degree.

THE SURGEON GENERAL'S CONSULTANT GROUP ON NURSING

Assuming office in January 1961, President John F. Kennedy declared in his televised inaugural that "the torch has been passed to a new generation of Americans—born in this century . . . and unwilling to witness or permit the slow undoing of those human rights to which this Nation has always been committed."[5] Nurses, physicians, and hospital administrators waited, complacently, on the whole, to see how the new generation would handle federal aid to nursing.

Postwar federal legislation to assist basic nursing education had long been backed by many hospital, nursing, and public health officials. It was not until 1961, however, that the surgeon general of the U.S. Public Health Service appointed the special Consultative Group on Nursing to advise him on nursing needs and to identify the appropriate role of the federal government in ensuring adequate nursing services for the country.[6]

In his foreword to the group's report, *Toward Quality in Nursing*, Chairman Alvin C. Eurich wrote: "In the opinion of the group, the nation faces a critical problem in ensuring adequate nursing services in the years ahead. The need for more nurses is urgent. . . . Lack of adequate financial resources is a basic prob-

lem. . . . In the judgment of the consultant group, if the nursing problem is to be solved, there is no alternative to federal aid."

The crux of the problem was contained in another paragraph of the foreword: "Today nursing education is at a crossroad. We need a careful examination of the existing types of nursing education programs, to determine how they can be merged into a pattern that will adequately prepare the nurse to render better patient care and allow her to advance professionally in an orderly manner." The passage went on to declare that "pending the outcomes of such an orderly study, we need immediate action to expand and improve nursing service within the evolving framework of education and patient care." Any timid, piecemeal approach to the nursing problem, warned Eurich, was "doomed to failure."[7]

As a basis for federal action, the major problems facing the nursing profession, according to the report, were identified as follows: (1) too few schools were providing adequate education for nursing; (2) not enough capable young people were being recruited to meet the demand; (3) too few college-bound young people were entering the nursing field; (4) more nursing schools were needed within colleges and universities; (5) the continuing lag in the social and economic status of nurses discouraged people from entering the field and remaining active in it; (6) available nursing personnel were not being fully used for effective patient care, including supervision and teaching as well as clinical care; and (7) too little research was being conducted on the advancement of nursing practice.

As a goal for the decade ahead, the consultants called for an estimated 680,000 professional nurses to be made available for practice by 1970—130,000 more than were then active. To reach the 1970 target, the consultants estimated that by 1969 the basic professional nursing schools should graduate 53,000 nurses annually, a 75% increase over the number of 1961 graduates. The estimates of the increased number of graduates needed, by type of basic nursing school, were as follows: basic baccalaureate-degree programs, 8000 (4039 in 1961); diploma programs, 40,000 (25,311 in 1961); and associate-degree programs, 5000 (917 in 1961).

The consultants also suggested a need for 3000 nurses with master's or higher degrees—a 194% increase over the comparable group in 1961—and 5000 post-RN baccalaureate graduates—an approximate 100% increase over comparable 1961 totals. The need for LPNs was estimated at 350,000 by 1970, an increase of more than 50% over the current level. More than 6% of the nation's female high-school graduates would have to be recruited into nursing, according to the consultant group, or an annual increase of at least 7000 over the existing recruitment rate.

To stimulate recruitment, the consultant group recommended that the Public Health Service

Toward
Quality in Nursing
Needs and Goals

Report of the Surgeon Generals'
Consultant Group on Nursing

Public Health Service   February 1963

U.S. DEPARTMENT OF HEALTH, EDUCATION, AND WELFARE

The report of the surgeon general's Consultant Group on Nursing established the framework for subsequent legislation. (The United States Public Health Service.)

expand financial and other aid to state, regional, and national agencies concerned with nursing recruitment. It also suggested that low-cost loans and scholarships, supported by federal funds, be provided by professional and practical nursing schools. To improve educational programs, the group recommended that federal funds be provided to construct additional nursing school facilities and to expand educational programs and services. It also suggested that the Public Health Service and the nursing profession develop prototypes of educational facilities most conducive to the effective teaching of nursing.

In addition, to assist professional nurses in obtaining advanced degrees, the group recommended that the federal program of Professional Nurse Traineeships be doubled within 5 years. They thought that this program should be expanded to provide for the preparation of nursing specialists in clinical fields. Other aspects of training for which the group recommended provision of federal funds were short-term traineeships and baccalaureate study for diploma graduates.

To help hospitals improve the utilization of nurses, the group suggested that federal funds be provided to conduct demonstrations, to experiment with new and improved methods, and to educate nurses in the use of these methods. Federal funds should be made available to expand consultative and other services designed to improve the quality and quantity of nursing care. Further, project grants should be made to nursing schools and other agencies to strengthen in-service education, on-the-job training, and continuing education of nurses. Finally, to increase support for nursing research, the consultant group recommended an immediate increase in funding for the Public Health Service nursing research fellowship program to finance the establishment of 100 new full-time research fellowships. The group also favored action that would double the funds for the Public Health Service's program of nursing research.

THE NURSE TRAINING ACT OF 1964

Based on these recommendations, a much-expanded program of federal aid for professional nursing education was proposed in a 1964 administration bill, H.R. 10042, the Nurse Training Act of 1964. The bill, incorporating White House proposals for nursing school construction grants as well as for student loans and scholarships, was introduced in February by Congressman Oren Harris of Arkansas. Witnesses for the Department of Health, Education, and Welfare strongly supported the bill. Boisfeuillent Jones, special assistant to the Department of Health, Education, and Welfare secretary, called H.R. 10042 "the logical next step in strengthening and coordinating existing programs aiding nurse education with a major new nationwide effort to alleviate critical shortages of nurses required for the health care of all citizens."[8]

Key supportive testimony at the House hearings came from the ANA. The ANA emphasized aid for collegiate schools of nursing, including construction grants, on the basis that these schools educated teachers, who in turn would be needed in greater numbers if the shortage of practicing nurses was to be alleviated. Nurses testifying at the House hearings seemed content to support the administration bill as drafted. It authorized $346 million, over 5 years, for nursing school construction, special projects and planning grants, student loans and merit scholarships, and a continuation of the professional nurse traineeship program.

The House considered the professional nurse education bill on July 21, 1964. During the House floor debate, discussion centered on the proposed $41 million formula grants to diploma nursing schools to help meet educational costs. Representative Kenneth A. Roberts of Alabama, a sponsor of the bill and its floor manager in the House debate, reported that the House Interstate and Foreign Commerce Committee had adopted this provision because "the committee was quite concerned by the trend that has been developing in recent years, under which the number of diploma schools of nursing has declined

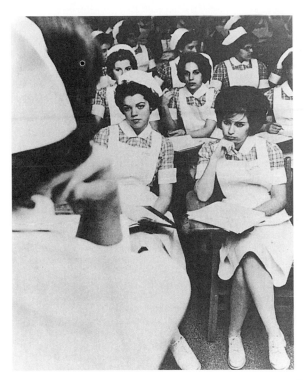

The Nurse Training Act of 1964 meant to rapidly expand enrollments in nursing schools.

from 1134 in 1949 to only 875 today." Representative Roberts added that "a number of these 875 schools face the very real possibility of having to close their doors because they are unable to meet the additional costs to them for training nurses [and that] these schools run a continuing deficit, which, of course, is borne by increased costs to patients at hospitals."[9]

The House-passed version of the Nurse Training Act of 1964 was approved by the Senate on August 12, with a few technical amendments and one other that incorporated recommendations made by the American Hospital Association. The latter amendment added diploma nursing schools to the 5-year, $17 million program for special project grants to aid schools in meeting the cost of improved or expanded nursing education. The House-passed version of the bill had limited these grants to public and nonprofit private collegiate and associate-degree nursing schools. This new assistance was made in addition to the House- and Senate-approved 5-year program of formula grants, totaling $11 million, for training costs of public and nonprofit private diploma nursing schools.

As finally approved for the president's signature, the 5-year legislation authorized $283 million for five programs and an additional $4.6 million for administration of the programs. Ninety million dollars was authorized for construction of nursing facilities, including new, renovated, or replacement buildings. Of this total, $55 million was for diploma and junior college programs, and $35 million was for collegiate programs. Another $17 million was authorized for "teaching improvement grants," or special projects, and would be available to all programs.[10]

Also authorized was $50 million for the continuance of existing traineeship programs that had been instituted to increase the number of graduate nursing students prepared for positions as administrators, supervisors, clinical specialists, and teachers in hospitals and related institutions, public health agencies, and nursing schools.[11] The bill provided $85 million for loans, not grants, to nursing students to

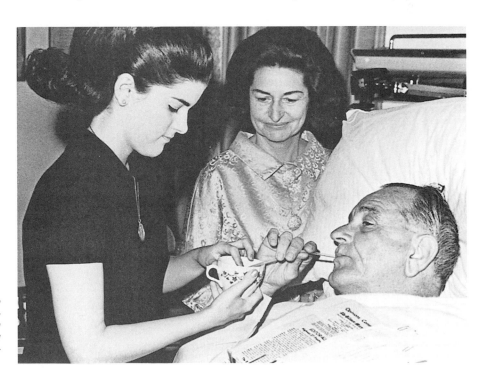

President Lyndon Johnson, who strongly supported the Nurse Training Act of 1964, received care from daughter Lucy, then enrolled as a nursing student at Georgetown University.

help defray the cost of nursing education. For those graduates who worked for 5 years after graduation, 50% of the loan was to be deferred.

Significant to those concerned about the future of hard-pressed hospital nursing schools was the authorization, specifically for diploma programs, of $41 million "to improve the quality of instruction." The maximum payment to any one program would be based on a formula granting $100 per year per student enrolled. The legislation was to cover the 5 fiscal years from 1965 to 1969, with the exception that construction grants were authorized to begin in fiscal year 1966. In the meantime, the Health Professions Educational Assistance Act of 1963 would continue to provide funds for the construction of collegiate facilities.

The loan program authorized by the Nurse Training Act of 1964 was designed to increase the number of nursing students by enabling the needy to finance their nursing education with long-term, low-interest loans. Nursing schools using loan funds requested and received allocation from the Public Health Service, determined the eligibility of student applicants for loans, decided the amount of the loans, administered the funds, and collected the repayments. The school was required to provide $1 for every $9 of federal contribution to the loan fund.

The dozen years from 1952 to 1964 were pivotal in the continued maturation of nursing. Fueled by biomedical advances, such as the wonder drugs, the number of hospital admissions soared; Hill Burton funds supported a concomitant increase in available hospital beds. The ongoing shortage of nurses and the resultant wide-scale employment of auxiliaries took the nurse further away from direct patient care

as she was required to assume managerial responsibilities. The student labor component of the total nurse staffing picture continued to diminish in importance. With the urging and assistance of the professional nursing associations, the federal government took important steps toward improving the quality of nursing education in America.

REFERENCES

1. Thomas Hales and Elizabeth A. Bell, "How Schools of Nursing Can Break Even," *Modern Hospital*, vol. 94 (April 1960): 103–106.
2. National League for Nursing, Department of Diploma and Associate Degree Programs, *Report on Hospital Schools of Nursing, 1957* (New York: The League, 1959), pp. 1–5.
3. National League for Nursing, Department of Diploma and Associate Degree Programs, *Today's Diploma Schools of Nursing: Report of the 1962 Survey of 728 Diploma Schools of Nursing* (New York: The League, 1963), pp. 3–4.
4. Margaret Bridgman, *Collegiate Education for Nursing* (New York: Russell Sage Foundation, 1953), pp. 185–197.
5. *New York Times*, January 21, 1961.
6. U.S. Public Health Service, *Toward Quality in Nursing: Needs and Goals. Report of the Surgeon General's Consultant Group on Nursing* (Washington, DC: Government Printing Office, 1963), p. xiii.
7. Ibid., p. xiv.
8. U.S. Congress, House, Committee on Interstate and Foreign Commerce, Subcommittee on Public Health and Safety, *Nurse Training Act of 1964*. Hearings Before the Subcommittee (Washington, DC: Government Printing Office, 1964), p. 27.
9. U.S. Congress, House, Committee on Interstate and Foreign Commerce, *Nurse Training Act of 1964*. Report to Accompany H.R. 11241 (Washington, DC: Government Printing Office, 1964), Report No. 1549, p. 3.
10. U.S. Congress, Senate, Committee on Labor and Public Welfare, *Nurse Training Act of 1964*. Report to Accompany H.R. 11241 (Washington, DC: Government Printing Office, 1964), Report No. 1378, pp. 1–24.
11. *Congressional Record*, August 12, 1964.

POLITICS, HEALTH, AND NURSES
The End of Innocence

19

By the mid-1960s, health care had evolved into a complex, rapidly changing technologic industry. Nursing practice had assumed progressively greater degrees of complexity and diversity as specialized roles, such as intensive and coronary care nursing, emerged and as the maturation of nursing as a scientific discipline affected new and traditional dimensions of patient care. Numerous diagnostic and therapeutic technologic medical advances—radioactive isotopes, ultrasound, and infrared machines, for example—also altered nursing practice and commanded the development of new modes of nursing practice.

THE RISE OF CORONARY CARE NURSING

At the turn of the century, the leading causes of death in the United States were acute and communicable diseases: the influenzas, tuberculosis, and gastritis. In 1900, these three diseases had a combined death rate of 540 per 100,000 and accounted for nearly one third of all deaths. In 1960, however, the top three killers were diseases of the heart, malignant neoplasms, and vascular lesions—such as strokes—affecting the central nervous system. Accidents followed closely in fourth place. The first three killers accounted for 693 deaths per 100,000 persons and 70% of all deaths in 1963.

A new role for the nurse in attacking heart disease, one of the nation's leading causes of death, had been developed under a Division of Nursing research grant during the mid-1960s. Remarkable success was achieved in an experimental coronary unit set up at Presbyterian Hospital in Philadelphia. The essence of the project was to continuously monitor patients with myocardial infarction with electrocardiographs, with specially prepared nurses providing needed intervention, without delay, until a physician could be summoned. Co-principal investigators for the project, Rose Pinneo, RN, and Lawrence E. Meltzer, M.D., reported that "the nurse is the most important factor in the

coronary care unit—even more important than the doctor or electronic equipment." They pointed out that nearly one third of all patients who were admitted to hospitals after an acute heart attack died during the period of hospitalization. The success of this experiment was underlined by the widespread acceptance of coronary care units by hospitals all across the nation.

Unnecessary duplication of hospital and medical facilities was evident. The director of New York's Montefiore Hospital stated that the city had twice as many centers for cardiac surgery as it needed, with results that were "astronomical" financially and "miserable" qualitatively. According to the President's Commission on Heart Disease, Cancer, and Strokes, 30% of the 777 hospitals equipped to do closed heart surgery had had no such cases during the year studied. Of the 548 that had cases, 87% had fewer than one operation a week, and 41% had fewer than one a month. Little of the surgery was of an emergency nature, and the mortality rate was higher in the institutions that performed such surgery relatively rarely, leading some to speculate that the reason for this might be that some of the expensive specialized units were not large enough or busy enough to give the staff practice in required techniques.

DILEMMAS IN HEALTH CARE

Over the years, most of the population of the United States had shifted to cities and towns. In 1910, about 65% of all Americans had lived in rural areas; by the 1960s, about 70% of all Americans lived in urban areas. Apart from congestion and pollution of the environment, perhaps the most serious problem associated with urbanization was that health services tended to be disproportionately concentrated and became less available to rural people. In rural areas, illness and disability had higher incidence rates, and, in terms of income, people living there could not afford the cost of health care. Because of the great middle-class exodus to the suburbs, many of the nation's cities had become ghettos for the poor, the aged, the uneducated, and other disadvantaged groups. These groups generally could not afford to pay for health care and were frightened of, and discouraged from, seeking it.

For low-income families, fee-for-service financing and the high cost of medical care acted as a deterrent to the early initiation of medical care. The tendency in many cases was to delay seeking care until the condition became intolerably serious; by the time care was sought, the benefits of early diagnosis and treatment had been lost. The disproportionate burden of the cost of health care for low-income people was demonstrated in a 1958 study of nationwide family health expenditures, which reported that the proportion of family income spent on health care decreased steadily from 13% among families earning less than $2000 per annum to 4% among families earning $7500 or more.

The American system of health care in 1965 was essentially a mosaic of public and private health programs that had grown, piece by piece, to meet national needs as they arose. For 200 million people there were 300,000 physicians in a variety of practices, 700,000 registered nurses, more than 3 million other health workers, 7000 hospitals, 20,000 long-term health facilities, and many other private and public institutions. Between 1956 and 1965, admissions to

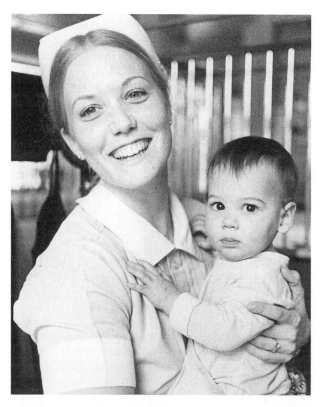

In 1965, about 700,000 RNs helped keep American families healthy.

short-term nonfederal hospitals rose from 120 per 1000 population to 138. Factors that had increased the demand for all forms of medical care included demographic changes, rising incomes, greater expectations from the health industry, and wider insurance coverage.

Annual national health expenditures in the late 1960s approached $50 billion, a figure representing roughly 6% of the gross national product (GNP) and, proportionally, the largest national health expenditure in the world. No other nation spent so high a proportion of its GNP on health. In Sweden and the United Kingdom, so-called welfare states, the proportion of the GNP directed to health was only 4.5% and 3.5%, respectively. Notwithstanding the large outlay, the pattern of financing in the United States had been predominantly private. Since the 1930s, the share from public sources had remained fairly steady at about one quarter of the total amount. This relationship was altered as a result of Medicare and Medicaid, which increased the government's contributions to total health outlays from 26% in 1966 to 34% in 1967.

Most experts agreed that several factors operated to increase the use of hospitals rather than relying on less expensive but perhaps equally effective forms of medical care. More people carried hospitalization insurance than coverage for other forms of care. A physician might choose to place his or her patient in the hospital rather than to treat the patient in the home or at the office, because hospitalization was covered by the patient's insurance and house and office calls were not. In many cases, hospitals were overutilized to suit the physicians, who found it convenient to have their patients available in one place. The relationship between physician and hospital was at the heart of the problem. Through real competence, seniority, or politics—usually a combination of all three—a physician became a member of a hospital staff, after which point, with almost no outside control, he or she could affect the largest component of hospital costs—labor—and seriously influence most other cost areas.

It was speculated that increased hospital use might be the result of increases in the number of hospital beds. Studies showed that physicians tended to keep patients in the hospital longer if beds were available and that the principal determinant of the level of hospital use was the availability of beds, not the price of the care or the characteristics of the patient population. In addition, demand for hospital beds varied with the seasons and the days of the week.

From 1946 to 1966, the average length of a hospital stay decreased from 9.1 to 7.9 days. Most of that decrease had occurred by 1950, however. Although from 1950 to 1966 daily costs had gone up and the length of stay had not changed appreciably, the number of bed-days per 1000 population had increased. In 1950, the average daily hospital census was 2.4 inpatients per 1000 population. By 1965 this figure

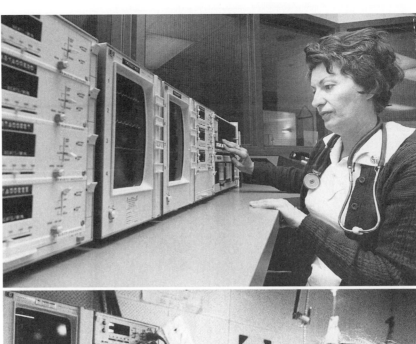

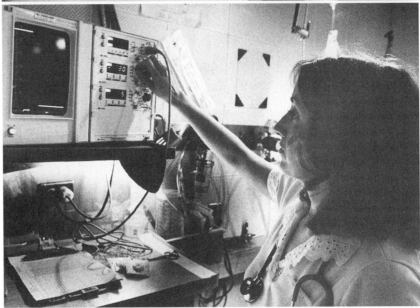

Advances in diagnostic devices created new nursing roles.

had risen to 2.9, an increase of about 12%. A more common measure of hospital use was admissions per 100,000. On this scale, the proportion had risen from 11,114 in 1947 to 13,885 in 1966, an increase of 25%. Although hospital use and daily costs were rising, lengths of stay and occupancy rates in general community hospitals had remained about the same. The occupancy rate of 72.1% in 1946 had declined to a low of 70.9% in 1954, climbing again to 76.5% in 1966.

MOVEMENT FOR NATIONAL HEALTH INSURANCE FOR THE ELDERLY

The elderly were twice as likely to have had one or more chronic conditions as were those younger than age 65. Although some of these conditions, such as sinusitis, hay fever, or bronchitis, were relatively minor, many more were serious: high blood pressure, heart disease, and diabetes. The incidence of chronic conditions increased from 74 per 100 people in the age group of 65 to 74 years of age to 84 per 100 people 75 years of age and older. Similarly, the extent of disability due to chronic illness increased with age. More than half of the aged with one or more chronic conditions had some limitation of activity, whereas, among younger people with chronic illness, only one of five had any such limitations.

Among the population 65 years of age and older during the period July 1957 to June 1959, 149 per 1000 had heart conditions, 129 had high blood pressure, and 266 had arthritis or rheumatism. In 1959, people age 65 years and older averaged 6.8 physician visits per year, 2 more than those averaged by

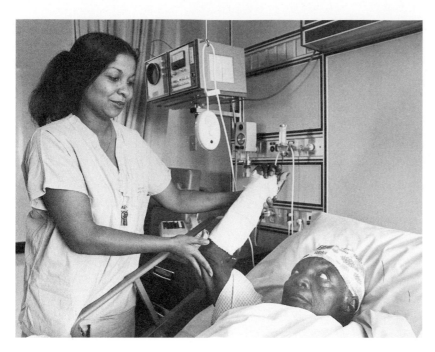

Soaring hospitalization costs were a growing concern.

younger people. The rate of physician visits was higher for women than for men and increased with the size of family income. Among the aged with equally severe limitations of activity or chronic illness, persons with high incomes visited physicians more often than those with lower incomes.

As might be expected, the elderly also used health facilities and medical services more than younger people, and they used a greater volume of physicians'

services and were admitted to hospitals more often and for longer periods. They were the primary users of nursing home and other long-term care facilities and received a greater amount of home care, part of which was provided by nurses. They needed and used more drugs.

The American Nurses Association (ANA) came out in favor of extension of social security to provide health insurance coverage for the aged along with

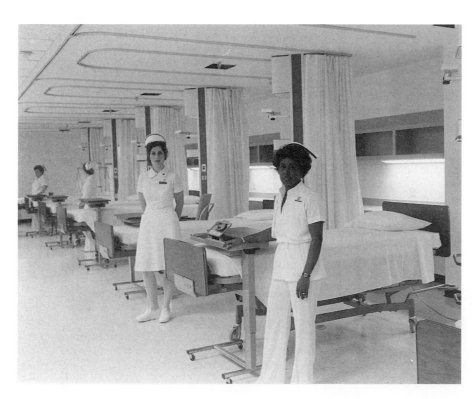

Increases in the numbers of hospital beds may have contributed to over-usage of hospitals.

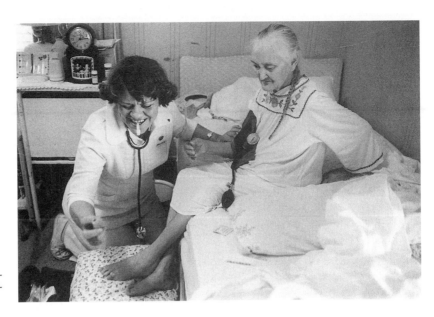

Older people were the primary users of long-term care facilities and required a disproportionate amount of home care.

inclusion of payments for private-duty and public health nursing care. The ANA also urged that careful attention be paid to the type of nursing home care covered to prevent the financing of substandard institutions. The ANA's position held that health insurance, especially for the aged, should cover more than the cost of hospital, nursing home, and surgical services. Nursing was an essential component of modern medical care and should be made available if the benefits of science were to be provided for the aged and disabled. Beneficiaries of any health insurance should be insured for needed private-duty nursing services no less than they were insured against surgical costs. Coverage should also include public health nursing care in the home as well as regular nursing home costs. This position had been established by the ANA House of Delegates at the 1958 convention, when the organization had moved from the neutral position on the broader question of compulsory health insurance adopted in 1952.

The American Medical Association (AMA) had gone on record, in 1957, in absolute opposition to use of social security for financing the health needs of the aged and had spared no words in doing so. President David B. Allman, addressing the AMA House of Delegates, had directed the opening barrage against the Forand bill. "This is socialized medicine," he said, adding that it was the beginning of the end of the private practice of medicine and the death knell for the young and growing voluntary health insurance industry. He further warned that the bill constituted a serious threat to the well being and local autonomy of the voluntary hospital at the community level and heralded the advent of federally sponsored socialism.

Allman charged that the Forand bill prescribed a course of treatment before there had been diagnoses of "(1) the economic resources of our older population; (2) the present and planned programs of voluntary insurance; (3) indigent care at the state level; (4) the incidence of hospitalization and illness by age groups and other complex research questions which they did not even try to find the answers to." Allman insisted that in the field of old-age coverage, the health insurance industry was beginning to make rapid and far-reaching strides and added that his own conviction was that "we are on the verge of giant achievements in furthering the well-being of our older population."[1]

An editorial in the *American Journal of Nursing* speculated on why nurses and physicians took opposite sides in this controversy:

> Day after day nurses watch the numbers of the chronically ill increase. Necessarily sensitive to their patients' needs, they are acutely aware of the fright of many patients—and their families—who cannot foresee how they can continue to pay for decent medical care for an uncertain future. They know many of these patients cannot begin to pay for medical expenses with the income limits placed on them when they are drawing social security. . . .
>
> Of less importance to them as nurses, but of equal importance as citizens, is the realization that they or members of their family might be facing the same situation.
>
> The vast majority of nurses are in the income bracket where high medical expenses can toss them into serious debt; and voluntary medical insurance—especially beyond the work years—is relatively costly, or impossible to buy. Though increased salaries might relieve this, [the nurses'] efforts at acquiring them are blocked by the shaky economy of those same voluntary

hospitals and public health agencies who are now subsidizing a large part of the cost of the care of the aging and chronically ill. And they are quite aware of the fact that the government is already in the health picture, for [it is] too often the inadequate reimbursement from local and state government—not to mention Blue Cross—which is the usual reason for denying their requests for salary increases. They know that all of this cannot help but affect the nursing care of the people.[2]

Pressure for a national compulsory health care plan, mainly from northern Democrats, labor, and liberal groups, had reached a high in 1949 and 1950. Hearings on the Wagner-Murray-Dingell bills, embodying the Truman proposals, had prompted criticism of the president and charges of socialism from the AMA. In the end, the opponents of Truman's proposals won. Congress failed to act again in 1950, but did move to help states provide medical care for welfare recipients under Old Age Assistance, Aid to Dependent Children, Aid to the Blind, and Aid to the Permanently and Totally Disabled. Although President Eisenhower had opposed compulsory health insurance during his 1952 campaign, in 1954, as president, he proposed that the federal government reinsure private insurance companies to protect them from losses on health insurance. The bill, supported by some insurance companies, was labeled inadequate by labor spokesmen, received criticism from the AMA, and underwent defeat that year.

Proponents of compulsory national health insurance had begun to suggest that an immediate step toward such an act would be payment, through Social Security Old Age Survivors Insurance (OASI), of hospitalization costs of people retired on OASI pensions. Such a bill was put forth in 1952, but no action was taken on it or similar bills during the next several years. In the late 1950s, in Congress, the OASI approach to health care for the elderly was sponsored by Representative Aimé J. Forand of Rhode Island. After a brief discussion, no action was taken on the 1957 Forand bill, but it was introduced again in 1959.

Although the 1959 version was defeated, the Forand bill had become a political issue. After much debate, in 1960, the House Ways and Means Committee rejected the Forand bill and an Eisenhower administration proposal calling for federal matching grants to the states to help the needy meet the costs of illness. Although similar legislation was turned back in both 1961 and 1962, the proponents kept fighting. During 1963 and 1964, more than 100 bills calling for provision of medical care for persons age 65 and older were introduced. In 1964 such a bill was passed by the Senate, representing for the first time passage of a health-care-for-the-aged bill by either house. The bill then went to conference committee, where a deadlock over its provisions lasted until Congress adjourned. Medicare, as it had come to be called, had once again failed to gain congressional approval.

When Lyndon B. Johnson was elected president in 1964, Medicare was high on his administration's priority list. Almost immediately after the 89th Congress had convened, the new Medicare proposals (H.R. 1 and S.1) were introduced. On March 29, 1965, the Ways and Means Committee reported its recommendations in the form of a new bill, H.R. 6675, which established two coordinated health insurance programs under the Social Security Act for people age 65 and older: (1) a basic plan of hospital insurance and related care under the social security program, with financing through a separate payroll tax and trust fund, and (2) a voluntary supplementary plan providing for physicians' fees and other medical and health services, financed by premium payments of $3 per month by each participant, matched from federal general revenues. Undergirding the two new insurance programs would be a greatly expanded medical care program, called Medicaid, for the financially and medically needy. The bill also provided for an across-the-board 7% increase in social security benefits, for an increase in the taxable wage base from $4800 to $6600 and for a 5-year program of "special project grants" to provide comprehensive health care and services for needy children.

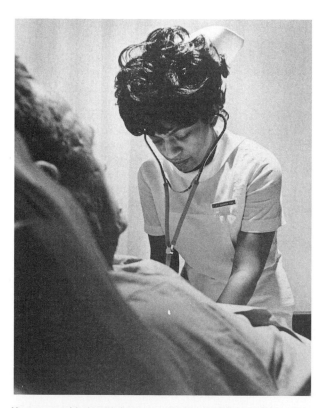

How to provide health insurance for the elderly became a major public issue.

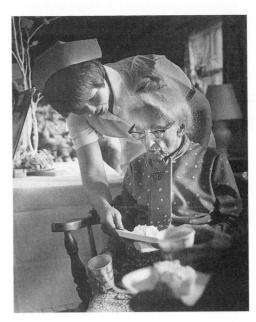

Medicare provided a comprehensive health insurance program for the elderly.

Congress was aware of the importance of this bill. Senator Russell B. Long, floor leader, opened debate on the measure:

> Mr. President, the pending bill will be the largest and most significant piece of social legislation ever to pass the Congress in the history of our country. It will do more immediate good for more people who need the attention of their government than any bill that the Congress has ever enacted. We measure our accomplishments here by our association with those few pieces of legislation which clearly move the American people toward a better life. . . .
>
> This Medicare program not only means dignity to the individual, but serves our country as an economic stabilizer while at the same time it provides for the whole of the free world a beacon reflecting the democratic way of achieving social progress. We are considering a bill which represents concern, consideration, and compromise in the best American tradition, and reflects the ideas of many men sitting here today.[3]

After action on numerous proposed amendments, the Senate passed the bill on July 9, 1965, by a vote of 68 to 21. The bill contained 513 changes from the version approved by the House. Most of them, however, were not substantial, and the major features of the two versions were the same.

The bill was sent to a conference committee for reconciliation of differences between the two versions. The conference committee convened on July 14 and promptly settled a major point of disagreement: 60 days of hospitalization would be provided, with the patient to pay a deductible of $40, and an additional 30 days would be added, with the patient to pay $10 a day. Agreement was also reached on the limits for nursing home or extended-care services and for home visits by nurses. The compromise bill, as signed by President Johnson, conformed in all basic respects to the administration's specifications for a comprehensive medical care program.

THE ANA POSITION PAPER ON EDUCATION FOR NURSING

During December 1965, a conflict over the future role of diploma schools intensified abruptly. "Education for those who work in nursing should take place in institutions of learning within the general system of education," stated the ANA's first Position Paper on Education for Nursing. Prepared by the ANA Committee on Education and adopted by the ANA board of directors in September 1965, the publication marked the beginning of what would become an ever-widening schism in nursing education. The statement pointed out that recognition of the need for improved nursing practice had led the association to conclude that

> The education for all of those who are licensed to practice nursing should take place in institutions of higher education; minimum preparation for beginning professional nursing practice should be a baccalaureate degree; minimum preparation for beginning technical nursing practice should be an associate degree in nursing; education for assistants in the health service occupations should be short, intensive preservice programs in vocational education rather than on-the-job training.[4]

In discussing the implications of the ANA position, the statement maintained that "responsibility for the education of nurses historically has been carried out by hospitals, and the graduates of hospital-based diploma programs comprise approximately 78 percent of nurses now in practice. However, economic pressures on the hospital, and other developments in society, are increasing the movement of nursing education programs into the colleges and universities. . . . It is reasonable to expect," the statement continued, "that many diploma schools of nursing will participate with colleges and universities in planning for the development of baccalaureate programs; others will participate with junior colleges in planning for the development of associate degree programs." Of course, senior and junior college programs would need hospitals and other community resources for use as laboratories. The statement also

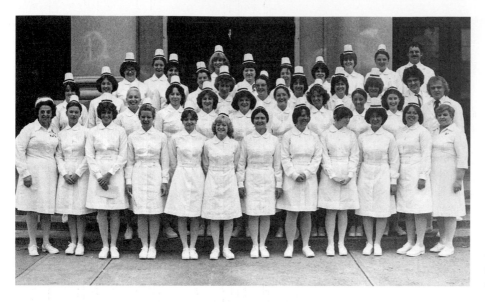

The 1965 ANA position paper favored moving all nurse preparation into colleges and universities.

noted that colleges and universities needed to provide improved education for nurses by offering new programs, expanding existing programs, determining the distinctions between programs of education that prepared either "technical" or "professional" nurses, and providing programs for continuing education, advanced study, and research.[5]

In line with the principle that all nursing education should take place in educational institutions, the ANA statement proposed that the nursing profession replace outside programs for practical nursing with junior college and community college programs in beginning-level technical nursing practice. The reasons given for this proposal were the major changes that had occurred in the nursing profession in the past few years: Increasingly complex activities were being delegated to practical nurses, many of whom were now expected to carry job responsibilities beyond those for which they had been educated.

CHANGES IN THE EDUCATIONAL SYSTEM

Only in the early 1960s did the effect of the relatively new associate-degree nursing program begin to be felt. In 1955, there had been only 16 schools with such programs; by 1964 the number had risen to 130. As this potential giant began to develop, the quality of some programs became suspect to some nurses because of what was perceived to be a drastic shortage of clinical experience in the curricula.

The trend in nursing education away from diploma schools and toward colleges and universities became even more pronounced during 1966. Statistics gathered by the National League for Nursing (NLN) indicated that the number of diploma programs had fallen from 821 in 1965 to 797 in 1966.

Simultaneously, associate-degree and baccalaureate programs had increased, respectively, from 174 to 218 and from 198 to 210. The decline in diploma programs was more than made up for by the increase in collegiate programs, with the total number of programs increasing in 1966 from 1193 to 1225. Of these programs, almost 61% were accredited by the NLN, including 72.4% of the diploma programs, 8.7% of the associate-degree programs, and 70% of the baccalaureate programs. Three fourths of all nursing students were enrolled in NLN-accredited programs.

The changing pattern in nurse education was reflected in student admission data. In 1966, diploma programs admitted 64.1% of the total 60,701 students newly enrolled in nursing programs, a decrease of 4.7% from the year before. Associate-degree programs showed a marked increase in students, admitting 14.2% of all students, compared with 10.7% in 1965. Total admissions to baccalaureate programs increased from 20.5% to 21.7%.

The trend away from diploma schools was even more marked when traced over the 10-year period beginning in 1956, when 82.8% of all nursing students had been receiving their education in hospital schools (94,920 diploma students of a total of 114,570). By 1966, the total number of students in diploma programs had decreased slightly to 90,651. In 1956, associate-degree programs had enrolled 1% of all nursing students—a total of 1132—compared with the 15,338 associate-degree students in 1966. Baccalaureate program enrollment also increased, although not as dramatically, growing from a total enrollment of 18,518 in 1956 to 33,081 in 1966.

According to a study published by the NLN in 1964, the operation of nursing schools cost hospitals in the United States an estimated $250 million a year. In a 6-year study on costs in nursing education made

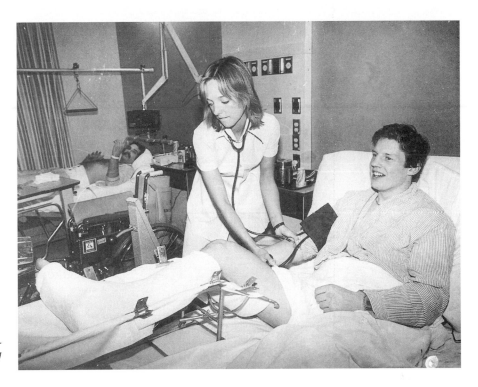

The quality of clinical experience re-mained a critical variable in nursing education.

under a grant from the Division of Nursing of the U.S. Public Health Service, the league had found that publicly controlled hospitals spent more money to educate nursing students than did privately controlled hospitals and that both types of schools spent more on noneducational functions, such as student maintenance, than they did on educational functions. By applying a uniform system of cost analysis to a representative sampling of the diploma program population, NLN researchers found that

the median gross cost of educating one student for one year in a diploma nursing program was $2,600; the median net cost was $2,300.

The median yearly income to the hospital per student to defray the cost of the program was $250. This included tuition, fees for room and board, health services and student insurance, and income from contributions and gifts. The estimated value of the student's clinical experience to the hospital and other

Nursing education programs began to slowly grow in number again in the mid-1960s.

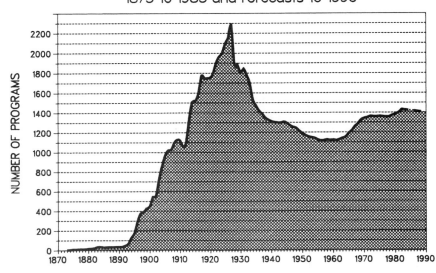

SCHOOL OF NURSING PROGRAMS
1873 to 1985 and Forecasts to 1990

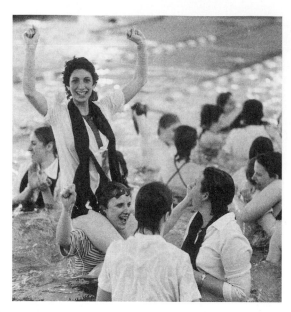

Nurses celebrating their completion of an increasingly costly education.

institutions in which she serves while learning was only $750.[6]

Of the $2600 gross cost of nursing education, $1500 went for noneducational school functions (including housing, meals, laundry, recreation, and separate health services), and $1100 went for educational functions (including the instructional program, counseling, libraries, and educational records). The investigators found that the cost of nursing education per student was highest in programs with fewer than 70 students enrolled and was lowest in programs with more than 120 students enrolled. The cost of instruction per student was higher in the Northeast than in any other region of the country, was greatest in tax-supported programs of municipal governments, and was least in programs controlled by religious institutions.

BROADENING THE TALENT BASE

Although there had been an impressive increase in the number of nurses with preparation for leadership during the 1960s, they were still in very short supply when considered in relation to need. These were the nurses responsible for teaching in all types of programs, for planning and directing the care given by all nursing personnel, for providing specialized care, and for the nursing research that would improve nursing practice and education. These were the nurses who would determine the quality of nursing care that patients received. Only 111,000 of the 748,000 registered nurses in practice in 1972 had at least a bachelor's degree. Of this group, those prepared

at the master's level or above were only 2.9% of the total employed registered nurses. Unlike that of other health professions, the cost of nursing education was not offset by one's eventual earning capacity. Because federal traineeships were awarded only for full-time academic study, nurses generally had to drop out of the work force to seek a master's degree. Virtually all had continuing financial obligations, and many had to support dependents.

A major thrust during the late 1960s and early 1970s was an attempt to broaden the base of potential nurses through recruitment efforts directed at minority groups, disadvantaged youth, men, and others who had not formerly considered nursing as a career. A college education was not a common goal for people from lower socioeconomic levels. Moreover, to recruit successfully from this group, nursing schools had to develop programs flexible enough to assist students hampered by inadequate elementary and high school educations. Imaginative ways to interest these young people in nursing, early counseling, and remedial and tutorial work that began in high school and continued through the nursing curriculum helped to increase the number of practicing nurses.

The rising expense of education placed an increasing burden on the students and their families. Many highly motivated and well-qualified students were prohibited from pursuing a career in the health fields because of the expense involved. With the increasing need for nurses, it was unfortunate that any qualified student should be turned away for economic reasons.

The Nursing Educational Opportunities Grants (scholarships) had been authorized by a 1966 amendment and initiated in the summer of 1967. During the 2 years that the program lasted, grants were awarded to an estimated 15,900 students who could not otherwise attend a nursing school. The individual grants ranged from $200 to $800. The average grant was $530. The awards totaled $8.4 million.

The Health Manpower Act of 1968, Title II, had established a new program of scholarship grants to nursing schools for full-time students of exceptional need. It provided greater support for the student than had the nursing educational opportunity grants and allowed the school greater flexibility in helping meet students' needs. The maximum annual amount of scholarship support a student could receive was $1500. No matching funds were required. The legislation provided no specific authorization of funds, because the allocation formula was based on enrollment. In 1971, 64% of all programs awarded scholarships to 10% of all enrolled students. Eighty-six percent of the students who were awarded scholarships came from families whose gross annual income was less than $10,000. The availability of scholarships remained a critical factor in recruitment and retention of students and in programs providing for career mobility. The Nurse Training Act of 1971 extended

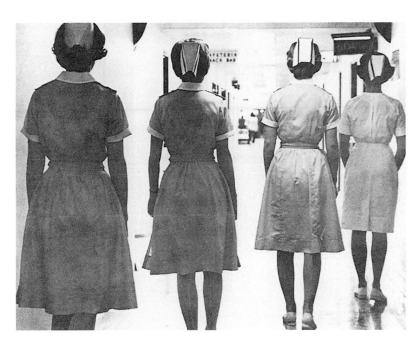

Federal loans and scholarships helped build and diversify nursing school enrollments.

the authority for scholarships and increased the maximum student scholarship per year to $2000 and revised the formula for scholarship grants to schools.

Meanwhile, the nursing student loan program had assisted students enrolled in diploma, associate-degree, baccalaureate, and graduate programs of nursing education. The program had begun in 1965, with 426 nursing education programs participating. In 1971, an estimated 943 programs participated, an increase of 121% in 6 years. In the same period, the number of students awarded loans increased from 3645 in 1965 (3% of the total enrollments in nursing schools) to an estimated 24,443 in 1971 (14% of the total enrollments). Seventy-seven percent of the students awarded nursing student loans came from families whose gross family income was less than $10,000.

In 1970, more than 5400 borrowers were taking advantage of the loan cancellation provision through full-time employment as registered nurses. With the graduation of borrowers from nursing schools, the number of borrowers canceling loans through employment had more than doubled each of the previous 2 years. Despite the benefits of this program, educational costs in all types of nursing education programs were increasing beyond the ability of students to meet them from their own or from their families' resources. The availability of this financial assistance was essential in making it possible for more persons to enter and remain in nursing schools.

NURSING IN THE VIETNAM ERA

Meanwhile, the 12-year-long American troop commitment to Vietnam had made that conflict the longest in U.S. history. American interest in Southeast Asia had begun in 1950, when President Truman sent a 35-man military advisory team to aid the French in their fight against the North Vietnamese. After the French garrison at Dien Bien Phu fell to communist forces in 1954, France and North Vietnam agreed to partition Vietnam, pending free reunification elections. The South Vietnamese government refused a North Vietnamese request to prepare for reunification elections on the grounds that free elections would be impossible in North Vietnam. The following year, President Eisenhower offered South Vietnam economic aid and agreed to help train the South Vietnamese army. In 1960, North Vietnam announced formation of the National Liberation Front (Viet Cong) of South Vietnam, and terrorism in the South increased. In response, the number of American military advisers in South Vietnam rose from about 2000 in December 1961 to more than 15,000 by the end of 1963.

It was at this stage that American military nurses arrived on the scene. Thirteen army nurses were included on the staff of the Eighth Field Hospital, arriving at Nha Trang in March 1962. Concomitantly, the first Navy Nurse Corps officers were assigned to duty at Station Hospital, Headquarters Support Activity, Saigon. The Vietnam conflict did not evoke widespread support from either the nation or the nursing profession. During the 1950s and 1960s, recruitment of nurses for the army posed recurrent difficulties. Professional nurses were in chronically short supply, and the military services were obliged to recruit in direct competition with civilian nurse employers.

Extraordinary incentives were offered. In 1956, the army established the Army Student Nurse Program. Student nurses received financial aid and in return

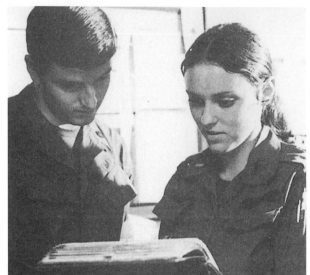

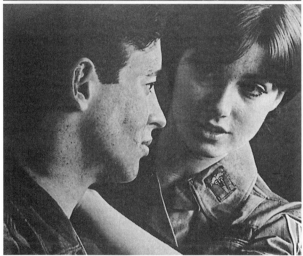

Army nurses in Vietnam.

It was thought that the difficulty encountered in recruiting army nurses reflected the general shortage of professional nurses in civilian life, but specialization, increased demands for health services, and the development of new fields of practice also contributed to the problem. Recruitment of military nurses had become increasingly competitive: Civilian hospitals were paying higher salaries, had improved working conditions and housing, and were offering other attractive inducements. The Army Medical Service had to employ hundreds of civilian nurses to fill military nursing requirements.

Within the context of a general military buildup, the Department of Defense, with congressional support, approved the establishment of the Walter Reed Army Institute of Nursing. It was stated that the army, by opening its vast resources to prepare qualified nurses, would make an important contribution to the fulfillment of military and civilian nursing needs. The goals of the new nursing school were to increase the army's number of degree-holding nurses and to increase the reenlistment rate of army nurses.

The first large contingent of air force nurses for Vietnam reported in February 1966 and was assigned to the Twelfth Air Force Hospital, Cam Ranh Bay. A rapid increase in the number of army nurses serving in Vietnam followed, from slightly more than 200 in June 1966 to more than 600 in June 1967, to a peak of 900 in January 1969. The military situation was discouraging, and by April 1966 more Americans than South Vietnamese were being killed in action: In July the number of American dead reached 4440—more than the number of Americans killed in the Revolution and 10 times more than in the Spanish-American

served in the army for a minimum of 2 years for a diploma in nursing or for 3 years for a degree. Students remained at their own nursing schools until they had completed the prescribed course and qualified for state licensure. Four months before completion of their nursing courses, the participants applied for commissions in the Army Nurse Corps Reserve. On receipt of notification of state licensure, they were commissioned and ordered to active duty.

Despite these incentives, the strength of the Army Nurse Corps dwindled, creating a gap between capability and mission. During the early days of the Vietnam conflict, the Army Student Nurse Program continued to be the major source for junior officers. Army Student Nurse Program participants represented 52% of the total nurse corps's growth in fiscal year 1962. Despite personnel policies disapproving resignations and voluntary requests for relief from active duty, the losses in the corps exceeded the gains for that year, and the downward trend continued.

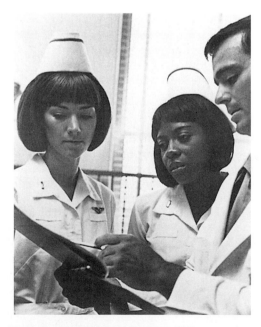

In contrast to World War II, nursing staffs were integrated during the Vietnam War.

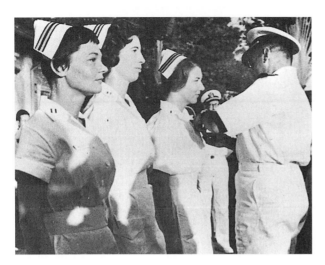

These three navy nurses rendered care to others, even though they were injured themselves, during the bombing of the Brink Bachelor Officer's Quarters in Saigon, Christmas Eve 1964. Here they received the Purple Heart for heroic action. (United States Navy.)

War. Four navy nurses were wounded during a Viet Cong attack on the Brink Bachelor Officers' Quarters and became the first women members of the armed forces to receive the Purple Heart for injuries sustained in Vietnam. In September 1966, Navy Nurse Corps officers were assigned to Danang. The navy hospital at Danang had become the largest combat-casualty treatment facility in the world. Designed originally as a 60-bed facility, it soon expanded to comprise 600 beds and eventually admitted more than 70,000 patients.

Two veteran hospital ships, U.S.S. *Repose* and *Sanctuary*, provided direct medical support, particularly to those units engaged in amphibious operations. *Repose* arrived at its assigned station in Vietnam in February 1966 and was joined by *Sanctuary* on April 12, 1967. Both ships were staffed with highly specialized personnel (including 30 nurses aboard each), were equipped with the most modern medical equipment, and could provide optimal medical care to the wounded. The hospital ships offered many advantages over fixed medical facilities, including versatility, mobility, a better environment, more efficient use of medical personnel, and greater support in amphibious operations. Although responsible mainly for providing medical service support to navy and marine corps personnel, the ships dispensed aid to all combat arms, and 28% of the workload involved patients other than members of the naval service.

A congressional bill authorizing appointment of male nurses to the regular forces of the Air Force, Army, and Navy Nurse Corps was signed by the president on September 20, 1966, and the roster of male nurses in all the services soon multiplied. By the close of the 1967 fiscal year, 1032 male Army Nurse Corps officers made up 22% of the army's nursing total. About half were in the clinical nursing specialties of anesthesia, operating room, and neuropsychiatry.

Meanwhile, the buildup of American forces in South Vietnam continued: By May 1965, troop strength had increased to 35,000; by January 1966, to more than 180,000; by December, to 380,000; and by the end of 1967, to nearly 500,000. As the fighting and the number of American casualties escalated, large-scale protests against the war erupted at home. Thousands of protesters marched in Washington in October 1967, and hundreds were arrested trying to storm the Pentagon. Although student unrest erupted into violence on campuses all across the country, nursing students in general did

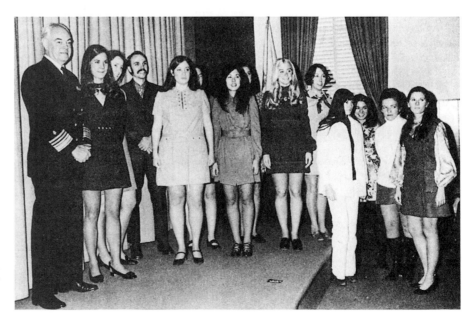

The surgeon general of the navy administers the oath of office to 13 student nurses on December 2, 1971. (United States Navy.)

not become involved. Despite mass protests at home, American troop commitment in Vietnam soon surpassed the peak reached in Korea 25 years earlier.

The peculiar nature of counterinsurgency operations in Vietnam required modification of the usual concepts of hospital usage in a combat area. Because the Viet Cong, using classic guerrilla strategy, declined to engage in set-piece battles against large enemy units, there was no "front" in the traditional sense. In reaction, American strategy dictated partitioning of the country into separate field zones, each patrolled from a central camp (fire base). Isolated and dependent on helicopter supply, the base camps, normally tranquil, were prey to night attack and envelopment by light infantry. Thus, with few exceptions, no large, dramatic battles took place during the Vietnam war.

Semipermanent, air-conditioned, fully equipped hospitals were constructed in Vietnam. In contrast to World War II and Korea, when overrun territory could be occupied and held, the Vietnam-era hospital could not follow in direct support of tactical operations. Operating on much the same principles as the fire base, all the army hospitals in Vietnam, including Medical Unit, Self-contained, Transportable (MUST) units, were fixed installations assigned to area-support missions. Because there was no secure road network in the combat areas of Vietnam, ground evacuation of the wounded was almost impossible.

Despite the obstacles, never before in the history of warfare had wounded received such complete, rapid health care. Even with the multitude of problems involved, including those of terrain and climate, almost 99% of the soldiers hospitalized for wounds, diseases, and injuries recovered, and about 90% returned to duty. Because of the courage and skill of nurses, physicians, medics, and helicopter and ambulance personnel, a soldier wounded in the jungles or rice paddies of Vietnam stood a much better chance of surviving, with the possibility of complete recovery, than the soldier in Korea or in any earlier war.

The ability of medical personnel to adapt recent medical advances to the situation in Vietnam showed clearly in statistics. For example, of all those Americans wounded and hospitalized in World War II, 4.5% died. The percentage had been reduced to 2.5 during the Korean conflict. In Vietnam, this was down to about 1.5%, marking a significant increase in the number of lives spared.

Between January 1965 and December 1970, 133,447 wounded were admitted to army medical treatment facilities in Vietnam; 97,659 of these were admitted to hospitals. The hospital mortality rate for this period was 2.6%. The very slight increase in hospital mortality in Vietnam over that in Korea (2.5%) was identified as the result of rapid helicopter evacuation, which brought into the hospital mortally wounded patients who by earlier, slower means of evacuation would have died en route. If one assumes that most of the hospitalized patients who died within the first 24 hours belonged to this class, the true rate would perhaps be much closer to 1%. The average length of stay per case for patients in Vietnam was considerably less than that in earlier conflicts, amounting to 63 days, compared with 75 days for those in World War II.

Despite the constant threat of enemy attack, the highest quality of nursing care was given. All the hospitals, from the northern highlands at Pleiku to the delta town of Vung Tau, were vulnerable to mortar, rocket, and small-arms fire. Several, such as the 45th Surgical Hospital at Tay Ninh, the Third Field Hospital in Saigon, and the 12th Evacuation Hospital at Chu Chi, were hit one or more times. First Lieutenant Sharon Anne Lane was killed by hostile fire on June 8, 1969, while on duty at the 312th Evacuation Hospital at Chu Lai.

The degree of sophistication of medical equipment and facilities everywhere in Vietnam permitted army nurses and physicians to make full use of their training and capability. As a result, the care that was available in army hospitals in Vietnam was far better than any that had ever been generally available for combat support. It was now possible to take a wounded man from the field to a hospital facility, perform surgery, close his wounds, and transport him to a hospital in the continental United

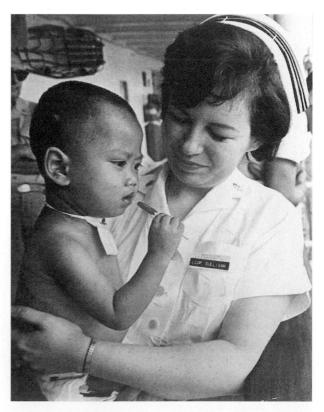

Navy nurse cares for Vietnamese child.

States within the same time it had taken to move a patient from France to a British hospital during World War I.

In the early 1970s, women began to assume more important roles in the federal government, including the Department of Defense, and became more active in the extension of national policy. In June 1970, Anna Mae Hays, chief of the Army Nurse Corps, was promoted to the rank of brigadier general. Nurses were indeed proud to welcome General Hays as the corps's first general officer and as one of the first two women in American history to have attained that rank. The navy and air force soon followed suit, and all the military nursing services were then headed by women generals or an admiral.

On January 25, 1972, President Nixon disclosed that secret peace negotiations had been conducted since the previous June by Secretary of State Henry Kissinger. After many interruptions, talks resumed January 8, 1973, and President Nixon ordered a halt to all offensive military operations against North Vietnam. Peace agreements were formally signed in Paris by the United States, North and South Vietnam, and the Viet Cong. A cease-fire was effected on January 28, 1973, and nearly 1600 American prisoners of war were released by the North Vietnamese. The last American troops left Vietnam on March 29, officially ending any direct American military role. There had been 46,079 American combat deaths, and the number of wounded totaled 304,000, the latter figure exceeded only during World War II.

Nurses in Veterans Administration hospitals noted that the uniqueness of the Vietnam War produced feelings in its veterans not experienced by veterans of other wars. No sooner had young recruits arrived in Vietnam than they became aware of the futility of American intervention. There was widespread resistance to fighting, extensive drug usage, and racial conflict among American troops. Profound guilt, feelings of stasis, impotence, psychic numbness, and a deeply embedded antiestablishment anger were common.

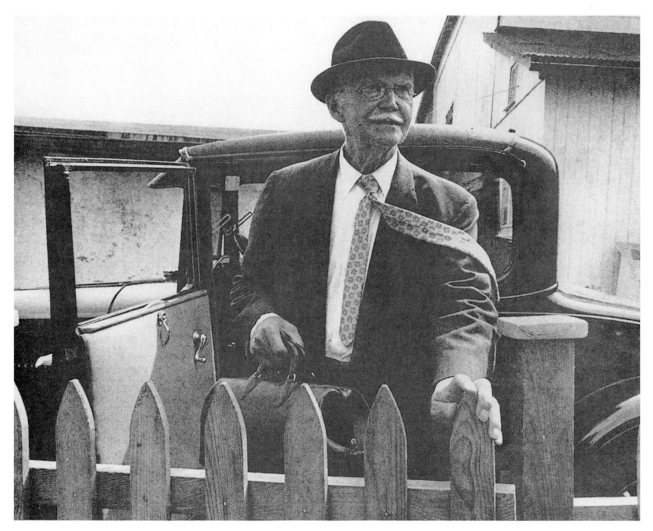

Although the "old country doctor" was nearly gone, the public continued to cherish him as a model health care provider.

The national trauma engendered by the Vietnam War signaled a transition from a heroic conception of the U.S. military as a bulwark against the spread of Communism toward a new ambivalence. The Cold War image of the American soldier as a noble fighter for freedom opposing the forces of totalitarianism had been irrevocably tarnished. Meanwhile, the social and technologic changes under way in the 1960s had begun to push another cherished image—that of the "old country doctor"—into the realm of nostalgia.

THE PASSING OF THE OLD COUNTRY DOCTOR

In earlier times, when most physicians were general practitioners and most graduate nurses served as private-duty specialists and when physician and nurse had known firsthand each personal and family history, they had been able to function reasonably well by treating their patients symptomatically, by supporting morale, and by observing the injunction, "First do no harm." There had been few barriers to access to the physician and the nurse who knew their patients and who were concerned with their needs and how they related to family and community. People did not expect miracles. They knew that tuberculosis and lobar pneumonia were dreadful diseases with high mortality rates; they knew that there was little that one could do about the childhood killers; and, in a prevailing spirit of fatalism toward those natural calamities, they accepted them, knowing that their physician and nurse were doing all that could be done.

The picture of the family doctor and the private-duty nurse had become idealized during the early decades of the century. The image of this "golden age" persisted in a nostalgic wish to return to the era of the family doctor and the private-duty nurse—good and all-knowing advisers embodied in countless novels, movies, and television shows.

The epitome of this image was forever implanted in the public conscience by the exploits of the radio and motion picture series, *Dr. Christian*, starring Jean Hersholt. The radio series, which introduced Dr. Paul Christian to the public, began on the CBS network in the 1937 season, and the half-hour show was heard every Wednesday night at 10:00 for 15 years. It was estimated that the show attracted a weekly listening audience of 20 million.

Like the radio series, the group of six black-and-white feature films centered on beloved Dr. Christian's practice in River's End, Minnesota, a storybook small midwestern town filled with all the homey virtues and stereotypes of pre–World War II America. Devoted to humanitarian causes, the wise Dr. Christian was not only a superb country doctor (with almost miraculous medical and surgical prowess) but also an unflagging optimist as to the goodness of mankind and the aspirations of his townfolk. Dr. Christian

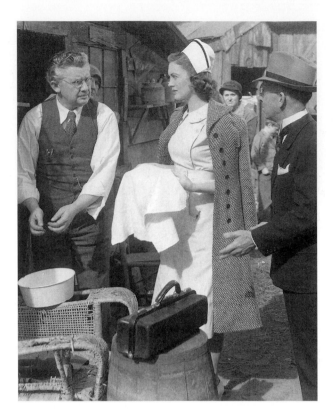

In "The Courageous Dr. Christian," one episode in the series of Dr. Christian movies, the good doctor (John Hersholt) and his loyal nurse (Dorothy Lovett) effectively combat an epidemic of spinal meningitis among River's End squatters. (RKO Pictures.)

maintained a simple professional office at home, unhampered by neopharmaceutical equipment or smart medical terminology. Probably his most essential basic tool was the constantly stoked pipe that allowed him to puff and meditate on the ramifications of his patients' medical and emotional problems.

Medical practice in the United States had changed markedly since that time. The number of specialists had increased and the number of general practitioners had declined. Although in 1934 85% of all practicing physicians had been general practitioners, only 45% filled this role in 1960 and only 37% in 1965. By the late 1960s, society had numerous medical specialists, such as internists, pediatricians, obstetricians, gynecologists, ophthalmologists, radiologists, pathologists, neurologists, and more than 30 other specialties.

Although the trend toward specialization produced many benefits, a widely held opinion maintained that the loss of general practitioners had created problems in the provision of health services. The concept of the family physician's office as the center of primary health care was no longer believed to be compatible with modern medicine. The physician of the 1960s believed that he needed ready, almost-immediate access to laboratory, radiologic, and other sophisticated facilities if he was to

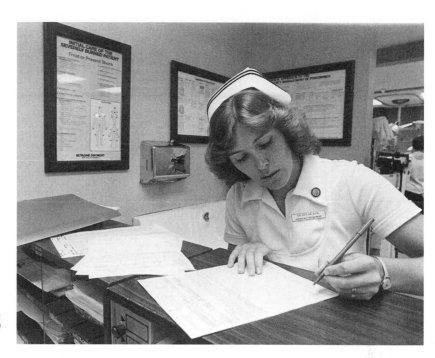

More and more of the professional nurse's time was consumed by documentation and administrative routine.

deliver high-quality medical care. Psychological needs of the patient, however, were not met as physicians concentrated their energies on biologic aspects of diagnosis and treatment and referred the patient from one specialist to another, leaving little or no time to deal with the patient's psychosocial problems.

The nurse of the 1960s was imbued with the concept of comprehensive patient care during her educational program but found on graduation that time and system constraints made it difficult, if not impossible, for her to fully meet the psychosocial needs of her patients. Sometimes even physical needs had to be ignored because of limited staff. Following in the trend that had been existent since the early 1950s, the professional nurse's time was increasingly being consumed with administrative routine. Many of the nurse's traditional duties had been delegated to licensed practical nurses, to nurses' aides, and to a host of newly developed specialized health care workers, such as respiratory therapists. Fragmented nursing and medical care prevailed, and the patient suffered the consequences. Furthermore, as nurses began to be offered fewer opportunities for direct patient care and clinical decision making, their personal satisfaction diminished. Many nurses felt a need to reclaim their professionalism in patient care and to reestablish the right and the opportunity to make, and act on, clinical decisions.

NEED FOR ROLE REALIGNMENT

The gradual evolution of the nurse's role strained her traditional relationship with the physician. Many physicians seemed unaware of nursing's move toward professionalization, or, if they were aware, they often ignored it in their working relationships with nurses. To fulfill the component of a profession, the professional person had to exercise independent judgment within his or her work; the function of professional education was to prepare the person to exercise such judgment. But many physicians still expected nurses to behave only as obedient extensions of their own professional judgment. The fiction seemed to be that the nurse was just the physician's helper.

So on the one hand, nursing schools and professional nursing associations reinforced the nurses' self-image of an autonomous, professional person, sharing with substantial equality in appropriate judgments about health care. Yet, on the other hand, physicians, reinforced perhaps by neglect of the study of nursing, if not by contrary indoctrination within their professional education, ignored or controverted this image of the professional person and colleague that many nurses presented. The results were inner tension within nurses and resentment, if not open conflict. The physician generally had little interest in seeing the optimal use of the full potentialities and skills of the nurse. He wanted an assistant who would do what he told her to do. The physician wanted to make use of an extra pair of eyes and ears and hands, but he was not concerned with developing a pattern of work that would allow the maximum combined output of a nurse and himself to achieve better health care for patients.

There was general agreement that the health care delivery system must be massively reorganized to increase efficiency and control soaring costs. In 1967, the Report of the National Advisory Commission on

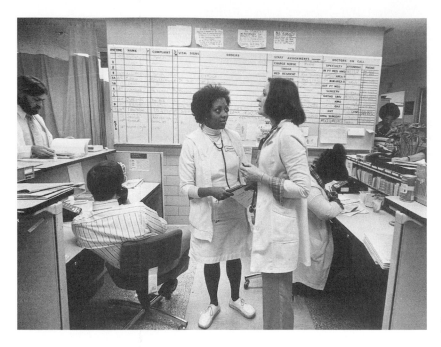

The thought of nurses exercising their own professional judgment unsettled some physicians.

Health Manpower summarized the case for reorganization:

> Many of the serious problems discussed in this Report arise from the lack of an organizational framework for the multitude of disparate

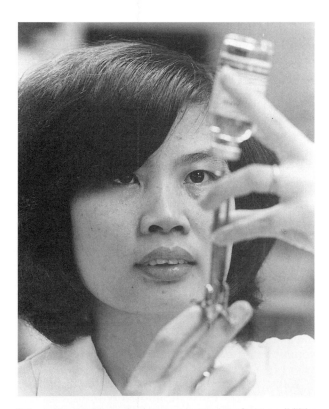

Role realignment brought the nurse a new set of responsibilities and degree of autonomy.

elements which provide medical care. Close cooperation and coordination among them is rare, and duplication of effort and actual conflict are all too common. Unfortunately, consumers of health care are unable to make the informed judgments required to assure an effectively operating market, and the sense of responsibility of most health professionals takes the form of concern for the individual patient rather than for society as a whole. As a result, there is limited effort to assure that resources are effectively coordinated and applied where they will be most useful.

In spite of the great complexity of modern medical care, independent practitioners and institutions continue to dominate the system. Individual practice has survived in medicine because it has features which are attractive both to the physician and to the public. We appreciate the advantages of independence but we are concerned about some of its associated disadvantages. Inadequate communication, coordination, and control links among practitioners and institutions contribute to gaps in quality and distribution, as well as to the inflation of medical costs.[7]

The years from the mid-1960s to the early 1970s, dominated by the domestic and foreign conflicts brought about by the Vietnam War, were years of controversy for the nursing profession as well. The issue of medical care for the aged saw the ANA clash with the AMA, while the ANA position paper on education for nursing brought to a crisis the deep-seated dispute over the future role of traditional hospital diploma programs. Although Congress accelerated its efforts to increase the supply of nurses, shortages continued unabated as the enlarged arena of health care created thousands of new nursing jobs.

REFERENCES

1. American Medical Association, House of Delegates, *Proceedings of the 105th Annual Session of the House of Delegates, June, 1957* (Chicago: The Association, 1957), pp. 15–24.
2. "Taking a Stand," *American Journal of Nursing*, vol. 59 (September 1959):1245.
3. *Congressional Record*, July 9, 1965.
4. "American Nurses' Association's First Position on Education for Nursing," *American Journal of Nursing*, vol. 66 (March 1966):515–517.
5. Ibid., pp. 516–517.
6. National League for Nursing, *Study on Cost of Nursing Education. Part I. Cost of Basic Diploma Programs* (New York: The League, 1964), pp. 1–7.
7. U.S. President, National Advisory Commission on Health Manpower, *Report of the National Advisory Commission on Health Manpower* (Washington, DC: Government Printing Office, 1967), vol. 1, p. 72.

20

NURSING IN TRANSITION
The Growth of the Health Care Industry

As the 1970s dawned, health care was the third largest industry in the United States. Along with a rise in the demand for medical services and a steady increase in the costs of those services, the number of workers employed in health services had grown at a rapid pace. As the 1970s opened, about 4.3 million persons were working in hospitals, convalescent institutions, physicians' and dentists' offices, or other health care facilities. By 1979 their number had grown to more than 6.7 million, an increase of 55%, whereas during the same period the total work force grew by only 23%. Median earnings of wage-and-salary workers in health services, however, were below the all-industry average throughout the decade. For full-time hospital employees (including staff nurses), median usual weekly earnings were 86% of the national average in 1979, up from 82% in 1970. In other segments of the health services industry, average wage-and-salary earnings remained at about three quarters of the all-industry average.

Hospitals employed most health service workers throughout the decade, with 3.7 of 6.7 million in 1979. However, the fastest employment growth was in other segments of the industry. Although employment in hospitals increased by 37% between 1970 and 1979, it nearly doubled in the rest of the industry. As a result, hospitals (with 62%) accounted for a smaller proportion of all health-industry workers in 1979 than in 1970. Employment rose at a less rapid rate in hospitals than in other segments of the industry because of decreases in the average length of a patient's stay, a lower birthrate (although childbirth remained the major reason for hospitalization in nonfederal short-stay hospitals, total maternal deliveries declined), and a growing substitution of ambulatory or outpatient care for hospital inpatient care. Outpatient visits increased by 62% between 1970 and 1979, compared with a 17% rise in inpatient admissions over the same period. The closing of many long-term hospitals (where patients stay an average of 30 days or more), especially government-owned

psychiatric facilities, also slowed the demand for hospital workers. Although the total number of beds in short-term hospitals (where patients usually stay fewer than 30 days) increased by about 10% during 1970–1979, the number in long-term hospitals decreased by 40%, as more of their patients were treated in outpatient facilities.

Hospitals in the 1970s were fairly well established and comfortable in their roles and missions. The main business of hospitals was to provide acute inpatient care, and the axiom that "a bed generates its own demand" was widely accepted. Hospitals were relatively independent of their external environment and could focus their planning efforts internally. In general, hospitals could reasonably function as they wanted, with a high degree of control over their own destinies. Hospitals attempted to meet the perceived health needs of their communities, but a hospital expected that it would provide services, programs, and facilities and that the public usually would accept whatever the hospital management decided was an appropriate scope of services.

THE FRUITS OF BIOMEDICAL RESEARCH

Since World War II, enormous strides had been made in biomedical research. Advances in physical, chemical, and engineering technology were quickly adapted for use in the biomedical fields and yielded extraordinary results in a better understanding of biologic processes, the analysis of various diseases, and the development of surgical and nonsurgical methods of patient care. In this short period, scientific breakthroughs, such as the development of cardiopulmonary bypass, open correction of congenital cardiovascular diseases, renal transplantation, replacement of arteries by graft, intravenous hyperalimentation, prosthetic heart valves, hemodialysis, microneurosurgery, total hip replacement, chemotherapy, development of compression plating for

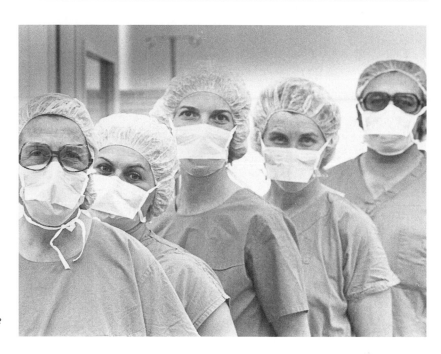

The number of active RNs skyrocketed in the 1970s.

fractures, and numerous other techniques, considerably alleviated the suffering of millions of human beings and prolonged life far beyond the expectations of three decades earlier. If one added to this list the development of antibiotics and antituberculosis drugs, the discovery of a polio vaccine, steroids and other hormones, and recent advances in immunology, the enormous impact of biomedical research on the lives of the American people was strikingly obvious.

Medical science had achieved spectacular successes, particularly in surgery, organ transplantation, the use of anesthetic agents, the development of oral contraceptives, the treatment of certain forms of cancer, and the use of psychopharmaceutical drugs in the treatment of mental disorders. These advances of modern medicine, however, had been made at a cost, for they all had side effects, some of which were serious. Moreover, these successes, which greatly increased the expectations of the patient, were partially responsible for the dilemma of modern medicine. Not only had the public conditioned itself to expect, quite unrealistically, a magic solution to every medical problem but also medical costs had skyrocketed as a result of technologic advances.

The dominant medical ideology in the United States in the 40 years after World War II was one that focused on cure rather than prevention and was driven by a view of the body as a machine, hospitals as repair shops, and physicians as master mechanics. It was a view that saw cost as no barrier and, to a certain extent, preferred to ignore the common or mundane in pursuit of the technical or engineering challenge. The 1970s witnessed the rapid expansion of chemotherapy, electronic fetal monitoring, renal dialysis, open-heart surgery, organ transplants, intensive care units, and computerized scanners. The initial outlay for such technology was extremely expensive. Moreover, once in place, additional personnel and other resources were needed for its operation and maintenance. Although new sophisticated machines dramatically improved hospital patient treatment and reduced diagnostic costs by shortening hospital stays and reducing the amount of exploratory surgery, lack of coordination in hospital facility planning resulted in expensive duplication and underutilization of services and equipment and hence increased hospital costs. The rate of obsolescence of such machines was very high; their life span was about 5 years, and they had very low resale value. Nevertheless, purchases of such equipment grew.

NURSING EDUCATION

As of 1982, there were 1432 programs of nursing education preparing their graduates for licensure as registered nurses: 288 leading to a diploma, 742 to an associate degree, and 402 to a baccalaureate degree. These numbers reflected a trend in nursing education toward preparation in academic institutions, with a corresponding decline in the number of hospital-based diploma programs. The steady decline in the number of diploma programs from 908 in 1960 to 288 in 1982 was the consequence of several social and economic factors.

The 1950s and 1960s witnessed marked efforts by hospital-based diploma programs to improve the quality of their educational programs. For example, many of the basic science courses, previously taught by nursing school faculty, were obtained instead through contractual arrangements with colleges and universities, and increased hours of classroom instruction reduced

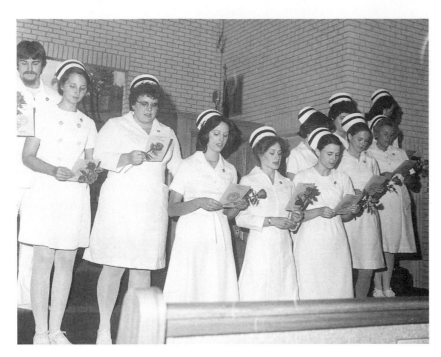

Hospital diploma programs improved in quality.

the amount of time spent by students in providing nursing service. As a result, the character of hospital-based programs became more general, preparing students for entry into the labor market as opposed to preparing them primarily for service in the hospital offering the training. To staff patient units, hospitals resorted to employing more registered nurses. The increased costs of providing an educational program coupled with the expense of staffing patient services made operation of hospital-based programs costly. Ultimately, a proportion of these costs was borne by the patient either directly or indirectly through third-party reimbursement mechanisms. Costs associated with operating educational programs in institutions whose primary mission was service precipitated the massive closing of hundreds of hospital-based programs. During the 1970s, the number decreased at a rate of approximately 30 to 40 programs each year. This drop reflected the preference of all students, including those whose career choice was nursing, for enrollment in programs that awarded academic credit. The decline was also attributable to the costliness of operating an educational program in a hospital in which income for the operation of the school was largely derived directly or indirectly from patient revenues.

As was true in the past, the only substantial source of money to carry the cost of hospital nursing education was patient fees, most of which were paid by insurance carriers. Acceptance of the principle of separating patient and education costs intensified, and new sources of financial support for hospital nursing schools had to be sought. Limits placed on allowable expenses by third-party reimbursement agencies probably had a greater impact on closing hospital nursing schools than any other single factor. A great

deterrent to the opening of new baccalaureate programs was their operating costs. Nursing programs were much more expensive to the college or university than were liberal arts or teacher education programs. They required a large number of laboratory courses in the physical and biologic sciences as well as close supervision in clinical courses that involved the care of sick people in hospitals and clinics, where patient safety mandated a low faculty–student ratio of about 1 to 10. Although innovative uses of educational technologies had been adapted to the needs of nursing programs, there was no substitute for supervised high-quality clinical practice.

Enrollment in baccalaureate programs increased substantially, however, reducing somewhat the reservoir of students from which hospital-based programs previously recruited. New baccalaureate programs, especially in public colleges and universities, were established in response to students' interest in a type of nurse preparation that combined general and professional education. In such educational linkages, affiliation agreements between universities and hospitals generally constituted legal arrangements that allowed academic units to pursue the placement of nursing students at either local hospitals or other health care agencies for clinical experience and education. The ties created by the affiliations often were strong and were essential to the fulfillment of the mission of both the university and the hospital or other health care agency. Hospitals that formerly offered their own nursing education programs moved to participate in affiliation agreements with colleges and universities for educational purposes.

Nursing education became increasingly integrated into academic settings during the late 1960s and early

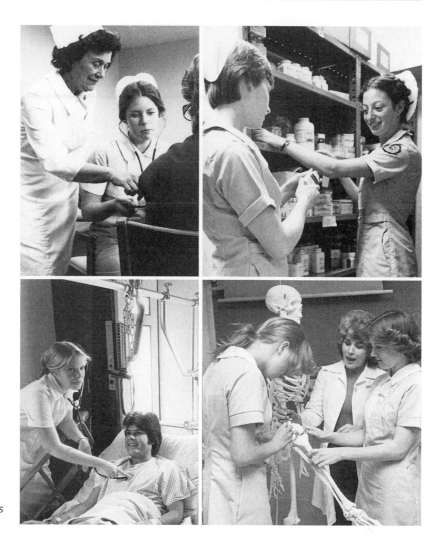

The high cost of nursing education programs slowed development in colleges.

1970s. The pool of nurses with baccalaureate degrees from high-quality college and university programs grew steadily. The number of nurses with master's and doctoral degrees, although still small compared with those in other professions, climbed sharply. Nursing became deeply involved in theory development and testing and in clinical research. A growing pool of well-educated nurses held powerful, well-paid, policymaking positions in health care service and educational institutions as well as in state and federal government agencies. As nursing matured, a growing segment of the profession saw itself as entirely different from the nurse of the bygone era: the dedicated, physician-dominated graduate of the past who accepted the widespread assumption that nursing was a lesser profession than medicine and entirely subservient to it.

GRADUATE EDUCATION FOR NURSES

Graduate programs in nursing also grew rapidly during the 1970s. Such study was undertaken at an institution of higher learning that offered major programs leading to the awarding of a master's or doctoral degree. Graduate education in nursing included specialization in a clinical area of interest and mastery of knowledge in that area as well as preparation in a functional role, such as teaching, administration, or research. Programs were designed to prepare nurses who would be capable of improving nursing practice and education through the advancement of nursing theory and science.

The roles for which nurses required graduate preparation included clinical nurse specialists, nurse practitioners, administrators, and teachers and researchers in nursing service and nursing education. The master's-prepared clinical nurse specialist was used by health care institutions and agencies to promote proficiency and effectiveness in clinical nursing. These nurses had knowledge and skills in a clinical field that allowed them to care for patients and their families who were experiencing health problems, such as patients in cardiac intensive care units or patients who had a terminal illness and were dying.

There were also nurse specialists in community health and in the care of the elderly. Clinical specialists

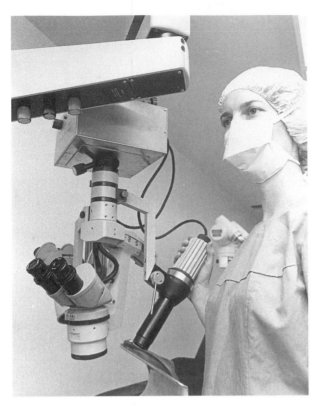

Advances in biomedical research had enormous consequences for patient care technology.

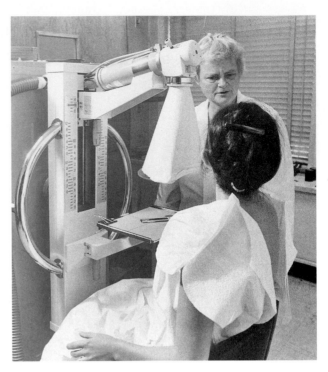

Medical science conceptualized the body as a machine and used sophisticated technologies in its repair.

provided expert care to patients who presented health problems and required modes of care consistent with specialized preparation. They were also resource persons to other nurses, physicians, students, and their clients and collaborated with these other providers in determining appropriate care and in resolving the patients' problems. Clinical specialists practiced interdependently with physicians and assumed authority and responsibility for the clinical practice of nursing in their area of expertise. Considerable evidence existed regarding the effectiveness of the clinical nurse specialist as a provider of high-quality care.

The importance of well-prepared nurse administrators became increasingly obvious during the 1970s. A 1977 study of approximately 7000 hospitals by the American Society for Nursing Service Administrators revealed that 46% of nursing service administrators held a diploma as their highest educational credential; 2.5% held an associate degree and another 23.6% a baccalaureate degree. Only 28% had preparation at the master's or doctoral level, the generally accepted level for management in nursing, as in other fields of endeavor. This was especially striking in considering that during 1979 the median salary of the top nurse administrator was $45,000 and that it was estimated to cost a hospital $50,000 to $55,000 a year to induce a top hospital nursing administrator to leave another institution.

The need for advanced preparation for the role of nurse administrator was underlined by the fact that the nursing service department was the largest single unit within the hospital. A study by Hospital Administrative Services, a division of the American Hospital

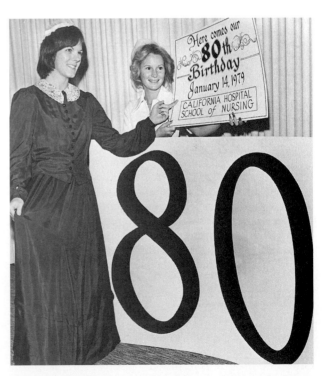

By the late 1970s, the future of diploma programs was increasingly doubtful.

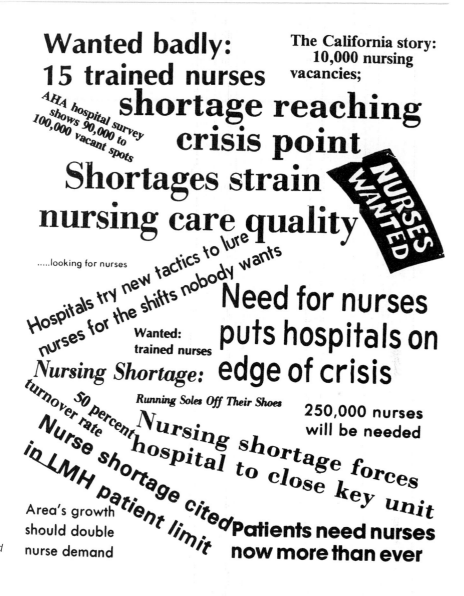

Wanted badly: 15 trained nurses

The California story: 10,000 nursing vacancies;

AHA hospital survey shows 90,000 to 100,000 vacant spots

shortage reaching crisis point

Shortages strain nursing care quality

NURSES WANTED

.....looking for nurses

Hospitals try new tactics to lure nurses for the shifts nobody wants

Wanted: trained nurses

Need for nurses puts hospitals on edge of crisis

Nursing Shortage:

turnover rate *50 percent*

Running Soles Off Their Shoes

250,000 nurses will be needed

Nurse shortage cited Nursing shortage forces hospital to close key unit

in LMH patient limit

Area's growth should double nurse demand

Patients need nurses now more than ever

Headlines of 1978 documenting the need for new nurses.

Association, reviewed data from more than 2000 hospitals to determine the relationship between salary and nonsalary costs in various departments. The study results showed that the nursing departments had the highest proportion of salary costs (95%). The well-educated nurse administrator of the 1980s, who was responsible for the most labor-intensive service provided by the hospital, was becoming extremely important in the cost-effective management of hospitals. The hospital nurse administrator was in transition from a time when her performance was measured solely by the quality of patient care to that of being evaluated on how well the nursing staff contributed to the hospital's productivity.

The importance of a nurse administrator to a facility's viability was a key factor inasmuch as the quality of nursing care could make or break a hospital's public image. In communities with competing hospitals with roughly equal facilities, the nursing director's effect on the nursing staff and how it dealt with patients and physicians could be the deciding factor in keeping hospital occupancy rates high. In some larger hospitals, even head nurses were required to have a master's degree. Consequently, graduate programs in nursing services administration (often with the cooperation of the school of nursing and the school of business administration) constituted one of the most important new graduate programs that a university could mount.

Nurse faculty in nursing schools as well as nurse researchers located in either universities or health care agencies also required graduate nursing education. The shortage of nurses prepared for these roles had greatly inhibited the quality education of nurses as well as the advancement of nursing knowledge to improve patient care. When nursing faculty did not measure up to the general university standards for promotion and tenure in terms of education, scholarly endeavors, and teaching, the very foundation of nursing education was jeopardized, because budgetary considerations sometimes resulted in severe cuts or even in the elimination of the school.

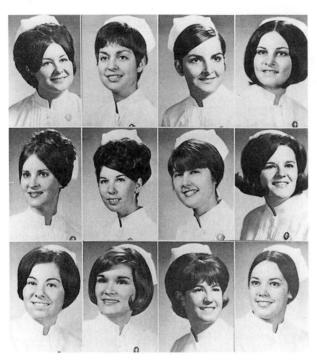

Nursing education became increasingly integrated into academic settings during the late 1960s and early 1970s.

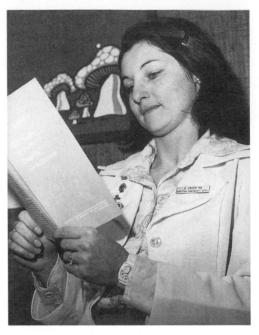

Clinical nurse specialists required graduate preparation.

NEED FOR NEW NURSE PRACTICE ACTS

Unlike the medical licensure laws, which had originally been necessary to combat widespread quackery, state licensure statutes for nursing personnel were not enacted to correct abuses of independent, entrepreneurial practice. Instead, they usually provided "friendly" regulation. Enacted with the cooperation of the nursing profession itself, they were designed to protect the regulated personnel and the public from unqualified, unethical practitioners. The forms of licensure, however, were generally similar to those for medical practice, except that in 20 states, licensure was permissive or optional rather than mandatory.

In 1970, every state licensed professional nurses. Whereas permissive licensure statutes merely prohibited unlicensed professional nurses from using the title "RN" or otherwise claiming to be licensed, mandatory licensure statutes established a precise definition of a licensed nurse and barred all unauthorized persons from nursing practice. By ensuring minimum personnel qualifications, mandatory licensure had the obvious advantage of facilitating resolution of scope-of-practice and delegation problems. Objection to it came chiefly from nurse employers, who feared that the loss of practicing unlicensed nurses would cause serious personnel shortages.

Even in those states where licensure was mandatory, the nursing practice acts were filled with exemptions from licensure requirements. Throughout the 51 jurisdictions, there were at least 13 different exemptions to the statutory definitions. Gratuitous nursing services were exempted from licensure in 46 jurisdictions; care provided by domestic servants was exempted in 23 states. Other exemptions included those for emergency care, federal employees, nursing students, recent graduates, nurses licensed in other states pending passage of the licensure examination, nurses licensed in neighboring states with overlapping practices, nursing in special facilities, services performed by auxiliary personnel, nursing under physicians' orders, and, in one state, nursing performed in a licensed facility.

In 1973, the efforts of the New York State Nurses' Association were instrumental in the passage of a revised nurse practice act that recognized nursing as an autonomous profession. This act distinguished between nursing practice and medical practice and described nurses' independent functions and defined nursing as "diagnosing and treating human responses to actual or potential health problems through such means as case finding, health teaching, and counseling." This definition was significant, because it established, for the first time, a statutory authority for the practice of nursing.

Owing to bitter opposition from the state medical society and the state hospital association, the new practice act for New York State was passed only after a prolonged struggle. Although the hostility of the medical society had been expected, that of the hospital association was surprising. At one point, it even issued a memorandum to state legislators charging that nurses were seeking unwarranted authority to practice medicine. Even though this memorandum temporarily killed the revised definition of nursing, the nurses persevered and finally obtained statutory independence for the nursing profession in New York State.

NEW NURSING ROLES

Expanding the role of the nurse could alleviate exorbitant health costs facing Americans. It was much less expensive for the public to train a nurse practitioner or midwife than it was to train a physician to perform the same services, and the quality of health care rendered could even be higher. It was especially important to raise the level of responsibility of the registered nurse, because combining the selected areas of expertise of nurses and physicians in the provision of primary health care would meet more of the health care needs of patients.

In the 1960s, numerous research studies had explored the potential for expanding and extending the nurse's role. Dr. John Hathaway of Yale University, for example, conducted a study of "The Role of the Nurse in the Preventive Services of a Student Health Clinic," which showed that a nurse in the college health service could safely replace the physician in taking the medical history. Charles Lewin, Barbara Resnik, and Thelma Ingles performed studies that lent additional credence to the view that traditional nursing roles could be expanded.

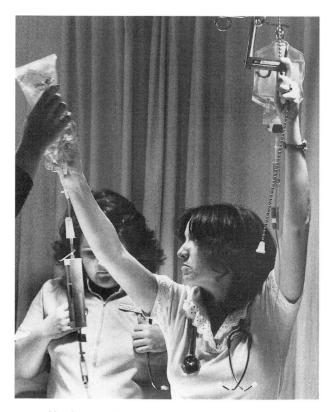

Nursing was ready to reach out for role expansion.

At the same time, the nursing profession, which was growing more concerned over the gaps in health care, began experimenting with the role of the clinical nurse specialist or nurse clinician. Emphasizing advanced nursing practice, in-depth knowledge, and a recognition of the full spectrum of patient needs, this new concept offered the nurse the opportunity to fully use her expertise. Unfortunately, the new role failed to achieve its objective of significantly upgrading the quality of patient care because hospital administrators and those who influenced them were frequently unwilling to pay for such services. Instead, hospitals often assigned the clinical nurse specialist with staff or head nurse responsibilities, which prevented her from discharging her clinician's role.

Another evolving role was that of the "nurse practitioner." This title was first used in a special demonstration funded by the Commonwealth Foundation at the University of Colorado in 1965. This demonstration was designed to prepare professional nurses to give comprehensive well-child care in ambulatory settings and to serve as a research study for future changes in traditional collegiate nursing programs. Nurses were taught to make sophisticated clinical judgments on conditions of acutely ill or chronically ill children and to perform adequately as primary practitioners in childhood emergencies.

The nurses received instructional theory and clinical practice in the assessment of the physical and psychosocial development of children; in the management of common childhood problems; in counseling and teaching patients; in the performance of certain developmental, immunologic, and evaluative procedures; and in the use of appropriate community resources. Emphasis on family dynamics and community cultural values formed an integral part of the program.

A study to evaluate the program, undertaken by the Bureau of Sociological Research at the University of Colorado, confirmed the value of the new role. Pediatric nurse practitioners were found to be highly competent in assessing normal and abnormal physical conditions in children and capable of caring for three fourths of the well and ill children coming to community health stations. Pediatricians in private practice who used pediatric nurse practitioners on their office staffs found that one third more patients could be seen.

By the late 1960s and early 1970s, the nurse practitioners had attained national visibility to consumers, other health professionals, and legislators. The nurse practitioner differed from the traditional nursing model in the autonomy of practice patterns, status in the provision of health care, and in relationship to patients, physicians, and health care agencies.

Actually, the concept of the expanded role for the nurse was not new. Some public health nurses had always engaged in many practices that belatedly came to be recognized as legitimate nursing functions. In

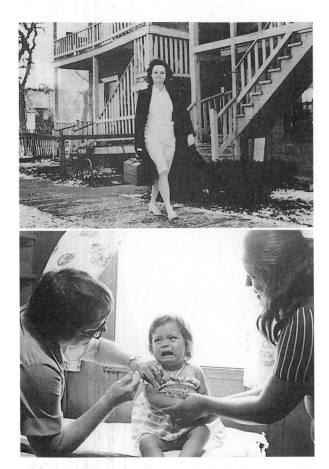

Nurse practitioners attained national visibility by the 1970s.

always respected their right to human dignity. And, as for reaching the disadvantaged, Lillian Wald went to live among them a good half-century before the Peace Corps and Vista were conceived.[1]

many public health agencies, especially in rural areas, nurses had traditionally functioned relatively independently, in collaboration with physicians. For example, since 1926, nurses in the Frontier Nursing Service in Kentucky had performed many functions commonly considered part of the physician's domain.

In a 1971 editorial, the editor of the *American Journal of Nursing* observed:

> The kind of health care Lillian Wald began preaching and practicing in 1893 is the kind the people of this country are still crying for. She demonstrated, with no need to rest on formal research, that nursing could serve as the entry point—not only for health care, but for dealing with many other social ills, of which sickness is only a part. She felt that nurses should go to the sick, instead of expecting the sick to come to them (and waiting for physicians to refer them); that care of persons in the home, especially children, was far more effective and much less expensive, except perhaps for those needing, to use her own word, "intensive" care; that the nurse was also a teacher, who respected the capacity of the disadvantaged to learn, just as she

This movement to expand the traditional nursing role gained speedy momentum in the early 1970s after Health, Education, and Welfare secretary Elliott Richardson requested a group of leaders in the field of health care to examine the possibilities of such an expansion. The resulting report, *Extending the Scope of Nursing Practice*, concluded that enlarging the nurse's role was essential for providing equal access to health services for all citizens. Despite widespread agreement among various health professionals that the scope of nursing practice should be extended, there was no consensus about how this could best be achieved. The committee admitted that "it would be naive to gloss over the fact that working relationships between physicians and nurses are often less than ideal, with results that are disadvantageous to both professions but, more important, to their patients." Moreover, many nurses were unprepared or reluctant to assume extended roles in patient care, and physicians were rarely trained to work with nurses who were qualified to function in such roles. "We are convinced, however, that attitudinal barriers can be lowered, educational deficiencies corrected, real and imaginary legal restrictions of nursing practice can be dealt with, and other impediments to the extension of nursing can be overcome," the committee said, urging establishment of curricular innovations by health education centers and increased financial support for nursing education.[2]

Although acknowledging that the implementation of expanded roles for nurses would require careful legal evaluation, the report noted that state licensure laws affecting nursing would not present an obstacle: "An orderly transfer of responsibilities between medicine and nursing has proceeded over many years, and there is no reason to assume that questions of law might impede this process."[3] The report also urged that the nursing profession undertake a study of recertification as a possible means of documenting new or changed skills among nurse practitioners and called for cost-benefit analyses and attitudinal surveys of providers and consumers to measure the effect of extended nursing practice on the health care delivery system.

In specifying how the roles of nurses could be extended, the committee pointed out that there were a number of primary care functions that many nurses were already performing and for which more nurses could be prepared. Such functions included (1) routine assessment of the health status of individuals and families; (2) provision of care during normal pregnancies and deliveries, provision of family-planning services, and supervision of health care of

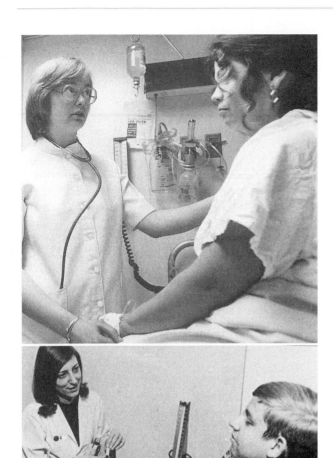

The federal government backed efforts to expand nursing into advanced practice.

Division of Nursing of the U.S. Public Health Service—supported these programs. The Nurse Training Act of 1971, which provided broadened authority for special project grants and contracts, specifically stated that funds could be used to "develop training programs for the training of pediatric nurse practitioners or other types of nurse practitioners."

During the 1970s, it was repeatedly demonstrated that nurse practitioners working cooperatively with physicians could increase the contribution that they both made to overall patient care. As a result, the nurse practitioner movement in the United States moved from a tenuous experiment as an alternate method of health care provision to one that received widespread acceptance by physicians and patients. Provision of care in ambulatory settings was revolutionized by the use of nurse practitioners who were effective, competent, and capable of providing high-quality, cost-effective care. By 1984, approximately 20,000 graduates of nurse practitioner programs were widely employed.

During the mid-1980s, most nurse practitioners were employed in the kinds of practices that the founders envisioned. They practiced in outpatient clinics, health maintenance organizations, health departments, neighborhood health centers, rural health centers, occupational health centers, schools, homes, and private medical practice settings.

Original intentions to supply primary care to world populations, however, had been hampered by

healthy children; (3) management of care for selected patients, including prescribing and providing care and making referrals as appropriate; (4) screening patients with problems requiring different medical diagnosis and medical therapy; and (5) consultation and collaboration with physicians, other health care professionals, and the public in planning and instituting health care programs.[4] Although the report observed that nurses had had a somewhat restricted role in clinical settings, it predicted that their increasing freedom from administrative functions would enable them to assume greater responsibility for the clinical management and care of patients.

The success of the initial programs and the financial support of federal and private funding agencies stimulated the development of training programs for the preparation of family nurse practitioners, school nurse practitioners, adult nurse practitioners, rural nurse practitioners, emergency nurse practitioners, geriatric nurse practitioners, obstetric/gynecologic nurse practitioners, and maternal nurse practitioners. Several federal agencies—Maternal and Child Health Service, Regional Medical Programs, and the

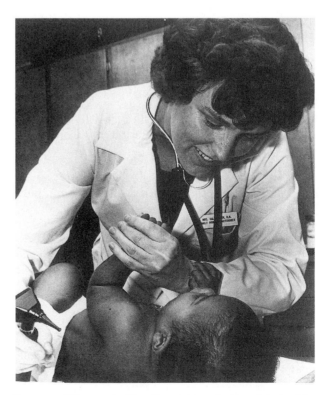

Nurse practitioners significantly overlapped generalist physician practice roles.

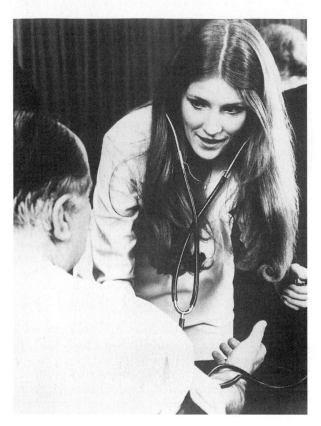

Nurse practitioners revolutionized care in various ambulatory settings.

the nonavailability of physician backup. Only about 12% of all nurse practitioners worked in remote or satellite clinics. In addition to the independent nursing functions of providing care, counseling, and teaching to individuals and patients, the nurse practitioners handled tasks formerly performed by physicians. Those functions included taking the medical history; performing a physical assessment; ordering laboratory and other diagnostic tests; making referrals to physical, social, and rehabilitative service agencies; and assuming responsibility for medical management in selected cases. Most nurse practitioners undertake routine and preventive health care, care of mild acute illnesses, and treatment of injuries in essentially well patients.

An increasing number of nurse practitioners was assuming responsibility for the chronically ill and elderly client. For example, at the Carle Clinic Association (a 125-physician group practice with five satellite clinics whose main campus is located in Urbana), the integration of expanded-role nurses (including nurse practitioners and clinicians) into a large multispecialty group practice in central Illinois had begun in 1978. A gradual change in the role and scope of nursing practice had produced a supportive, congenial relationship between the physicians and these nurses and a high degree of patient satisfaction.

The addition of a health maintenance organization in 1980 brought increased demands for service and provided impetus toward the development of expanded nursing roles. By 1984, there were 120 physicians and 27 expanded-role nurses practicing in Urbana, with more than 20 medical specialties represented. Nurse practitioners worked as primary care providers in collaboration with on-site physicians in many locations throughout the main complex and at the five satellite facilities.

Beginning in 1971, when Idaho became the first state to authorize an expanded role for registered nurses, all states except Ohio and Rhode Island had revised their nurse practice acts or had issued regulations to extend the functions that qualified nurses might perform. Several approaches had been used to accomplish this. First, there were the "nonamended statutes," where the state legislature had left the original definition of nursing unamended. Some states within this category had decided to interpret the statute liberally, and others had substituted words or phrases to accommodate more autonomous functions, especially diagnosis and treatment.

Second, some states used amended new authorization statutes, where the state altered the statute by inserting clauses or completely redefining nursing practice to include the expanded role. Third, several states used new administrative regulations to provide an approach where the state statute redefined nursing by allowing nurses to perform additional tasks such as may be authorized by appropriate state regulatory agencies, usually the state board of nursing and/or the state board of medicine.

In addition to redefining nursing, some states mandated additional acts necessary for functioning in the expanded role. Examples included formal education, continuing education, pharmacology courses, specified previous clinical practice, possession of a master's degree, and professional certification.

In the area of prescriptive authority, many nurse practitioners functioned under a delegable prescriptive authority and could prescribe according to authority found in the medical practice act. When functioning under a physician's delegation, the nurse could prescribe according to standing orders or protocols and provide a patient-specific alternative drug. The other type of prescriptive authority originated from specific mention in the state nurse practice act.

However, unless the authority was mentioned in the statute, prescribing by the nurse might be incompatible with state pharmacy and state medical practice acts and be invalid. "Dependent" or "independent" prescriptive authority was derived from nursing legislation. In dependent authority, the physician retained ultimate authority over what the nurse might prescribe, and the nurse's name had to be on the prescription blank. Nurses documented pharmacology courses, had a list of medications to be approved by a physician, and identified how often the physician would review the prescriptions they had written. Idaho was one of the first states to grant this type of authority.

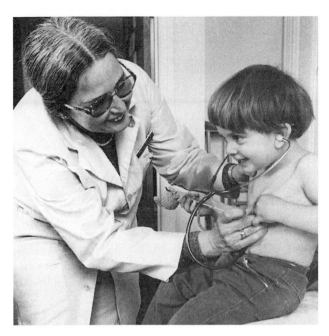

There was wide variation among states in relation to prescriptive authority for NPs.

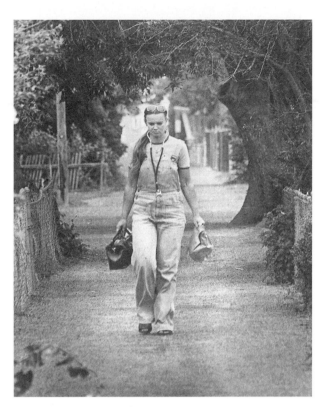

State medical societies bitterly opposed state legislation to expand the prescriptive authority of nurse practitioners.

In 1983, only Oregon and Washington gave nurses independent prescriptive authority—the ability to prescribe alone. In Oregon, qualified nurses prescribed drugs listed in a formulary. In Washington, certified registered nurses must have practiced for a year as such and have had at least 30 additional hours of pharmacology education. The nurse practitioners had dependent or independent prescribing authority in approximately 16 states. In addition, they could recommend nonprescription drugs.

Barriers affected the legislative processes that define nursing practice. In some locations, bitterness among nurses, physicians, and other health care providers centered on the debate about how much independence nurses should be allowed. Many nurse practitioners believed that physicians expected them to perform many more independent functions than the physicians were willing to legally support in nurse practice acts. Some nurses wanted an independent role in the primary care of selected patients, and others did not want the responsibilities associated with greater independence. In 1984, lawsuits were in progress in several states against nurses accused of practicing medicine without a license, even though the nurses functioned within the realm of their job descriptions.

Nurse practitioner legislation under consideration in New York in 1983 and 1984 became the focal point of a particularly heated debate. Under the proposed bill, the responsibilities of nurse practitioners would include the "diagnosis of illness or other physical conditions and performance of therapeutic and corrective measures." The law would also allow nurse practitioners to prescribe certain medications. According

to the Medical Society of the State of New York, which was vehemently opposed to the bill, no other state "has ever proposed, let alone enacted, a nurse practice law which even approaches the present proposal in terms of the scope of the approved practice and the lack of a defined nurse-physician relationship." The medical society maintained that the bill not only failed to specify a minimum program of study for the nurse practitioner, but also that its definition of nursing was virtually "indistinguishable from the present statutory definition of the practice of medicine." As one observer noted, "Ten years ago a nurse practitioner was someone who practiced nursing, but in the current context, it is someone who is a quasi-doctor." Nevertheless, an editorial by the *New York Times* supported the legislation, with suggestions for only minor changes in language.[5]

NURSING AND MEDICAL TECHNOLOGY

The importance of the nurse in the provision of patient care increasingly faces the challenge of medical technology. Every year, hundreds of new technologies enter the hospital, including procedures, devices, drugs, and instrumentation. Although many of these technologies contribute to the improvement of patient care, their benefits are sometimes more apparent than real. Invisible indicators of alleged benefits and costs are associated with the "high tech," but the identification of the benefits and costs derived from the "high touch" of nursing is often absent from policy considerations.

Before the 1960s, medical technologic advances contributed substantially to reducing medical costs, because they reduced the amount of care required to treat patients with tuberculosis, typhoid fever, diphtheria, rubella, lobar pneumonia, and poliomyelitis. As medical advances developed cures for these infectious diseases, more people survived long enough to develop degenerative diseases, such as heart disease and arthritis, that were costly to treat. During the 1960s and early 1970s, new technologies, such as renal dialysis, cancer chemotherapy, and open-heart surgery, achieved dramatic effects in particular cases but made only marginal improvements in general indexes of health. Whereas the earlier advances tended to be physician saving, the later ones were characteristically physician using.

The intensive care unit was the hallmark of the modern hospital of the 1970s and 1980s. Intensive care was and is in large part an organizational innovation, built on the simple idea that critically ill patients need close observation, constant nursing, and quick action in a crisis and that the most efficient way to provide this kind of care is not to disperse these patients throughout wards, but to bring them together in one place with the most sophisticated equipment and highly trained people in the hospital. Historically, intensive care has been the natural consequence of new methods of patient monitoring and life support and the stimulus for their invention.

Intensive care first appeared about the time of the Second World War in the form of the postoperative recovery room. Located near the operating rooms, the recovery room was a place where patients who had just undergone surgery were cared for until they had come safely through the anesthesia and the immediate aftereffects of the surgery itself. In 1951, only about 20% of all community hospitals with 100 beds or more had recovery rooms. In the manner typical of hospital technologies, recovery rooms spread first and fastest through the largest hospitals and more slowly through successively smaller ones. By the early 1960s, virtually all hospitals of more than 100 beds reported recovery rooms.

With its strong appeal to common sense, the philosophy of intensive care quickly found wider application. The average hospital saw many patients during the course of a year who were in critical condition. Many of them were suffering from heart attacks or other coronary conditions. Suicide attempts, severe asthma, gastrointestinal bleeding, acute kidney or liver failure, and other such conditions appeared frequently. The development of new and more extensive types of surgery, particularly open-heart surgery, created a need for care of a much higher order and over a much longer period than was required by the usual surgical patient. The

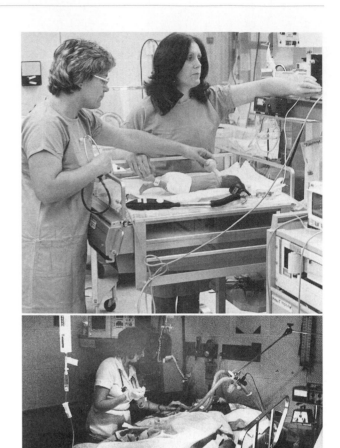

Intensive care became the hallmark of the modern hospital.

mixed intensive care unit (ICU), designed to accommodate all these patients, followed the recovery room by about a decade.

As new equipment and techniques for treating patients with heart conditions appeared—the defibrillator, the pacemaker, anticoagulant therapy, and others—a new unit was created specifically for these patients. In 1962, the first coronary care units (CCUs) were established independently, and almost simultaneously, in at least three urban medical centers in North America. Evidence was accumulating to show that irregularities in heart rhythm often preceded more serious crises in the coronary patient, and the hope was that by watching closely for these irregularities and trying to correct them at once, the nursing staff of the unit could reduce the death rate from heart attacks. By 1976, most hospitals with 300 or more beds had separate CCUs for heart patients, as did 57% of community hospitals with 200 to 299 beds, 29% of those with 100 to 199 beds, and 18% of those with fewer than 100 beds. Some hospitals had gone a step further and spun off intermediate coronary care units for patients believed to need the attention of people trained in the treatment of heart conditions but not as much attention as provided in the CCU.

The refinement and extension of intensive-care philosophy had not stopped with coronary units. The larger the hospital, the more likely it is to have additional units and subunits: separate units for medical and surgical patients, stroke units, respiratory units, renal units, burn units, neonatal units for the intensive care of newborns, and pediatric units. Although many patients benefited greatly from intensive care, several studies suggested that 20% to 25% of admitted patients were either "too healthy" or "too ill" to benefit from these unique services. Nevertheless, the number of admissions to ICUs continued to rise, as did the number of ICU beds, from a handful in the 1970s to more than 66,000 in 1984. With the addition of these beds came bigger bills, triple the number of laboratory tests given on the hospital floor, and more consultations with specialists. Although ICU beds made up 6% of the total hospital beds, they accounted for 20% of all health care costs, an amount equal to 1% of the gross national product.

The health care community was becoming increasingly aware that medical costs must become

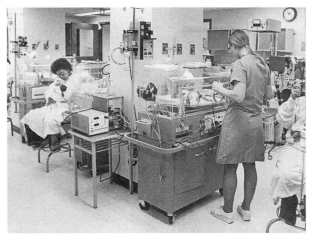

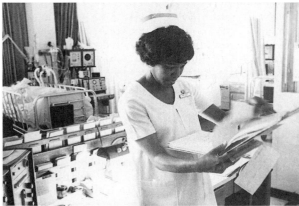

Although accounting for only 6% of all hospital beds, ICUs created 20% of all health care costs.

more efficient; one area that had been criticized for inefficiency was intensive care. Hospitals tended to concentrate their most skilled staff members in these units, reducing the experience of the general staff in caring for the very sick. The artificial atmosphere of an ICU could disrupt sleep, cause severe disorientation, and expose patients to the needless infection that could result from invasive monitoring, such as the use of heart catheters. Substantial savings could be achieved by better defining which patients to admit to these special units and which ones were in need of the monitoring equipment and the intervention procedures that they provide.

ECONOMIC AND GENERAL WELFARE

In the period before the Depression, various employers had effectively used several antilabor instruments developed before World War I. They used discriminatory hiring and firing practices against employees who had joined organized unions. The "yellow-dog contract" (which forbade an employee from joining a union) was commonly used to prevent union membership and as a basis for civil suits against unions that persuaded employees to violate their contracts. The most useful of all weapons was the injunction by which a court could forbid, at least temporarily, practices such as picketing, secondary boycotts, and the feeding of strikers by the union.

Section 7a of the National Industrial Recovery Act of 1933 contained the first positive assertion of the right of labor to bargain collectively but provided no means of enforcing this principle. Two years later, when the National Industrial Recovery Act was declared unconstitutional for reasons that had nothing to do with the labor section, Congress replaced Section 7a with the much more elaborate National Labor Relations Act of 1935, usually referred to as the Wagner Act after its sponsor, Senator Robert F. Wagner of New York.

The Wagner Act proceeded from the premises that inequality of bargaining power between individual employees and large business units depressed "the purchasing power of wage earners in industry" and prevented "stabilization of competitive wage rates and working conditions" and that denial of the right to self-organization created industrial strife.[6] The Wagner Act established the principle of collective bargaining as the cornerstone of industrial relations in the United States and imposed on management the obligation to recognize and deal with a legitimate labor organization in good faith. Furthermore, it guaranteed workers the right to form and join labor organizations, to engage in collective bargaining, to select their own representatives, and to engage in labor organization activities. The Wagner Act also outlawed a list of managerial practices that had had the effect of denying workers their rights. Henceforth, employers could not interfere with, restrain, or coerce employees in the exercise of their rights of self-organization and collective bargaining; dominate or interfere with the formation or administration of any labor organization or contribute financial or other support to it; encourage or discourage union membership by discrimination in regard to hiring or tenure of employment or condition of work, except such discrimination as might be involved in a closed-shop agreement with a bona fide union enjoying majority status; discharge or otherwise discriminate against an employee for filing charges or testifying under the act; refuse to bargain collectively.[7]

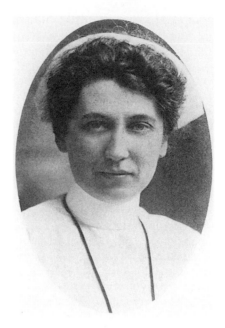

Shirley C. Titus. (Bentley Historical Library, University of Michigan.)

The Wagner Act established the three-member National Labor Relations Board to enforce the above-mentioned clauses. After conducting hearings to determine the validity of union complaints, the board could issue cease-and-desist orders to employers judged guilty of unfair labor practices. If employers did not comply with these orders, the National Labor Relations Board could turn to a U.S. Circuit Court of Appeals for enforcement. The board also had the power, on its own initiative or at the request of a union, to supervise a free, secret election among a company's employees to determine which union, if any, should represent the workers.

A decade later, in 1946, the American Nurses Association (ANA) took a step forward by adopting an economic security program, which endorsed state professional nurses' associations as exclusive representatives for their members in all matters affecting employment conditions and as their collective bargaining agents. According to the platform adopted at that time, the ANA was committed to obtaining wider acceptance of the 40-hour workweek with no decrease in salary, minimum salaries sufficient to attract and retain nurses of quality and to enable them to maintain standards of living comparable with those of other professions, and the expansion of nurses' professional associations as exclusive representatives for nurses in all questions affecting their employment and economic security. "Such a development," it was stated, "should be based on past successful experience of professional nurses' organizations in collective bargaining and negotiation."[8]

One of the main principles of this economic security program was its exclusive control by nurses. Nurses would represent themselves through state nurses' associations in collective bargaining with their employers. Immediately after acceptance of this principle, several state nurses' associations adopted programs and were fairly successful in representing their members in collective bargaining.

The most successful of these early efforts to obtain economic security occurred in California under the leadership of Shirley C. Titus, executive director of the California State Nurses' Association. A Cali-

fornia native, Titus was born in 1892 and spent her early years in San Francisco, where she received a diploma from St. Luke's Hospital School of Nursing in 1915. Immediately thereafter, she assumed the position of assistant principal of her training school. Two years later she went to Washington, DC, to work with Julia Lathrop as assistant in the Prevention of Infant and Maternal Mortality in the U.S. Children's Bureau. After World War I, she worked as assistant superintendent of nurses at Barnes and St. Louis Children's Hospitals.

In 1924, Titus entered Teachers College, Columbia University, where she earned a bachelor's degree in nursing in 1925. Immediately thereafter, she assumed the position of director of the School of Nursing and director of Nursing Services at the University of Michigan Hospital. Despite working long hours at this job, she still found time to pursue a master's degree in philosophy at Michigan, where she developed a deep sense of responsibility for the social and economic conditions of student and graduate nurses. This commitment inspired her to produce a flood of articles with titles such as "Is the Hospital Administrator Fulfilling His Responsibilities Toward His Nurses?" which advocated using public taxes to support nursing schools, and "The Pre-professional Education of the Nurse," which sought to explain why physicians objected to the establishment of minimum standards for nursing school admissions.

During her tenure as dean of the School of Nursing at Vanderbilt University from 1930 to 1939, Titus embarked on a campaign to realize some of her ideals. After becoming executive director of the California State Nurses' Association in 1940, she launched a vigorous campaign to improve the economic status of nurses. It was largely due to her efforts that the ANA economic security resolution won acceptance at the 1946 convention. Afterward, she made the following comment about this new nurses' movement:

> Although the workweek of all other workers has been markedly reduced during the past two or three decades, the professional nurse in many states today still works a forty-eight hour week or even longer. On the whole, because of long hours, the nurse's life is still pivoted on work, and this has tended to restrict her social horizon. Also, her low income has further restricted her social experience and her social outlook on life. Both organized medicine and the hospital have always sought to assume active and positive direction of nursing affairs in order that both nurses and nursing should function in a way that would best serve their special interests. These controls have prevented nurses from securing that background and experience which would have prepared them to live more fully and function more effectively in the present social scene. These controls have also seriously retarded and deflected the normal evolution of nursing from the status of a craft to that of a profession.
>
> Because the nurse spends most of her waking hours in an environment which is dominated by hospital management and the doctors, she has remained far more docile, if not actually subservient, than perhaps any other American worker. Hospital management and organized medicine have not only shaped in part the world of nursing but they have also conditioned the thinking of nurses. And the nurse has accepted the thinking of these two groups—especially in regard to her status, her function, and her social and economic welfare—with amazingly little demur or question.
>
> The result has been that during the last twenty-five or fifty years when other groups have been demanding their "place in the sun" and have been insistently and persistently striving to improve their economic world, nurses have continued to accept the status quo and to embrace the laissez-faire philosophy of life that rests on the principle that things as they are, however unsatisfactory and disagreeable they may be, must be accepted.
>
> As I have given thought to the situation, it has seemed to me that the nurse within the four walls of her job—and her job has practically constituted her whole waking life—has been like a sleeper who has slept serenely on while a great battle—a battle for human freedom and the rights of the common man—was being waged. But eventually the sleeper awakens.[9]

THE TAFT-HARTLEY ACT

During the postwar era, however, the fortunes of labor took a turn for the worse, and the hospital lobby succeeded in blocking the nurses' drive to secure greater economic benefits. In 1947, Representative Fred Hartley introduced into the House a bill to exempt from the provisions of the 1935 Labor Relations Act "institutions that qualify as charities under our tax laws," such as churches, hospitals, schools, colleges, and societies for the care of the needy. The only opposition to this proposal came from Representative Arthur Klein of New York, who objected to excluding charitable and educational organizations from the ranks of "employers." Although the number of workers who would thus be deprived of Wagner Act protection was not large, Klein considered it ironic to exempt organizations devoted to social welfare from bargaining with their own, often underpaid, employees. Despite his opposition, however, the bill passed the House and went to the Senate, where there was no comparable committee report or proposal. Instead, Senator Joseph Tydings of Maryland simply offered a floor amendment to release nonprofit hospitals from the restrictions of the Wagner Act. During the scant debate that ensued, Senator Tydings justified his amendment as "designed merely to help a great number of hospitals which are having very difficult times. They are eleemosynary institutions, no profit is involved in their operations, and I understand from the Hospital Association that this amendment would be very helpful in their efforts to serve those who have not the means to pay for hospital service." Senator Robert Taft then explained that his Labor and Public Welfare Committee "considered this amendment, but did not act on it, because we felt it was unnecessary. The committee felt that hospitals were not engaged in interstate commerce and that their business should not be so construed. We felt it would open up the question of making further exemptions. That is why the committee did not act upon the amendment as it was proposed."

The remainder of the debate, between Senators Glenn Taylor of Idaho and Joseph Tydings, was very brief:

> *Mr. Taylor:* What does the amendment do? Does it prevent hospitals' employees, particularly nurses, from organizing? Is that the sense of the amendment?
> *Mr. Tydings:* It simply makes a hospital not an "employer" in the commercial sense of the term.
> *Mr. Taylor:* Would nurses be prevented from organizing—they are poorly paid.
> *Mr. Tydings:* I don't think so. They [the hospitals] should not have to come to the National Labor Relations Board. . . . A charitable institution is a way beyond the scope of labor management relations in which profit is involved.

Mr. Taylor: These may not be profit-making institutions, but even so I feel that simply because an institution, even one like the Red Cross, is kept up by popular subscription, the professional workers being employees of the Red Cross should be permitted a decent living and should not be hamstrung in their efforts to obtain it.

Mr. Tydings: I agree with the Senator.[10]

The bill then passed the Senate. The conference committee accepted the Senate version, which became part of Section 2 of the National Labor Relations Act. Passage of the Taft-Hartley Act, with its provision exempting nonprofit hospitals from the obligation to bargain collectively, encouraged many employers to refuse to meet with their nurse employees to discuss working conditions or other matters affecting patient care. Some hospitals interpreted this exemption as a legal sanction for their *refusal* to engage in collective bargaining with nurses, a view that had been expressly denied on the floor of the Senate. At other times, hospitals seemed to regard the exemption as the equivalent of an outright prohibition of collective bargaining.

THE FIGHT FOR COLLECTIVE BARGAINING

As soon as this exemption became law, the ANA began efforts to secure its repeal. In 1949, two bills relating to the Taft-Hartley Act were introduced in Congress. The ANA presented testimony before the Senate Committee on Labor and Public Welfare, and ANA representatives personally contacted many influential senators of both parties. Both bills as well as a compromise proposal that finally passed the Senate would have repealed the exemption of nonprofit hospitals and included them in the provisions of an amended National Labor Relations Act. Unfortunately, the House of Representatives killed this compromise bill by failing to act on it before the adjournment of the 81st Congress.

Five years later, improvement of working conditions through strengthened economic security programs and extension of the Federal Social Security Act shared the spotlight as key planks in an 18-point platform adopted by the ANA at its 1954 convention in Chicago. More than 9400 registered graduate nurses and students witnessed the defeat of a motion that would have struck the phrases "collective bargaining" and "labor legislation" from a platform supposedly endorsing a stronger economic security program. In voting against the motion, the ANA's House of Delegates pointed out that the economic security program had too often been regarded as an emergency tool to be used only as requested by small groups of nurses in crisis situations. The House of

Delegates appealed to the states nurses' associations to organize movements for the improvement of personnel conditions for nurses.

In the following year, a study comparing the earnings and working conditions of nurses with those of other professional and nonprofessional groups amply demonstrated the inferior economic status of nurses. In 1955, the average gross monthly starting salary for a general-duty nurse amounted to $253, which included the estimated cash value of any maintenance items provided by hospitals. Nurses' incomes fell below those of accountants, draftsmen, teachers, social welfare and recreation workers, and librarians. In some cases, nurses' educational requirements and professional responsibilities exceeded those of higher-paid groups. Most startling was that the average factory worker earned about $70 more per month than the average nurse. Nursing also suffered in economic comparison with secretarial workers, who earned approximately $62 per month more than the average general-duty nurse. Besides lower salaries, nurses received far fewer benefits than most other employees and often worked longer hours, which in many cases surpassed the then-standard 40-hour workweek.

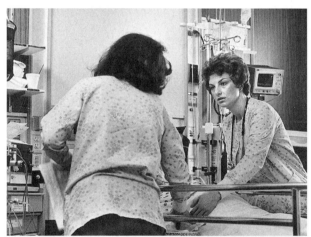

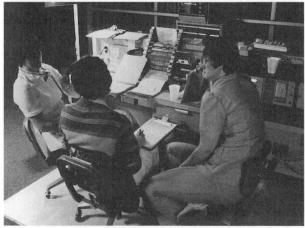

Nurses' wages were below those of comparable occupations.

Two years later, resolutions urging the amendment of state and national labor laws were adopted in Chicago at the 40th convention of the ANA. The House of Delegates unanimously passed a resolution advocating amendment of the Taft-Hartley Act of 1947 "to remove the exemption granted to nonprofit hospitals in order that the protections and benefits of the act can be extended without discrimination to hospital employees." Nonprofit hospitals had "relied on the exemption to refuse to meet salary and other demands of nurses over the bargaining table," the resolution stated. An accompanying resolution urging state associations to take similar action regarding state labor laws also passed unanimously.[11]

At that time, on the assumption that employers would deal with them fairly, the ANA publicly announced that nurses had voluntarily relinquished the right to strike. However, as Barbara Schutt, chairman of the Committee on Economic and General Welfare, pointed out to the delegates, many hospital administrators were refusing to discuss working conditions with nurses.

In 1959, the American Hospital Association House of Delegates approved a statement reaffirming the AHA position that voluntary nonprofit hospitals remain exempt from the provisions of the Taft-Hartley Act and from all laws requiring compulsory collective bargaining. This statement also reiterated the AHA position "upholding a strong and positive personnel policy in hospitals to provide for all hospital employees compensation, working conditions, and other personnel practices at least at levels prevailing for equivalent work in the community."[12] This position had previously been expressed in the AHA *Statement on Hospital Management-Employee Relations* of 1956.

A hospital wage survey conducted by the Bureau of Labor Statistics revealed that salaries for general-duty nurses in 1960 ranged from $65 per week in Atlanta to $89 per week in the Los Angeles area. The city average was $79.50 per week. Nurses earned $25 to $30 less per week than office, clerical, and maintenance crew employees in the 15 cities covered by the survey. Accounting clerks and secretaries with skills usually acquired in high school or on the job averaged $4 to $8 per week more than the general-duty nurse. Such hard economic facts provided little encouragement for prospective nurses.

The outlook was no more promising for the registered nurse who had obtained a baccalaureate degree. The highest salaries for female college graduates went to beginning chemists, mathematicians, and statisticians, who earned an average of $95 to $98 per week. Nurses with baccalaureate degrees commanded salaries identical to those for home economists, research workers, and therapists—approximately $78 per week. In contrast to those entering these other professions, however, most college-educated nurses were by no means untried beginners. After acquiring their basic nursing educa-

tion in diploma schools, they usually completed a year or more of nursing practice before starting college programs leading to degrees.

Inadequate levels of compensation obviously discouraged the practicing nurse from acquiring further education. Although the growing complexity of the health care delivery system and the expansion of medical knowledge made additional academic training imperative, such advanced study was usually beyond a nurse's financial means. Moreover, the slight salary differential hardly made this financial investment worthwhile. Significantly, even a director of nursing with administrative responsibility for all nursing care in a hospital earned only from $118 to $158.50 per week in the cities surveyed by the Bureau of Labor Statistics—only $59 a week more than a general-duty nurse.

REINVIGORATION OF ECONOMIC AND GENERAL WELFARE PROGRAMS

In 1960, the ANA continued to push its economic security program by approving a resolution introduced by the Michigan State Nurses' Association, the purpose of which was to initiate a strong public information campaign for the economic security program. In her call for action, Anne Zimmerman, chairman of the ANA Committee on Economic and General Welfare, urged the delegates to have "enough humility to acknowledge the economic poor health of the nursing profession and to continue to speak out courageously through our professional organizations to improve it." Supporting this position, Matilda Young, a member of Zimmerman's committee, urged the House of Delegates to fight for the elimination of "legislative discrimination against nurses." It was shocking, she said, that 40% of nongovernmental hospitals in the United States were not covered by the Old Age Survivors Insurance System. Arguing for collective bargaining, Young reminded the audience that the efforts of the ANA would be greatly facilitated "if each state nurses' association would make it clear to their congressmen that the exemption of nonprofit hospitals from the Taft-Hartley Act has created a most unfavorable climate."[13]

The proposed ANA platform for 1960–1962 was fortified by the retention of a plank committing the ANA "to assist nurses to improve their working conditions through strengthening economic security programs, using group techniques such as collective bargaining."[14] All attempts to amend the plank from the floor, including a proposed deletion of the words "using group techniques such as collective bargaining," were defeated after a heated debate.

During the 1960s, nurses' salary raises continued to lag behind general increases around the country. The Bureau of Labor Statistics' survey figures for 1963–1964 showed that teachers averaged $6325; secretaries, $5170; factory workers, $5075; and the general-duty nurse in nonfederal city hospitals, $4500.

NURSES ON STRIKE

In 1966, approximately 2000 dissatisfied nurses in 33 San Francisco Bay area hospitals resigned during a dispute over salary demands. This dispute was temporarily resolved when the hospitals and representatives of the California Nurses' Association agreed to submit the question of nurses' salaries to a fact-finding committee. This kind of militant action on the part of the nurses placed the California Nurses' Association in an untenable position. "If we put our foot down about the mass resignation technique, they would go ahead anyway," remarked an association executive. "We firmly believe that resignations on the part of nurses are a more serious step than strike," she added.[15]

Soon afterward, the board of directors of the California Nurses' Association broke with tradition and with the policy of the national organization by endorsing the strike as a weapon for attaining economic objectives. It was not an easy decision to make according to the associate executive director of the California Nurses' Association, A. Lionne Conta, who observed that there had been a "total change in the attitude of the nurses" in recent months. Referring to "powerful and active" unions in California, she noted, "We felt that if we did not take action, they [the nurses] would turn to other organizations."[16]

Nursing incomes improved somewhat in the late 1960s. A survey made by the Bureau of Labor Statistics in March 1969 reported an average hourly wage of $2.44 for nonsupervisory employees in nongovernmental hospitals, ranging from a high of $2.67 in the West to $2.13 in the South. National averages of earnings for a 40-hour week for selected occupations in nonfederal city hospitals on that date were as follows:[17]

Full-time general duty nurses	$141.00
X-ray technicians	120.50
Switchboard operators-receptionists	78.00
LPNs	99.00
Nursing aides	76.00

These figures could be compared with the $129.51 weekly average of all American production workers in the same year, 1969. Nurses achieved additional gains in starting salaries during the early 1970s, although the increases were moderate compared with the successes of the nation's school teachers. Nurses could not expect any substantial salary increments for longevity of service, even in the best-paying hospitals.

Because of the belief that nurses should be represented by their professional association rather than by outside labor unions, late in 1973 the ANA launched an aggressive campaign to organize the nation's 800,000 registered nurses. Several months later, in June 1974, 2 days before a record ANA conference crowd of more than 10,000 nurses gathered in San Francisco, 4400 members of the California Nurses' Association walked off their jobs at 43 Bay-area hospitals and clinics when contract negotiations broke down between the California Nurses' Association and Kaiser Foundation Hospitals, Affiliated Hospitals in San Francisco, and Associated Hospitals of San Francisco and the East Bay. Responding to the opportunity to dramatize the ANA's new cohesion and militancy, convention attenders manned picket lines and donned blue armbands in support of the striking nurses. "Take a striking nurse to lunch!" was the battle cry as convention goers lent moral and financial support to their picketing colleagues.

The San Francisco strike attracted national attention and focused interest on the issues involved in collective bargaining with health care agencies. The ANA's 980-member House of Delegates passed a resolution stating that "[the ANA] fully supports and encourages actions of the California Nurses' Association . . . in strike action" and that the walkout did not endanger "the safety and well-being of hospital patients." A fund was created for voluntary strike support donations.[18]

Six weeks later, on July 26, 1974, President Nixon signed into law amendments to the Taft-Hartley Act that permitted nurses in 3500 nonprofit hospitals to engage in collective bargaining. They joined employees in profit-making hospitals and nursing homes, which had come under National Labor Relations Board jurisdiction in 1967, and those in nonprofit nursing homes, which had come under board jurisdiction in 1970. Federal employees, including those in federal health care institutions, had had the right to bargain collectively since 1962, under provisions of an executive order signed by President Kennedy. Moreover, in 1967, the federal government had granted the ANA and its constituent state associations the right to represent registered nurses in Veterans Administration hospitals during collective bargaining. In August of that year, the Iowa Nurses' Association had signed the first contract with the Veterans Administration in Des Moines.

As soon as Congress repealed the exemption of nonprofit hospitals from provisions of the National Labor Relations Act in 1974, the ANA embarked on an energetic campaign to organize the nurses in the nation's hospitals. By raising additional sums of money, increasing the number of field workers, enlarging staff at its Kansas City headquarters, and conducting a series of educational collective bargaining programs for its 53 constituent state and territorial nursing associations, the ANA succeeded in greatly revitalizing its economic and general welfare program. Under the banner of "collective professional action," the ANA began striving for recognition as a distinct professional group and as the primary advocate for the patient. One year later, in 1975, the ANA groups represented 200,000 of the 800,000 practicing RNs, including 70,000 RNs for whom state nursing associations had negotiated 515 bargaining contracts.

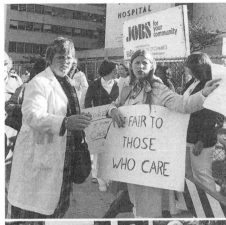
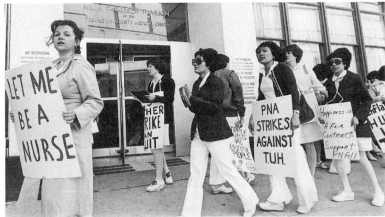
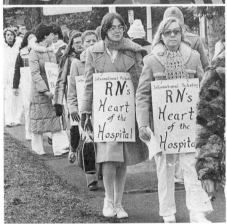
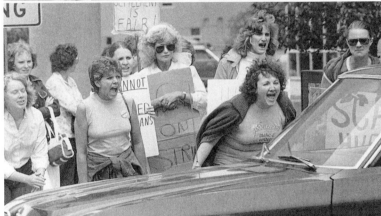

Nurse union activity was inspired by the women's movement.

Both the Taft-Hartley amendment and the women's liberation movement, which instilled in nurses a sense of worth as individuals and as professionals, promised to accelerate this process of change within the nursing profession.

NURSES AND NURSING HOMES

"Nursing home" is a generic term covering a wide variety of institutions providing health care of various levels to people with health problems ranging from minimal to very serious. The origin of nursing homes in the United States can be traced to the Social Security Act of 1935. Because of the tremendous public outcry against the public poorhouses of the Depression era, Congress stipulated that persons in public institutions should not receive old-age assistance funds. Such funds were still available, however, to the aged in private boarding homes. As a result there ensued a sharp increase in the number of boarding homes throughout America. After these homes began hiring nurses to care for the infirm aged, they were increasingly referred to as "nursing homes." Because physicians tended to overlook nursing-home patients, many of whom had been transferred as

chronic cases from hospitals, they imposed a heavy burden on nurses working in these homes.

The number of nursing-home employees increased 405% from 1960 to 1970. In 1970, about 215,000 (43%) were aides and orderlies, 7% were professional nurses, and 8% were licensed practical nurses. The annual turnover for nursing-home employees averaged 60%. In 1970, nursing homes employed a disproportionate number of aides (26% of the 830,000 national total), few licensed practical nurses (10% of the nation's 370,000), and a minuscule number of the nation's registered nurses (0.05% of 700,000). That same year, registered nurses received an average wage of $3.75 per hour and had a turnover rate of 71%.

There were many reasons for the limited number of professional nurses in nursing homes. Federal regulations required the presence of registered nurses in approximately 7300 skilled nursing facilities, and even then, with exceptions in rural areas, only one registered nurse was required to be on duty at all times. Significantly, about 90% of the nation's nursing homes were being operated as profit-making business ventures, in sharp contrast to the overwhelming nonprofit nature of short-term care facilities. Some nursing-home operators, intent on reducing

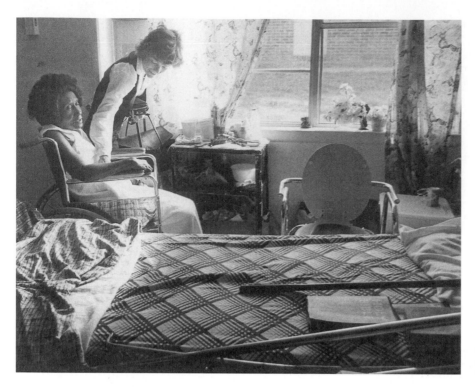

Aides rather than professional nurses provided the vast majority of nursing care in nursing homes.

costs and increasing profits, refused to hire more than the minimum number of nurses required by law. Instead, they sought to "make do" with unlicensed aides and orderlies, whom they paid only the minimum wage. Other reasons for the comparative absence of nurses in nursing homes included the poor image of these homes, wretched working conditions, low job satisfaction, inadequate wages, and few fringe benefits. At the same time, nursing schools and federal government programs had failed to stress geriatrics in nursing education.

Federal investigations disclosed that routine medical and nursing procedures, designed to ensure the maintenance and well-being of the patient, were not being carried out. A 1971 study of 75 nursing homes conducted by the Department of Health, Education, and Welfare revealed the following:

> Thirty-seven percent of the patients taking cardiovascular drugs (digitalis or diuretics or both) had not had a blood pressure reading in over a year, and for 25 percent of these there was no diagnosis of heart disease on the chart.
>
> Most of the patients reviewed were on one to four different drugs and many were taking from seven to twelve drugs; some were on both psychotropic "uppers" and "downers" at the same time.
>
> Revised treatment of medication orders had been written for only 18 percent of the patients in the past thirty days, and 40 percent had not been seen by a physician for over three months.

> Eight percent of the patients had decubitus ulcers, and 15 percent were visibly unclean.
>
> Thirty-nine percent of the patients reviewed were inappropriately classified and placed.
>
> No nursing care plans existed with respect to diets and fluids for 19 percent of the patients; personal care for 23 percent; activities for 14 percent; and individual treatment needs for 18 percent.[19]

By the end of the 1970s, there were approximately 18,300 nursing homes (including nursing care homes, personal care homes, and domiciliaries), with a total of 1,383,600 beds, serving about 1,287,400 residents annually. About 71% of these residents were female, 85% were 65 years of age and older, 58% were widowed, and 92% were white. The mean age was 78; the mean length of stay, 2.7 years; and the median stay, 1.6 years.

Expenditures for nursing-home care had soared from $480 million in 1960 to $31 billion in 1983 and were expected to reach $82 billion by 1990. Nursing homes were operated largely (95%) by privately owned organizations. Most of these (81%) were operated for profit.

Although many factors contributed to the rapid growth of nursing homes, the single greatest factor was the aging of the population. The proportion of the population age 65 and older had more than doubled from 5.4% in 1930 to 11.3% in 1980. This trend was expected to continue, nearly doubling again the proportion of persons older than age 65 to 20% by the year 2030. Within the older-than-65 age group, the growth spurt was even more accelerated for people older than age 75.

Medicaid had become the nation's primary payer of nursing-home care. Medicare and private insurance supported only a negligible proportion of nursing-home services, because the catastrophic cost of long-term institutional care often exceeded the financial resources of elderly persons. Within the Medicaid program, expenditures for nursing-home care represented the largest single expenditure category. Medicaid covered long-term care, but only for the elderly who had completely exhausted their financial resources. In 1984, state Medicaid programs were the largest purchasers of nursing-home care, providing more than one half of nursing homes' revenues.

About 60% of nursing-home residents were supported by Medicaid, either in total or as a supplement to their limited incomes. Medicaid set the rate paid by patients who received any Medicaid support. The elderly who became eligible for Medicaid through a "spend-down process" exhausted most of their assets. They had to pay most of their income toward the cost of care but were protected from nursing-home expenses that exceeded their income. Medicaid policies largely shaped the character of the nursing-home market—where homes were located, how many beds were supplied, and the type of care provided. A 1984 analysis indicated that some states clearly spent more Medicaid nursing-home dollars per elderly resident than other states. Even when state and local expenditures are adjusted for differences in nursing-home wages, the state spending the most for nursing-home services per elderly resident spent eight times as much as the state spending the least.

Most of the nursing care in nursing homes was given by personnel prepared at below the professional nurse level. Only 22% of nursing homes had a registered nurse on duty around the clock, and 71% of nursing personnel in skilled nursing facilities were aides, 14% were licensed practical nurses, and 15% were registered nurses. Nurses' aides, generally minimally prepared for their responsibilities, performed complex nursing tasks. Full-time registered nurses per 100 nursing-home beds ranged from 1.2 in Texas to 9.6 in Alaska. Registered nurses had little time to spend with patients—12.5 minutes of care per day in skilled nursing facilities assuming that professional time was entirely devoted to bedside care. Most of the registered nurse's time was taken up by administrative and supervisory functions. Aides constituted by far the largest proportion of nursing-service personnel in skilled nursing facilities and combined skilled-nursing and intermediate-care facilities. Licensed nurses were responsible for their supervision as well as for the direct care of patients, record keeping, and decisions about emergency medical situations, because physicians were rarely in attendance.

The assurance of quality nursing-home care was important for this vulnerable population. This was especially critical at a time when a patient's care needs might be increasing and becoming potentially more costly, while states, because of difficulties in financing their Medicaid nursing-home services, were trying to reduce the growth of their reimbursement rates. Attempted solutions to this problem were complex, and their effectiveness had yet to be determined. These attempts included providing reimbursement incentives to nursing homes to admit hospital backup patients, expanding nursing-home bed supply, and using excess hospital capacity for long-term care. All three proposals would increase Medicaid expenditures.

Federal nurse staffing standards in nursing homes, although they are intended to establish only a minimum requirement, had been interpreted by Medicaid programs in some states to represent a maximum limit on licensed nurse hours. Mandatory strengthening of the staffing standards, therefore, appeared to be required to correct this situation and to avoid penalizing through the payment system those homes that choose to provide better services to their patients. More than two thirds of the nonprofit nursing homes represented by the American Association of Homes for the Aging recommended strengthening the standard to 24-hour coverage by licensed nurses. However, under the current Medicaid reimbursement system, facilities appeared to be faced with a choice of paying high salaries to a few nurses or paying low wages to a greater number of unskilled aides.

REVOLUTION IN HOSPITAL REIMBURSEMENT

In short-term-care facilities in the early 1970s, rapidly increasing hospital costs became a concern of the public and the federal government. Until then, the health care industry and the federal government had encouraged the construction and modernization of facilities and the purchasing of new equipment to provide the public with better services. Cost containment was not an issue until increasing Medicare expenditures brought the federal government into the health care market as a major third-party payer. Subsequently, massive regulation of the health care industry was instituted, with the overriding goal of controlling health care costs. Generally, it was believed that increasing costs would bring some form of comprehensive national health insurance. Hospitals were cognizant of this expectation and attempted to control costs as well as they could. The financial environment at that time included retrospective cost (or charge-based) reimbursement, readily available capital for expansion or renovation of facilities, limited consideration of price in purchasing hospital services, and franchises for hospitals to deliver services through the certificate-of-need process.

Numerous federal, state, and private-sector cost containment initiatives were attempted with varying degrees of success. Although no one pattern emerged as a reliable prototype for the system as a whole, these initiatives offered some important lessons on the limitations of arbitrary government controls and private-sector initiatives. Evaluation of hospital cost-control statutes in Connecticut, Maryland, Massachusetts, New Jersey, New York, Washington, and Wisconsin tended to measure state program effectiveness by contrasting the rate of increase in the national average with the state's cost per capita, cost per admission, or cost per equivalent inpatient days. When data were adjusted for important variables, such as an increase in the supply of acute general hospital beds, it was clear that greater cost-effectiveness was achieved in the states with cost-control programs. Although these state programs differed in detail and mechanics, they all had the following characteristics:

A statewide prospective budget review process for all hospitals in the state.

Incentives and penalties for hospitals designed to encourage cost-effective management.

Equality of treatment as to payment for all patients regardless of the third-party payer (private or governmental) involved.

A system of payer discounts based on objective factors that result in actual cost savings to the hospital.

Utilization review for all patients in the hospital.

Uniform cost and utilization reporting requirements for all hospitals.

In addition, the Massachusetts and New York programs established relief funds for hospitals that incurred large losses due to bad debt and charity care.

In 1977, President Carter again tried to control runaway health care costs. Recognizing that hospital costs represented a major portion of the total health bill (40%), he concentrated his efforts there. The vehicle was Hospital Cost Containment, a proposal that would have capped the amount of a hospital's annual increased costs. The legislation did not pass, but hospitals responded with the *voluntary effort*, under which hospitals attempted to trim costs by keeping staff levels and the number of beds constant. Unfortunately, this effort did not show long-term results. Although the rate of increase dropped from 13.8% in 1977 to 11.3% in 1979, hospital costs were back up to 18.4% in 1981.

Despite a decline in the overall rate of inflation, health care costs continued to compound at an alarming rate. Because of persistent annual increases of 15% to 17% for hospital costs, there was a growing consensus that the status quo in hospital reimbursement was unacceptable. Overall health insurance premiums for business were rising at rates ranging from 20% to 40%, depending on the size and location of the business. This reflected not only 15% to 17% increases in the daily room rate, but

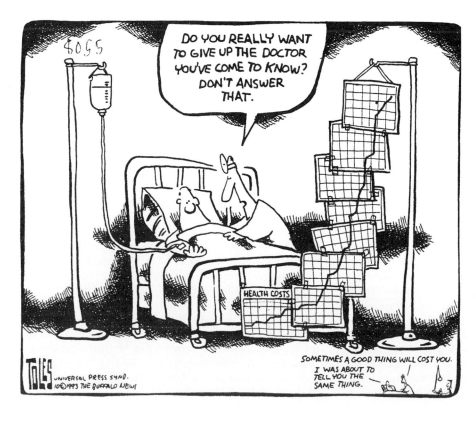

The escalating costs of health care have prompted much concern among providers and patients. (Buffalo News.)

also increased use, total cost increases, and cost shifting—all of which had to be passed on to employees and consumers.

Higher product prices due to rising health care costs left many other industries more vulnerable to competition from foreign manufacturers, reduced their operating margins, and added to their difficulty of attracting investment capital to finance plant expansion and new ventures. Labor was increasingly alarmed, because premium increases reduced funds available for wages and forced some employers to reduce coverage and employee protection. Higher premiums and higher deductibles and co-insurance further increased the economic burden on workers and their families at a time when overall inflation was eroding the size of take-home pay. Something had to be done about these soaring health care costs, particularly the hospital portion, and the first step appeared to be prospective reimbursement.

The growth of third-party payment had been most extensive for hospital care. In 1950, between 40% and 50% of hospital costs had been paid through third-party payers, with the rest paid directly by the patient. In the years that followed, more people bought private insurance or received it as a fringe benefit of employment. Medicare and Medicaid were passed in 1965 to help the aged and the poor, two groups whose high medical expenses and low incomes made insurance difficult to buy. By the mid-1970s, 90% of all hospital costs were paid through third-party payers and only 10% directly by patients.

Motivated by the necessity of coping with historic budget deficits and faced with the projected bankruptcy of the Medicare program, Congress included stringent cost limits on hospital payments in the Tax Equity and Fiscal Responsibility Act of 1982. As a result of a directive of this act, in early 1983 the federal government, moving with unusual speed and unanimity, enacted Medicare legislation that reverses key economic incentives that have traditionally driven the behavior of hospitals. The government replaced the system of reasonable cost reimbursement with a policy requiring that Medicare establish and fix prices in advance on a cost-per-case basis, using as a measure 467 categories of diagnosis-related groups.

To reduce unnecessary institutional care and decrease health care costs, the United States was in the process of changing its approach to health care from that of a predominantly inpatient orientation to one with increasing emphasis on ambulatory care and community health facilities for primary care and disease prevention. The provision of health care services in the home was one aspect of the health care delivery process that was being fostered as an alternative to costly nursing-home and extended hospital stays. Besides the presumed cost benefits, care provided in the individual's residence was believed to be qualitatively better and more humane than that typically provided in the institutional setting. Given a disease or disability that was relatively stable in its

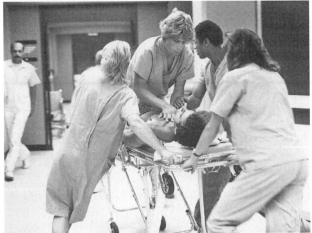

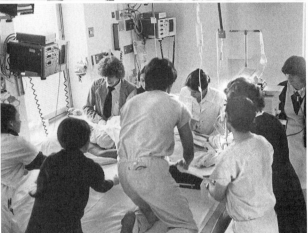

Expenditures for health care continued to extract a larger share of the national economy.

course and given a responsible "other person" within the home to render basic care, personal care and most medical services for the patient could be provided in the client's home, including attention to health maintenance and disease prevention.

To further complicate the scenario, traditional roles of other players in the field were also changing. Active participation by the business community in health care cost containment, the entry of the health care products industry into the delivery arena, and a more price-conscious public had created new dimensions to issues of accountability and competition.

The health care industry appeared to be undergoing forms of production expansion and horizontal integration in response to the increasing demand pressures on the sector. Hospitals were expanding services offered to include greater emphasis on ambulatory care (such as hemodialysis, physical therapy, and treatment for alcoholism and chemical dependency), home health services, hospice care, and skilled nursing care. Horizontal integration appeared to be taking place with the increased formation of multihospital chains. In addition, there was a shift toward the for-profit sector. Between 1970 and

1984, investor-owned (for-profit) community hospital beds increased at an average annual rate of four times faster than total community hospital beds. The American health care system was caught in a tightening bind between the nation's limited resources and its open-ended commitment to provide the elderly and the poor ready access to tax-financed care through Medicare and Medicaid.

REFERENCES

1. "A Prophet Honored," *American Journal of Nursing*, vol. 71 (January 1971):53.
2. U.S. Department of Health, Education, and Welfare, Secretary's Committee to Study Extended Roles for Nurses, *Extending the Scope of Nursing Practice: A Report of the Secretary's Committee* (Washington, DC: Government Printing Office, 1972), pp. 3–6.
3. Ibid., pp. 7–9.
4. Ibid., pp. 3–9.
5. *New York Times*, November 16, 1983.
6. U.S. Congress, House, Committee on Labor, *Labor Disputes Act. Hearings Held March 13–April 4, 1935* (Washington, DC: Government Printing Office, 1935), pp. 1–9.
7. Ibid., pp. 5–12.
8. "The Biennial," *American Journal of Nursing*, vol. 46 (November 1946):729.
9. Shirley C. Titus, "Economic Facts of Life for Nurses," *American Journal of Nursing*, vol. 52 (September 1952):1109–1110.
10. *Congressional Record*, May 12, 1947.
11. "ANA Platform for 1956–1958," *American Journal of Nursing*, vol. 56 (July 1956):882.
12. "Statement of AHA Concerning Collective Bargaining in Hospitals," *Hospitals*, vol. 33 (September 16, 1959):98.
13. "ANA Platform, 1960–1962," *American Journal of Nursing*, vol. 60 (August 1960):1100.
14. Ibid.
15. M. D. Kossoris, "San Francisco Bay Area 1966 Nurses' Negotiations," *Monthly Labor Review*, vol. 90 (June 1967):8–12.
16. "California Nurse Group Endorses Strike as Acceptable Bargaining Technique," *Hospitals*, vol. 40 (September 15, 1966):201.
17. U.S. Department of Labor, Bureau of Labor Statistics, *Industry Wage Survey—Hospitals: March, 1969* (Washington, DC: Government Printing Office, 1971), pp. 1–11.
18. "American Nurses' Association Convention '74," *Nursing Outlook*, vol. 22 (August 1974):506–514.
19. U.S. Congress, Senate, Special Committee on Aging, *Nursing Home Care in the United States: Failure in Public Policy; Supporting Paper No. 4—Nurses in Nursing Homes: The Heavy Burden* (Washington, DC: Government Printing Office, 1975), p. 369.

DANGER AND OPPORTUNITY
Health Care Reform and Nursing

21

By the mid-1990s, as it became obvious to nurses and other Americans that slow economic growth was continuing into its third decade, a feeling of apprehension began to grow. At the end of the 1980s, statisticians called attention to a troubling economic trend: This was the first postwar recovery period in which economic inequality continued to worsen. During the years 1989 to 1992, the unlucky administration of President George Bush presided over the lowest economic growth rate of any 4-year term since Herbert Hoover's.

For nurses and others, the American dream had rarely slowed for so long without a clear sign of revitalization. Real household incomes were stagnating. When adjusted for inflation and taxes, the median family income for the early 1990s fell back to the levels of the late 1970s. Members of the 35-to-45 age group, collectively, were little more than half as wealthy (in constant dollars) as their parents had been at the same age. Those younger were worse off, and it was widely predicted that the disparity would widen as the baby boomers reached retirement age in the years around 2020.

Demographers offered yet another warning. Millions of women had entered the work force during the 1980s, sacrificing time with their children to provide additional paychecks essential to keeping their families afloat. Many of these women had been inactive nurses, and they now felt obliged to enter the work force to maintain their families' standard of living or to support their halves of broken families. By the mid-1990s, however, few families still had nonworking women available to bolster purchasing power for yet another economically weak decade.

NEW INFECTIOUS AGENTS AND HIGH-RISK HABITS

At the beginning of the 1990s, mortality in the United States was characterized by many diseases associated with preventable causes. Approximately 2,148,000 U.S. residents died in the year 1990. The most common causes of death were heart disease (720,000), cancer (505,000), cerebral vascular disease (144,000), accidents (92,000), chronic obstructive pulmonary disease (87,000), pneumonia and influenza (80,000), diabetes (48,000), suicide (31,000), chronic liver disease and cirrhosis (26,000), and human immunodeficiency virus (HIV) infection (25,000).

Numerous factors contributed to these specific diseases and causes of death. Tobacco use was associated with an estimated 400,000 deaths; diet and activity patterns, with 300,000. Other contributors to mortality included alcohol abuse (100,000), microbial agents (90,000), toxic agents (60,000), firearms (35,000), sexual behavior (30,000), motor vehicle accidents (25,000), and drug abuse (20,000). Socioeconomic status and access to health care also had a significant influence on mortality rates but were difficult to quantify independent of other factors.

The way in which citizens of the United States viewed health and disease had changed dramatically over the course of the 20th century. People once considered chronic diseases, for example, as the inevitable consequences of the aging process. During the 1970s and 1980s, however, epidemiologic studies and clinical trials, which began to reveal the effects of risk factors such as tobacco use, high blood pressure, and blood cholesterol levels on the development of chronic disease, also suggested strategies for combating these diseases. This scientific progress prompted a new focus on disease prevention and health promotion, particularly within schools of nursing and schools of public health. New research findings lent momentum to the campaign against tobacco use and also encouraged the development of national educational programs on factors such as high blood pressure.

The onset of AIDS put the greatest new demand on the health care and nursing delivery systems of the 1980s and 1990s. Despite advances in nursing

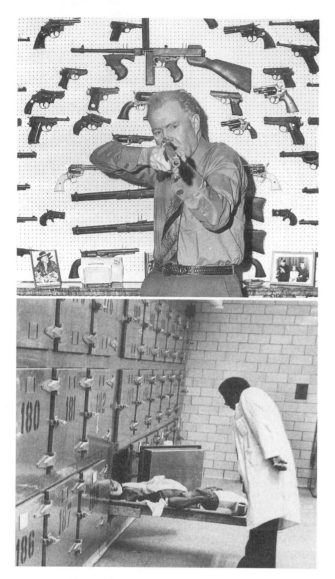

Firearms caused 35,000 deaths in 1990.

people diagnosed with AIDS was expected to reach about 500,000, up from 340,000 in September 1993. The cumulative number of deaths from the disease was projected to top 320,000 in 1993 and reach 385,000 in 1994. AIDS was now the leading cause of death among men age 25 to 44 and the sixth leading cause among men and women age 15 to 24.

While the epidemic grew, treatment efforts suffered a setback in 1993 when long-term studies released at the International AIDS Conference in Berlin showed that nucleoside analogs such as AZT and ddC did not improve survival rates among asymptomatic patients. The findings, though controversial, prompted the National Institutes of Health to rescind its recommendation that physicians routinely prescribe these drugs to newly diagnosed patients.

The AIDS epidemic also brought new awareness to the importance of infection control within hospitals and other health care institutions. In the late 1980s, several nurses were among a small group of health workers who acquired HIV in the course of their duties, usually through accidental needle sticks. In addition, nurses faced increasing threats from work-place exposure to AIDS patients with infectious tuberculosis (TB). A related concern involved exposure to aerosolized pentamidine, the drug used to prevent infections in HIV-positive patients, some of whom also had TB. While administering the drug, nurses could be exposed to TB—at times undiagnosed—as well as to pentamidine, itself a potent substance and airway irritant.

The resurgence of TB was especially troublesome considering the advances in health care over the previous century. In 1962, the International Union Against Tuberculosis had declared TB "conquered." No one imagined that 30 years later, in fiscal year 1994, the federal government would be spending nearly $70 million to combat the disease. Nor did anyone expect that isolating patients in specialized TB treatment facilities—an updated version of the old-time sanitarium—would resurface as a serious option. But the appearance of new TB strains unresponsive to standard therapy posed a new and unexpected problem. Nurses caring for TB patients infected with drug-resistant strains knew that treatment resembled that of 100 years earlier, in the days before chemotherapy, when patients had to be placed where they could be cared for and not infect others.

The surge in TB cases, nearly 30,000 more than expected over the preceding 5 years, was traced mainly to the AIDS epidemic and the low resistance of AIDS patients to TB and other infections. The rise of the drug-resistant strains that had nurses and public health officials most concerned stemmed largely from patient failure to complete 6 to 9 months of standard drug therapy.

The inability of physicians and nurses to prevent mortality in patients with AIDS reminded the two

practice, AIDS defied efforts at prevention or cure, remaining invariably fatal. An increasing number of nurses devoted themselves to battling the epidemic, which was first recognized in 1981 as a disease in homosexual men. AIDS evolved into a broad spectrum of illnesses, however, and afflicted heterosexuals as well. Though incidence remained highest among homosexuals, the proportion of AIDS cases attributed to heterosexual contact increased by 17% from 1991 to 1992 to 7% of all cases. The rate of new infections grew fastest among young heterosexual women, who accounted for 14% of all cases in 1992, an increase of 9% over 1991. AIDS cases related to the use of intravenous drugs represented about 25% of cases in 1992.

The cost of the epidemic, in human and financial terms, proved staggering. By 1993, an estimated 1 million Americans—about 1 in every 250—were infected with HIV. By the end of 1994, the number of

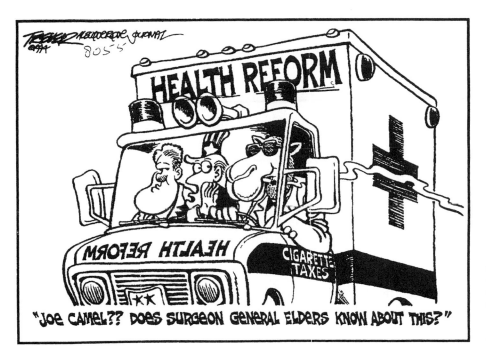

"JOE CAMEL?? DOES SURGEON GENERAL ELDERS KNOW ABOUT THIS?"

As the toll of tobacco on the nation's health became clear, the social climate began to turn against smoking, and an increase in the tax on cigarettes was proposed as a means to help finance health care reform. (Orlando Sentinel.)

professions of their joint responsibility to care as well as to cure. Growing reliance on medical technology during the previous 30 years had led to more and more impersonal treatment within medicine, and nurse observers described a crisis in the physician–patient relationship. This observation was bolstered by studies that found that patients filed malpractice suits more because of what they perceived as unfeeling treatment from their physicians than because of bad outcomes from their medical care.

LEGAL CHALLENGES

Malpractice activity increasingly encouraged the practice of defensive medicine. The threat of lawsuits gave American physicians a powerful incentive to

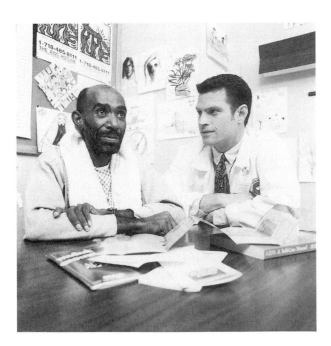

Nurses provided counseling and education as a crucial component of AIDS care. (Nursing Spectrum, July 13, 1992. Photo credit: Meryl Alexander-Tihanyi.)

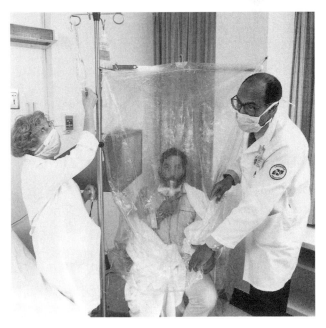

The reappearance of tuberculosis required new infection-control procedures. Here an isolation chamber is used when inducing sputum for TB testing. (Nursing Spectrum, October 18, 1993. Photo credit: Sandor Acs.)

provide numerous procedures and tests. As a direct result of the fear of litigation, an estimated 70% of physicians ordered more consultations, 66% ordered more diagnostic tests, and about 55% ordered more follow-up visits than they would have otherwise. This impetus created by the malpractice liability system further compounded incentives elsewhere in the U.S. health care system to overuse services and supply excessive medical intervention.

On another legal front, the nation was introduced to the physician who pioneered the medical role of managing deaths. His business card read:

> Jack Kevorkian, M.D.
> Bioethics and Obitiatry
> Special Death Counseling
> By Appointment Only

Dr. Kevorkian (who later lost his license) invented the specialty obitiatry, which he tried for the first time in 1990 on a 54-year-old patient from Portland, Oregon. Kevorkian invented and used a "self-execution machine" that allowed the patient, in the back of a Volkswagen van, to kill herself by flipping the intravenous switch from saline to thiopental and then to potassium chloride. The procedure took less than 6 minutes.

Called "Dr. Death" by his detractors and the "Great Pioneer" by his supporters, this 62-year-old pathologist became a popular figure on television talk shows and in other forms of mass media. Images of Kevorkian posing with his death machine circulated throughout the nation. Kevorkian spoke of his disdain for the American medical profession and snubbed the medical press, which had consistently refused to publish his ideas, including his proposal to experiment on death-row prisoners by killing them in such a manner that their organs might be retrieved and used. While some thought Kevorkian a prophet, others saw him as mentally deranged. By the mid-1990s, public opinion over Kevorkian was sharply divided.

WAR PREPARATIONS

On another front altogether, in late 1990 several thousand nurses were deployed with Operation Desert Storm to provide nursing care for the 500,000 troops sent to Saudi Arabia and the Persian Gulf in an effort to force Saddam Hussein's Iraqi army out of Kuwait. The nurses were equipped to handle at least 15,000 casualties daily. The fighting capacity of the Iraqi forces was overestimated, however, and a stunning ground war lasted but 100 hours, with the allies spared extensive casualties. Despite the low number of allied fatalities, the engagement still brought progress in health care. For the first time, frozen blood was prepared for transfusing to the injured, and stocks of monoclonal antibody treatment were on hand for large wounds and multiple-system trauma. In addition, stockpiles of improved antichemical treatments stood ready, including some never before used, such as pyridostigmine. The large-scale mobilization also enabled military planners to update reserve staffing requirements for physicians and nurses.

A NEW NURSE SHORTAGE

By the mid-1990s, the U.S. health care industry employed more than 10 million people, including 2,200,000 nurses, 650,000 physicians, and 150,000 dentists. Moreover, the industry—now the nation's largest—encompassed 126 medical schools, 1300 nursing schools, 6600 hospitals, and 26,000 nursing care facilities.

Now the leading labor sector in the entire U.S. economy, health care employment increased during the early 1990s at an average annual rate of 3.8%, despite the effects of the recession and the slow economic recovery that followed. The highest growth rate occurred in home health care services, where employment rose at an annual pace of nearly 18%, to a total work force of more than 500,000 by the end of 1994. Hospitals experienced the lowest rate of growth, but they still accounted for more than half of total employment in the health care industry.

Meanwhile, the supply and demand for nurses fluctuated wildly during the 10 years from 1985 through 1994. Although a 1983 Institute of Medicine study concluded that the national nurse shortage of 1978 to 1982 had ended and that federal support for nursing education should be scaled back, in a few years the shortage conditions returned with a vengeance. An American Hospital Association survey taken in 1987 found that 79% of hospitals needed more nurses. Almost one fifth of large urban hospitals claimed that they had to take beds out of service temporarily due to the shortage, and 14% reported shortage-caused closings of emergency rooms. In addition, three quarters of all hospitals relied on overtime work from temporary nurses hired from agencies.

Additionally, more than 10% of hospitals turned to hiring foreign nurses when they could not find an adequate supply from the domestic work force. In New York City hospitals, the registered nurse (RN) vacancy rate reached 15%; when per diem nurses and nurses working on agency registries were taken into account, however, the vacancy rate climbed to 20%. On any given day, New York City needed 5000 additional RNs. A Greater New York Hospital Association survey substantiated the reliance on foreign nurses when it found that 26% of the nurses then employed by hospitals and nursing homes had been trained overseas.

The U.S. Department of Health and Human Services set up a special commission to study the nurse shortage. After holding extensive hearings and analyzing a massive amount of evidence, the Secretary's Commission on Nursing issued its final report in December 1988. The report documented shortages in virtually every sector of the health care industry and warned that the health of the nation would be at risk unless the federal government as well as health care organizations made specific changes to increase the nurse supply.

Former University of Michigan School of Nursing dean and the most recent administrator of the Health Care Financing Administration, Carolyne K. Davis, headed the 19-member commission. Dr. Davis said that up to 200,000 more nurses were needed to meet the demands of the nation's health care system. She noted that although the number of RNs in the United States had increased by roughly 100,000 since 1983, demand still far exceeded supply because of changes in the nature of health care delivery. These changes included the advent of AIDS, which required much hands-on nursing care; the increased use of sophisticated technology; and the aging of the population, because older people were generally much more likely to need health care. In addition, the panel noted that between 1983 and 1986 health care organizations nationwide had laid off 125,000 licensed practical nurses and nurses' aides, thus leaving RNs to perform work previously handled by these support personnel.

Specifically, the report highlighted that in hospitals the average vacancy rate for RNs had risen from 4.4% in 1983 to 11.3% in 1987. The study also found that nursing homes faced a high RN vacancy rate and long recruitment times. In home care, 40% of the agencies surveyed by the secretary's commission reported RN recruitment and retention problems. Health maintenance organizations (HMOs) reported vacancy rates of about 10%.

Near the top of the commission's list of recommendations stood a call for increasing nurses' wages and salaries and expanding their pay ranges. Wage compression—the lack of a meaningful series of wage steps from entry into the profession to retirement—had been identified as a major problem in retaining nurses. The commission noted that although the beginning salary for nurses, between $22,000 and $23,000 per year, compared favorably with that in similar jobs, the salary did not increase proportionately. Higher wages and salaries thus seemed the best means to increase nurse retention. Moreover, higher levels of compensation were expected to actually cost employers less in the end, because they would no longer have to expend large sums of money—approximately $20,000 per nurse—to recruit and train replacements for nurses who left.

The panel also suggested ways to enhance the image and position of nurses to attract more entrants into the profession. One suggestion urged increased RN involvement in patient-care decisions and the appointment of RNs to policymaking boards. A further

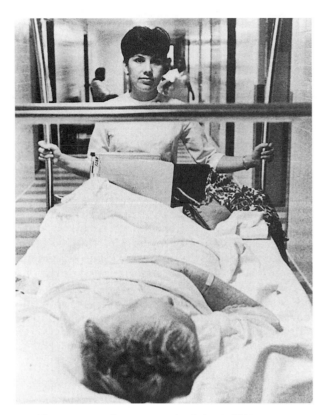

Wage compression was a major factor in RN turnover.

recommendation advised that health care organizations consider switching to automated clinical information systems as a way to reduce the excessive time demands made on the nursing staff by unnecessary documentation.

The shortage of nurses moved hospitals and other employers to consider radical ways of restructuring the patient-care work force to foster greater productivity. Health care organizations focused on how to best use the time of nurses already on staff. Increasingly, nurses' aides and other nurse extenders took on duties traditionally done by RNs. Studies estimated that 30% to 40% of the tasks on many nursing units could be delegated to and performed by these less-educated and less-expensive workers.

A REGISTERED CARE TECHNOLOGIST?

At the height of the nurse shortage, the American Medical Association (AMA) determined that because the inadequate supply of nurses was precipitating a health care crisis, the time had come to introduce a new type of bedside-care giver. Acting independently of organized nursing, the president of the AMA, James E. Davis, M.D., attacked nursing leaders for wanting to turn the registered care technologist (RCT) idea into a "turf" issue. Traditionalists in the AMA held that modern nurses had moved away from bedside care toward an overemphasis on book learning, thus creating a gap that could be filled by a new RCT. The AMA board approved plans for four RCT pilot projects and announced that the first class would commence in July 1989. Applicants would need a high school diploma and would earn $5 to $7 per hour while training. Nine months of preparation would lead to the basic RCT, with an additional 9 months required to become an advanced RCT. Basic RCTs would transport patients, care for wounds, and learn some higher-level skills, such as administering oral medications under supervision. Advanced RCTs would learn to administer routine intravenous medication under supervision, care for ventilators and cardiac monitors, and recognize changes in patient status.

Enormous opposition to the RCT proposal came from the professional nursing associations as well as the American Osteopathic Association—which voted unanimously against it—and the Florida Medical Association. As a result of this pressure, only one pilot program was initiated, at a Kentucky nursing home, and the first class of RCTs apparently never completed their training and certification.

DECLINE IN HOSPITAL PRODUCTIVITY

As the nurse shortage slowly abated during 1991 and 1992 and economic pressures increased, hospitals began to look at ways to cut labor costs, an expense representing more than half of an institution's total budget. In 1991, hospital payroll and benefit costs constituted 54% of overall hospital expenses for full-time equivalent employees in acute-care hospitals. RNs constituted 24% of that year's 841,000 employees. Between 1985 and 1991, the total hospital work force, including nurses, increased by nearly 18%, to more than 3.5 million. This growth in the number of hospital workers occurred despite a decline in hospital occupancy. The number of acute-care hospitals fell by 7% from 1985 to 1991, and the number of staffed beds dropped nearly 8%.

One measure of hospital productivity, at least on the surface, was the ratio of full-time equivalent employees to patients, and by this yardstick productivity had taken a nosedive. In 1982, hospitals employed 353 full-time equivalents per 100 patients, but by 1991 that figure had jumped 22% to 431. Many experts saw the increasing employee/patient ratio as a reflection of the fact that hospitals treated sicker patients who required a higher intensity of care. Indeed, some evidence supported the contention that the overall acuity of the hospital inpatient population had risen as less acutely ill patients received treatment in other settings. For example, the Medicare-patient case mix index (the disease-specific makeup of the inpatient Medicare workload) for all acute-care hospitals increased from 1.17 in 1985 to 1.39 in 1992. This index gauges the acuity of Medicare inpatients, with 1.0 being average; a rise in

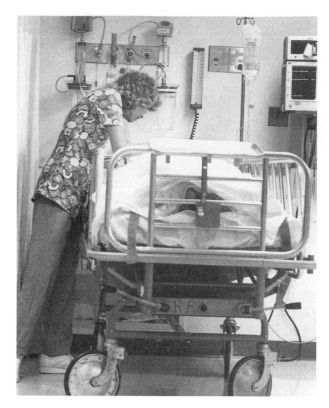

Hospitals experienced a productivity decline.

the index indicates greater severity of illness among patients. Other factors cited for the decline in hospital productivity included the addition or expansion of services, the opening of more intensive-care units, the purchase of new medical technology, and the increase in specialization among physicians.

THE COMPUTER ENTERS HEALTH CARE

One glaring omission in the efforts to improve productivity in the early 1990s pertained to the use of new information technologies. By 1993, only an estimated 15% of hospitals had a clinical information system. Experts calculated that computerizing the entire health care system could cut from $4 billion to $30 billion from the nation's trillion-dollar annual health care bill. Some health care organizations had already installed computer systems for a variety of purposes: to quickly retrieve patient histories; to record diagnoses and patient care; to order tests, x-rays, and supplies; to assign beds and nursing staff; to gather statistics on patients, illnesses, and care; and to generate bills and insurance claims. Making such a system work, however, required that nurses, physicians, and patients trust it to record and store essential, confidential details about patient care.

Computerization did speed up hospital work processes dramatically. Pharmacy and supply orders, for example, could be accelerated by replacing phone calls or written requests with computer messages. When nurses, physicians, or technicians typed information or orders on a keyboard, the data automatically became part of the patient's record, accessible from any other terminal in the system. Pharmacists, surgeons, and nurses could retrieve needed information quickly, and no one had to spend time transcribing physicians' notes.

Strategies to save time loomed ever more important. Experts estimated that paperwork consumed half of all nurses' time and about one third of all physicians' time—mostly to record diagnoses and treatment. Without a computer, information often had to be written more than once: on a notepad, in greater detail on the patient's chart, in a letter to a consulting physician, on a prescription, and on a bill. Computers could reduce that process to a single entry.

Despite the obvious benefits of computerization to the health care industry, medical personnel often resisted the installation of computers. A 1992 survey of residents revealed that only 13% would choose to use computers. Furthermore, the survey determined that computer use actually declined during the residency period for medical staff, possibly because the residents perceived themselves as too busy to bother with it. This finding illustrated a message that echoed throughout the health care industry in the mid-1990s: Although improved computer capabilities had removed the technical barriers to computerizing patient records, behavioral, professional, and institutional obstacles remained.

A survey of 1000 health care system developers conducted by Ohio State University in 1993 found that four of the five most serious barriers to the implementation of computerized records were organizational rather than technical. The most troublesome deterrents to computer use were, in descending order, insufficient funding, inadequate interfaces, muddled objectives, absence of definitions or standards, and the fragmented environment of health care.

Overall resistance by physicians to computerized records ran high because many feared they would have to relinquish their dictation systems, memorize a list of codes or passwords, and spend valuable time typing data. Some of these fears were justified. Certain computerized record systems proved difficult for some physicians to master, required more time than manual systems, and detracted from interactions with patients. A time-and-motion study at one Indiana hospital, for example, measured work patterns of 24 internal medicine interns who used computers to enter orders and drug information and conduct rounds. The interns took almost twice as long to enter admission orders electronically than by hand and almost three times as long to enter daily orders.

Another study videotaped four physicians before and after the introduction of a computerized medical-record system at a hospital. After examining 132 patient encounters, the researchers concluded that the system demanded more time than traditional written records, even though it required little typing. With the new system, the amount of interaction time between physicians and patients also decreased significantly. Thus, the adoption and diffusion of computerization in business offices across all industries was not readily repeated in medicine. Unlike professionals in other fields, such as engineering and the sciences, many physicians believed they had little to gain from the effort that computerized records could require of them. Nurses, however, tended to view the benefits of applying computerization to hospital work more positively. The largest stumbling block among medical personnel appeared to be the perception that computer use demanded extra time and thus reduced opportunities.

By the mid-1990s, however, computerization had acquired irresistible momentum. Hospitals, insurance companies, payers, and regulators all saw benefits in computerizing medical and patient information data. As computers facilitated the processes of managing care, controlling costs, and measuring outcomes, the users of these data became the primary proponents of computerized patient records.

HEALTH CARE EXPENDITURES SOAR

Large-scale changes in economic realities constituted the primary driving forces behind the most far-reaching developments in nursing and health care during the 10 years from 1985 through 1994. With overall health care costs soaring and the elderly population burgeoning, the federal government had acted in 1983 to contain the growth of its Medicare budget by introducing diagnosis-related groups, which capped hospital reimbursements. Following the government's lead, private insurers also imposed reimbursement controls. Before long, utilization review, preapproval of admissions, second opinions for surgery, and other cost-containment measures became an integral part of nurses' and physicians' daily practices. As indemnity insurers increasingly adopted so-called managed care techniques, HMOs, preferred provider organizations (PPOs), and other managed care options moved into the mainstream of the health care industry. Physician autonomy diminished in the face of oversight by third-party payers, and a highly traditional medical staff expressed much disenchantment with the emerging world of health care practice.

The ability of most Americans to meet household health care costs remained relatively constant for most of the period from World War II up through the early 1980s. During the decade ending in 1994, however, health care costs began to claim steadily increasing shares of household incomes. By 1994, American families spent (largely through their employee benefits payments) an average of $5000 yearly

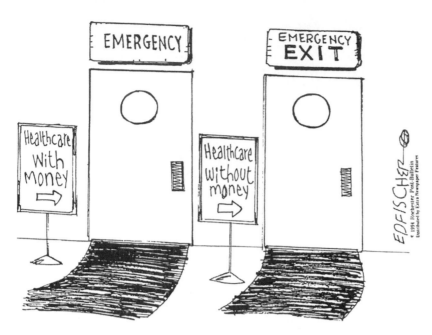

A lack of financial resources barred millions of uninsured Americans from access to adequate health care. (Rochester Post-Bulletin.)

on health care, or 15% of the total family budget, up from 7% in 1980. Several factors worked to fuel the escalating expense of health care: (1) the price of health care increased much faster than most other goods and services during the 1980s and early 1990s, (2) increased use of health care services continued to add to the overall health cost burden, (3) employer- and government-based health benefits programs ceased to shield households from increasing costs as they had in the 1960s and 1970s, and (4) wages declined in inflation-adjusted terms rather than increasing as they had during previous decades.

Most significant was the finding that health care prices soared above overall economic inflation. For the early part of the period after World War II, health prices rose only somewhat more rapidly than other prices in the economy. From 1950 to 1980, all prices advanced at an average rate of about 4.2% per year, while health care prices increased at a 5.5% average annual rate. During the 1980s and early 1990s, however, the rate of real yearly health care inflation more than doubled, jumping 8.1% per year while overall prices in the U.S. economy rose at a 4.7% yearly rate. As a result, a medical procedure that cost $1000 in 1980 could by 1994 be expected to cost $1625 in inflation-adjusted dollars.

These health care price increases over and above the general rate of inflation drove up the nation's health care bill by more than $150 billion and accounted for well over 55% of the increase in real health spending during the period. Inflation in health prices contributed more to the nation's total health bill than did the combined effect of a larger population, an aging population, and new medical technologies.

Health care payments rose much more rapidly for businesses during the 1980s and early 1990s than for governments or households. But these higher payments fell unevenly among the nation's businesses. During this period, many employers elected not to offer employee health benefits. As a result, such employers experienced no increase in health care expenses. Many other businesses decided to significantly expand their use of part-time employees and exclude such workers from health care and other benefits, thus minimizing the steady upward growth in corporate health costs. In addition, some businesses passed all or most of the increased premiums demanded by insurance companies onto their employees.

EXPERIENCE-RATED HEALTH INSURANCE TAKES OVER

A further problem involved the shift by the health insurance industry from community rating to experience rating. Until the most recent several decades, community-rated policy had dominated the private health insurance market. With these policies, insurers charged all purchasers in a geographic region the same rate. Under community rating, premiums were based on the average cost of anticipated health care for all purchasers, thus spreading the risks of high health care expenses throughout the community. Community rating constituted one of the principles fundamental to the operation of Blue Cross and Blue Shield plans from the 1930s through the 1960s.

As commercial insurers established a significant presence in the health insurance marketplace in the 1960s, 1970s, and 1980s, they began to compete for group customers by means of experience rating. In this approach, insurers offered rates to a firm based on the particular experience of that firm. By offering rates to firms based on their own claims record—rates lower than those of comparable Blue Cross and Blue Shield policies—many commercial insurers managed to siphon from the community pool large firms with younger and healthier work forces. This phenomenon went unnoticed by most nurses, but as commercial insurers pulled more and more low-cost, low-risk groups out of community pools, only older and sicker individuals remained. Thus, by the end of the 1980s, community-rated health insurance policies had become virtually extinct.

Although at least originally beneficial to many large companies with young, healthy workers, experience rating had a devastating effect on the availability of health insurance to small businesses. When insurance premiums reflect the experience of one small firm, even a single employee with high health expenses could cause the firm's insurance premiums to skyrocket.

EXCLUSIONARY PRACTICES BY HEALTH INSURERS

The 1980s witnessed another ominous change in the practices of the insurance industry: Health insurers began to exclude not only high-risk individuals but entire occupations and industries based on the insurer's profit-and-loss experiences with such groups. Some large commercial insurers listed more than 40 industries as ineligible for health insurance. High-risk industries included those such as logging, mining, and oil drilling, whose workers had a history of frequent accidents or illnesses. Health insurers also increasingly excluded businesses with seasonal work and many low-paying jobs—such as motels, restaurants, and beauty salons—because transient employees might be in poor health to begin with and had health histories difficult to verify.

Ironically, insurance companies began to exclude more and more workers in the health care industry, such as nurses, physicians, dentists, and others, because experience had shown that health care providers tended to use health services frequently, apparently because they were highly aware of their own health care needs. Finally, insurers moved to exclude groups that required high administrative expenses, such as local governments, which practiced annual open bidding and switched insurers frequently.

The lack of health insurance effectively barred access to medical care. Millions of people found themselves unable to obtain health care because they did not have adequate financial resources. Moreover, evidence indicated that the uninsured commonly delayed seeking medical care, which often led to a more serious and otherwise avoidable illness. Growing evidence also showed that, even when admitted to a hospital, the uninsured received care very different from the insured. For example, a study released

in 1991 of 600,000 patient records from around the country found that hospital patients with and without health insurance received distinctly different treatment. The uninsured were far less likely to undergo high-cost medical procedures or key diagnostic tests. The study concluded that differences in care on the basis of insurance appeared to make the uninsured 1.2 to 3.2 times more likely than the insured to die during their stay.

By 1994, at any one time, an estimated 38 million Americans (around 18% of the population) carried no health insurance. Because health insurance in the United States is largely employment based, people who moved in and out of jobs also tended to move in and out of health coverage. Thus, more than 38 million Americans lacked *continuous* health insurance coverage. A 1990 Census Bureau study estimated that 63 million Americans—about 28% of the population—lacked health insurance protection for at least 1 month during the previous 28-month period.

CONSEQUENCES OF LIMITED ACCESS TO HEALTH CARE

That large segments of the U.S. population found themselves saddled with the problem of how to obtain and pay for health care was well known to nurses. According to surveys, around 17% of Americans had inadequate access to physicians, a troubling reality reflected in such statistics as high rates of infant and child mortality and premature death and disability due to controllable illnesses. The indigent faced especially acute access problems. Nurses in inner-city hospitals noticed that the poor were more likely to be seriously ill on admittance to the hospital and to receive less aggressive medical care when hospitalized. The poor also more often experienced injury by substandard medical care and were more likely to die during their hospitalization. When indigent patients lost health coverage as a result of government budget cuts, their health care decreased markedly and the outcomes of their hospital stays worsened. Minority populations among the poor were especially vulnerable; inner-city neighborhoods with large black populations experienced a risk of mortality double that of other Americans.

The absence of health insurance coverage imposed perhaps the largest barrier between the poor and the health care they needed. In addition, health insurance was becoming unaffordable for many Americans not considered to be poor. Absence of health insurance did not always translate into a lack of access to health care, but it did affect usage patterns. Compared with the insured, people without insurance reported up to 47% fewer visits to physicians and fewer hospitalizations, even though they endured more health problems. Each year an estimated million or more people attempted but failed to obtain health care for economic reasons. The extent of the problem increased steadily from 1985 to 1994. More than half of the population living in poverty—by the government's own definition of poverty—were not eligible for federal health care systems, and this population consisted disproportionately of women and children. The consequences of growing up without receiving needed health care services can be profound.

Exclusion from health care services, particularly primary and preventive care, had pronounced consequences for the health care system and for society in general. Many nurses noted that when the poor could not obtain health care in clinics, physicians' offices, or other settings, they ultimately sought care in hospital emergency departments.

This behavior led to two consequences. First, many patients who did not need emergency treatment but who nevertheless went to emergency departments added to the costs and strains of an already overloaded system. Second, those patients who had to defer health care often presented more severe problems and suffered worse outcomes. As a result, systemic health care costs mounted and the misuse of scarce resources continued while patients' health care outcomes deteriorated.

In short, a significant share of the U.S. population could not obtain adequate health care because they lacked the resources. This problem was not randomly distributed; it disproportionately affected social and ethnic groups disadvantaged in other ways as well. Numerous and extensive consequences attended the inadequate and unequal availability of health care, ranging from the wasting of scarce resources to the raising of philosophical questions about the moral worth of specific socioeconomic groups.

Many people who lived in the inner cities of the United States suffered poverty, overcrowding, crime, and unemployment. Low-income minority populations in urban areas had as much as a fourfold higher incidence of diabetes, hypertension, heart disease, and stroke than the general population. These chronic diseases were also more likely to be poorly controlled and to be the cause of death in poor urban populations than among other Americans. Cancer, moreover, was diagnosed at late stages in inner-city populations, often when no longer treatable. In the Harlem area of New York City, for example, only 5% of women with breast cancer were diagnosed at an early stage, compared with 42% of black women and 52% of white women nationwide.

Births among girls 15 to 17 years of age were three times higher for blacks than for whites, and for girls 14 years of age and younger, the rate was six times higher. The incidence of low-birth-weight infant mortality was twice as high for all black mothers compared with white mothers. Severe problems involving early pregnancy and high infant mortality also occurred in certain rural poverty areas and in places without health care facilities, physicians, or nurse practitioners.

To assist the poor and underserved, health departments at local, state, and federal levels carried out programs in family planning and maternal and child health. The agencies provided community and migrant health centers, health care for the homeless, and substance abuse and mental health clinics. However, under the current system, a single mother of one or several children who was pregnant, drug addicted, and heading her family alone might have to go to four or five locations to obtain appropriate care for herself and her children.

A SHRINKING HOSPITAL INDUSTRY

By the mid-1990s, the hospital industry had become considerably smaller compared with 20 years earlier. Health care costs, just beginning to become an issue at the close of the 1970s, grew into an overriding concern by the end of the 1980s. The 1970s had been a period of expansive increases in hospital costs, services, payments, technology, and intensity of care. When the 1980s began, the hospital sector looked as if it would follow the same course. But driven by financial concerns, advances in technology, and a rise in patient expectations, the hospital sector, which employed most of the nation's nurses, made a dramatic shift toward ambulatory care. This strong movement away from the inpatient side of the hospital industry was a major phenomenon that marked the decade, and many nursing jobs moved to outpatient settings.

At the beginning of the 1990s, the United States had about 5800 short-stay hospitals: 31% governmental (mostly local), 56% nongovernmental (not for profit), and 13% for profit. These short-stay hospitals represented a total of about 1 million beds, with state governmental and nongovernmental, nonprofit hospitals accounting for a somewhat disproportionate share. Although for-profit hospitals controlled only 10% of the beds, this was double the share of the market they had controlled 30 years earlier.

Hospital use peaked in 1981 at about 280 million patient days. By the mid-1990s, this number had fallen by 100 million patient days and was continuing to fall. In 1985, the number of hospital beds crested at almost 1 million, but that number dropped to about 900,000 in the mid-1990s, continuing a downward trend that actually began as early as 1977.

The decline in beds marked a significant turning point for hospitals. By the mid-1990s the traditional acute-care hospital had clearly entered a process of rapid change, and many questions arose as to just how many beds of what type would ultimately remain. An increase in outpatient visits to hospitals made up for some of the decline, but hospital market share fell overall, losing out to home care, physician offices, clinics, HMOs, and numerous other provision sites.

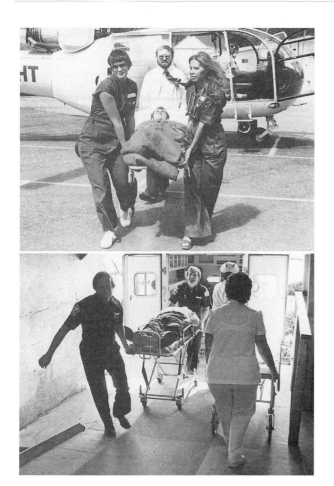

Fewer people overall were entering the hospital, but trauma admissions remained strong.

DEMOGRAPHIC CHANGE AMONG PATIENT POPULATIONS

With the aging of the U.S. population, the growth in numbers of patients older than 65 continued through the 1980s and early 1990s. When Medicare was established in the mid-1960s, the aged represented about 10% of the U.S. population, 20% of hospital admissions, and 30% of patient days. By the early 1990s, the aged constituted about 14% of the U.S. population, 33% of hospital admissions, and more than 50% of patient days. Hospitals were becoming increasingly geriatric. The Medicare program accounted for about half of all hospital revenues by the mid-1990s. Industry representatives claimed that about 55% of all hospitals lost money on Medicare, and they considered its prospective payment system a factor in the large number of hospital closings that had characterized the previous decade.

The most common surgical operations performed in hospitals during the early 1990s were cardiac catheterization, prostatectomy, fracture reduction, and coronary bypass. Cardiac catheterization rates more than doubled during the decade before 1994, whereas the frequency for each of the other operations declined slightly. For females, the most frequent operations were birth related, with normal delivery most frequent (17.3 per 1000 population), followed by cesarean section (6.6) and episiotomy (5.5). Other frequent operations in women were hysterectomy (4.3), removal of the ovary (3.4), tubal ligation (2.8), and dilation and curettage (0.8). Cesarean section rates had increased by more than 25% since 1980.

THE RISE OF INTEGRATED HEALTH CARE SYSTEMS

Hospitals came under attack when several studies showed bloating administrative costs. One study published in the *New England Journal of Medicine* claimed that administrative costs accounted for about 25% of hospital spending in fiscal year 1990; 22.4% of hospital salaries went to administrators. One factor behind this rising cost was an increase in the number of administrators even as the number of patients was declining. In addition, a far-reaching reorganization within the hospital industry had begun, motivated by the need for economic survival. This reorganization involved vertical and horizontal integration among hospitals and sharply reduced the number of stand-alone hospitals in a given community. Hospitals, physicians, and insurers were joining forces to protect or increase their incomes and market share. To do this, they sought ways to exert control over each other and to use economies of scope and economies of scale.

By the mid-1990s, some of the most advanced of the integrated health care marketplaces were dominated by a small number of integrated systems. Rapidly consolidating markets characterized cities such as Albuquerque, San Diego, Portland, Sacramento, and Minneapolis–St. Paul. In Albuquerque, for example, three integrated systems—St. Joseph's, Presbyterian's Southwest, and the Lovelace Clinic—had tied up the market. There were no nonsystem hospitals. In Portland, most hospitals belonged to the Kaiser Permanente, Sisters of Mercy, or Legacy system. By the end of 1994, Portland had no non-aligned hospitals. In Sacramento, California Kaiser captured about one third of the market, and the Sutter Health System and Sisters of Mercy controlled most of the rest. For San Diego, Kaiser dominated the market but with strong competition from Sharp Health System and the recently merged Scripps Clinic/Scripps Memorial Hospital. In the Twin Cities area, mergers produced three regional delivery systems. Group Health aligned with Methodist Hospital, whereas HealthOne and LifeSpan formed the Alina System, referring tertiary care patients to Abbotts-Northwestern.

As hospitals lost inpatient days, home-delivered nursing and medical services became increasingly recognized as vital components of the newly integrated systems. High hospital and nursing-home costs underlined the need for alternative, less-expensive ways to treat patients who did not require continuous institutional care. If some type of nursing and support services were available, it was found that many people with chronic illnesses could be adequately cared for in a home setting. Home care agencies began to meet this need. The estimated 12,500 home care agencies in the United States by 1993 included more than 6000 Medicare-certificate home health agencies and more than 1000 certified hospices. The remaining 5000 organizations—home health agencies, home care aid organizations, and hospices—did not participate in the Medicare program.

TOO MANY SPECIALISTS, TOO FEW PRIMARY-CARE PROVIDERS

A fundamental flaw in the American health care industry was the overspecialization of the medical profession. The health care systems of all other industrialized nations relied on work forces with far higher proportions of generalists than existed in the United States. In countries such as Canada, Great Britain, and Germany, as well as in cost-efficient, physician-salaried-model HMOs in the United States, generalist physicians constituted more than 50% of the medical pool.

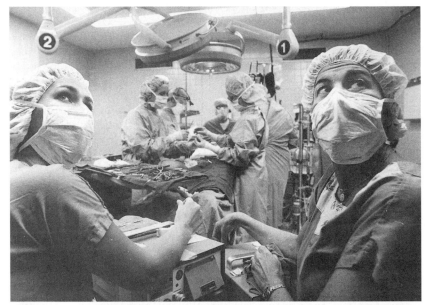

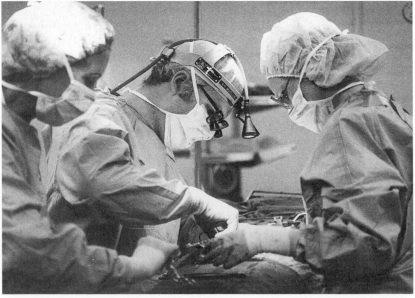

Too many medical specialists created an imbalance in the American health care system.

In 1950, more than half of all U.S. physicians had been generalists, but since then the proportion of generalists had declined dramatically to about one third, with 14% in general internal medicine, 13% in family practice, and 6% in general pediatrics. Concurrently, many nonprimary specialties and subspecialties experienced significant growth. Between 1980 and 1990, major increases occurred in emergency medicine (up 150%), radiology (118%), radiation oncology (78%), and anesthesiology (63%).

All projections suggested that unless the structure of residency training within American medical schools underwent drastic alteration, the proportion of generalists would continue to decline as smaller and smaller percentages of medical school graduates planned generalist careers. Medical students interested in family practice, general internal medicine, and general pediatrics dropped from 36% in 1982 to 15% in 1992. The increasing generalist-to-specialist imbalance among America's physicians undermined the nation's ability to provide affordable health care for its citizens and especially limited the capability to meet the needs of underserved urban and rural Americans.

A high proportion of medical specialists led to higher health care costs, because specialists tended to practice a much more intensive, expensive style of medicine than did generalists. In addition, highly paid specialists in the United States often performed tasks executed adequately and less expensively by primary-care physicians or nurses in other nations. Other countries not only monitored the number of specialists trained but also tended to control their reimbursement. Germany and Japan, for example, erected a strict demarcation between physicians providing inpatient care and those providing outpatient care. Generalists usually worked outside the hospital on a fee-for-service basis, whereas specialists usually worked inside the hospital on a salary basis. Thus, as salaried employees, most specialists in countries like Germany and Japan had none of the incentives for excessive medical intervention and unnecessary procedures and tests that influenced their American counterparts.

The major shortcoming of the American health care system appeared to be the growing vacuum around primary care. The health care systems of most industrialized countries—but not the United States'—were organized so that primary care formed the foundation for all health care services. In such countries, primary care offered first-contact, longitudinal care that was comprehensive and person-centered rather than disease or organ-system specific. The full range of personal health care needs was addressed directly through preventive, curative, and rehabilitative care or, when necessary, through referral to other services. The U.S. health care system, by contrast, did not have a clearly defined mode of primary-care provision. A pluralistic approach to seeking and providing health care described the situation

in the United States, with overlapping services by different kinds of health care practitioners in a wide variety of settings. This patchwork of provisional modes resulted in little system-wide accountability for primary-care provision.

NURSES WORK TO EXPAND THEIR SCOPE OF PRACTICE; THE AMA RESISTS

The complexity of the U.S. health care system also made a satisfactory definition of primary care elusive. Perhaps the leading opportunity for the nursing profession in the mid 1990s was to move aggressively into the void of primary-care providers. Nurse practitioners, physicians' assistants, and nurse-midwives were highly cost-effective in providing high-quality primary-care services, although they were often required to do so in conjunction with a physician and in facilities offering care for the underserved in inner-city and rural areas.

In 1986, a study by the Congressional Office of Technology Assessment observed that within their areas of competence, nurse practitioners and certified nurse-midwives provided care of quality equivalent to that dispensed by physicians. The Office of Technology Assessment study suggested that these nurses were cost-efficient substitutes for physicians in providing many health care services, and they could potentially lower costs to third-party payers and patients and thus for society as a whole. Some studies showed that 60% to 80% of primary-care services traditionally rendered by physicians could be provided by nurse practitioners and nurse-midwives. Nurses appeared ready, willing, and able to fill the gap in primary care left by physicians in their search for specialization. In addition, nurses emphasized primary and preventive health care rather than acute, high-tech medical intervention and were more likely to practice in areas with disadvantaged socioeconomic groups.

By 1994, almost 100,000 RNs were considered advanced-practice nurses with special authority to treat patients, usually with physician supervision. This group included 30,000 nurse practitioners certified in neonatal, geriatric, obstetric-gynecologic, pediatric, and adult fields whose average pay was around $44,000; 6000 certified nurse-midwives who did low-risk obstetric care, delivering 3.6% of all babies, and whose pay averaged $43,500; 35,000 clinical nurse specialists usually employed in hospital or high-tech settings with a pay range of $30,000 to $80,000 per year; and about 25,000 registered nurse-anesthetists who most often worked in smaller hospitals, especially rural ones, at an average pay of $77,500.

State by state, these advanced-practice nurses looked to broaden their clinical authority but were challenged in this quest by the state medical societies. Physicians' associations argued that nurses should always work under a physician's authority,

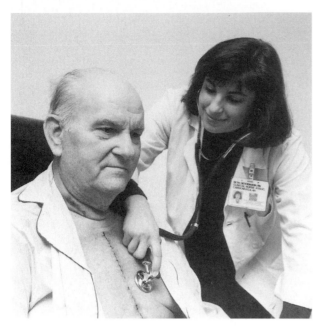

Advance-practice nurses, like this clinical nurse associate, look to broaden their authority to provide primary care independently. (Nursing Spectrum, February 7, 1994. Photo credit: Sandor Acs.)

claiming that nurses did not have the training that physicians had and thus needed oversight on their extended practices. Organized nursing, meanwhile, asserted that appropriately educated nurses should be able to practice independently, consulting physicians the same way generalists consulted specialists in medicine. Nurses did not consider collaboration as necessarily meaning supervision and argued that nurses provided care safely and responsibly.

Organized nursing began the process of lobbying states to relax the historically strict physician supervision and use of protocols for nurses, and some states responded favorably. Oregon and Alaska granted advanced-practice nurses a great deal of independence in diagnosing and prescribing, whereas Illinois and Pennsylvania held back and defeated proposals to loosen the strictures on advanced-practice nursing.

Nursing groups argued that physicians lost interest in providing basic care as they became more specialized, opening a useful opportunity for nurses to fill an unmet social need. Physician groups disputed claims that advanced-practice nurses could provide up to 80% of primary care and dismissed the studies cited as inconclusive. Physicians also denied the charge that medicine was merely defending its economic interest in opposing greater independence for nurses. In the struggle between physicians and nurses over this issue, the battleground soon shifted from the states to Congress.

Physicians expressed concern that a number of policymakers might embrace the claims of organized nursing that advanced-practice nurses could take over certain physicians' duties and perform them at a lower cost. Federal health reformers faced having to control costs while increasing access to health care and began to examine seriously the possibility of expanding the nonphysician scope of practice by preempting restrictive state laws through federal legislation. Many state nursing boards had already granted greater license privileges to nurse practitioners. In some states, for example, nurses could prescribe from a limited drug formulary. But physicians worried that an extravagant use of nonphysicians, though cheaper, would reduce the quality of care. The debate flared with the release of a 1992 study conducted by the American Nurses Association (ANA) that declared that nurses performed as well or better than physicians in providing primary care.

The AMA appointed a special committee to make a recommendation on the nurse practitioner–physician controversy. At a meeting in December 1993, the AMA's House of Delegates endorsed a toughly worded board-of-trustees report that defied the quest of advanced-practice nurses to become independent primary-care providers. During discussion of the issue, many physicians contended that nurses wanted to practice medicine rather than nursing. The president of the ANA, Virginia Trotter Betts, challenged this assumption, stating that nurses were charting their own course. Rather than attempting to imitate medicine, she said, nursing would offer a new paradigm in health care. Betts maintained that the biomedical model was not necessarily the most effective way to provide health care. Instead, she explained, nursing strove to be holistic in emphasizing wellness over acute, episodic care. By citing the profession's role in the identification, diagnosis, and referral of individuals' physical and mental problems, Betts supported nursing's claim to primary care.

The report of the AMA board took issue with Betts' position. "Nurses' education does not prepare them to serve as the first point of contact for all of the patient's medical and health care needs," the report stated. The board also lashed out at what it called "the narrow segment of the nursing community" pushing for greater autonomy and a broader scope of practice. The document attacked nurses' educational qualifications for primary care, criticized the variable requirements for certification, and argued that projected cost savings from the use of advanced-practice nurses were in fact illusory. The report insisted that to use unsupervised nurse practitioners and thereby jeopardize patient safety was irrational.

The trustees of the AMA maintained that they had searched diligently but in vain for evidence that nurse practitioners could independently substitute for physicians or that they were more likely than physicians to work in rural areas or that direct reimbursement and prescribing privileges for nurse practitioners would improve the availability of health care for underserved groups. Costs would only be

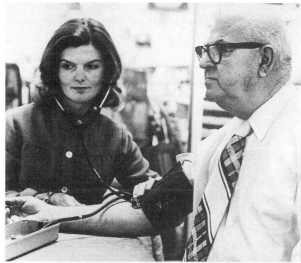

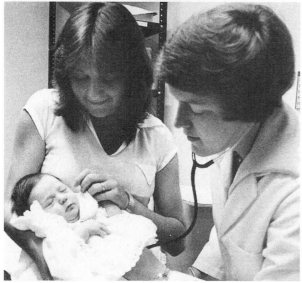

The scope of advanced practice was significantly expanded despite medical opposition.

increased, the AMA argued, by creating a separate level of providers who would refer complex cases to physicians. ANA president Betts charged that the report used inaccurate information and innuendo to undermine the 25-year record of high-quality and cost-effective primary care on the part of nurse practitioners. The debate was sure to continue.

NURSE PRACTITIONERS GAIN NEW AUTHORITY

Despite such controversy, the advancement of nurse practitioners continued into the mid-1990s. Health system reform supplied the key to an expanded scope of practice. In reviewing nurse practice acts, legislators began to rethink the role of nursing in health care delivery. Many of the old laws had been written a decade or two after nurse practitioners

emerged in the 1960s. Reflecting concerns about granting new duties to untested professionals, these laws contained tight restrictions proposed by organized medicine. Now, however, policymakers seemed more trusting of nurses' knowledge and skills and were less impressed with physicians' advice about the proper role for nurse practitioners. Legislators also appeared more inclined toward health promotion and disease prevention, which nurses had championed, and less influenced by physicians' high-tech, disease-oriented medicine. Some critics even suggested that medicine's opposition to enlarging the range of nursing practice had its roots in a desire to protect income or reflected a pervasive sexism, charges that representatives of medical societies strongly denied.

One example of the new climate created by health care reform occurred in Tennessee. Many legislators hoped that nurse practitioners would assume a larger role in caring for the underserved, but they discovered that due to Tennessee's restrictive nurse practice act, most graduates of the state's nurse practitioner programs were leaving for states with fewer limitations. With that in mind, the state broadened the nurses' range of practice soon after starting TennCare, a new law to privatize Medicaid. Under a 1980 law—which the governor thought no longer met the needs of the state's residents—nurse practitioners could prescribe drugs only at specific sites in underserved areas, but under TennCare, they could do so at any location. In reaction, the president of the Tennessee Medical Association characterized the law expanding nursing practice as yet another retaliatory move by the state against organized medicine, pointing out that the medical group was seeking to block TennCare in court by contending that the program did not have sufficient input from providers.

Meanwhile, a new law in California extended the ability of nurses with advanced training to prescribe drugs and devices. Taking effect in 1992, the law applied to nurse practitioners and certified nurse-midwives who provided routine health care, prenatal care, and family planning services. The law covered about 6500 advanced-practice nurses in acute-care hospitals, maternity hospitals, outpatient departments, clinics, physicians' offices, and student health centers.

The California Medical Association forcefully opposed the legislation. A California Medical Association letter to the governor stated that the measure would probably restrict access to perinatal services, reduce quality of care while increasing the potential for serious harm to patients, and raise significantly the cost of medical liability insurance and the cost of health care services overall.

Nurses praised the new law, saying that it would make prenatal care and other services more widely available. To acquire privileges under the new regulations—which did not cover the prescription of controlled substances—nurses first had to complete a pharmacology course and a 6-month preceptorship with a physician. Patients had to be "essentially healthy" before a nurse could prescribe to them. In addition, a physician had to design the protocol and supply specific instructions. Legislators saw the primary intent of the bill as making prenatal care obtainable for more people.

THE CLINTON PLAN AND THE POLITICS OF HEALTH CARE REFORM

The idea that health care reform might become one of the most important voting issues of the 1990s emerged from the results of a special senatorial election in Pennsylvania in November 1991. In that race, voter interest in reform of the American health care system played a central role in the come-from-behind victory of Democratic senator Harris Wofford over Republican candidate Richard Thornburgh. A post-election poll of Pennsylvania voters showed that 50% identified national health insurance as one of the two issues that mattered most in deciding their vote, whereas 21% cited the issue as the single most important factor. The results of the Pennsylvania senate race suggested that health care had arrived as a major political issue, one that could decide the outcome of key elections. Senator Wofford had demonstrated that talking about health care elicited concerns people harbored about a precarious economic future.

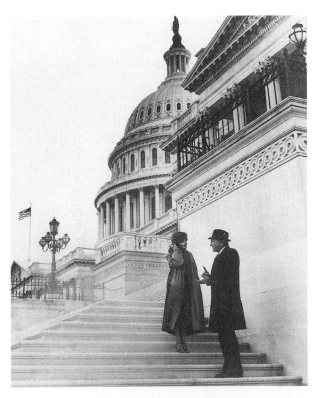

National health insurance again took center stage in the new Clinton presidency.

This message was put effectively into action by candidate Bill Clinton during the presidential election of 1992. Clinton perceived that in winning the election he had received a general mandate to expand health coverage and contain costs. He did not, however, have a mandate for a particular plan and thus faced the formidable challenge of building consensus for a specific program of health reform. Opinion surveys showed that most Americans were dissatisfied with one or more aspects of the nation's health care system. Older Americans and their families worried about the out-of-pocket costs associated with long-term care. Residents of many rural areas expressed dismay over the disappearance of rural hospitals and clinics. The meteoric rise of health insurance costs upset businesses. Some families were disturbed when they discovered that insurance covered surprisingly little of their ordinary health care costs. In addition, governmental policymakers worried that the escalating costs of providing health care to the nation's elderly and destitute would crowd out the government's capacity to act in a host of other areas.

Released in late 1993, President Clinton's sweeping proposal to overhaul the American health care system centered on an ambitious promise to furnish affordable and permanent health insurance coverage for everyone. Not since the New Deal had a president proposed such a grand plan that appeared to offer so much to ordinary citizens at such great expense. The financing of the reform would be dauntingly difficult for a nation struggling with an unmanageable deficit and a sluggish economy. Under Clinton's proposal, the government would set in motion new market forces that would eventually steer the health care system. His plan intended to reorganize the market to give consumers the power to control their health care costs. But to do that, Clinton would require consumers to enter into new financial relationships with health care providers, and he would restrict the power and profitability of the health care industry. Clinton's plan relied on competitive forces to reduce prices and improve services, but it was backed up by government regulation, including a tight cap on annual increases in insurance premiums.

The Clinton plan would radically restructure the current health care system by setting up a series of state-regulated purchasing cooperatives—or alliances—as quasi-regulatory bodies to oversee insurance companies and health care providers. Moreover, a national health board would stand over the alliances, help set national health policy, and enforce the nation's health budget restrictions. The plan was designed to control growth and costs through various mechanisms, including managed competition, a system that would gather most people into regional alliances for the purpose of purchasing health insurance and then ask health plans, physicians, hospitals, and others to compete for subscribers.

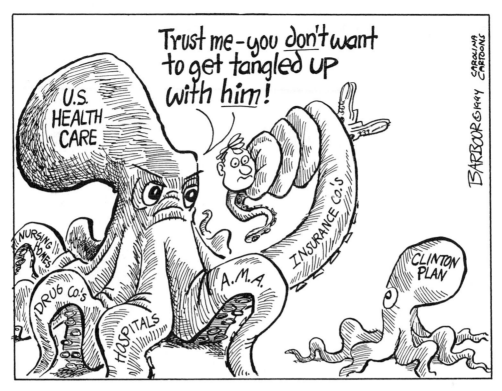

An array of powerful interest groups—businesses, insurers, drug companies, physicians—worked force-fully to shape the outcome of health care reform. (Carolina Cartoons, 1994, Barbour.)

In theory, the competition among plans would limit increases in health costs as subscribers made choices based on quality, price, services, or extra benefits, such as the guarantee that they would have to wait no more than half an hour to see a physician or nurse practitioner. The most successful plans would be those that spent the least on administrative overhead and trained their medical staff to limit the use of expensive tests, surgical procedures, and referrals to specialists. As a fail-safe plan in the event managed competition and other mechanisms did not produce the desired savings, the Clinton proposal would establish a global budget for overall health care spending nationwide. The lid on spending would be enforced by capping the premiums consumers paid through the regional alliances. Alliances could compel compliance with the premium caps by barring offending health plans from competing for consumers or by assessing all health plans in the alliance a charge for any excess above the premium ceiling.

Taking many of its ideas from the president's task force on health care reform, which completed its work late in the summer of 1993, Clinton's proposed health plan initiated an important national debate that came to play a commanding role in the agenda of Congress and the nation. The concept of managed competition involved designing a health-services purchasing strategy in the market that would promote competition and reward providers and insurers for efficient and effective health care delivery in terms of cost, accessibility, quality, and consumer satisfaction. Consumers would receive information on health care prices and quality and would be able to make choices annually as to which plan to purchase. The system would be nondiscriminatory, so that high-risk people could obtain health care coverage at a reasonable price. The plan was meant to be affordable for small businesses, which would supply coverage for employees who might otherwise have gone uninsured. Major national corporations would be allowed to organize their own corporate health alliances and continue to cover their employees through these. Corporations would have to comply, however, with national guarantees relating to the provision of a comprehensive benefits package, quality of care, and other critical factors.

A significant feature distinguishing this debate from earlier ones was that the president had not simply endorsed health reform but had empowered his administration to carry it through. The enormous forces of the American presidency were being mobilized to convince Americans that their health protection was precarious and that although reform required sacrifice, it promised the peace of mind that comes with security.

Surveys repeatedly described the American public as significantly dissatisfied with the health care system, although less so with their personal health care. Although a majority expressed a willingness to pay

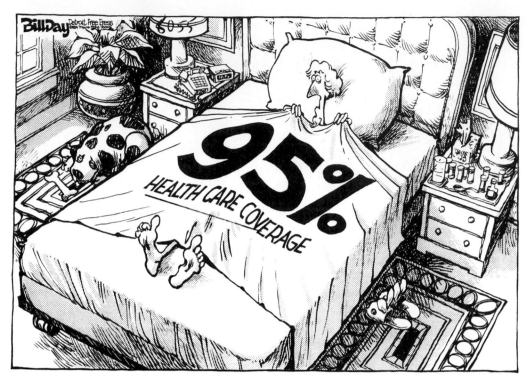

In mid-1994 President Clinton's plan for blanket coverage of all citizens began shrinking. (Detroit Free Press, *August 10, 1994, Bill Day.*)

somewhat more in taxes for a more equitable and better-functioning system, most were not ready to consent to pay enough to implement the comprehensive changes the Clinton plan envisioned. Moreover, there was little agreement on preferred health reform initiatives. Forging consensus among the public and especially in Congress presented the administration with a thorny task.

The reforms now contemplated by the Clinton plan as well as by the several other bills under consideration looked likely to give managed competition a chance to demonstrate its ability to please patients and control costs. The proposed reform of the nation's health care system also prompted many nurses to contemplate their employment future in the industry, especially within hospital settings. Although the extension of health care to an additional 38 million uninsured people would create more nursing jobs, many of these jobs would shift from hospitals to home care.

COST CONSCIOUSNESS PROLIFERATES

Even without federal health care reform, drastic changes were occurring within the employment structure of the health industry. Much of the shake-up resulted from large corporations steering their employees out of fee-for-service insurance into managed-care plans, particularly HMOs. This lowered insurance premiums for the employers. HMO membership had more than doubled from 25 million people in 1986 to more than 50 million in 1994. Not only were HMOs less expensive than fee-for-service plans, but also their premium hikes had fallen for 5 straight years, from 16% in 1990 to 5.6% in 1994. A 1993 study concluded that if all Americans belonged to HMOs, the 19% chunk of the gross national product projected for health care by the year 2000 would shrink to 15%. As a consequence of the surge toward managed care, fewer patients were hospitalized and many fewer physician specialists were used.

As the locus of care moved out of hospitals, nurses had to reorient themselves. Ethical dilemmas demanded of nurses the wisdom of a philosopher, while economic exigencies required sophisticated business expertise. For the first time, the nursing profession acquired a business side. Clinical nursing was now beginning to incorporate content from traditional MBA programs, including economics, finance, accounting, and strategic planning. The new business aspect of nursing and of health care in general was the upshot of an alarming growth in health care costs. Per capita spending for health care in the United States far exceeded that of any other nation, both in absolute terms and as a percentage of income. Nonetheless, 38 million Americans carried no health insurance. Others had insurance too stingy to ensure adequate access to needed care; still others felt deep insecurity at the prospect of losing their health coverage.

At its best, the U.S. health care system of 1994 provided outstanding quality of care to those who had outstanding insurance. At its worst, the U.S. system imposed barriers to health care and sometimes provided care more likely to harm than to help. Whatever the case, current health care industry arrangements looked ever more economically, socially, and politically unsustainable. Most Americans believed that everyone should have the right to receive the best possible care, and most found it unfair that some people had more comprehensive coverage than others.

THE RUSH TO MANAGED CARE

The most common approach being implemented in the early 1990s to solve the problem of high health care costs was the movement toward managed care. Once in the quiet backwaters of health insurance, managed care had swelled to a powerful current. As a system of prepaid plans providing comprehensive coverage to voluntarily enrolled members, managed care continued to consume an increasingly greater proportion of health insurance enrollment.

Managed care encompassed various forms of HMOs and PPOs. HMO plans and enrollments had risen dramatically over the past 20 years in sharp contrast to their slow evolution during the preceding 40 years. By 1994, more than 135 million Americans had enrolled in managed care plans. Total enrollment in HMOs reached 40 million by 1994, whereas the number of employees covered by PPOs grew from zero in the late 1970s to an estimated 90 million.

Managed care comprised many forms, including the following:

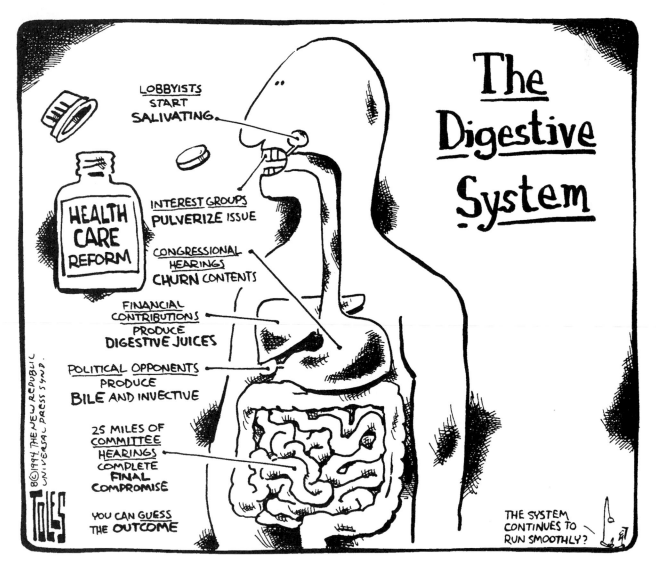

The process of enacting health care reform legislation was suggestive of the workings of the digestive system. (Courtesy of The Buffalo News *and Tom Toles.)*

HMOs consisting of allied clinics and hospitals that enrolled patients as members, charged a fixed fee per year, and for that fee provided all health care services deemed necessary.

PPOs in the form of a collective of private physicians and hospitals that contract with a private indemnity insurance company to provide health care at a discounted fee. The incentive to control use of medical services is weaker in PPOs than in HMOs. Efforts to reduce patient use of unnecessary services under PPOs involve various management programs, such as recertification, concurrent review, and discharge planning.

Individual practice associations as a sort of decentralized HMO in which physicians are not salaried employees of the plan but instead band together to share risks and profits while contracting to provide patients with services for a discounted fee. Physicians may receive 50% to 80% of their customary fees, with about 15% to 20% of this withheld as an incentive to meet quality standards and stay within budget. Physicians meeting such criteria receive the withholdings at the end of the year; those who do not satisfactorily limit tests, referrals, and hospitalizations lose the compensation.

Point-of-service systems are open-ended HMOs that allow enrollees to go outside the system to physicians not in the plan's network. For example, a woman might use the plan's internists and pediatricians but go elsewhere for gynecologic care. If she uses providers outside the network, however, the patient may pay 30% of the medical bill with a deductible running as high as $1000.

Some health care critics had misgivings about the quality of care provided by managed care organizations, although no hard evidence indicated that the trend toward managed care compromised quality of service. Others maintained that managed care might actually improve the quality of care compared with traditional fee-for-service indemnity insurance. Moreover, managed care plans offered more coverage than indemnity plans, especially in terms of preventive health care services, where HMOs had ongoing wellness programs addressed to smoking cessation, prenatal care, and diet and nutrition counseling.

The tools of managed care—case management, utilization review, innovative use of information systems, and efficiency through total quality management—were used selectively to improve quality and lower costs through a more rational use of scarce resources. Such a development seemed almost inevitable. Payers had snapped to attention when RAND Corporation researchers reported in the early 1980s that HMOs were achieving 40% fewer hospital days than indemnity insurers by requiring prior authorization for admissions. Employers began offering HMOs along with their indemnity plans. Many

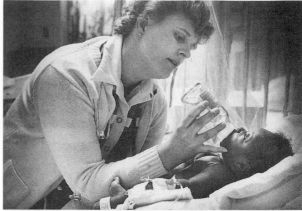
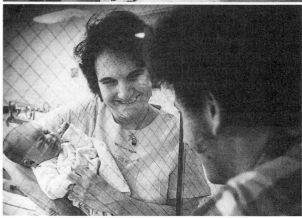

A hot debate emerged about the quality of managed care plans and their requirements.

workers, saddled with greater cost sharing in benefit plans, appreciated the first-dollar coverage of HMOs and switched over.

Indeed, in some markets most employers offered the HMO option—96% of large Los Angeles corporations did so—and 70% of their employees were choosing it. HMO penetration was also high in certain regions of the Midwest, such as Minneapolis–St. Paul, where more than 75% of employers provided managed care and 62% of their workers opted for it. Even in the Northeast, in cities like Boston, roughly 95% of all large employers extended the managed care option to their employees, two thirds of whom chose it. Managed care appeared to be the most economical form of health care, in part because it was the only system of payment that did not reward overtreatment. Under a prepaid managed care plan, an employer set a fixed amount to provide health care for a certain number of employees over the course of a year. No incentive existed to order extra tests or procedures, because neither the physician nor the hospital would be paid more. Physicians working for the plan would receive a predetermined fee in one of three ways: (1) according to the number of patients they cared for; (2) as a fixed, discounted fee for service; or (3) in the form of a salary, as at Kaiser Permanente, one of the oldest and most successful West Coast plans.

Experts agreed that the winners in the growing dominance of HMOs were primary-care physicians and certain nurse practitioners who served as the cost-saving gatekeepers in managed care, because these people were in short supply and could command higher salaries. Increasingly, medical specialists were perceived as the losers in the HMO-dominated environment. Some specialists watched their incomes drop and found themselves with fewer patients. The federal government's Bureau of Health Professions predicted that by the year 2000 the nation would face an oversupply of more than 100,000 medical specialists and a shortage of as many as 50,000 generalists.

Research showed that well-managed HMOs averaged 1 physician for every 800 members, about half the ratio of U.S. physicians to the general population. The HMO physician staff was weighted more heavily toward primary care than was the overall physician supply: Where the United States as a whole had about 250 physicians per 100,000 patients, HMOs used only half as many physicians, or a ratio of around 125 per 100,000 patient population.

Perhaps the alliances and mergers among hospitals, clinics, and physicians to sell their services to cost-conscious insurance companies would lead to a reduction in the number of hospital beds, a curtailment in needless duplication of services, and an end to the medical arms race.

The debate on how to reform the American health care system raged on during the mid-1990s. It was clear that changes in health care would greatly affect the financial and clinical sides of nursing. The remainder of the decade would challenge nurses more than any other time in history, and the ability of the profession to deal successfully with the changes resulting from reform would draw much of its inspiration from a proud history and a promising future.

22

NURSING IS HEALTH CARE: THE DAWN OF THE 21ST CENTURY

More than 30 years ago, in 1972, a prophetic nursing leader, Rozella Schlotfeldt, Dean of the Frances Payne Bolton School of Nursing at Case Western Reserve University in Cleveland, stated that nursing "as a field of professional endeavor is to help people attain, retain, and regain health. The phenomena with which nurses are concerned are man's health-seeking and coping behaviors as he strives to attain health. Nurses are independent, professional practitioners whose field of work is health care."[1]

As we write in mid-2003, the last year has been appalling in terms of national and world events. Overseas, nurses watched as a short but controversial war with Iraq was waged, along with continued fear of terrorism, the lethal risk in North Korea's atomic capability, the continued confusion in Afghanistan, the powder kegs of the West Bank, and the global spread of anti-Americanism, along with the rise of anti-Semitism and the economic collapse of much of South America. In addition, the massive AIDS epidemic in sub-Saharan Africa and the SARS epidemic in China and Toronto, as well as worries about global warming and other environmental disasters created insecurity.

Domestically, there was the scandal within the Catholic Church, shocking corporate malfeasance and the ensuing loss of faith in many of our business leaders, blizzards of pink slips from a continuing recession and an ugly stock market, rancid politics, growing ranks of the homeless, and much talk but little action about improving the health care system.

Also on the minds of nurses was a torrent of images pertaining to the attack on the World Trade Center nearly two years earlier. Over and over, the image of the two towers wearing a cloak of dense smoke and the grotesque shapes of the ruins that followed so swiftly created additional stress and uncertainty. Nurses were among the volunteers that focused on the plight of humans dealing with the aftermath.

The attack on the World Trade Center revealed the awesome power of pure caprice. And it continued to cause hearts to quicken, because it told Americans that they had been deluding themselves in thinking that everything was under control. This led to a significant upswing in depression and stress, with a new demand for pharmaceutical solutions.

Prescriptions soared for antidepressants such as Zoloft, Paxil, Celexa, and Prozac, among others. The increase amounted to over 20% for the year following. Use of anxiety drugs and sleeping aids also was on the rise, as attempts were made to find relief from the pressure. Others were fearful of bioterrorism attacks and also asked for sleeping aids.[2]

A nursing career offered one of the few safe havens for secure employment in the earliest years of the 21st century. For most Americans, the collapse of the stock market in March of 2000 delivered a crushing blow not only to their investment accounts, but also to their plans—indeed, to their present way of life. Many people lost a quarter to a half of their savings in the following 2 or 3 years.

For baby boomers and Generation X-ers, who had been working in the past half-dozen years, this event was as seminal as the Great Depression. The stock market demise was likely to be a defining event for the current generations.

Especially hard hit was the technology sector, including the promising biotech industry. The tech industry's incredible growth, where 25% jumps in annual earnings and 50% to 100% increases in stock valuations were common, represented much more than simply an adolescent sector experiencing its years of hyperexpansion. In the United States, tech companies were doing the heaviest lifting of the entire economy in the late 1990s and much of the year 2000. Much like the gold rush that hit California more than 150 years earlier, the tech boom had seemed to be changing the rules regarding everything.[3]

Nurses were largely on the sidelines as entrepreneurial activity was glorified and the smell of money was everywhere, especially in anything related to the Internet. Hordes of millionaires were created, both inside and outside the tech sector, and just about everybody seemed to be taking a shot at making a lot of money in a short period of time.

Tech workers often inspired bidding wars, and hopped from job to job in search of better pay or equity stakes in companies that might soon go public, be acquired, or just take off on their own. Start-ups, some of which had yet to make a single sale, attracted millions from venture capitalists and investors, using business plans that were no more than a paragraph in length. More mature companies often went public, garnering market capitalizations valued in the billions without ever turning a profit—or even offering much hope that any black ink was on the horizon. Meanwhile, nurses and other private investors, often using their retirement funds, jumped into the stock market via mutual funds to buy stakes in start-ups and load up on tech stocks rated highly by industry analysts, as overnight double-digit returns became commonplace during the long-running bull market period. Many others outside the sector, including real estate agents, car dealers, and investment bankers, also benefited from the boom as their businesses took off. It was a period when practical questions did not apply because it was believed they didn't matter, and no one predicted that the whole phenomenon was no more than a bubble.

Like many crazy rides, however, the tech bonanza ended with a crash. Many of the dot-coms the companies had tried to make money by selling online were the first to go. Their bubble burst in early 2000, as investors became increasingly skeptical that online retailing would ever produce profits. Many other corners of the tech sector, including telecommunications, ran into trouble later in the year, as many markets became flooded with competitors and venture capitalists started to tighten their belts. The September 11 terrorist attacks caused a business pause that contributed to the problems.

The downturn was also made worse because lots of companies believed the industry analysts and the corporate customers who said the rapid growth would continue indefinitely. The downturn was supposed to be brief. With the industry now over 3 years into what has become a severe meltdown, however, major questions continue to linger in mid-2003 about both the tech sector's future and the stock market as a whole.

The effects of the stock market meltdown touched just about everybody, including nurses. Virtually anyone with an equity portfolio had been hit, while countless investors had been battered to the point that their retirement plans had been pushed back a number of years. Thousands of companies went out of business, chief executive officers have for the most part lost their iconic status, and millions of workers have lost their jobs.

A GLOBAL PERSPECTIVE FOR NURSING

Meanwhile, as population statistics for both the world and the United States became available in the very early years of the new millennium, a number of trends have tremendous significance for nursing abroad and at home. Indeed, nursing itself was becoming increasingly global in its perspective. The broadening of the nursing honor society, Sigma Theta Tau, to include nations on other continents, as well as the continued activities of U.S. nurses in the International Council of Nurses and numerous partnerships between nurses in the U.S. and nurses in foreign countries, all bode well for a much broader and much more active interchange among nurses worldwide.

At the beginning of the 21st century, world population had experienced an unprecedented increase from 1.7 billion 100 years earlier in 1900 to more than 6.2 billion in the year 2000. Of these, 1.19 billion were in the developed countries and about 5 billion were in the less developed regions. The United Nations Population Fund estimated that world population would reach 7 billion in 2013 and 8 billion in 2028.[4]

World population growth had fallen from its peak of 2% per year to around 1.2% in 2002. Even so, global fertility was still above replacement level, that is, the number of children needed to replace people who die, despite an increasing number of countries with below-average fertility rates. Of the 76 million people added to the world in 2002, 95% were in

Worldwide Killer Diseases, 2000		
CAUSE	ESTIMATED DEATHS	PERCENT OF TOTAL
Cardiovascular diseases	16,701,000	30.0
Ischemic heart disease	6,894,000	12.4
Cerebrovascular disease	5,101,000	9.2
Cancer	6,930,000	12.4
Trachea/bronchus/lung	1,213,000	2.2
Stomach	744,000	1.3
Liver	626,000	1.1
Colon/rectum	579,000	1.0
Breast	459,000	0.8
Esophagus	413,000	0.7
Mouth/oropharynx	340,000	0.6
Acute lower respiratory infections[1]	3,866,000	6.9
Respiratory infections	3,941,000	7.1
HIV/AIDS	2,943,000	5.3
Diarrheal diseases	2,124,000	3.8
Perinatal conditions	2,439,000	4.4
Tuberculosis	1,660,000	3.0
Childhood diseases	1,385,000	2.5
Malaria	1,080,000	1.9

[1]Includes chronic obstructive pulmonary disease, asthma, and other respiratory diseases.
Source: World Health Organization, *The World Health Report 2001* (2002).

Leading Worldwide Causes of Death, 2000

CAUSE	ESTIMATED DEATHS (MILLIONS)	PERCENT OF TOTAL
World total deaths	**55.7**	**100.0**
Communicable diseases, maternal and perinatal conditions, and nutritional deficiencies	17.8	31.9
Infectious and parasitic diseases	10.5	18.8
Respiratory infections	4.0	7.1
Noncommunicable conditions	32.9	59.0
Cardiovascular diseases	16.7	30.0
Cancers	7.0	12.4
Injuries	5.0	9.1
Respiratory diseases	3.6	6.4
Digestive diseases	2.0	3.5

Source: World Health Organization, *The World Health Report 2001.*

less developed regions of Africa, Asia, and Latin America. Six countries contributed half of the annual increase: India at 21%, China at 12%, Pakistan at 5%, Nigeria at 4%, Bangladesh at 4%, and Indonesia at 3%.[5]

China and India each had more than a billion people. China had about 1.3 billion, and India was close behind with about 1.05 billion. The United States had the third-largest population in the world with 289 million people, followed by Indonesia with 218 million and Brazil with 175 million.[6]

By 2016, the United Nations estimated, India would have a population of 1.22 billion, making it larger than all the more developed countries, including Australia, New Zealand, Japan, Canada, the United States, and all of Europe combined. The UN also predicted that India would surpass China in population by 2045, and would have a total of 1.5 billion compared with 1.4 billion for China.[7]

World population growth reflected a remarkable decline in fertility in the developing world, from an average of six children to less than four children between 1965 and 2000. An unprecedented pace of decline had been experienced in much of Asia and Latin America. Slower declines were witnessed in South Asia and the Middle East, while little or no decline was experienced in sub-Saharan Africa, although there was evidence that fertility had finally begun to decline in about four African countries. Around North America and western, central, and eastern Europe, fertility had been near or even below replacement levels. The fertility declines had been associated with a marked increase in the prevalence of contraceptive use, from 9% to over 50% in the developed world.[8]

THE CHANGING CHARACTER OF AMERICA

The 2000 United States Census reported a total population of 281,421,806, a growth rate of 13.2% over the last decade. There had been just under 250 million in 1990. In addition, the U.S. population had increased

Infant Mortality and Life Expectancy for Selected Countries, 2002

COUNTRY	INFANT MORTALITY[1]	LIFE EXPECTANCY[2]	COUNTRY	INFANT MORTALITY[1]	LIFE EXPECTANCY[2]	COUNTRY	INFANT MORTALITY[1]	LIFE EXPECTANCY[2]
Albania	38.6	72.1	Germany	4.7	77.8	Panama	19.6	75.9
Angola	191.7	38.9	Greece	6.3	78.7	Peru	38.2	70.6
Australia	4.9	80.0	Guatemala	44.5	66.8	Poland	9.2	73.7
Austria	4.4	78.0	Hungary	8.8	71.9	Portugal	5.8	76.1
Bangladesh	68.0	60.9	India	61.5	63.2	Russia	19.8	67.5
Brazil	35.9	63.5	Iran	28.1	70.2	Slovakia	8.8	74.2
Canada	5.0	79.7	Ireland	5.4	77.2	South Africa	61.8	45.4
Chile	9.1	76.1	Israel	7.5	78.9	Spain	4.8	79.1
China	27.3	71.9	Italy	5.8	79.2	Sri Lanka	15.7	72.3
Costa Rica	10.9	76.2	Japan	3.8	80.9	Sweden	3.4	79.8
Cyprus	7.7	77.1	Kenya	67.2	47.0	Switzerland	4.4	79.9
Czech Republic	5.5	75.0	Korea, South	7.6	74.9	Syria	32.7	69.1
Denmark	5.0	76.9	Mexico	24.5	72.0	United Kingdom	5.5	78.0
Ecuador	33.0	71.6	Mozambique	138.5	35.5	United States	6.7	77.4
Egypt	58.6	64.0	New Zealand	6.2	78.2	Venezuela	24.6	73.6
Finland	3.8	77.8	Norway	3.9	78.9	Zimbabwe	63.0	36.5
France	4.4	79.0	Pakistan	78.5	61.8			

[1] Infant deaths per 1,000 live births.
[2] Life expectancy at birth, in years, both sexes.
Source: U.S. Census Bureau, International Database.

World's Largest Countries by Population, 2002, 2025, and 2050						
	2002		2025		2050	
COUNTRY	RANK	POPULATION	RANK	POPULATION	RANK	POPULATION
China	1	1,294,000,000	1	1,480,400,000	2	1,462,100,000
India	2	1,041,100,000	2	1,330,400,000	1	1,572,100,000
United States	3	288,500,000	3	332,500,000	3	397,100,000
Indonesia	4	217,500,000	4	273,400,000	5	311,300,000
Brazil	5	174,700,000	6	217,900,000	8	247,200,000
Pakistan	6	148,700,000	5	263,000,000	4	344,200,000
Russia	7	143,800,000	9	137,900,000	16	104,300,000
Bangladesh	8	143,400,000	8	170,000,000	7	265,400,000
Japan	9	127,500,000	11	121,200,000	15	109,200,000
Nigeria	10	120,000,000	7	183,000,000	6	278,800,000
Mexico	11	101,800,000	10	130,200,000	10	146,700,000
Germany	12	82,000,000	18	80,200,000	19	70,800,000
Vietnam	13	80,200,000	14	108,000,000	12	123,800,000
Philippines	14	78,600,000	13	108,300,000	11	128,400,000
Iran	15	72,400,000	16	94,500,000	13	121,400,000
Egypt	16	70,300,000	15	95,600,000	14	113,800,000
Turkey	17	68,600,000	17	87,900,000	17	98,800,000
Ethiopia	18	66,000,000	12	115,400,000	9	186,500,000
Thailand	19	64,300,000	19	72,700,000	18	82,500,000
France	20	59,700,000	20	61,700,000	20	61,800,000

Source: United Nations Population Fund, *The State of World Population 2002* (2002), United Nations Population Division, *World Population Prospects The 2000 Revision: Highlights* (2001).

by more than 100 million since 1960, and had doubled since 1940.[9]

Across the nation, the greatest population growth occurred in the West and the South and added to many pressures regarding the recruitment of an adequate supply of nurses. The five fastest growing states were all in the West, with Nevada growing at 66% since 1990, Arizona at 40%, Colorado at 31%, Utah at 30%, and Idaho at 29%. Overall, the West grew by over 10 million people to a total of 63 million. The South increased by nearly 15 million, or 17%, with Georgia being the fastest growing state at 26%. The Midwest grew by about 8%, while the Northeast experienced growth of 5.5%.[10]

The United States was also growing increasingly diverse. Although the population remained largely white, non-Hispanic at 73%, the Hispanic, African American, Asian, and Native American populations were all growing faster than the population as a whole. This trend was driven by both higher immigration and higher birth rates among these groups.[11]

By 2010, it was estimated, minority ethnic and racial groups would account for 32% of the population, up from 20% in 1980. Looking ahead, if one assumes high rates of immigration, the ethnic composition of Americans from 1950 to 2050 would undergo two striking changes. Anglo-Americans will be a minority group, and the Hispanic population will grow to become almost twice the size of the African American population between 2000 and 2050. Medium and low levels of immigration might mute some of these changes, but the directions would remain constant.[12]

Even in 2003, the demand for Hispanic nurses was at an all-time high as hospitals and other health providers tried to meet the needs of America's largest emerging minority population. Hispanics were the most underrepresented ethnic group in the registered nursing ranks, according to the Health Resources and

Years to Reach Population Milestones					
MILESTONE	YEAR REACHED	YEARS TO REACH	MILESTONE	YEAR REACHED	YEARS TO REACH
1 billion	1804	N.A.	6 billion	1999	12
2 billion	1927	123	7 billion	2012	13
3 billion	1960	33	8 billion	2026	14
4 billion	1974	14	9 billion	2043	17
5 billion	1987	13			

Source: U.S. Census Bureau, *World Population Profile: 1998* (1999).

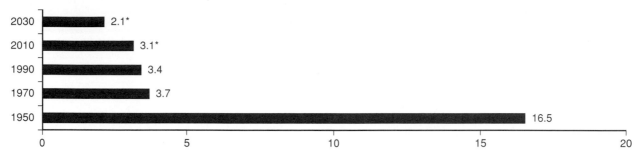

Social Security contributors vs. beneficiaries, 1950–2030. The ratio of covered workers to those drawing Social Security benefits has decreased sharply since 1950, and is projected to decrease further in the 21st century. By 2030 there will only be 2 workers for every beneficiary. (Asterisks indicate projected values.) (Source: Social Security Administration.)

Services Administration of the federal government. For example, in Texas, despite its large population, the group made up only 7% of registered nurses. In addition to being able to break down cultural and language barriers, Hispanic nurses acted as consultants to the medical profession. It was important to have professional nurses who understood every aspect of Hispanic life, including immigration, foods, religions, beliefs, and how those beliefs shaped patients' feelings about health care.[13]

Another acute shortage of nurses was caused by the rapid growth in the elderly population of the United States. The number of Americans aged 65 and older climbed to about 35 million in 2000, compared with 3.1 million in 1900. For the same years, the ratio of elderly Americans to the total population jumped from 1 in 25 to 1 in 8. This trend was guaranteed to continue for the rest of the new century, as the baby boom generation grew older. Between 1990 and 2020, the population aged 65 to 74 was projected to grow 74%.[14]

The elderly population explosion was a result of impressive increases in life expectancy. At the time of the Revolutionary War in 1776, the average American could expect to live to no more than age 35. Life expectancy at birth had increased to 47.3 by 1900, and in 2000 stood at 77 years.[15]

Along with the growth of the general elderly population was a remarkable increase in the number of Americans reaching age 100. In 2000, there were more than 50,000 centenarians, or people aged 100 or over, representing 1 out of every 5578 people.[16]

Few nurses were interested in careers in gerontologic nursing, unfortunately, even though as a group, the elderly had greater health risks for physical, mental, socioeconomic, and societal reasons. American society continued to be youth oriented, and the attitudes and values that characterized it played an important role in the way that nurses and other health care providers related to elderly people. Perhaps part of it was fear of growing old and becoming vulnerable themselves. Compounding the problem were the poor wage and benefit packages available in many long-term care institutions.

Another important implication for nurses was the fact that by the year 2020, the United States will have more than 20% of its population older than 65 years, higher than today's most aged society, Sweden, at 18%. Meanwhile, Japan and China, the latter with its one-child-per-family policy, will experience similar aging processes. Among the aged, the proportion of those who are "very old" (over 75) will also increase. Aging raises concerns not only about the economic and social aspects of nursing care for the elderly, but also about the ratio of elderly dependents to productive adults, whose caring responsibilities will shift increasingly from children to the elderly.[17]

The "old-old," those over 85 years, are the fastest-growing segment of the senior population and are often called the "frail elderly" because they are also the most likely to suffer from chronic disease and disability. Although only about 5% of people over 65 are institutionalized, the frail elderly have such

U.S. Elderly Population by Age, 2000–2040									
	65–74 YEARS		**75–84**		**85+**		**65+**		
CENSUS YEAR	*Number in Thousands*	*% of Total Pop.*	*Number in Thousands*	*% of Total Pop.*	*Number in Thousands*	*% of Total Pop.*	*Number in Thousands*	*% of Total Pop.*	**TOTAL, ALL AGES**
2000	18,391	6.5	12,361	4.4	4,240	1.5	34,992	12.4	281,422
2020	30,910	9.5	15,480	4.7	6,959	2.1	53,348	16.4	325,942
2040	33,968	9.1	29,206	7.9	13,840	3.7	77,014	20.7	371,505

Source: Administration on Aging, U.S. Department of Health and Human Services; Bureau of the Census, U.S. Department of Commerce.

15 Leading Causes of Death in the U.S., 2000[1]

RANK[2]	CAUSE OF DEATH	NUMBER	DEATHS PER 100,000
	All causes	2,404,624	873.6
1	Diseases of heart	709,894	257.9
2	Malignant neoplasms (cancer)	551,833	200.5
3	Cerebrovascular diseases (stroke)	166,028	60.3
4	Chronic lower respiratory diseases	123,550	44.9
5	Accidents (unintentional injuries)	93,592	34.0
	Motor vehicle accidents	41,804	15.2
	All other accidents	51,788	18.8
6	Diabetes mellitus	68,662	24.9
7	Pneumonia and influenza	67,024	24.3
8	Alzheimer's disease	49,044	17.8
9	Nephritis, nephrotic syndrome, and nephrosis	37,672	13.7
10	Septicemia	31,613	11.5
11	Suicide	28,332	10.3
12	Chronic liver disease and cirrhosis	26,219	9.5
13	Hypertension and hypertensive renal disease	17,964	6.5
14	Pneumonitis due to solids and liquids	16,659	6.1
15	Homicide	16,137	5.9
	All other causes	400,401	145.5

[1]Preliminary.
[2]Rank based on number of deaths.
Source: U.S. National Center for Health Statistics, *National Vital Statistics Reports*, vol. 49, no. 12, Oct. 9, 2001. Web: www.cdc.gov/nchs.

significant losses of function that the rate goes up to 20%. As a group, they are vulnerable to disability and loss of independence, and consequently their quality of life becomes compromised.[18]

The troubled health care institution of the nursing home requires substantial attention in the United States. A study by the United States Department of Health and Human Services reported that people aged 65 or older face a 40% lifetime risk of entering a nursing home. In 2002, approximately 1.6 million older adults were receiving care in some 17,000 nursing homes across the United States, approximately 75% of which were for-profit operations. Because of the dramatic growth in the number of Americans over age 75, the nursing home population is frailer than ever before and requires more specialized care. There is a desperate need for gerontologic nurse practitioner services in many nursing homes in the United States, but the need to make a profit and inadequate reimbursements conspire to make such hires all too rare.[19]

Nursing home prices are dependent on supply and demand and on the cost of living, with average charges higher in the Northeast and the West and lower in the Midwest and the South. According to statistics from 2002, the average cost of a nursing home stay in the United States was $168 per day for a private room. However, there were large variations from one metropolitan area to another. The costliest area surveyed was Stamford, Connecticut at $347 per day, whereas Shreveport, Louisiana was lowest at $88 per day.[20]

Americans spent $800 million on nursing home care in 1960, $4.2 billion in 1970, $17.6 billion in 1980, and $51 billion in 1990. By 2000, the figure had reached over $90 billion. Out-of-pocket payments,

Data and Death Rates for Leading Causes for Americans 65+, 2001*

CAUSE OF DEATH	NUMBER	RATE	CAUSE OF DEATH	NUMBER	RATE
All Causes	1,805,187	5,190.8	Alzheimer's disease	48,492	139.4
Heart disease	595,440	1,712.2	Kidney disease	31,588	90.8
Cancer	392,082	1,127.4	Accidents	31,332	90.1
Cerebrovascular disease	146,725	421.9	Motor vehicle accidents	7,165	20.6
Chronic lower respiratory diseases	107,888	310.2	All other accidents	24,167	69.5
Influenza and pneumonia	60,261	173.3	Blood poisoning	25,143	72.3
Diabetes	52,102	149.8			

* Preliminary data; rates are per 100,000 people 65 and older.
Source: National Center for Health Statistics, U.S. Department of Health and Human Services.

including personal savings and Social Security benefits, covered about one-third of this cost; Medicare and Medicaid especially covered most of the remaining costs.[21]

An increasing number of institutionalized elderly were suffering from Alzheimer's disease, a progressively degenerative condition characterized by forgetfulness in early stages and, as the disease progresses, increasingly severe, debilitating symptoms that create demanding nursing needs. An estimated 4 million Americans, most of them elderly, had Alzheimer's disease, and it caused over 49,000 deaths in 2000, making it the eighth leading cause of death in the United States that year. Many more women than men die from Alzheimer's, but this mainly reflects the larger number of women alive at older ages. Death rates are much higher for whites than blacks, but the risk of acquiring Alzheimer's is higher for blacks than whites.[22]

A CRISIS OF COST: CRACKS IN THE U.S. HEALTH INSURANCE SYSTEM

Meanwhile, health care was in the process of literally pricing itself out of the market for many Americans. Indeed, after being held in check in the mid- and late 1990s, due to aggressive managed care plans, health care costs began soaring, with employers facing increases of 10% to 20% even as the economic slump continued and profits plummeted for many businesses. It will be recalled that the U.S. health insurance system developed out of a need for hospitals and physicians to make their services affordable during the Great Depression. Health insurance had become a reality in the 1930s with the creation of specialized health insurance companies, initially the Blue Cross and Blue Shield plans. This system was given impetus during World War II when a government ruling exempted health insurance from wage and price controls and also from the income tax. Thus a solid link between employment and health insurance was established in the United States. From a strictly financial point of view, employer-paid, private health insurance was subsidized by the government, in the sense that employers were able to take the expenses as full tax deductions from their profits.

Medicare for the elderly and Medicaid for the poor were created in 1965. Thus it was this indemnity-based system of mixed public and private insurance sources that constituted the mainstream of health care for most Americans until the early 1980s. Only in some regions, especially in the West, was there any substantial number of people enrolled in prepaid health plans, later known as health maintenance organizations (HMOs).

During the 1970s and 1980s, a series of legislative and court decisions encouraged the growth of selective contracting. Selective contracting allowed insurance plans, which came to be known as preferred provider organizations (PPOs), and HMOs to contract with networks of providers. The plans could arrange for contracts at a predetermined price and reimburse providers for their services in a number of different ways, still including—but not limited to—the traditional fee-for-service model. By the early 1990s, the cost advantages that HMOs and PPOs afforded employers were great enough that most large employers moved their employees to this type of insurance arrangement. This caused a rapid growth in the number of people enrolled in HMOs and PPOs, and later

The State of Managed Care—HMO Market Penetration by State, 2001

STATE	PERCENTAGE	STATE	PERCENTAGE	STATE	PERCENTAGE
Alabama	5.7	Kentucky	29.8	North Dakota	0.7
Alaska	0.0	Louisiana	15.3	Ohio	22.8
Arizona	29.6	Maine	29.2	Oklahoma	13.8
Arkansas	10.7	Maryland*	33.9	Oregon	31.4
California	51.6	Massachusetts	44.7	Pennsylvania	32.3
Colorado	33.9	Michigan	25.2	Rhode Island	34.6
Connecticut	39.7	Minnesota	27.7	South Carolina	8.8
Delaware	23.3	Mississippi	1.4	South Dakota	10.3
District of Columbia	31.2	Missouri	30.4	Tennessee	30.9
Florida	29.7	Montana	7.5	Texas	16.4
Georgia	15.0	Nebraska	9.5	Utah	31.5
Hawaii	33.1	Nevada	19.4	Vermont	4.2
Idaho	3.9	New Hampshire	38.1	Virginia*	15.4
Illinois	18.8	New Jersey	31.4	Washington	16.8
Indiana	11.8	New Mexico	28.6	West Virginia*	10.9
Iowa	5.9	New York	34.8	Wisconsin	29.5
Kansas	13.2	North Carolina	15.5	Wyoming	2.2

* Includes partial enrollment reported for five plans serving the District of Columbia.
Source: InterStudy Publications, 2610 University Ave. W., St. Paul, MN 55114, Phone: 800-844-3351, www.hmodata.com.

in hybrid models such as point-of-service (POS) programs. By 2003 most companies had moved their workers away from indemnity plans, and more than 73 million people were enrolled in HMO plans.[23]

In 2003, there was worry that the $1.4 trillion health economy was in a state of erosion. Employers were passing an ever-increasing share of soaring health care costs to employees. As a result, many workers were dropping coverage. The burgeoning ranks of uninsured were overwhelming already stressed public and community hospitals, emergency rooms, and clinics with demand for care they could not pay for, leading to financial problems for these facilities. Some experts predicted that the number of uninsured working Americans could reach 30% of the labor force by 2009. That would be an increase from 23% in 1999.[24]

The U.S. health care industry continued to be an anomaly on the world stage. The nation spent more on health care than any other nation, yet had millions of citizens without access to even the most basic health care services. Despite an enormous investment in health care—over $1.4 trillion in 2003 (or one-seventh of the economy)—health care's status as measured by such conventional measures as longevity, morbidity, and mortality was only fair, lagging far behind nations that invested much smaller shares of their national wealth in health objectives.

American health care had, of course, evolved along a path quite different from that taken by all other industrialized nations. Although health occupied much of the national interest and wealth, the basic strategy for delivering care had largely been left to the vagaries of chance and self-interest. Not only was the United States without an organized national health service, it also lacked any financing mechanism to ensure that individuals could obtain needed health care without plunging into poverty. Health care policy was determined primarily by groups that profited from decisions that they made, namely, insurance and pharmaceutical companies, hospitals, physicians, and other health care professionals.

Many nurses were increasingly concerned that health care in the United States was too much of a business market–oriented system that was nowhere near as efficient and effective in providing health for the vast majority of people as it could be. Not only was the medical enterprise continuing to move forward without any master plan, there was also considerable debate as to whether the activities on which most of the time and money was spent contributed to the health of either the individual patient or the society as a whole.

It was clearly evident that the rate of increase in spending for health could not continue indefinitely. Health services were a valuable commodity, but money spent for health meant less money available to purchase other important services and products. The amount the nation spent on health affected all other parts of the economy. As health insurance was a continually increasing expense for business, the competitiveness of U.S. enterprise in the global economy was diminished, because all other competitive nations had nationalized health systems with general revenues from taxation supporting their operations. The annual increase in the rate of spending in the U.S. health care industry had averaged about 10% since 1950. At that rate, spending doubles in 7 years. Health care services were now accounting for more than the nation spent on either education or national defense—in fact, more than was spent on education and defense combined.

Thus, workers, already nervous about the sagging economy, had added a new concern to the list, and that was worry that the employer-based health care system that they had depended on for decades was in a state of erosion. Especially employees of smaller firms noticed the trend toward dropping or sharply diluting the benefit package in health care coverage. Many larger employers were passing on the significant insurance rate hikes to employees. Additionally, a small group of employers was opening up troublesome new options.

Since the business sector's once-fond hopes for cost containment through managed care had begun to die out, many companies were looking for a new model. The emerging idea was that instead of picking a health plan and paying whatever it cost to provide care for workers, a company would instead give its workers a fixed amount of money to spend on coverage. Workers would be responsible for choosing their own health plan, and those who wanted more generous plans would put up some of their own money to fund it.

These companies offered "defined contribution plans." And they appeared to be the most effective cost-saving option on the horizon. The worry was that employers would be tempted to take shortcuts that would leave their workers as vulnerable as the uninsured. They might choose low-cost plans with their defined contribution, and be unprotected if insurance refused to cover chronic illnesses and other preexisting health problems, or if insurers drastically hiked rates for an employee who encountered an expensive illness. Inflation could also quickly erode the value of the benefit, leaving workers unable to afford more than bare-bones coverage, if any.

These new plans took different forms. In some, the employers paid a fixed amount, for example, the cost of a single person's policy, and told employees that if they wanted family coverage they would have to pay the difference. In many cases, that difference amounted to $500 to $600 a month. Another popular strategy was raising the deductible. Policies that made individuals responsible for the first $500 or $1000 of health care expenses were becoming more common, and in some instances even $2500 deductibles were catching on in the small business market. High deductibles held down premiums, and they also shifted risk from the business to the employee.

The individual market for health insurance was a difficult one, especially for those who had experienced significant illness. As nurses who worked for many temporary staffing agencies or worked on a per diem basis without benefits understood, insurance companies desired to sell policies to individuals when they could avoid those with medical conditions that made them bad financial risks. But even people without serious health problems might not be able to get coverage or afford it if they were offered the plans. It was not uncommon for individuals with hay fever, temporary depression, asthma, and other conditions to be turned down, along with those with such risks as cancer, high blood pressure, or AIDS.

Over 16 million Americans purchased their own coverage in the individual market. These people tended to be between jobs or to have lost coverage through divorce or the death of a spouse, or were part-time workers, contract workers, early retirees, or those whose employers did not offer coverage. Unless they were self-employed, most got no tax credit for purchasing health insurance, and coverage became more difficult to obtain as they aged, because health problems increased.[25]

A study by Georgetown University in 2002 asked 19 insurance companies in 8 cities to consider applications from 7 people for policies with $500 annual deductibles and $20 co-pays for physician office visits. The insurers knew the applicants were fictional, but were asked to underwrite them as if they were real. One applicant had hay fever, another had injured his knee in college, and a family of 4 was healthy except for one son who had asthma. One

woman had survived breast cancer; another was depressed after the death of her husband. One man smoked, was overweight, and had high blood pressure. Another was HIV positive.[26]

Every single applicant, no matter how healthy, was turned down at least some of the time. The HIV-positive individual was turned down every time, and the 24-year-old waitress with hay fever was turned down 8% of the time and offered substandard plans 87% of the time. These substandard plans limited coverage for certain conditions or required a premium surcharge because of a health condition. The waitress's plan limited coverage for allergies.[27]

The widow with depression was rejected 23% of the time. In 80% of the policies offered to the family of 4, limits were placed on the son's asthma treatment, and the son was excluded entirely in 15% of the policies. The overweight smoker was rejected 55% of the time, but did get offered some coverage with premiums ranging from $2928 a year to $30,048. The five single applicants were quoted premiums that averaged $3996 per year, but had they been in perfect health the premium would have been $2988 annually, according to the study.[28]

Tying health care insurance to employers had made sense during World War II and after, when most workers aspired to lifetime jobs with one firm. But now the average job tenure in the United States was only 3 to 5 years, and there was serious question as to whether it still made sense. Replacing this antiquated link between employers and health insurance with a new citizen-based system could make basic health benefits universal and

Percent of Americans Without Health Insurance by State, 2000

STATE	PERCENTAGE	STATE	PERCENTAGE	STATE	PERCENTAGE
Alabama	13.6	Louisiana	18.9	Oklahoma	19.3
Alaska	19.3	Maine	11.8	Oregon	13.8
Arizona	16.0	Maryland	9.9	Pennsylvania	7.5
Arkansas	13.7	Massachusetts	9.5	Rhode Island	6.2
California	17.9	Michigan	9.8	South Carolina	12.0
Colorado	13.3	Minnesota	9.0	South Dakota	11.7
Connecticut	8.5	Mississippi	12.9	Tennessee	10.3
Delaware	10.6	Missouri	10.8	Texas	21.4
District of Columbia	14.5	Montana	18.4	Utah	13.4
Florida	17.2	Nebraska	10.0	Vermont	11.0
Georgia	14.4	Nevada	15.7	Virginia	12.7
Hawaii	10.2	New Hampshire	6.8	Washington	13.7
Idaho	15.5	New Jersey	12.5	West Virginia	14.3
Illinois	13.4	New Mexico	23.8	Wisconsin	7.4
Indiana	11.9	New York	15.1	Wyoming	14.4
Iowa	8.8	North Carolina	12.9		
Kansas	11.7	North Dakota	11.5		
Kentucky	13.0	Ohio	10.8	**Total U.S.**	**14.0**

Note: These estimates should not be used to rank the states. Results from different samplings could easily show different estimates and rankings because of small sampling sizes. For example, the high noncoverage for Texas is not statistically different from that of New Mexico.
Source: U.S. Census Bureau, *March 2001 Current Population Survey*.

fully portable, both from job to job and during periods of unemployment.

The nation's more than 40 million people without health insurance represented a huge dilemma. Managed care plans had cut the profits in most facilities, and expenses for indigents stood out as a huge problem. According to the Census Bureau, about 15% of Americans were without health insurance. Young adults from 18 to 24 years of age remained the group least likely to have coverage, with more than 28% in this age group without health insurance.[29]

The fastest-growing health care expenditure was for prescription drugs. The Centers for Medicare and Medicaid Services reported that the rate of growth in prescription drug spending in 2001 exceeded that of other health services by a wide margin, jumping over 21%. Increasing demand for drugs was related to an aging population, the introduction of new therapies for chronic conditions, and a shift in payment from out-of-pocket sources to third parties that had paid for only 41% of prescription drugs in 1990 but now paid for nearly 70%.[30]

In addition, widespread advertising by pharmaceutical companies stimulated consumer interest in these modern miracles. From early morning until late at night on television and radio, prescription drug makers were flooding the airwaves with pitches

Healthiest and Unhealthiest States

Ranked using a composite of 17 criteria measuring demographic and lifestyle factors, access to healthcare, occupational safety, and disease/mortality rates, 2002 data.

RANK	STATE	RANK	STATE
1	New Hampshire	50	Louisiana
2	Minnesota	49	Mississippi
3	Massachusetts	48	South Carolina
4	Utah	47	Arkansas
5	Connecticut	46	Oklahoma
6	Vermont	45	Alabama
7	Iowa	44	Tennessee
8	Colorado	43	Florida
9	North Dakota	42	New Mexico
10	Maine	41	West Virginia

Source: America's Health: UnitedHealth Foundation State Health Rankings, 2002 Edition; UnitedHealth Foundation, 9900 Bren Road East, Minnetonka, MN 55343, www.unitedhealthfoundation.org.

aimed at the nation's aches and pains, health worries, and phobias. Newspapers and magazines and other forms of advertising direct to the public contributed to creating mass awareness of the benefits of a specific drug.

The Food and Drug Administration had opened the door in 1997 to direct-to-consumer drug advertising, and the annual advertising expenditures

Drugs Most Frequently Prescribed in Physicians' Offices, 2000 (in Thousands)

RANK	NAME OF DRUG (PRINCIPAL GENERIC SUBSTANCE)*	TIMES PRESCRIBED	THERAPEUTIC USE
1	Claritin (loratadine)	17,145	Antihistamine
2	Lipitor (atorvastatin calcium)	16,267	Lowers cholesterol
3	Synthroid (levothyroxine)	15,999	Thyroid hormone therapy
4	Premarin (estrogens)	14,775	Estrogen replacement therapy
5	Amoxicillin	13,068	Antibiotic
6	Tylenol (acetaminophen)	12,789	Analgesic (for pain relief)
7	Lasix (furosemide)	12,577	Diuretic, antihypertensive
8	Celebrex (celecoxib)	12,161	Anti-inflammatory agent
9	Glucophage (metformin)	11,468	Blood glucose regulator
10	Albuterol sulfate	10,862	Antiasthmatic/bronchodilator
11	Vioxx (rofecoxib)	10,801	Anti-inflammatory agent
12	Prilosec (omeprazole)	10,751	For duodenal or gastric ulcer
13	Norvasc (amlodipine besylate)	10,635	For high blood pressure
14	Atenolol	10,372	For high blood pressure
15	Influenza virus vaccine	10,197	Vaccine
16	Prednisone	10,049	Steroid replacement therapy, anti-inflammatory agent
17	Amoxil (amoxicillin)	9,719	Antibiotic
18	Prevacid (lansoprazole)	9,268	For duodenal or gastric ulcer
19	Zocor (simvastatin)	9,202	Lowers cholesterol
20	Zoloft (sertaline hydrochloride)	9,183	Antidepressant
	All other	1,026,216	

*The trade or generic name used by the physician on the prescription or other medical records. The use of trade names is for identification only and does not imply endorsement by the Public Health Service or the U.S. Department of Health and Human Services.
Source: National Center for Health Statistics, U.S. Dept. of Health and Human Services; *Physicians' Desk Reference.*

reached over $3 billion a year by 2001, roughly two-thirds on television and radio. Consumer advertising of drugs had been authorized on the premise that it would make people aware of potential treatments for ailments they were suffering in silence.[31]

All these factors contributed to the annual number of retail prescriptions per capita, rising to about 11 per person in 2001, up from just 8 per person in 1995. The 50 top selling drugs in 2001 accounted for more than 30% of all prescriptions and were about twice as expensive as all other drugs. Retail pharmacies filled over 3 billion prescriptions in 2001, an increase of 8% over 2000, but the number of prescriptions for the 50 best-selling drugs jumped almost 20%, to about 900 million.[32]

Especially squeezed in terms of pharmaceutical expenses were the 40 million Medicare beneficiaries. Although prescription drugs were covered during hospitalizations, once discharged, the seniors were on their own. Medicare beneficiaries spent an average of $1051 annually in out-of-pocket prescription drug costs in 2002. Although older Americans were 13% of the population, they accounted for 34% of all prescriptions. For many years there had been discussion of extending Social Security coverage to prescription drug costs out of the hospital, but the pharmaceutical lobby had successfully staved this off. The pharmaceutical industry in 2002 employed 623 lobbyists, 23 of whom were former members of Congress, and 32 of them former staffers for the two House committees charged with oversight of the Medicare program. The drug industry was threatened with the prospect that adding a drug benefit to traditional Medicare would inevitably lead to government price controls. And price controls, industry officials argued, would hurt research that had created many wonder drugs in the past 10 years, as well as profits.[33]

Meanwhile, the forces transforming the health care delivery system during the previous decade had significantly affected nursing work environments. Not only had biologic sciences advanced at a dizzying pace, new drugs and chemical entities had been discovered, and the nation was on the threshold of using gene transfer for therapeutic purposes. Along with vaccines, gene transfers showed considerable promise for controlling certain cancers, and this marked the nation's entrance into an entirely new phase of therapeutics.

Cerebrovascular and cardiovascular diseases were on the decline, thanks to advances in anesthesiology and critical care medicine. We were capable of saving neonates who would not have survived 2 decades earlier. Older patients had a much-improved chance to survive surgical procedures, and the ability to return people to productive work was also unprecedented.

Because sophisticated laboratory tests and novel functional imaging techniques had eliminated most invasive diagnostic methods, and a significant percentage of surgical procedures were performed with laparoscopic techniques that required brief hospitalization or none at all, the majority of patients were now treated as outpatients. Even though hospital stays in the United States were the shortest in the world, the cost of inpatient care continued to rise, because only the most severely ill—those with multiple organ failures, multiple life-threatening injuries, or cancers refractory to traditional treatments—were hospitalized.

In 2002, spending for hospital care reached over $420 billion, up from $392 billion in 1999. However, hospital care comprised a steadily smaller share of overall health care spending. In 2002 it accounted for about 30% of national health expenditures, down from slightly over 47% in 1980. This decline came as hospitals cut costs with shorter lengths of stay and moved to increasing treatment on an outpatient basis.[34]

In 2002, the average adult stay in community hospitals (excluding federal, psychiatric, and long-term-care hospitals) was about 5.8 days. The average cost to the hospital was about $1200 per day, and about $7000 per stay. In contrast, the average stay in 1980 was close to 8 days, and average costs were $245 per day and about $1900 per stay.[35]

People age 65 and older were still the major consumers of inpatient care. They represented less than 13% of the population but accounted for over 40% of the estimated 33 million patient discharges from community hospitals in 2002. Their average length of stay, at 6.1 days, was higher than any other age group.[36]

NURSING IN 2003: CRISIS AND OPPORTUNITY

Registered nurses remained the largest single group of health care providers by far, numbering over 2.7 million. Hospitals were still the primary places of employment, and although there had been significant growth of other points of the care continuum, nearly two thirds of RNs continued to work in the hospital setting. That ratio had remained fairly steady over the past 15 years.[37]

The current RN work force included about 25% with diplomas, 34% with associate degrees, 31% with baccalaureate degrees, and 10% with master's or PhD degrees. Although about one third of all students enrolled in BSN programs were associate-degree or diploma-prepared RNs acquiring the BSN, these students represented less than 3% of all RNs without the BSN. Only about 16% of RNs prepared initially at the associate-degree level were acquiring a baccalaureate or higher degree in nursing.[38]

Fewer than 60 hospital-owned diploma programs remained from the over 2500 such programs that had existed back in the late 1920s. These few had evolved to include college coursework in the social and physical sciences along with hospital-based instruction.

Health Care Employment Trends, 2000, and Projections for 2010

Ranked by projected amount of growth for selected positions

OCCUPATION	2000 NUMBER	2010 NUMBER	EMPLOYMENT CHANGE, 2000–2010
Registered nurses	2,194,224	2,755,325	561,101
Nursing aides, orderlies, and attendants	1,373,206	1,696,579	323,374
Home health aides	615,381	906,633	291,253
Medical assistants	328,649	515,846	187,197
Licensed practical and licensed vocational nurses	699,600	841,924	142,324
Physicians and surgeons	597,852	704,956	107,104
Pharmacy technicians	109,847	258,998	69,151
Medical records and health information technicians	135,733	202,206	66,473
Dental hygienists	146,629	201,033	54,403
Pharmacists	216,865	269,560	52,695
Physical therapists	131,822	175,682	43,861
Radiologic technologists and technicians	167,413	206,052	38,638
Physician assistants	57,813	88,720	30,907
Medical transcriptionists	101,864	132,260	30,396
Respiratory therapists	83,010	111,902	28,892
Surgical technologists	71,185	95,884	24,700
Physical therapist aides	35,902	52,539	16,637
Cardiovascular technologists and technicians	38,663	52,174	13,511
Respiratory therapy technicians	26,818	36,085	9,267
Nuclear medicine technologists	18,219	22,305	4,086

Source: Office of Occupational Statistics and Employment Projections, U.S. Department of Labor, Bureau of Labor Statistics, 2 Massachusetts Ave. N.E., Room 2135, Washington, DC 20212, 202-691-5712, www.bls.gov/emp.

Associate-degree programs, which were established in the early 1950s in response to the postwar shortages, dominated the preparation of entry into the practice of nursing. There were slightly fewer than 900 such programs in 2003, and they accounted for over 60% of new entry-level graduates. These graduates were, on the average, nearly 34 years of age versus 28 years for graduates of basic baccalaureate programs. BSN programs were offered in 661 four-year colleges and universities, and the graduates represented about 37% of all new entry-level RNs.[39]

As the nation moved into the earliest years of the 21st century, it was clear that one of the greatest shortages of nurses in U.S. history was in the process of formation. While more than 2 million RNs dominated the health care industry in terms of professional talent, the growth factor had slowed to just a 5.4% increase from 1996 to 2000. This was the lowest rate of increase since the federal government had been conducting surveys of the nursing profession back in 1980. The survey results from 2000 also showed that the average age of nurses continued to rise, while the rate of new nurses entering the profession continued to drop. The projected shortage threatened the health of the nation and the integrity of the nursing profession.[40]

What is more, the 2000 National Sample Survey of Registered Nurses, which identified specific characteristics of the population, reported that only 9.1%

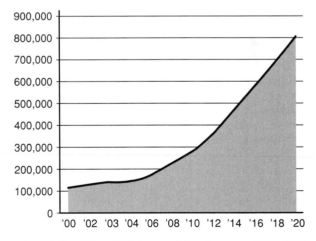

Projected shortfalls of full-time registered nurses, 2000–2020. (Projections based on July 2002 data; Source: HHS, Health Resources and Services Administration, Bureau of Health Professions, 5600 Fishers Lane, Rockville, MD 20857; 301-443-3376; www.bhpr.hrsa.gov.)

of RNs were younger than 30 years of age, down from 25% in 1980. And the average age of RNs was now slightly over 45 years.[41]

For the first time in the history of American nursing, there was widespread disillusionment and

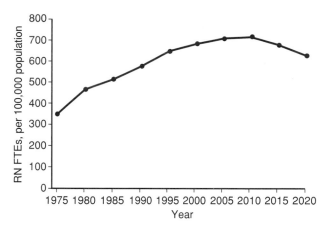

Supply of active registered nurses per 100,000 population in the United States. (FTE = full-time equivalent.)

dissatisfaction with the wages, salaries, and working conditions associated with active service. This demoralization included the common practice of RNs themselves now discouraging friends, relatives, and students from going into the field and admitting to others that they had made the wrong career choice, as well as advising recent graduates to escape from bedside care as quickly as possible.

Part of the problem was that nursing was still a single-sex, woman-dominated profession (93% female) by large, and gender barriers to access for most of the other professions had systematically come down over the years, providing many more options for women. Women now constituted about 50% of admissions to medical, dental, veterinary medicine, and law schools, and dominated admissions to pharmacy programs. Many of these women used to be attracted to nursing careers. All of this was exacerbated by the poor quality of public information about nurses and nursing work. The image of nursing continued to be dominated by a few ancient stereotypes associated with following doctors' orders, taking temperatures, giving medications, and doing a significant amount of housekeeping work. Perception served as reality for many young women and men as well as their parents and high school counselors.

In addition, the intensity of nursing work had climbed dramatically. The level of acuity of patients was up significantly: patients were older and sicker, and the length of stay was down, making for rapid turnover of patients on nursing units.

Turnover rates for hospital nurses had been increasing dramatically in recent years, which was partly the result of increasing pressure on nurses from higher productivity expectations in managed care environments, as well as the still heavily bureaucratic structures of hospital management systems. Improving nurse retention was a difficult challenge because the bureaucratic cultural norms of hospitals, with their hierarchical structures, rules and regulations, and heavy emphasis on cost control were not conducive to enhancing nurse job satisfaction and commitment.

In early 2003, a survey conducted by the United American Nurses called for radical changes in nurses' wages, working conditions, and staffing. The solution to the hospital nurse staffing shortage, which was projected as high as 800,000 to 1 million in coming years, was said to be associated with paying nurses more and decreasing the number of patients each nurse cared for. These conclusions came from a poll of 600 hospital staff nurses providing direct nursing care that was conducted via telephone by a research firm. Eighty-two percent of those surveyed responded that increased pay was a top solution to the nurse shortage; 85% responded that a reduced nurse-patient ratio would improve the shortage. Other highly rated solutions included greater autonomy and control for staff nurses (66%) and safer working conditions (65%).[42]

Eight out of 10 survey respondents felt that there was a serious shortage of RNs in their hospital, and 3 out of 10 respondents said it was unlikely they would be a hospital staff nurse in 5 years. Work-related stress, patient load, and inadequate pay were identified as the three top reasons nurses left the profession. A majority of the group felt that their hospitals were only doing a fair to poor job attracting and retaining nurses.

Discrepancy between the problems and solutions identified by respondents was particularly stark in the area of nurse wages. Six out of 10 nurses surveyed made less than $46,000 a year, and 55% of staff nurses with more than 10 years of experience also made less than $46,000. Two-thirds of those polled felt they made less money than the demands of their job warranted. Of those who felt they made a lot less, a third believed their appropriate annual income should be $70,000 or more.[43]

At the same time that nursing enrollments were declining, there was an increasing amount of evidence demonstrating a significant association between the quality of health care provided and the educational level of nursing staff, as well as the number of RNs in a critical setting and the perceived value placed on nursing in a practice setting. These findings had been documented by the American Nurses Credentialing Center, in its move to identify outstanding facilities as "magnet hospitals." The magnet hospital program was a mechanism for recognizing excellence in nursing care, and hospitals seeking the designation had to meet 14 standards through a process that required both written documentation and the facility's ability to meet the standards with an on-site evaluation review.

The seeds for the program had been planted in the mid-1980s, during one of the previous nursing shortages, when a national study was conducted to determine why some hospitals were more successful than others in recruiting and retaining nurses. A report to the American Academy of Nursing identified the 14 key attributes of a successful nursing workplace as including competitive salaries and benefits; a cooperative and professional relationship with physicians; a decentralized organization that provided recommendations from nurses; the quality of nursing leadership; participatory management style; and a strong emphasis on professional development.

Using these 14 factors as measurement criteria, the Credentialing Center launched a pilot program in the early 1990s; as a result of that project, the University of Washington Medical Center in Seattle was named in 1994 as the first magnet hospital in America. By 2003, statistics indicated that the more than 50 magnet hospitals were more successful than most in several key outcomes, including retention rates and some quality indicators. Nurses at magnet hospitals remained on the job an average of 8.6 years, compared with a national average of about 3.5 years. Meanwhile, about 95% of nurses in magnet hospitals took continuing education classes, and 100% of the chief nurse executives held at least a master's degree. In addition, magnet hospitals had nurse-to-patient ratios that were almost 50% higher than the national average of about 109 RNs per 100 patients, and 89% of the nurses reported excellent or good patient care.[44]

Advocates of the magnet hospital movement argued that it did not cost any more to operate a magnet-designated hospital, despite the typically higher nurse staffing ratios. The hospital would save money through lower turnover, much lower recruitment costs, and fewer adverse events that often led to increased use of high-cost intensive care units, respiratory assistance, or additional drugs. In fact, some asserted that there was no evidence that magnet hospitals cost more than conventional hospitals, and that they might even cost less while achieving better outcomes.

These conclusions were buttressed when the Joint Commission on Accreditation of Healthcare Organizations released a study in late 2002 showing that an absence of qualified nurses contributed to one in every four unexpected hospital deaths since 1996. This report immediately triggered renewed calls for more nurses, higher wages, and an elevated status for the profession, as well as including an expansion of the magnet program. The Joint Commission looked at the magnet hospital movement as a complementary accreditation program that examined distinctly different elements of health care facilities but worked toward the same goal.[45]

Two months later, in October 2002, another important study found that the number of patients a nurse had to care for could in fact be a matter of life and death. This National Institute of Nursing Research–sponsored study at the University of Pennsylvania concluded that patients had a greater chance of dying following surgery in hospitals where nurses had to take care of more patients. A heavy workload also meant nurses were more likely to be burned out and unhappy with their job. The researchers found that each additional patient in a nurse's workload translated to about a 7% increase in the likelihood the patient would die within 30 days of admission. For example, the difference between four and six patients per nurse translated to a 14% increase in mortality, while a difference between four and eight patients increased the likelihood of dying by 31%.[46]

Yet a third study on nurse staffing levels and the quality of care in hospitals found evidence that a higher proportion of hours of nursing care correlated with better patient care in hospitals. Specifically, a higher proportion of hours of care per day and a greater absolute number of hours of care per day provided by RNs were associated with shorter lengths of stay; fewer urinary tract infections and incidences of upper gastrointestinal bleeding; and lower rates of pneumonia, shock, and cardiac arrest. In addition, longer hours of RN care resulted in fewer "failure to rescue" deaths from pneumonia, shock or cardiac arrest, upper gastrointestinal bleeding, sepsis, and deep venous thrombosis. Among surgical patients particularly, a greater number of hours of care per day by RNs was associated with lower incidence of urinary tract infections and lower rates of "failure to rescue."[47]

Finally, a study released in January 2003 by Lynn Unruh examined hospitals in Pennsylvania from 1991 to 1997, and concluded that a greater incidence of nearly all adverse events occurred in hospitals with fewer licensed nurses, whereas a greater incidence of decubitus ulcers and pneumonia occurred in hospitals with a lower proportion of licensed nurses.[48]

The prospects for alleviating the nation's increasingly acute shortage of nurses improved somewhat with approval of the Nurses Reinvestment Act, which President George W. Bush signed in August 2002. This act would fund an expanded scholarship and loan repayment program for nurses who agreed to work in underserved areas, mandate studies to generate additional solutions to the nurse shortage, and promote the field of nursing through national awareness campaigns. There were also grants to improve working conditions, bolster recruiting programs, and provide stipends for poor students.

In addition to nursing organizations, the American Hospital Association supported this legislation, noting that the mean vacancy rate for hospital nurses was 13%, and one in seven hospitals was dealing with nursing vacancies exceeding 20%. Vacancy rates had worsened at 60% of U.S. hospitals since 1999, and the shortage commonly led to emergency department overcrowding and diversions, a reduced number of staffed beds, severe budget problems, cancellations, and increased wait times for surgeries.[49]

TAKING CONTROL: PATIENTS INVERT THE TOP-DOWN MODEL OF HEALTH CARE

Meanwhile, consumers were becoming much more actively engaged in their own health care than previously. Up until the mid-1980s, consumers generally had been passive recipients of care, submitting to whatever procedures a physician recommended, asking few questions and willing to let the system take responsibility for almost all decisions about their options. This was due to the fact that most people revered physicians and trusted them, and nurses were expected to remain in the background and not become involved in patient decision making. This gap was sustained by the significant difference in clinical information that physicians had as opposed to the average patient. In addition, the patient's perspective was virtually ignored because employers and government entities, not patients, were the true purchasers of health care for the majority of adults.

Now, a growing number of patients were turning to the Internet, where health care sites maintained huge amounts of general information on countless diseases. Some of the Web sites had begun to offer tools to help patients make better treatment decisions tailored to their conditions.

For instance, visitors could watch video clips of patients with similar conditions explain how they made their own treatment decisions. Web visitors could also get detailed information on treatment options and outcomes that were specific to their conditions, or join community sessions or chat rooms to share their concerns and experiences with other patients.

This type of information sharing, unique to the Internet, helped new patients make more informed and better treatment decisions. The Internet sites could deliver more information more effectively than even the best clinician could during an office visit, and did so completely and with the patients' perspectives. This could also be augmented by disease-specific chat sessions among current and former patients. It was also available to anyone at home or at work, all hours of the day and night. More than 70 million Americans went online in search of health information in 2002, and about 70% of them said that what they found influenced their treatment decision making.[50]

Another consumer-driven initiative in the health care industry was associated with the alternative and complementary medicine movement. Complementary and alternative medicine (CAM) comprised a large number of healing philosophies, approaches, and therapies. It included treatments and health care practices not widely taught in nursing schools or medical schools; not generally used in hospitals; and not usually reimbursed by health insurance companies. Although some scientific evidence existed regarding some of the therapies, for the most part there were key questions that had not yet been answered through well-designed scientific studies, questions such as whether they were safe and whether they worked for the diseases or health conditions for which they were used. Both nurses and physicians spearheaded the complementary and alternative medicine movement, and several journals devoted to the field carried articles contributed by members of both professions. The National Center for Complementary and Alternative Medicine was created at the National Institutes of Health to bring scientific study to the field. This organization distinguished between complementary medicine, which was used together with conventional medicine (as, for instance, the use of aromatherapy to lessen discomfort after surgery), and alternative medicine, used in place of conventional medicine (as, for instance, adopting a special diet to treat cancer instead of using the conventional approaches of chemotherapy, radiation, or surgery). The list of what was considered to be CAM changed continually, as therapies proven to be safe and effective became adopted into conventional health care and as new approaches to health care emerged.[51]

Worldwide, only about 20% of health care was provided by conventional practitioners; the remaining 80% involved alternative practices of some type. An estimated one in three Americans used some form of alternative medicine, and the field was in a steady growth mode. Complementary and alternative medicine was classified into five categories as follows:

1. Alternative medical systems were built upon complete systems of theory and practice, often having evolved apart from and earlier than the conventional medical approach used in the United States. Examples of alternative medical systems that had developed in Western cultures included homeopathic medicine and naturopathic medicine. Systems that had developed in non-Western cultures included traditional Chinese medicine and Ayurveda.
2. Mind-body medicines use a variety of techniques developed to enhance the mind's capacity to affect body functions and symptoms. Some techniques that had been considered CAM in the past had become mainstream (for example, patient support groups and cognitive behavioral therapy). Other mind-body techniques were still considered CAM, including meditation, prayer, mental healing, and therapies that used creative outlets such as art, music, dance, or pet therapy.
3. Biologically based therapies in CAM used substances found in nature, such as herbs, food, and vitamins. Some examples included

the booming dietary supplement industry, with its herbal products, and other so-called natural but yet scientifically unproven therapies such as using shark cartilage to treat cancer.

4. Manipulative and body-based methods in CAM were based on manipulation and/or the movement of one or more parts of the body. Some examples included chiropractic or osteopathic manipulation and massage therapy.

5. Energy therapies involved the use of energy fields and were of two types. Biofield therapies were intended to affect energy fields that surrounded and penetrated the human body. Although existence of such fields had not yet been scientifically proven, some forms of energy therapy manipulate biofields by applying pressure and/or manipulating a body by placing the hands in or through these fields. A number of nurses were active in this area, using Qi Gong, Reiki, and Theraputic Touch. Bioelectromagnetic-based therapies involved the unconventional use of electromagnetic fields such as pulse fields, magnetic fields, or alternating current or direct current fields. Magnet therapy had been popular for over a century in parts of Europe as well as the United States.

The most popular traditional herbs in the United States in 2001 were echinacea, ginkgo biloba, garlic, ginseng, saw palmetto, Noni-Morinda, St. John's wort, soy, ma huang, and milk thistle. A number of nurses had achieved licensure in alternative health fields, including massage therapy, homeopathy, naturopathy, and traditional Oriental medicine.

In 2002, the National Institutes of Health spent more than $100 million to study alternative remedies such as ginkgo biloba to prevent Alzheimer's disease, yoga for insomnia, massage for lower back pain, and the use of garlic and other dietary supplements for a wide variety of ailments. Several studies were attempting to cure high blood pressure with acupuncture. Researchers were hoping to sort out what worked and what was ineffective, and they were also playing catch-up with the American public, which spent over $30 billion on alternative dietary products and medical treatments in 2002, most of it out of pocket and mostly without consulting their physicians.[52]

Led by an increasingly health-conscious public and a generation of baby boomers who were bent on delaying the effects of aging as much as possible, the health care industry was confronting a mandate to move beyond the biomedical model and become much more engaged in preserving health and preventing illness and disease. Dependence on the biomedical model to define disease and health had been rendered insufficient by a growing body of

evidence that health involved much more than freedom from active disease or illness, and that lifestyle, environmental, and psychosocial determinants of disease deserve parity with conventional biologic theories.

As the U.S. population increasingly ages and the burden of morbidity and mortality from diseases that affect the elderly continues to grow, the public focus on both individual and environmental risk factors became much more important. This concern stimulated the development of a number of federally sponsored programs in the areas of health promotion and disease prevention. Among the best known were several long-term studies of cardiovascular risk factors sponsored by the National Heart, Lung, and Blood Institute.

In addition, the publication of *Healthy People 2000: National Health Promotion and Disease Prevention Objectives*, and its update 10 years later with the addition of new information in *Healthy People 2010*, highlighted the individual responsibility and its centrality to the promotion of healthy living habits and the avoidance of behaviors and exposures that contribute to the presence of chronic and degenerative diseases. Emphasizing health promotion and disease prevention was especially important for the nursing profession, which was rich in a nursing theory that had so far experienced limited opportunities for implementation in everyday practice across the health care continuum. Preventing an illness was much less expensive and more humane than attempting to either cure illness or manage the long-term complications that might follow. It was difficult to understand why disease prevention as a cost-containment strategy had not gained wider acceptance, other than the fact that it was not perceived as a source of significant profitability due to archaic reimbursement practices that tied significant payments to acute stages of disease and heroic interventions. Approximately one half of the health care dollar was now being spent on the care of patients in the last months of their lives. As new and more expensive technologies become available, this figure will certainly increase, yet only a small fraction of this large sum is being invested in programs to maintain health and prevent disease.

Healthy People 2010 offered a vision characterized by significant reductions in premature mortality and preventable morbidity, increases in healthy life spans, greatly reduced disparities in the health status of specific populations, particularly the poor, elderly, and minorities, and expanded access to basic health services. These health promotion and disease and injury prevention objectives considerably expanded the concept of health. The objectives emphasized that health was not just the absence of disease and disability, but included the promotion of health and improvement in the quality of life.

In terms of which health care practitioners should engage in health promotion activities, especially health education, counseling, and patient teaching, research indicated that physicians' attitudes, skills, and compensation compromised such activities. The literature was replete with articles suggesting that registered nurses should play the major role in health promotion and prevention because they were better trained for it, more willing than other health professionals to do it, and tended to be more successful than others in this area.

It was clear that significant forces were promoting the idea of preventive behavior as a major deterrent to disease, death, and disability, and that the biopsychosocial model of health care was in the process of replacing the more limited and traditional biomedical model. There were increased expectations that people must change aspects of their lifestyle if their physical health was to be made optimal. Such behavior change ran the gamut from smoking cessation to prevent cancer to the use of seat belts to reduce the risk of injury from motor vehicle accidents or the use of home smoke detectors to avoid burns. The role of the individual had been expanded from a passive receptor of medical interventions to an active partner in preventing disease and disability.

A change in the underlying philosophy of intervention helped explain how government regulation in the 1990s extended to the advertising and sale of tobacco and alcohol, the use of seat belts and motorcycle helmets, and the disposal of toxic substances and solid waste. Coupled with these changes had been the major demographic shifts, specifically the aging of the American population and a reorientation in public perceptions due to the self-help and wellness programs and the physical fitness activities, along with growing concern for healthy lifestyles.

Implementation of health promotion and disease and injury prevention objectives was requiring innovations and creative partnerships for nursing programs, as well as collaborative educational activities between those traditionally concerned with populations and those traditionally concerned with the individual. There were growing opportunities for closer linkages among schools of nursing, schools of public health, and schools of medicine. Of the competencies thought to be required of practitioners, a number were skills related to populations, such as care for a community's health, an emphasis on primary care, and a team approach to care, ensuring cost-effective and appropriate care. In addition, such activities as practicing prevention, involving patients and families in the decision-making process, promoting healthy lifestyles, improving the health care system at large, and participating in a racially and culturally diverse society were all deemed essential.

THE ADVANCED-PRACTICE NURSING SOLUTION

This new vision of health care for the dawn of the 21st century was especially important for the fast-growing numbers of advanced-practice nurses. About 8% of all RNs in the United States had obtained advanced-practice education, including nurse practitioners, clinical nurse specialists, nurse anesthetists, and certified nurse midwives. The approximately 100,000 nurse practitioners represented the single largest group of the nearly 200,000 advanced-practice nurses (APNs) in 2003.[53]

It was obvious that the growth in the role of advanced-practice nurses was the most cost-effective solution to many of the nation's health care problems. Many studies pointed to the approximate 80% overlap between nurse practitioners and primary care physicians, with nurse practitioners having equal or better outcomes, especially in terms of health promotion, prevention, and patient education. What is more, an APN could be educated at about one fourteenth of the cost of an average physician. However, this success was bringing increased efforts by state medical societies to limit or slow down the growth in the scope of nurse practitioner activities.

Much remained to be done to continue to broaden laws, rules, and regulations regarding state nurse practice acts, insurance reimbursement policies, hospital staff privileges, and full prescriptive privileges. Many MDs were worried that advanced-practice nurses were a threat in terms of the continued growth of their own practices, and it was common to see medical societies and associations warning that nurse practitioners were providing services beyond the scope of their abilities, although there were no studies to prove that this was an actual risk.

Perhaps the most important public policy rationale for the utilization of advanced-practice nurses was their effectiveness in addressing access issues of poor, rural, and inner-city populations. These locations continued to see an exodus of office-based physicians, and the only hope of replacement was associated with the nurse practitioners who might be able to locate in such settings and provide services that would otherwise require the use of hospital emergency rooms or, in many cases, no services at all.

While the nurse-practitioner movement was gaining ground in the delivery of health services, public support for biomedical research was facing some significant questions. Much of this research was based on the expectation that it would lead to improved health, and not just to new knowledge. Although the nation's biomedical research program had been enormously successful in generating new knowledge and had made the United States the world leader in such research, it had been less obviously successful in improving health. It was this relative lack of success in its applied mission that had placed serious concern on the difficulties of capitalizing on discoveries in basic research.

More than 60% of all Americans who died each year did so prematurely, that is, before age 65. As many as three quarters of these premature deaths could be prevented were people more successful in adopting healthier behaviors. Through early detection and intervention, immunization, and motivating change in individual behavior, the utilization of large numbers of nurse practitioners and other clinicians could eliminate an estimated 45% of cardiovascular deaths, 23% of cancer cases, and over 50% of the disabling complications of diabetes. These three conditions dominated much of the current practice of health care and, with the enormous potential for prevention, offered an ideal entrée for greater nurse practitioner involvement in health promotion and disease prevention.[54]

Health promotion services provided by nurse practitioners in a clinical setting were not the exclusive nor by any means the most effective way for nurse practitioners to help Americans modify their risks. Evidence from community-based interventions demonstrated that radio and TV spot announcements; labeling of food products in grocery stores; health education programs in the schools; and peer counseling programs by middle school students to teach them to say no to cigarette smoking, drug experimentation, and other habits had proved more effective in changing behavior than most interventions using a purely medical model. The traditional medical model was much better suited to secondary and tertiary prevention than to health promotion.

Nurse practitioners were using their power to empower a patient or client by providing information with which the individual could make an informed choice, exploring that person's values and preferences, respecting their autonomy, and finding means to help them achieve desired behavior change. This did not involve simply a transfer of power from the nurse practitioner to the patient or client (as would be the case in the consumer model of patient-nurse practitioner relationships), but rather a sharing of power to the extent possible to achieve a good outcome as defined by the client and by the nurse practitioner. Nurse practitioners could also act in their traditional advocacy role, using their knowledge of useful services that were potentially available to the client.

OBESITY EPIDEMIC

Perhaps the most difficult new major health challenge to face nurses in general was the rapidly growing epidemic of obesity in the United States. Sixty-one percent of U.S. adults and 13% of children were either overweight or obese. The incidence of obesity had risen 21% from 1990 to 2000, while diabetes rose 49% during the same period. This was not a coincidence, and nurses had stopped referring to Type B diabetes as adult-onset diabetes because so many children were now developing it.

The surgeon-general of the U.S. Public Health Service identified being overweight as an epidemic that threatened to overtake smoking as the nation's leading contributor of preventable deaths in 2002. Smoking-related illnesses claimed 400,000 Americans

a year, but the annual death toll from obesity-related illness was estimated at well over 300,000, and was growing more rapidly than cigarette-related deaths.[55]

The overall economic costs of obesity in the United States were estimated at about $120 billion in direct health care costs and indirect costs such as productivity losses, according to a report by the surgeon-general. Overweight and obese adults in the workplace were estimated to cost employers more than 39 million days of work time each year.[56]

A growing number of health insurance plans were developing disease management programs with which nurses would work more closely with individuals to control their illnesses and hopefully prevent further deterioration of their health. The design of these programs varied, depending on the health plan and the individual. Some, for example, tried to identify those who had been diagnosed with diabetes and put them in a disease registry. They were then targeted for intervention depending on their determined risk factor. If they were extremely high risk, a visiting nurse was sent to their home and they were called every day or every other day. If they were not at high risk, they might be called every 1 or 2 weeks. These kinds of programs worked by reducing the risk factors of participants.

Usually, however, people who were overweight and obese did not receive intervention until they had developed one of the diseases that qualified them for a disease management program. Then almost always managing weight was an integral part of managing the disease, and the patient was educated about diet and exercise. Some plans provided classes in nutrition and exercise to members in the disease management program.

There was a growing debate about whether obesity, technically defined as a BMI of 30 or more, should be classified, like cancer or emphysema, as an illness that should be covered by insurance companies and the federal Medicare and Medicaid programs.

Some of the leading advocacy groups for obesity issues were pushing for such classification. They claimed that more people would seek help if obesity were recognized as an illness and pointed to the health benefits produced by even modest improvements in weight. They claimed that such preventive programs would save money in the long run, and most nurses tended to agree.

The opponents said that treating obesity like cancer would force insurers to provide a wide range of treatments, from nurse practitioner and physician visits and nutrition counseling to exercise programs and psychiatric counseling. They were afraid that would cost billions of dollars, which would translate into even higher health insurance premiums, something no one wanted.

The Centers for Medicare and Medicaid was considering whether to characterize obesity as an illness for Medicare coverage. Current language specifically excluded obesity as an illness. Ultimately, however, the debate about obesity did not address the more complicated issue of preventing weight gain and, consequently, the health care ills associated with excess weight. Insurers still took the position that the matter essentially rested with the individual and started well before they became a worker insured by an employer.

A report in the January 8, 2003, *Journal of the American Medical Association* concluded that obesity appeared to lessen the life expectancy of all adults, but particularly younger adults. Researchers found that younger adults generally had greater years of life lost due to obesity than did older adults. White men age zero to 30 years with a severe level of obesity could lose up to 13 years of life, and white women, 8 years. Severely obese black men and black women under 60 had a maximum of 20 years of life lost for men and 5 for women. Again, the findings indicated that obesity would soon overtake smoking as the primary preventable cause of death.

At the same time, the Centers for Disease Control reported that obesity (not including just overweight) had climbed from 19.8% of American adults in 2000 to 20.9% of American adults in 2001, and diagnosed diabetes increased from 7.3% to 7.9% during the same year.[57] The obesity epidemic also resulted in various publications identifying the most overweight cities in the United States. An annual list compiled by *Men's Fitness* magazine identified Houston, Texas as the most overweight city in the United States, followed by Chicago, Detroit, Philadelphia, and Dallas. In contrast, the fittest cities in the country were Colorado Springs, Denver, San Diego, Seattle, and San Francisco. The magazine's goal was not to pick on any particular city, according to the editor, but to get the nation moving and thinking about obesity. To come up with the list, the magazine evaluated the nation's 50 largest cities with 16 equally weighted categories: overweight and obesity rates, junk food outlets, gyms/sporting goods retailers, fruit and vegetable consumption, participation in exercise/sports, alcohol use, smoking, TV viewing, air quality, water quality, climate index, geography, commute time, parks/open spaces, recreation facilities, and health care access. Americans were characterized as the fattest of the major nations on earth, and growing fatter by the day.[58] And to expect a nation that was grossly overweight to be combat ready, prepared to engage in 21st-century struggles, whether the enemy was terrorism, organized military force, or environmental hazards, was simply foolhardy.

INTERNATIONAL CONFLICT AND COOPERATION

The terrorist attacks of September 11, 2001, and the subsequent discovery of letters laced with anthrax heightened concerns about the possibility of terrorist or state-sponsored attacks using biologic or chemical agents. A variety of microorganisms and chemicals, many of them extremely difficult to detect, could be employed for that purpose. Some, such as the virus that causes the highly contagious smallpox disease, could be considered weapons of mass destruction because of their power to kill thousands, even millions. Experts estimated that if terrorists can infect 100,000 individuals with highly contagious smallpox, as many as 30 million deaths could ensue within 4 months. This led to a nationwide campaign to provide the smallpox vaccine for most of the nation's nurses and other clinicians.

Most harmful biologic and chemical agents did not match smallpox in their capacity to cause widespread illness and death, but many might still fit the needs of terrorists who aim to weaken their enemy by generating panic among the population or sabotaging its economy. Shortly after the September 11 attacks, a few individuals in the media, Congress, and elsewhere received envelopes containing spores of the bacterium that caused anthrax, sent by some unknown person or group. Fewer than two dozen confirmed or suspected cases resulted, and five people died, one a worker at a New York City hospital. Nonetheless, the anthrax cases precipitated widespread social disruption, and special concern about the safety in processing the U.S. mail. Public health agencies were inundated with samples of spore-like powder, and with worried people describing suspicious symptoms.

The Bush administration's goal to topple President Saddam Hussein and disarm Iraq of its chemical, nuclear, and biological weaponry, by force if necessary, triggered a national debate and an international diplomatic struggle. Nervous allies in the Persian Gulf and Europe warned that attacking Iraq could ignite a wider Middle East war or prompt Hussein to launch chemical weapons at American-led troops in the region. Critics contended that Iraq was agreeing to United Nations weapons inspections, even if belatedly, and that there was no immediate threat at this time. However, the war with Iraq was carried out with quick military victory but lingering problems associated with occupation and the installation of a new government remained.

America's health in the third year of the 21st century was thus attempting to wrestle successfully with perceived international threats, a declining economy, and the challenge of providing health care for all spectrums of the public from the young to the aged and among the various social and ethnic groups. It was clear that the aging of the nation's population would have enormous social implications for health care costs, family structures, and caretaking of the elderly. We were moving into a time when the voting population would be made up of more than one third who were older than age 65. The ability to continue to support Medicare and Social Security at the current levels was increasingly being questioned. The politics of health care access was also accentuated by immigration and the changing ethnic

Wars of the United States and Casualties

WAR	BRANCH OF SERVICE	NUMBER SERVING	CASUALTIES			TOTAL
			Battle Deaths	*Other Deaths*	*Wounds Not Mortal*	
Revolutionary War	Total	—	**4,435**	—	**6,188**	**10,623**
1775–1783	Army	184,000	4,044	—	6,044	10,048
	Navy	to	342	—	114	456
	Marines	250,000	49	—	70	119
War of 1812	Total	**286,730**	**2,260**	—	**4,505**	**6,765**
1812–1815	Army	—	1,950	—	4,000	5,950
	Navy	—	265	—	439	704
	Marines	—	45	—	66	111
Mexican War	Total	**78,789**	**1,733**	**11,550**	**4,152**	**17,435**
1846–1848	Army	—	1,950	11,550	4,102	17,373
	Navy	—	1	—	3	4
	Marines	—	11	—	47	58
	Coast Guard	71 off.	—	—	—	—
Civil War						
Union forces	Total	**2,213,363**	**140,415**	**224,097**	**281,881**	**646,392**
1861–1865	Army	2,128,948	138,154	221,374	280,040	639,568
	Navy	—	2,112	2,411	1,710	6,233
	Marines	84,415	148	312	131	591
Confederate forces	Total	—	**74,524**	**59,297**	—	**133,821**
(estimate)	Army	600,000	—	—	—	—
1863–1866	Navy	to	—	—	—	—
	Marines	1,500,000	—	—	—	—
	Coast Guard	219 off.	1	—	—	1
Spanish-American War	Total	**307,420**	**385**	**2,061**	**1,662**	**4,108**
1898	Army	280,564	369	2,061	1,594	4,024
	Navy	22,875	10	0	47	57
	Marines	3,321	6	0	21	27
	Coast Guard	660	0	—	—	—
World War I	Total	**4,743,826**	**53,513**	**63,195**	**204,002**	**320,710**
April 6, 1917–	Army	4,057,101	50,510	55,868	193,663	300,041
Nov. 11, 1918	Navy	599,051	431	6,856	819	8,106
	Marines	78,839	2,461	390	9,520	12,371
	Coast Guard	8,835	111	81	—	192
World War II	Total	**16,353,659**	**292,131**	**115,185**	**671,846**	**1,079,162**
Dec. 7, 1941–	Army	11,260,000	234,874	83,400	565,861	884,135
Dec. 31, 1946	Navy	4,183,466	36,950	25,664	37,778	100,392
	Marines	669,100	19,733	4,778	68,207	91,718
	Coast Guard	241,093	574	1,343	—	1,917
Korean War	Total	**5,764,143**	**33.667**	**3,249**	**103,284**	**140,200**
June 25, 1950–	Army	2,834,000	27,709	2,452	77,596	107,757
July 27, 1953	Navy	1,177,000	493	160	1,576	2,226
	Marines	424,000	4,267	339	23,744	28,353
	Air Force	1,285,000	1,198	298	368	1,864
	Coast Guard	44,143	—	—	—	—
Vietnam War	Total	**8,752,000**	**47,393**	**10,800**	**153,363**	**211,556**
Aug. 4, 1964–	Army	4,368,000	30,929	7,272	96,802	135,003
Jan. 27, 1973	Navy	1,842,000	1,631	931	4,178	6,740
	Marines	794,000	13,085	1,753	51,392	66,230
	Air Force	1,740,000	1,741	842	931	3,514
	Coast Guard	8,000	7	2	60	69
Persian Gulf War	Total	**467,939**	**148**	**151**	**467**	**766**
1991	Army	246,682	98	105	354	557
	Navy	98,852	6	14	12	32
	Marines	71,254	24	26	92	142
	Air Force	50,751	20	6	9	35
	Coast Guard	400	—	—	—	—

composition of America's population, as the Anglo majority declined and Hispanic and other minority groups increased. How the poor and the disadvantaged in the nation would gain access to high-quality health services was very much a part of the debate about national priorities and responsibilities.

Finally, it was more and more obvious that America's health and its nurses in the 21st century were already inextricably linked to world population, world events, and world health. We were now a part of a global health village, because of health interdependence and the transnationalization of disease and risk. Most health problems were commonly shared, and many health risks clearly had transnational properties. The imperative for international cooperation was intensifying, and the world view of most nurses was becoming broader, as it was clear that no longer could the nursing profession view itself as a singular entity in the United States; rather, it was a profession that had sisters and brothers throughout the world, all seeking with the resources at their disposal to provide nursing care demands that were growing ever larger.

REFERENCES

1. Rozella M. Schlotfeldt, "This I Believe...Nursing is Health Care," *Nursing Outlook*, vol. 20 (April 1972):245.
2. "Drug Pitches Resonate with Edgy Public," *Wall Street Journal* (January 14, 2003), p. B7.
3. "Battered Market Threatens Many Americans' Dream," *Boston Sunday Globe* (July 14, 2002), p. 1.
4. United Nations Population Fund, *The State of World Population* (2002), pp. 1-9.
5. Ibid., p. 5.
6. Ibid., p. 21.
7. United Nations Population Division, *World Population Prospects: The 2000 Revision* (2001), pp. 1-8.
8. "World-wide Baby Bust has Profound Implications," *Wall Street Journal* (January 24, 2003), pp. B1, B4.
9. "A Nation Ablaze with Change," *USA Today* (July 3, 2001), p. 4A.
10. Ibid.
11. "U.S. Now More Diverse, Ethically and Racially," *New York Times* (April 1, 2001), p. 18.
12. Ibid.
13. "Demand for Spanish-speaking Nurses at All-time High," *Chicago Tribune* (September 30, 2001), p. 6.
14. U.S. Census Bureau, *Census 2000: General Population Characteristics* (2001), pp. 1-12.
15. Ibid., p. 8.
16. Ibid., p. 3.
17. U.S. Census Bureau, *International Data Base* (2002).
18. "Persons 65 Years Old and Over—Characteristics By Sex," *U.S. Census Brureau: Current Populations Reports* (2001), (www.census.gov).
19. www.medicare.gov/nursing/overview.asp.
20. U.S. Department of Health and Human Services, National Center for Health Statistics, *Health, United States, 2002*, p. 58.
21. Ibid., p. 63.
22. U.S. National Center for Health Statistics, *National Vital Statistics Report*, vol. 49, no. 12 (October 9, 2001), www.cdc.gov/nchs.
23. "Spending on Healthcare Rose 10 Percent Last Year," *USA Today* (September 25, 2002), p. B1.
24. "The 39 Million Who Musn't Get Sick," *Wall Street Journal* (December 27, 2001), p.1.
25. "Need Health Insurance? Good Luck," *USA Today* (July 31, 2001), p. 1.
26. "Individual Health Insurance Study," Kaiser Family Foundation, Menlo Park, California (2002), pp. 1-3 (press release).
27. Ibid., p. 12.
28. Ibid., p. 15.
29. U.S. Bureau of Census, *Current Population Survey* (March 2002), p. 1-3.
30. "Spending on Healthcare Rose 10 Percent Last Year," *USA Today* (September 25, 2002), p. B1.
31. "Misleading Drug Ads Slip Under Regulators' Radar," *USA Today* (January 6, 2003), p. 12A.
32. "Big Pharma Real Enemy in War on Drug Costs," *Toronto Star* (August 3, 2002), p. C1.
33. Ibid.
34. U.S. Department of Health and Human Services, National Center for Health Statistics, *Health, United States, 2002*, pp. 1-2.
35. Ibid., p. 23.
36. Ibid., p. 62.
37. U.S. Department of Health and Human Services, *The Registered Nurse Population: National Sample Survey of Registered Nurses—March 2000* (Washington, D.C., 2001), pp. 1-16.
38. Ibid., p. 12.
39. Ibid., p. 3.
40. "Area Short of Nurses; Care Suffers," *Detroit News* (January 11, 2001), p. 1.
41. *The Registered Nurse Population*, p. 6.
42. United American Nurses, AFL-CIO, *Poll of Registered Nurses Conducted by Lake Snell Perry and Associates* (January 16, 2003), pp. 1-3 (press release).
43. Ibid., pp. 1-2.
44. American Nurses Credentialing Center, *Magnet Nursing Recognition Program for Excellence in Nursing Service—Acute Care* (Washington, DC: American Nurses Credentialing Center, 2003).
45. Joint Commission on Accreditation of Healthcare Organizations (November 2, 2002) (press release).
46. "Nursing Shortage Can Often Prove Fatal," *Detroit News* (October 23, 2002), p. 3A.
47. "Shortage of Nurses Hurts Patient Care, Study Finds," *Boston Globe* (May 30, 2002), p. 3.
48. University of Pennsylvania (January 10, 2003) (press release).
49. "ANA Addresses the Impact of the Nursing Shortage at Senate Committee Hearing" (June 23, 2002) (press release).
50. For example, see www.mayoclinic.com; www.healthdialog.com; www.nexcura.com; chess.chsra.wisc.edu.
51. Personal communication, National Center for Complementary and Alternative Medicine, National Institutes of Health (Bethesda, Maryland: February 14, 2003).
52. Ibid.
53. Personal communication, Health Resources and Services Administration, Bureau of Health Professions (Rockville, Maryland: March 3, 2003), www.bhpr.hrsa.gov.
54. "Advanced Practice Nursing Today," *RN*, vol. 63 (September 2000), pp. 57-62.
55. "Eating Health Away," *Detroit Free Press* (March 26, 2002), p. 1A.
56. Ibid., p. 3A.
57. "Health Hazards Continue to Grow," *Ann Arbor News* (January 12, 2003), p. E4.
58. "Fat or Fit: How You Look, Feel May Depend on Where You Live," *USA Today* (January 8, 2001), p. 7D.

INDEX

Note: Page numbers followed by t indicate tables.